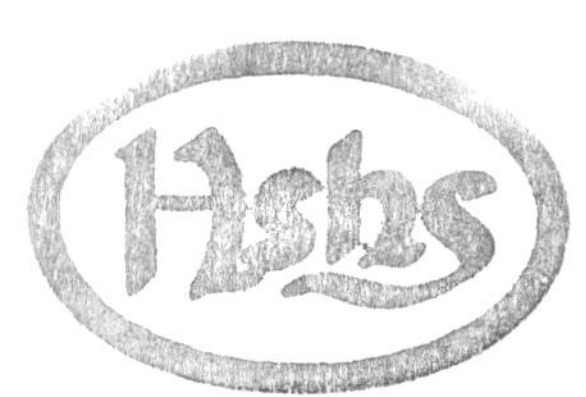

THORACIC ONCOLOGY

Cancer Treatment and Research
Steven T. Rosen, M.D., *Series Editor*

Goldstein, L.J., Ozols, R. F. (eds.): Anticancer Drug Resistance. Advances in Molecular and Clinical Research. 1994. ISBN 0-7923-2836-1.

Hong, W.K., Weber, R.S. (eds.): Head and Neck Cancer. Basic and Clinical Aspects. 1994. ISBN 0-7923-3015-3.

Thall, P.F. (ed): Recent Advances in Clinical Trial Design and Analysis. 1995. ISBN 0-7923-3235-0.

Buckner, C. D. (ed): Technical and Biological Components of Marrow Transplantation. 1995. ISBN 0-7923-3394-2.

Winter, J.N. (ed.): Blood Stem Cell Transplantation. 1997. ISBN 0-7923-4260-7.

Muggia, F.M. (ed): Concepts, Mechanisms, and New Targets for Chemotherapy. 1995. ISBN 0-7923-3525-2.

Klastersky, J. (ed): Infectious Complications of Cancer. 1995. ISBN 0-7923-3598-8.

Kurzrock, R., Talpaz, M. (eds): Cytokines: Interleukins and Their Receptors. 1995. ISBN 0-7923-3636-4.

Sugarbaker, P. (ed): Peritoneal Carcinomatosis: Drugs and Diseases. 1995. ISBN 0-7923-3726-3.

Sugarbaker, P. (ed): Peritoneal Carcinomatosis: Principles of Management. 1995. ISBN 0-7923-3727-1.

Dickson, R.B., Lippman, M.E. (eds.): Mammary Tumor Cell Cycle, Differentiation and Metastasis. 1995. ISBN 0-7923-3905-3.

Freireich, E.J, Kantarjian, H. (eds.): Molecular Genetics and Therapy of Leukemia. 1995. ISBN 0-7923-3912-6.

Cabanillas, F., Rodriguez, M.A. (eds.): Advances in Lymphoma Research. 1996. ISBN 0-7923-3929-0.

Miller, A.B. (ed.): Advances in Cancer Screening. 1996. ISBN 0-7923-4019-1.

Hait , W.N. (ed.): Drug Resistance. 1996. ISBN 0-7923-4022-1.

Pienta, K.J. (ed.): Diagnosis and Treatment of Genitourinary Malignancies. 1996. ISBN 0-7923-4164-3.

Arnold, A.J. (ed.): Endocrine Neoplasms. 1997. ISBN 0-7923-4354-9.

Pollock, R.E. (ed.): Surgical Oncology. 1997. ISBN 0-7923-9900-5.

Verweij, J., Pinedo, H.M., Suit, H.D. (eds.): Soft Tissue Sarcomas: Present Achievements and Future Prospects. 1997. ISBN 0-7923-9913-7.

Walterhouse, D.O., Cohn, S. L. (eds.): Diagnostic and Therapeutic Advances in Pediatric Oncology. 1997. ISBN 0-7923-9978-1.

Mittal, B.B., Purdy, J.A., Ang, K.K. (eds.): Radiation Therapy. 1998. ISBN 0-7923-9981-1.

Foon, K.A., Muss, H.B. (eds.): Biological and Hormonal Therapies of Cancer. 1998. ISBN 0-7923-9997-8.

Ozols, R.F. (ed.): Gynecologic Oncology. 1998. ISBN 0-7923-8070-3.

Noskin, G. A. (ed.): Management of Infectious Complications in Cancer Patients. 1998. ISBN 0-7923-8150-5

Bennett, C. L. (ed.): Cancer Policy. 1998. ISBN 0-7923-8203-X

Benson, A. B. (ed.): Gastrointestinal Oncology. 1998. ISBN 0-7923-8205-6

Tallman, M.S. , Gordon, L.I. (eds.): Diagnostic and Therapeutic Advances in Hematologic Malignancies. 1998. ISBN 0-7923-8206-4

von Gunten, C.F. (ed.): Palliative Care and Rehabilitation of Cancer Patients. 1999. ISBN 0-7923-8525-X

Burt, R.K., Brush, M.M. (eds): Advances in Allogeneic Hematopoietic Stem Cell Transplantation. 1999. ISBN 0-7923-7714-1

Angelos, P. (ed): Ethical Issues in Cancer Patient Care 2000. ISBN 0-7923-7726-5

Gradishar, W.J., Wood, W.C. (eds): Advances in Breast Cancer Management. 2000. ISBN 0-7923-7890-3

Sparano, Joseph A. (ed.): HIV & HTLV-I Associated Malignancies. 2001. ISBN 0-7923-7220-4.

Ettinger, David S. (ed.): Thoracic Oncology. 2001. ISBN 0-7923-7248-4.

THORACIC ONCOLOGY

edited by

David S. Ettinger, MD
The Johns Hopkins Oncology Center
Bunting Blaustein Cancer Research Building
Baltimore, Maryland, USA

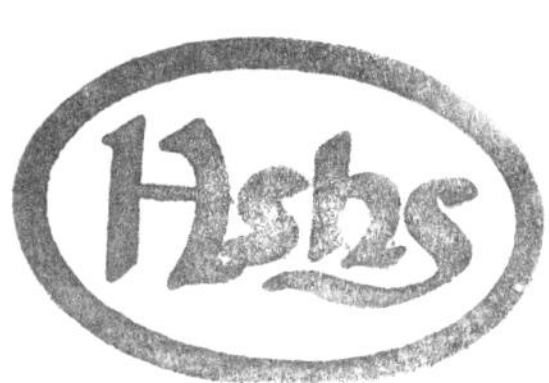

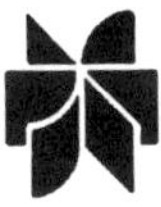

KLUWER ACADEMIC PUBLISHERS
Boston / Dordrecht / London

Distributors for North, Central and South America:
Kluwer Academic Publishers
101 Philip Drive
Assinippi Park
Norwell, Massachusetts 02061 USA

Distributors for all other countries:
Kluwer Academic Publishers Group
Distribution Centre
Post Office Box 322
3300 AH Dordrecht, THE NETHERLANDS

Library of Congress Cataloging-in-Publication Data

Thoracic oncology / edited by David S. Ettinger.
    p. ; cm. – (Cancer treatment and research ; v. 105)
    Includes index.
    ISBN 0-7923-7248-4 (alk. paper)
    1. Chest--Cancer. I. Ettinger, David S. II. Series.
    [DNLM: 1. Thoracic Neoplasms. WF 970 T4876 2001]
    RC280.C5 . T482 2001
    616.99'494--dc21
                                      00-051456

DEDICATION

To my wife, Phyllis, and children, Laura, Daniel and Kathryn, for their love, understanding and support.

ACKNOWLEDGEMENT

I would like to thank my administrative assistant, Angela Liggins, for all the hours she spent making this book a reality.

Table of Contents

List of Contributors
Preface

List of Contributors

Kathy S. Albain, M.D.
Cancer Center, Loyola University Medical Center, Illinois, USA

Bond Almand, B.S.
Department of Medicine, Vanderbilt Cancer Center, Tennessee, USA

Chandra P. Belani, M.D.
Division of Medical Oncology, University of Pittsburgh,
Pennsylvania, USA

Alejandro R. Calvo, M.D.
Division of Medical Oncology, University of Pittsburgh,
Pennsylvania, USA

Joseph Clark, M.D.
Cancer Center, Loyola University Medical Center, Illinois, USA

David Carbone, M.D., Ph.D.
Department of Medicine, Vanderbilt Cancer Center, Tennessee, USA

Anuradha Chakravarthy, M.D.
Vanderbilt University School of Medicine, Tennessee, USA

Hak Choy, M.D.
Vanderbilt Center for Radiation Oncology, Tennessee, USA

Walter J. Curran, M.D.
Department of Radiation Oncology, Thomas Jefferson Hospital,
Pennsylvania, USA

Arlene A. Forastiere, M.D.
The Johns Oncology Center, Maryland, USA

F. Anthony Greco, M.D.
Sarah Cannon Cancer Center, Tennessee, USA

John D. Hainsworth, M.D.
Sarah Cannon Cancer Center, Tennessee, USA

Elisabeth I. Heath, M.D.
The Johns Oncology Center, Maryland, USA

Richard F. Heitmiller, M.D.
Johns Hopkins Medical Institutions, Maryland, USA

Linus Ho, M.D., Ph.D.
Brigham and Women's Hospital, Massachusetts, USA

Jae-Sung Kim, M.D.
Vanderbilt University School of Medicine, Tennessee, USA

Karen Kelly, M.D.
University of Colorado Health Sciences Center, Colorado, USA

Corey J. Langer, M.D.
Fox Chase Cancer Center, Pennsylvania, USA

Patrick J. Loehrer, M.D.
Indiana Cancer Pavilion, Indiana USA

Jocelyne Martin, M.D.
Memorial-Sloan Kettering Cancer Center, New York, USA

Valerie W. Rusch, M.D.
Memorial-Sloan Kettering Cancer Center, New York, USA

Alan Sandler, M.D.
Vanderbilt University Medical Center, Tennessee, USA

Wasif Shirazi, M.D.
Rush Medical College, Illinois, USA

Arthur T. Skarin, M.D.
Brigham and Women's Hospital, Massachusetts, USA

David Sugarbaker, M.D.
Brigham and Women's Hospital, Massachusetts, USA

Mark R. Wick, M.D.
Brigham and Women's Hospital, Massachusetts, USA

Mark D. Williams, M.D.
Indiana Cancer Pavilion, Indiana USA

PREFACE

In the United States today, the incidence of new cases of thoracic neoplasms is over 180,000. Each year, over 170,000 individuals are expected to die of their cancer. Lung cancer is the most common of the thoracic neoplasms. It is the leading cause of death in both men and women accounting for 28% of all cancer deaths in the United States.

Other thoracic neoplasms include mesothelioma, esophageal carcinoma and the rare cancers – thymoma, mediastinal tumors such as germ cell neoplasms and lymphoma.

In recent years, there has been significant increase in knowledge of the biology of thoracic neoplasms as well as improvement in the diagnosis, prevention, early detection and treatment of these diseases. These advances have been made by individuals working collaboratively in a multidisciplinary approach that includes translational researchers, epidemiologists, pulmononlogists, radiologists, pathologists, thoracic surgeons, radiation and medical oncologists.

In this volume, *Thoracic Oncology*, a part of the Cancer Treatment and Research Series", the contributors provide an up-to-date, concise review of the various thoracic neoplasms to allow the reader to have a better understanding of the biology, natural history, diagnosis and treatment of these malignancies. Since lung cancer is the most common and most deadly of all the thoracic neoplasms, ten of the fifteen chapters in the book deal with it including an important chapter on the biologic considerations in lung cancer. The chapter on malignant mesothelioma provides a comprehensive state-of-the-art review of the disease. Two chapters discuss an up-to-date review of the epidemiology, diagnosis, staging and therapy of esophageal cancer. The two chapters dealing with the rarely occurring thymic malignancies, germ cell neoplasms and other malignancies of the mediastinum, emphasize the various treatment options for these cancers.

I believe that the contributors to this volume provide the reader with an understandable, concise and comprehensive review of thoracic oncology. It is hoped that this book will assist those clinicians interested in thoracic neoplasms, to better understand and treat them.

David S. Ettinger, Editor

Biological Considerations in Lung Cancer

Bond Almand, B.S.
Vanderbilt Ingram Cancer Center, Nashville, TN 37232 USA

David P. Carbone, M.D., Ph.D.
Vanderbilt Ingram Cancer Center, Nashville, TN 37232 USA

INTRODUCTION

Despite recent advances in treatment, lung cancer remains one of the deadliest human malignancies with little change in prognosis or overall survival rates in the past 20 years. Approximately 90% of patients diagnosed with lung cancer eventually die of their disease resulting in lung cancer having by far the worst overall cure rate of the common solid tumors in the United States (1). Thus, while it is not the most common type of cancer, lung cancer causes the largest number of cancer deaths in both men and women in the USA.

While the cure rate of lung cancer has improved only slightly in recent decades, our knowledge of the genetic and molecular changes in lung cancer as well as our understanding of tumor-host interactions has greatly increased. This knowledge has resulted in new therapeutic strategies targeting both the molecular machinery involved in tumorigenesis and the immune cells involved in tumor-host interactions.

In this chapter we will briefly review the molecular biology of lung cancer and the recent advances in our understanding of tumorigenesis and tumor-host interactions.

THE GENETIC BASIS OF LUNG CANCER

Lung cancer is unique among the most common human solid cancers in that the majority of cases can be linked to a single, although complex, environmental factor, i.e. tobacco smoke (2, 3). Many known carcinogens in tobacco smoke directly damage DNA. This DNA damage causes somatic mutations in growth regulatory genes leading to the dysregulated growth seen in cancer. Current opinion holds that multiple genetic hits are required to push a cell from normal cell cycle control to cancer, and that these lesions must occur in a certain order to escape host protection mechanisms including cell cycle arrest, immune recognition, and tumor-suppressor-mediated apoptosis.

GENETICS OF PRENEOPLASIA AND THE DEVELOPMENT OF LUNG CANCER

Chronic exposure to cigarette smoke causes a progression of preneoplastic histologic changes that herald the development of lung cancer that are best described for the squamous subtype. This progression begins with epithelial hyperplasia and metaplasia, followed by mild, moderate, and severe dysplasia; carcinoma in situ; invasive cancer; and metastatic disease. Recent studies have attempted to identify genetic alterations previously found in invasive and metastatic lesions in preneoplastic lesions. Investigators have found many of the same alterations in preneoplastic lesions, and Gazdar et al have shown that loss of heterozygosity of 3p and 9p may be some of the earliest events in the pathogenesis of lung cancer (4). Loss of genetic material from the short arm of chromosome 3 and p53 mutations have been detected in carcinoma in situ (5). Additionally, cytogenetic changes and the overexpression of growth factors have been described in morphologically normal epithelium from patients with lung cancer (6).

Unfortunately, the genetic and histologic events leading up to adenocarcinoma and small cell carcinoma are less well defined as often no clear preneoplastic sequence is seen by light microscopy. Clearly, our ability to detect preneoplastic changes histologically lags far behind our ability to detect genetic changes that may be associated with the development of cancer. Bridging this gap in our ability to detect the earliest steps in tumorigenesis will extend our understanding of the molecular pathogeneisis of lung cancer and possibly create the ability to detect such lesions for earlier intervention.

Once a cell accumulates the changes needed to become malignant, additional changes may occur during tumor evolution. Some authors have reported that early stage lung tumors have a lower incidence of p53 abnormalities, but this may reflect the differing underlying behavior of tumors with different genetic compositions. Most studies demonstrate that metastases always have the same p53 mutations as other metastases as well as the primary (7, 8). Some mutations, such as those found with the oncogene ras are stable with disease progression (9) while others may develop during treatment, as is seen for the oncogene myc whose amplification has been found to be associated with recurrent SCLCs after cytotoxic therapy (10).

Inherited predisposition to lung cancer

Although the great majority of lung cancers are associated with smoking, there is a small population of patients that develop lung cancer without any known environmental risk factors. Case studies of such patients has provided evidence that hereditary and genetic influences play an important role in host susceptibility to lung cancer (11). Multivariate analyses of clinical data on lung cancer incidences have demonstrated a significant excess of deaths related to lung and other cancers among relatives of patients compared with the general population, even when adjusted for tobacco exposure (12).

The Rb gene is the classic example of a tumor susceptibility gene that can be inherited and somatically mutated in some cases of lung cancer. Survivors of hereditary retinoblastoma are at higher risk of developing lung cancer as adults, and they develop lung tumors at an earlier age than the general population (13). Further, relatives that are carriers of the Rb gene have a 15 fold higher risk of developing lung cancers as compared to the general population (14).

Although the tumor suppressor p53 is frequently mutated in lung cancer, there have only been rare cases in which lung cancer developed in an individual carrying a mutant allele. This finding suggests that p53 is not an early hit in the development of lung cancer and that some as yet unknown gene may be the primary susceptibility gene.

Chromosomal alterations in lung cancer

Cytogenetic analysis of lung tumors indicates that both SCLC and NSCLC have multiple genetic alterations. The chromosomal alterations seen in lung cancer includes an unstable number of chromosomes as well as chromosomal abnormalities including interstitial and terminal deletions, duplications, balanced and unbalanced translocations, ring chromosomes, and centromereless chromosome fragments. New techniques such as fluorescent in situ hybridization (FISH) and comparative genomic hybridization have led to the discovery of novel genes in lung cancer by aiding in the identification of chromosomal fragments and the rapid screening of the entire human genome for both losses and gains in genetic material. The new comprehensive analytical technologies including the cDNA microarray and protein mass spectrometry hold great promise in the identification of new genes or gene clusters responsible for tumorigenesis, invasion, metastasis and response to therapy. These technologies use advanced computer software to analyze tissue samples for DNA, RNA, or protein expression and correlate these with the behavior of interest. These studies will allow the differential detection of genetic abnormalities between different tumors as well as within a given tumor as it invades and metastasizes and will give us additional insight into the genetic basis for these behaviors that should lead to improved strategies for prevention, diagnosis, and treatment.

The most common cytogenetic abnormality found in lung cancer is a loss of genetic material from the short arm of chromosome 3 (15-21). Loss of all of part of chromosome 3p has been reported to occur in 25-100% of cases examined (15, 22-26). Adding weight to the role of 3p in lung cancer is the fact that 3p has been found to be altered in several other types of human solid tumors including renal cell carcinoma, mesothelioma, ovarian carcinoma, and breast carcinoma. Several candidate tumor suppressor genes have been proposed to account for this association, but due to the large amount of DNA material involved, progress has been slow. The presence of a tumor suppressor gene in this region is supported by the observation that transfection of genetic material from the short arm of chromosome 3 into mouse A9 cells results in reduced tumorigenicity (27). Other research that has found homozygous deletions of chromosomes 3p12-13, 3p14.2, 3p21.31, and 3p21.33 suggests that more than one tumor suppressor gene may be located in this region (17, 28-33).

Another commonly implicated cytogenetic abnormality in lung cancer involves loss of heterozygosity for chromosome 9p21 (34, 35). Both the p15 and p16 cdk inhibitor genes have been mapped to a deleted region of 9p21 and have been frequently found to be inactivated in NSCLC (36). Others have found additional candidate regions on 9p21 homozygously deleted suggesting that, like chromosome 3p, multiple tumor suppressor genes my be located in this region (35).

Frequent loss of chromosome 5q in SCLC has been reported (37). D'Amico et al have found frequent loss of heterozygosity at the loci of two genes commonly implicated in colorectal cancer, MCC and APC, which are located at 5q21 (38). Several regulatory genes are located on 5q including p85a, phosphatidyl inositol 3-kinase associated protein (39) and the RASA locus (40). p85a has been shown to modulate interactions between certain activated receptors and the phophatidylinositol 3-kinase (41) while RASA encodes the GTP-activating protein involved in signal transduction.

Additional chromosomal alterations implicated in the pathogenesis of lung cancer involve chromosomes 11q, 13q, and 17p. Raiso et al has suggested that chromosome 11q may be the locus for one or several tumor suppressor genes due based on the finding of frequent LOH in lung cancer (42). Additionally, loss of chromosome 13 has been reported in SCLC (43, 37). The tumor suppressor gene Rb1 which has been shown to be absent or expressed in low levels in nearly 80% of SCLC's (44) is located on 13q suggesting that some of these alterations unmask an inactivated Rb1 on the remaining, karyotypically normal 13q. Finally, several authors have reported abnormalities of chromosome 17. Yokota et al found LOH in 17p in 5 of 5 SCLC cases (23) while Testa has reported on loss of part of all of 17p in 14 of 17 SCLC specimens (20). Additionally, DNA losses from 17p are a frequent finding in NSCLC (24). The tumor suppressor gene p53 is located at 17p13 and has been frequently shown to be altered in lung cancer (45). This loss of the p53 locus may lead to neoplasia by uncovering a mutated p53 at the remaining allele.

Genetic instability in lung cancer

Instability and loss of genetic material are recognized events in the development of cancer. In addition to the alterations of genes directly involved in the cell cycle, abnormalities in genes involved in the detection and repair of DNA mismatches may predispose individuals carrying these abnormal genes to cancer. This is just the case with two such genes, mutl (hMLH1) and muts (hMSH2), which have been shown to cause hereditary nonpolyposis colon cancer (HNPCC) (46-49). The tumors seen in HNPCC have difficulty in replicating DNA, especially across stretches of dinucleotide repeats. HNPCC tumor cells have been found to have different numbers of these repeats (50, 51) and this same phenomenon has been observed in lung cancer (52). Of note, the locus for hMLH1 is 3p21.3 which is commonly deleted in SCLC. The role, if any, of these DNA mismatch detection and repair enzymes in the molecular pathogenesis of lung cancer remains to be demonstrated.

Dominant oncogenes in lung cancer

Dominant oncogenes actively promote cancer development by loss of regulation or overexpression, and thus only one of the two alleles needs to be altered in the cancer. Oncogenes can be activated by mutation, gene amplification, or inappropriate expression.

Ras

The ras family of genes encode for 21kDa proteins which attach to the inner surface of the cytoplasmic membrane via a post-translationally added farnesyl group. Ras genes are homologous to G proteins and are thought to mediate signal transduction by a similar mechanism. G proteins exist in 2 states, guanosine diphosphate (GDP)-bound and guanosine triphosphate (GTP)-bound. The GTP-bound state is the active state that is capable of transducing a response from cell surface receptors. Growth stimuli such as mitogens and growth factors cause the substitution of GDP for GTP resulting in ras activation. Ras is converted to its inactive form, ras-GDP, by intrinsic GTPase activity. Ras mutations in human solid tumors usually lock the ras protein into its active, GTP bound, state by mutating its GTP-ase activity. Mutations typically occur at codons 12, 13 or 61. Work by Mitsudomi et al. (53) suggests that ras mutations are limited to NSCLC. In a series of 77 non-small cell lung cancers and 42 small cell lung cancers, ras mutations were found exclusively in NSCLC, predominantly in codon 12. Most authors find mutations in about 25% of lung adenocarcinomas, with lower frequencies in the other subtypes of NSCLC. The lack of ras mutations in SCLC suggests a molecular specificity to this genetic abnormality that may reflect different pathogenetic mechanisms. An inverse relationship may exist between the presence of ras mutations and abnormalities of p53, pRb, or p16 (54, 55). On the other hand, ras gene amplification in lung cancer is uncommon (56, 57), but when present is stable and present in both primary and metastatic tissues (9).

The ras protein must be bound to the inside of the cell membrane to promote tumor growth, and this is accomplished by post-translational lipid modification by a farnesyl group. Selective inhibitors of the enzyme responsible for adding this lipid group, the farnesyl protein transferase, have been developed by several companies and are currently in clinical trials.

Myc

The myc family of oncogenes includes c-myc, N-myc, and L-myc. The myc gene encodes for a nuclear phosphoprotein that functions in the regulation of transcription. The myc genes are rarely mutated and are found to be activated by overexpression, either by up-regulation or gene amplification. L-myc has been found to be amplified in SCLC (58). In a study of SCLC tumor samples taken before chemotherapy, Johnson et al. found N-myc and L-myc gene amplification in 10% to 20% of SCLC samples (59). In cell lines established after chemotherapy and clinical relapse this number increased to 44% with 11 out of 25 samples containing myc amplification (10). Others have found c-myc gene amplification to be associated with the variant phenotype of SCLC (60) and with a decreased survival (10). When RNA expression of myc genes in SCLC samples is compared to normal fetal lung tissue, 80% to 90% of tumors show overexpression of the myc genes (61). In contrast, NSCLC rarely contains amplification of c-myc (only 2 of 47 tumors), and these 2 were adenocarcinomas with normal ras genes (62). These findings demonstrate that myc amplification is associated with a class of lung cancer (SCLC), exposure to chemotherapy, a particular subtype (variant phenotype), and poor survival. Newer techniques of comparative genomic hybridization and arbitrarily primed PCR have confirmed the amplification of myc family members in lung cancer (63, 64).

Tumor Suppressor Genes

Tumor suppressor genes are those that normally function to down-regulate cell division, and tumors are frequently found to bypass this function by their deletion or mutational inactivation. Thus typically both copies of a tumor suppressor gene need to be inactivated before a phenotype is evident. The tumor suppressor gene retinoblastoma (Rb) and p53 have been implicated in human tumors including lung cancer. Rb and p53 are intimately associated with the network of proteins involved in the regulation of cell growth and division. Mutation of Rb, p53, or alteration of many proteins upstream or downstream of these key proteins can lead cancer by dysregulating cell cycle and apoptotic regulatory mechanisms.

Retinoblastoma

The retinoblastoma (Rb) gene encodes for a nuclear phosphoprotein that is involved in cell cycle regulation through binding to G1 cyclins and transcription factors such as E2F1 (reviewed in 65-67). The Rb protein is inactive in its bound form, and the binding of E2F1 to Rb is dependent on phosphorylation. Interestingly, several tumor virus gene products including the SV40 large T antigen, adenovirus E1A, and human papilloma virus E7 have evolved to take advantage of this by binding and inactivating the Rb protein forcing cells from G0 into the cell cycle to facilitate viral replication.

The vast majority (nearly 80%) of SCLC's studied have absent or abnormal Rb protein while only a small percentage of NSCLC's have structural defects in Rb (44). Not suprisingly, most of these mutations involve the pocket region of Rb which disrupts binding of Rb to other proteins. It has recently been found that the cyclin-dependent kinase inhibitor p16 is inactivated in many of the NSCLC that appear to have wild-type Rb (68). In the absence of this inhibitor, Rb stays in its phosphorylated activating state, releasing E2F and promoting cell cycle progression. Thus, most NSCLCs have somatically inactivated some component of the Rb pathway. Studies of individuals who are carriers for abnormal Rb genes further support the role of Rb in lung tumorigenesis. These individuals develop non-ocular tumors at 10 times the expected rate with SCLC being prominent among these with a 15-fold increase in incidence in this population (14). A central and perhaps necessary step in lung tumorigenesis is the presence of defective Rb. Supporting this is the fact that when normal Rb gene is re-introduced into Rb negative human lung cancer cells via retroviral transduction, these cells lose tumorigenicity in nude mice despite the fact that these tumors contain multiple genetic lesions (69).

p53

Like Rb, p53 is a nuclear phosphoprotein that has been the subject of intense research since its discovery. p53 binds to DNA and functions in transcriptional regulation. The p53 gene is the most frequently mutated gene in human cancer. p53 normally functions as a tumor suppressor gene, but when mutated may also function as a dominant oncogene. The physiologic role of p53 as a tumor suppressor comes from evidence of its induction by DNA damage as well as it apparent role in programmed cell death or apoptosis (70).

Studies of cell cycle control after radiation induced DNA damage indicate a link between p53-mediated transcriptional activation and apoptosis. If DNA damage is induced in normal cells they arrest at the G1-S phase of the cell cycle. However, in cells with mutated p53, this damage fails to arrest cell growth and cells proceed through the S phase (71). This pause in G1-S seen in normal cells is believed to allow for DNA repair before proceeding with replication or to induce apoptosis. Thus, in cells with mutant p53 that lack this checkpoint, the DNA damage is incorporated into the genome of the daughter cells and may serve as a key step in the cascade of genetic alterations in tumorigenesis.

p53 is very commonly abnormal in lung cancer with nearly 50% of NSCLCs and nearly 90% of SCLCs demonstrating abnormalities in p53 (72, 73). These abnormalities consist of several types of alterations and occur throughout the open reading frame. The most commonly identified mutations are missense mutations that occur in exons 5 through 8 (72) and are associated with prolonged protein half-life resulting in an increased steady-state protein level. Normal cells express low levels of p53 but abnormal proteins with prolonged half-lives accumulate and are readily detectable. As such, most tumors with abnormal p53 gene products can be identified with immunohistochemistry although this misses about one-third of p53 abnormalities, mostly splicing and nonsense mutations and sometimes stains tumors with no structural p53 abnormalities (74).

Inactivation of the p16 (INK4A)/retinoblastoma (RB) or p53 biochemical pathway is a frequent event in most human cancers. An alternative mechanism for p53 inactivation involves binding to the protein mdm2, which is in turn modulated by a newly discovered protein ARF. Recent evidence has shown that P14ARF binds to MDM2 leading to an increased availability of wild type p53 protein. Recent studies have shown that inactivation of the INK4a/ARF locus frequently coexists with p53 mutations in NSCLCs suggesting that p14ARF inactivation is not functionally equivalent to abrogation of the p53 pathway by p53 mutation. (75). Others have shown that p16INK4a and p19ARF expression is altered in about half of NSCLCs, and that there is an inverse association between p19ARF and p53 expression suggesting a linked pathway (76).

Growth factors
In the process of tumorigenesis cells may develop alterations that lead to altered expression of growth factors and/or their receptors. These abnormalities can lead to changes in cell cycle regulation through autocrine or paracrine loops. Furthermore, tumor expression of certain growth factors may have profound systemic biological effects.

The oncogene c-erbB-1 encodes the EGF receptor and c-erbB-2 (HER2neu) encodes a protein with structural similarity to EGFr. Schneider et al have reported that erb-B-2 alterations are rare (2 of 60 specimens) in NSCLCs (77). However, among lung cancer cell lines, 4 of 4 SCLC cell line demonstrated minimal or non-detectable expression of c-erb-B-2 mRNA compared with high levels of expression in NSCLC cell lines (77). The highest expression levels of erb-B-2 were seen in 4 of 4 adenocarcinomas. Further, overexpression of erb-B-2 as has been shown to be a poor prognostic indicator in

NSCLC (78), and overexpression may be associated with metastases (79). Antibody to HER2 has been shown to inhibit lung cancer cell growth (80), and this is currently being tested in a human clinical trial.   The vast majority of NSCLCs are positive for EGFrs (81), and the expression of EGF raises the possibility of EGFr acting in an autocrine loop to promote cell growth and perhaps metastases. Further, Garcia de Palazzo et al have reported that some NSCLCs express a mutated form of the EGFr (82). Small molecule inhibitors of the EGF receptor that compete with ATP for its binding site in the kinase domain or blocking antibodies show promise in early phase lung cancer trials (83, 84). Other growth factor receptors implicated in the pathogenesis of lung cancer include c-myb and c-raf. c-myb is a nuclear oncogene whose level has been shown to be inversely associated with differentiation and is expressed in SCLC but not NSCLC (85). c-raf is an oncogene that is frequently deleted in NSCLC and SCLC including every case of SCLC examined (86).   Further, c-kit, a tyrosine kinase receptor involved in hematopoiesis, and its ligand, stem cell factor (SCF), or co-expressed in SCLC but not in NSCLC (87, 88). The mitogen platelet derived growth factor (PDGF) and its receptor have been found to be expressed in both primary lung cancers and cell lines (89, 90). Both c-kit and PDGF may act in autocrine loops to promote cell growth. Finally, Plummer has demonstrated a correlation between c-kit levels and the overexpression of myc (91).

Molecular approaches to improving lung cancer outcomes

Knowledge of the specific molecular abnormalities in lung cancer should allow improved prevention and early detection strategies, and lead to the design of therapeutics specifically targeting these abnormalities. Molecular damage can be detected in bronchial epithelial cells of non-smokers (92) and the relationship of this damage to lung cancer risk is currently being assessed.   It is possible that minimally invasive technologies involving peripheral blood or sputum could be used to screen for the presence of clonal abnormalities preceding the development of clinically apparent lung cancer (93-95). Molecularly-targeted therapeutics should be more effective and less toxic. Antibodies or small molecules that block growth factor receptors have already been mentioned. Other examples include anti-angiogenics, antisense and gene therapies, metalloproteinase inhibitors and immunotherapy.   We will briefly review these approaches as they apply to lung cancer.

Targeting of tumor vasculature

The tumor vasculature is an extremely attractive therapeutic target for many reasons. Tumors are thought to induce and require the ingrowth of blood vessels in order to reach macroscopic size. While tumors themselves are genetically unstable and able to mutate in the face of selection pressure applied by cancer therapeutics, tumor neovasculature is comprised (in general) of normal endothelial cells whose behavior and responses to agents is much more stable and predictable. These tumor-induced blood vessels are different enough from blood vessels in normal tissues to allow selective therapeutic targeting. In addition, these blood vessels are induced by specific tumor-derived factors such as VEGF and FGF that can be inhibited directly.

Vascular endothelial growth factor (VEGF) is an angiogenic factor induced by hypoxia and known to be essential for tumor neo-vascularization. High levels of VEGF expression have been shown to predict poor survival and to be inversely correlated with wild type p53 (96). In vivo preclinical trials have shown that anti-VEGF monoclonal antibodies inhibit tumor growth in a dose-dependent manner and the results of phase II trials in lung cancer have been promising. There is an ongoing phase III trial evaluating anti-VEGF in combination with paclitaxel/carboplatin in NSCLC.

Metalloproteinase Inhibitors

The metalloproteinases are specific proteases involved in a variety of tissue remodeling processes, including pathologic cancer invasion and metastasis. MMP-2 and MMP-9 are frequently expressed in non-small cell lung cancer (97), Gelatinases can be expressed by small cell lung cancer (98), and MMP-9 can even be elevated in the blood of cancer patients (99). Their expression is associated with metastasis and angiogenesis (100). MMPs can be expressed by the tumor directly or can be induced by the tumor to be expressed in surrounding stromal cells. Their expression is associated with the formation of scarring and sclerosis in lung tumors (101). Endogenous protease inhibitors called "Tissue Inhibitors of MetalloProteases" or TIMPs can also be expressed in some NSCLC (102). Specific drugs that inhibit these enzymes have been developed and are effective in animal models in inhibiting tumor angiogenesis and metastasis (103). Several of these are being tested in human clinical trials (104, 105).

Gene Therapy Approaches for Lung Cancer

The fact that cancer appears to arise as a result of an accumulation of genetic damage suggests that direct introduction of the damaged genes or genetic approaches to therapy may be useful. Gene therapy is the use of DNA or RNA as a therapeutic agent. Approaches fall into 4 main categories: 1) replacement of a deleted, mutated, or under-expressed gene, 2) inactivation of an overexpressed gene, 3) the use of a suicide gene selectively targeted to tumor cells, and 4) immune inducing gene therapies. Examples of each are given below.

Gene replacement

Recently, the use of wild type p53 (wtp53) as a gene therapeutic approach has received significant attention. Several authors have reported that restoration of wtp53 function in cancer cells be gene transfer is sufficient to cause cell cycle arrest or apoptosis (106-110). This observation suggests that restoration of function of a single gene, p53 in this case, is capable of causing arrest in tumor growth and even cell death. This set the stage for recent trials of gene therapy for lung cancer aimed at reintroducing wtp53. Roth et al have reported on 9 patients with recurrent or metastatic NSCLC treated with the retroviral p53 expression vector ITRp53A (111). Of the seven patients evaluated, three showed evidence of tumor regression at the treatment site and six patients showed an increase in apoptosis of tumor cells at post-treatment biopsies. Many hundreds of patients have now been treated with a recombinant adenovirus expressing wild-type p53 delivered by direct injection into tumors. In lung cancer, clinical responses have been observed for this approach (112). Gene delivery is a major problem with directly injected gene therapy vectors, so biologically confined tumors such as mesothelioma and ovarian cancer are being targeted in increasing numbers of studies. We are currently conducting a trial of Ad-p53 delivered by bronchoalveolar lavage for bronchioloalveolar lung cancer (BAC). BAC characteristically grows as a thin layer of tumor cells lining the alveoli and small airways and appears to spread by direct extension. It should thus be readily accessible to delivery of therapeutics via the airway. To date we have treated 14 patients on this study and have seen both pathological responses and improvements in diffusing capacity.

Gene inhibition

Inhibition of any dominantly acting gene might be a reasonable therapeutic strategy. As previously mentioned HER-2neu overexpression has been found to be associated with malignant transformation and present in 30% of lung adenocarcinomas (78). Deshane et al. have demonstrated the feasibility of functionally disabling the HER2 receptor by using a vector encoding an intracellular single chain antibody fragment directed against HER2neu. The gene vector expresses the antibody inside the cell and this binds and inactivates HER2neu, resulting in cell arrest (113). Also, approximately 30% of NSCLCs have abnormalities in expression of K-ras (114). Several authors have shown the potential efficacy of neutralizing the mutated dominant negative K-ras oncogene using a vector encoding the antisense transcript (115, 116). Another interesting approach involves the antisense inhibition of bcl-2 (117).

Suicide gene therapies

The approach of suicide gene therapy is based on the transduction of tumor cells with a vector encoding a gene that sensitizes cells to an otherwise non-toxic drug (118). This approach involves selective transcriptional targeting of cancer cells by regulating the expression of the suicide gene (119). Since tumor transduction is never complete, effective cytoreduction by this approach requires a significant bystander effect (120). The efficacy of such approaches has been hypothesized to be in part due the bystander effect. This refers to the ability of transfected tumor cells to mediate killing of adjacent non-transfected (120, 109). Several authors have reported in the success of this approach in lung cancer both in vitro and in vivo using nonselective promoters driving the herpes simplex virus thymidine kinase (HSV-tk) gene followed by gancyclovir therapy (121-124). Additionally, there is the possible role of an immune-mediated response to the transgene or contributing to tumor cell death (125, 126).

The Immunology of Lung Cancer

The underlying principle of cancer immunotherapy is that cancer cells differ from normal cells either in the number and/or type of antigens they express. It is now clear that all cancers, including lung cancer, express antigens that represent potential immunotherapeutic targets. These antigenic differences are due to abnormal post-translational modification of surface proteins or the expression of viral, mutated, or overexpressed oncogenes or differentiation products. Attempts to induce therapeutic immunity can be grouped into "non-specific" immunostimulation, specific immunization with uncharacterized antigens, and specific immunization with defined antigens.

BCG and bacterial products - "non-specific" immunostimulants

In the early 1970's, the observation was made that empyema improved the outcome of resected lung cancer patients. In an attempt to safely mimic this effect, a number of studies utilized either the vaccine strain of mycobacteria (bacille Calmette Guerin, or BCG) or various bacterial cell products such as *Nocardia rubra* cell wall skeleton. McKneally and co-workers conducted a randomized trial of intrapleural BCG versus no treatment in surgically resected stage I and II non-small cell lung cancer (127). This study showed a small but statistically significant prolongation of remission and survival for stage I patients only. A trial was conducted to confirm these findings by the Lung Cancer Study Group (128). In this study, 141 patients with resected stage II and III adenocarcinoma and large cell carcinoma were randomized to receive either chemotherapy or intrapleural BCG. No untreated control arm was included. The chemotherapy arm was found to be statistically significantly superior to the BCG arm, and the BCG arm was not significantly different from historical controls. This trial is taken as proof of the lack of efficacy of BCG, and by many as evidence that immunotherapy will not work for lung cancer, even though comparison with placebo was not made directly.

A randomized study on SCLC was performed by the Southwest Oncology Group (SWOG) randomizing between two different chemotherapy regimens and either BCG (during chemotherapy) or no additional treatment (129). Of the 114 patients who survived more than one year after registration, there was a statistically significantly improved survival in patients who received BCG, with a 35% versus 5% survival after an additional 2 years. The authors concluded that the magnitude of this benefit was not sufficient to warrant further investigation. In addition, immunotherapy during full dose chemotherapy may not have been an optimal study design. However, these data may support the hypothesis that there is some actual benefit, though small, to adjuvant BCG in lung cancer, and that more focussed immune manipulation might result in improved therapeutic efficacy.

Other studies have evaluated a bacterial cell wall component from *Nocardia rubra* (Nocardia cell wall skeleton, or N-CWS) administered intrapleurally or intradermally. In a randomized study of 87 patients with completely resected NSCLC treated with adjuvant chemotherapy or chemotherapy followed by N-CWS therapy, a significantly prolonged survival was noted in the immunotherapy group (130). This observation has not been seriously pursued.

"Specific" Immunotherapy for lung cancer

The term "specific" immunotherapy applies to the use of tumor cells (either autologous or allogeneic) or purified tumor antigens in an attempt to boost antigen-specific responses to shared antigens (common between individual tumors) or unique tumor antigens present in each patients tumor. Takita and coworkers conducted a randomized trial of 86 resectable NSCLC patients who received either no postoperative treatment or two arms with different doses of tumor antigen in adjuvant. A significantly improved survival was observed in the subset of N0 patients in the "low dose" antigen group. Analysis of data from another 3 trials involving 234 stage I and II resected NSCLC patients found a 5 year survival benefit (p = 0.0002) in patients treated with specific tumor antigen extracts (131). No follow-up study has been reported.

Tumor infiltrating lymphocytes, or TIL, are presumably enriched for those effector cells with tumor specificity (132). These cells are harvested from a tumor biopsy and expanded *in vitro* in the presence of cytokines and the absence of potential tumor-derived immunosuppressive factors. Tan and coworkers (133) harvested TIL from 10 lung cancer patients with malignant pleural effusions, introduced the IL-2 gene into them with a recombinant retrovirus, and expanded them *in vitro*. The patients were then treated with 1-6 X 10^{10} TIL intrapleurally. No reaccumulation was observed for at least 4 weeks in 6 of 10 patients, and one patient had a lasting resolution of the effusion and an objective response of the primary tumor mass. Even more intriguing is a randomized study conducted by Ratto and collegues in Italy (134). In this study, 113 patients with resected stage II, IIIA and IIIB NSCLC were randomized to receive autologous TIL intravenously 6-8 weeks after surgery with subcutaneous IL-2 for 3 months or control therapy. Stage II patients received either immunotherapy or no treatment, and stage III patients were randomized to receive immunotherapy plus radiation or chemotherapy plus radiation. This study demonstrated a statistically significant improvement in survival for the group as a whole, but interestingly, the largest benefit was for immunotherapy plus radiation therapy in patients with stage IIIB disease. In this study, only T4 IIIB patients were eligible, and not patients with N3 disease. Also, perhaps unexpectedly, among these patients the benefit was almost entirely from reduction in local relapse rather than reduced development of metastatic disease.

These trials suggest that there may be some benefit to adjuvant immunotherapy in lung cancer, but definitive trials are lacking. A major problem with historical immunotherapeutic approaches has been the lack of a clear and practical path to follow. Many of these treatments were laborious, specialized, difficult to standardize, and difficult to assess. These issues are being overcome in some of the newer approaches to immunotherapy to be discussed next.

Therapy with defined tumor antigens
Many potential tumor specific antigens have been postulated in tumor cells including viral antigens, fetal genes, and mutated oncogene or tumor suppressor gene products (135). Intensive studies of tumor specific antigens during the last decade resulted in the identification of numerous antigens associated with different types of cancer, including melanoma, cervical cancer, colon cancer, and lung cancer (rev. in 136, 137). During carcinogenesis, it is clear that multiple genetic and protein structural changes occur. The inactivation of tumor suppressor genes and activation of oncogenes through mutation and/or dysregulated expression are examples of these genetic alterations. These alterations represent differences between cancer cells and normal cells. Most cancer cells are thus likely to have protein structural features or patterns of protein expression which could allow immune detection and elimination.

As has been discussed above, mutations in the p53 tumor suppressor gene are common in lung cancer. In most cases the mutant p53 protein product is also overexpressed (74).

There are a few 'hotspots' for mutations in p53 (such as codons 175, 248 and 273); however, these make up only a small fraction of the mutations observed. This complicates mutation-specific immunotargeting, as each patient is likely to have a different mutation.

Mutant-specific epitope targeting may, however, not be necessary, as several authors have demonstrated efficient recognition of wild-type p53 sequences in murine models (138, 139) or human cells *in vitro* (140). This occurs in spite of the fact that every normal cell in normal individuals expresses a low level of structurally identical p53 protein. The typically massive overexpression of the mutant protein may allow sufficient tumor-normal discrimination to be of clinical utility. The major practical advantage of targeting a wild-type epitope is that a single vaccine preparation can be used to target a wide variety of tumors producing different mutated p53 proteins, and these sequences can be selected to match the peptide-binding preferences of large classes of patients with common MHC antigens.

Animal studies have demonstrated the induction of effective CTL responses against the mutant p53 protein (139). Using peptides that span mutation sites in mutant p53 to immunize animals, it is possible to show the development of p53-specific CTL. Some of these CTL recognized the mutant peptide sequence and not the corresponding wild-type one (141). It is remarkable that a CTL response can be generated in such animals that is specific for the presence of a single amino acid substitution in the p53 protein. This underscores the specificity achievable when a finely tuned biological process, such as the cellular immune system, is evoked, as opposed to the lack of specificity observed for standard chemotherapeutic agents. This CTL response provided tumor protection of control mice against subsequent challenge with tumor cells bearing specific mutation (141-144). A recent study in animals demonstrated the enhancement of the immunogenicity of a mutant p53 epitope after transduction of the costimulatory molecule B7 via recombinant adenovirus (145). This underscores the fact that appropriate antigens may be present and not recognized without therapeutic manipulation.

Anti-p53 immune responses in cancer patients

Immune responses in cancer patients against p53 can occur in the absence of specific vaccination. Anti-p53 antibodies have detected in the serum of human lung cancer patients and correlate with the presence of missense mutations in p53 (146). Cellular immune responses specific for p53 have also been observed in humans. CD4$^+$ T cells (those which produce cytokines and proliferate in response to antigen) that respond to p53 peptides have been reported in breast cancer patients (147). All of the patients from which helper T cell responses could be detected also had antibodies against p53, demonstrating the existence of a combined cellular and humoral response in these patients. Kast and Melief showed *in vitro* induction of human CTL to both normal and mutant p53 epitopes (140). In breast cancer patients, significant CTL responses specific for the mutant p53 in a cancer patient's tumor have been observed (148). In most cases, these CTL recognized mutant, but not the corresponding wild-type p53 sequences. Therefore, p53 protein can behave as an antigenic target for CTL during the natural process of tumorigenesis without external immunization or other immunotherapy. The role of these CTL in affecting the clinical course of the cancer is unclear, but the majority of patients with these responses in this study were apparently cured of their disease with surgery alone. A human clinical trial attempting to induce CTL in cancer patients using custom p53- or ras-derived peptide corresponding to the mutant p53 or ras sequence in the particular patient's tumor has recently found induction of responses in 19 of 33 treated patients. With rapidly improving technology, inexpensive and rapid genetic analysis of tumors is a real possibility, but a vaccine composed of a collection of mutant peptides may be impractical given the huge number of different mutant sequences observed in most naturally occurring tumors.

Another promising protein in the search for cancer antigens capable of inducing CTL's is the recently discovered testicular cancer antigen NY-ESO-1. Lee et al. have reported expression of NY-ESO-1 in 11 of 16 SCLC's and 3 of 7 NSCLC's tested. Further, this antigen is capable of inducing HLA-restricted CTL's and may have promise as a lung cancer immunotherapy target.

Others have reported that the presence of anti-GM2 ganglioside antibodies is associated with a prolonged disease-free survival in patients with melanoma, and that SCLC patients immunized with BEC2, an anti-idiotypic monoclonal antibody that mimics the ganglioside GD3, had a prolonged survival compared with historical controls. (149). The same group has recently shown that the Fuc-GM1 ganglioside is present on most SCLC's and of 10 patients treated with at least 5 vaccinations with Fuc-GM1, all patients demonstrated a serological response with the induction of both IgG and IgM.. These novel lung tumor antigens may serve as targets in developing future immunotherapies.

A variety of genetic approaches have been demonstrated in model systems to assist in the induction of immunity. Allogenic and syngenic major histocompatibility complex (MHC) class I and II genes, costimulatory molecule genes (e.g. B7), and cytokine genes have all been inserted into tumor cells to alter the immunological environment and to overcome the defective induction of immunity in tumor-bearing hosts. In a murine lung cancer system (3LL/3) from C57BL/6 mice (MHC type $H-2^b$), transfection of the allogeneic MHC molecule $H-2L^d$ caused a reduction in tumorigenicity and protection against unmodified 3LL/3 (150). Plautz et al. (151) showed that expression of a murine class I $H-2K^s$ gene in CT26 mouse colon adenocarcinoma ($H-2K^d$) or MCA 106 fibrosarcoma ($H-2K^d$) induced a cytotoxic T cell response to $H-2K^d$ and, more importantly, to other antigens present on unmodified tumor cells which hadn't been recognized previously. Recently, allogenic MHC transfection has been applied to humans with HLA-B7 gene transfer. Nabel et al. (152) reported the reduction of tumor size in a melanoma patient after the direct gene transfer of an HLA-B7 gene in a liposome complex. Clinical protocols of HLA-B7 gene transfer by lipofection in advanced cancers are under way.

Effective antitumor immunity is usually dependent on T-cell mediated responses. Two kinds of signals are required for the activation of T cells. The first signal is the antigen-specific binding of a peptide antigen-MHC complex on the surface of antigen presenting cells with antigen specific T cell receptors. The second signal is transmitted by the antigen-independent binding of costimulatory molecules on antigen presenting cells with their corresponding receptors on T cells. A number of molecules have been found to mediate this second signal, including the B7 family (unrelated to the HLA-B7 class I molecule described above), which interact with the CD28 receptor on T cells (153, 154). B7 transduction via recombinant adenovirus into murine tumors expressing mutant p53 resulted in the induction of mutant p53 specific CTL and loss of tumorigenicity as well as protective immunity against challenge by untransduced tumor (145). Another recent study demonstrated that B7 and CD28 interaction provided costimulatory signals not only for T cells but also for natural killer (NK) cells (155). In contrast to defined antigen vaccine approaches, another important aspect of B7 gene therapy is the potential ability to increase the immunogenicity of all tumor specific antigens, whether or not they have been identified.

To avoid systemic side effects and to better approximate normal physiological conditions, gene therapy has been used to insert cytokine genes into tumor cells and induce the production of cytokines in the vicinity of tumor. Local production of cytokines from tumors can modify the tumor's interactions with the host immune system. Many cytokines have been tested for efficacy in animal models of cytokine gene therapy. IL-2, IL-4, IL-6, IL-7, IL-12, IFN-γ, TNFα-, G-CSF and GM-CSF among others have been investigated. Using a highly malignant and poorly immunogenic Lewis lung carcinoma, IL-2 production by retrovirally transduced tumor cells induced antitumor CTL and eliminated the generation of lung metastasis (156). Retroviral IFN-γ gene insertion into poorly immunogenic 3LL-D122 showed a significant decrease in tumorigenicity and metastatic potential and induced tumor specific CTL when modified tumor cells were injected after irradiation (157).

GM-CSF appears to be one of the most active cytokines in the induction of antitumor immunity. In a comparison of the efficacy of a number of cytokines using retroviral vectors, GM-CSF demonstrated the most potent, specific and long lasting antitumor immunity (158). The antitumor immunity induction after gene therapy with GM-CSF was dependent on both CD4$^+$ and CD8$^+$ T cells. This activity may be related to its ability to promote the differentiation of hematopoietic precursors to dendritic cells and other professional antigen presenting cells (159). We have designed and produced an adenovirus-GM-CSF vector that also overcomes many of the limitations of *in vitro* culture of primary human tumors. Transduction of 3LL with this adenovirus-GM CSF vector eliminated its tumorigenicity, induced tumor specific CTL and the cure of established Lewis Lung carcinoma tumors(160). Furthermore, we showed that this was associated with an increased number of dendritic cells in the tumor vaccine injection site.

Immune defects in cancer patients
Demonstration of antitumor responses induced by peptide immunization in animals bearing pre-existing tumors has been much more difficult than demonstrating tumor protection, presumably due to tumor associated immune dysfunction to be discussed in the next section. However, when repeated immunizations with p53 peptide-pulsed dendritic cells were used in animals bearing palpable tumors, clinically significant antitumor effects were observed (161). The combination of this approach with the

cytokine IL-12 yields further improvement in the antitumor effect (162). In these studies, repeated immunizations were important, and this stresses the difference between the common prophylactic immunization for infectious diseases and antigen-specific immunotherapy. The prior presence of the tumor appears to inhibit the ability of the individual to maintain a response and repeated antigen exposure is essential. The development of clinically evident tumors implies a failure of the immune system to detect and reject cancer cells as foreign. We have recently demonstrated a clear defect in DC function in patients with advanced cancer (163), but that DC from these patients function normally after growth from precursors *in vitro*, free from the influence of tumor derived factors. We have gone on to demonstrate that tumor-derived Vascular Endothelial Growth factor (VEGF), a factor produced by most tumors and known to be important for tumor angiogenesis, is an important factor in the induction of this DC defect (164) and that inhibiting VEGF improves the efficacy of immunotherapy (165). A multi-modality approach which utilizes optimal standard therapeutic modalities, followed by anti-angiogenic and immunotherapeutic strategies may well ultimately prove to be superior to the traditional modalities of chemotherapy, radiation and surgery alone.

SUMMARY

Our understanding of lung cancer biology has rapidly expanded in recent years. Lung cancer, unlike most human cancers, can be traced to an environmental risk factor in the majority of cases, and this fact is reflected in the vast number of genetic alterations discovered in lung tumors whose pathogenesis is believed to be mediated by carcinogen exposure. The discovery of these alterations has led to a greater understanding of tumor development. The dramatic progress in the understanding of the genetic and molecular basis of oncogenesis and the induction of immunity has led to a rejuvenation of efforts to apply this new knowledge to this common and refractory disease. Further, the resurgent interest in cancer immunology and tumor-host interactions holds promise for the development of new approaches to treatment based on harvesting the immune systems ability to recognize these alterations. Hopefully, this understanding will lead to novel approaches with real and convincing clinical efficacy once some of these strategies are tested in carefully performed randomized clinical trials with appropriate power to detect meaningful differences.

REFERENCES

1.   "Cancer Facts and Figures - 2000." 2000 American Cancer Society. Atlanta.

2.   Doll R, Gray R, Hafner B and Peto R. Mortality in relation to smoking: 22 years' observations on female British doctors. Br Med J 280: 967-71, 1980.

3.   Doll R and Hill A. Lung cancer and other causes of death in relation to smoking. A second report on the mortality of British doctors. Br Med J 2: 1071-1081, 1956.

4. Gazdar A F, Bader S, Hung J, Kishimoto Y, Sekido Y, Sugio K, Virmani A, Fleming J, Carbone D P and Minna J D. Molecular genetic changes found in human lung cancer and its precursor lesions. Cold Spring Harbor Symposia on Quantitative Biology 59:565-72, 1994.

5. Sundaresan V, Ganly P, Hasleton P, Rudd R, Sinha G, Bleehan N M and Rabbitts, P. p53 and chromosome 3 abnormalities, characteristic of malignant lung tumours, are detectable in pre-invasive lesions of the bronchus. Oncogene. 7:1989-1997, 1992.

6. Sozzi G, Miozzo M, Tagliabue E, Calderone C, Lombardi L, Pilotti S, Pastorino U, Pierotti MA and Della Porta G. Cytogenetic abnormalities and overexpression of receptors for growth factors in normal bronchial epithelium and tumor samples of lung cancer patients. Cancer Res 51:400-4, 1991.

7. Li X, Liu J, Park JK, Hamilton TA, Rayman P, Klein E, Edinger M, Tubbs R, Bukowski R and Finke J. T cells from renal cell carcinoma patients exhibit an abnormal pattern of kappa B-specific DNA-binding activity: a preliminary report. Cancer Research 54:5424-9, 1994.

8. Sameshima Y, Matsuno Y, Hirohashi S, Shimosato Y, Mizoguchi H, Sugimura T, Terada M and Yokota J. Alterations of the p53 gene are common and critical events for the maintenance of malignant phenotypes in small-cell lung carcinoma. Oncogene 7:451-7, 1992.

9. Li S, Rosell R, Urban A, Font A, Ariza A, Armengol P, Abad A, Navas JJ and Monzo M. K-ras point mutation: a stable tumor marker in non-small cell lung carcinoma. Lung Cancer 11:19-27, 1994.

10. Johnson BE, Ihde DC, Makuch RW, Gazdar AF, Carney DN, Oie H, Russell E, Nau MM and Minna J D. *myc* family oncogene amplification in tumor cell lines established from small cell lung cancer patients and its relationship to clinical status and course. J Clin Invest 79:1629-1634, 1987.

11. Tokuhata G. Familial factors in human lung cancer and smoking. Am J Public Health 54:25-32, 1964.

12. Sellers T, Ooi W and Elston R. Increased familial risk for non-lung cancer among relatives of lung cancer patients. Am J Epidemiol. 126:237-246, 1987.

13. Leonard R, MacKay T, Brown A, Gregor A, Crompton G and Smyth J. Small-cell lung cancer after retinoblastoma. Lancet 2:1503, 1988.

14. Sanders, B., Jay, M., Draper, G. and Roberts, E. Non-ocular cancer in relatives of retinoblastoma patients. Br J Cancer. 60:358-365, 1989.

15. Brauch H, Johnson B, Hovis J, Yano T, Gazdar A, Pettengill OS, Graziano S, Sorenson GD, Poiesz BJ, Minna J, et al. Molecular analysis of the short arm of chromosome 3 in small-cell and non-small-cell carcinoma of the lung. N Engl J Med 317:1109-13, 1987.

16. Johnson BE, Sakaguchi AY, Gazdar AF, Minna JD, Burch D, Marshall A and Naylor SL. Restriction fragment length polymorphism studies show consistent

loss of chromosome 3p alleles in small cell lung cancer patients' tumors. J Clin Invest 82:502-507, 1988.

17.   Kok K, van den Berg A, Veldhuis PM, van der Veen AY, Franke M, Schoenmakers EF, Hulsbeek MM, van der Hout AH, de Leij L, van de Ven W, et al. A homozygous deletion in a small cell lung cancer cell line involving a 3p21 region with a marked instability in yeast artificial chromosomes. Cancer Res 54:4183-7, 1994.

18.   Naylor S, Johnson B, Minna J and Sakaguchi A. Loss of heterozygosity of chromosome 3p markers in small-cell lung cancer. Nature (London). 329:451-454, 1987.

19.   Whang-Peng, J, Kao-Shan C, Lee E, Bunn P, Jr, Carney D, Gazdar A and Minna J. A specific chromosome defect associated with human small-cell lung cancer: deletion 3p (14-23). Science. 215:181-182, 1982.

20.   Testa, J. R. and Graziano, S. L. Molecular implications of recurrent cytogenetic alterations in human small cell lung cancer. Cancer Detect Prev 17:267-77, 1993.

21.   Miura I, Siegfried JM, Resau J, Keller SM, Zhou JY and Testa J R. Chromosome alterations in 21 non-small cell lung carcinomas. Genes Chromosomes Cancer. 2: 328-38, 1990.

22.   Kok K, Osinga J, Carritt B, Davis M, van der Hout A, van der Veen A, Landsvater R, de Leij L, Berendsen H, Postmus P, Poppema S and Buys C. Deletion of a DNA sequence at the chromosomal region 3p21 in all major types of lung cancer. Nature 330:578-581, 1987.

23.   Yokota T, Coffman RL, Hagiwara H, Rennick DM, Takebe Y, Yokota K, Gemmell L, Shrader B, Yang G, Meyerson P, Luh J, Hoy P, Pene J, Briere F, Spits H, Banchereau J, de Vries JE, Lee F, Arai N and Arai K. Isolation and characterization of lymphokine cDNA clones encoding mouse and human IgA-enhancing factor and eosinophil colony-stimulating factor activities: relationship to interleukin 5. Proceedings of the National Academy of Sciences of the United States of America 84:7388-92, 1987.

24.   Weston A, Willey JC, Modali R, Sugimura H, McDowell EM, Resau J, Light B, Haugen A, Mann DL, Trump BF, et al. Differential DNA sequence deletions from chromosomes 3, 11, 13, and 17 in squamous-cell carcinoma, large-cell carcinoma, and adenocarcinoma of the human lung. Proc Natl Acad Sci U S A. 86:5099-103, 1989.

25.   Rabbitts P, Douglas J, Daly M, Sundaresan V, Fox B, Haselton P, Wells F, Albertson D, Waters J and Bergh J. Frequency and extent of allelic loss in the short arm of chromosome 3 in nonsmall-cell lung cancer. Genes Chromosom Cancer. 1:95-105, 1989.

26.   Viallet J and Minna JD. Dominant oncogenes and tumor suppressor genes in the pathogenesis of lung cancer. Am J Respir Cell Mol Biol 2:225-32, 1990.

27.   Daly MC, Xiang RH, Buchhagen D, Hensel CH, Garcia DK, Killary AM, Minna JD and Naylor, SL. A homozygous deletion on chromosome 3 in a small cell lung

cancer cell line correlates with a region of tumor suppressor activity. Oncogene. 8:1721-9, 1993.

28.   Daly, M. C., Douglas, J. B., Bleehen, N. M., Hastleton, P., Twentyman, P. R., Sundaresan, V., Carritt, B., Bergh, J. and Rabbitts, P. H. An unusually proximal deletion on the short arm of chromosome 3 in a patient with small cell lung cancer. Genomics. 9:113-9, 1991.

29.   Drabkin HA, Mendez MJ, Rabbitts PH, Varkony T, Bergh J, Schlessinger J, Erickson P and Gemmill RM. Characterization of the submicroscopic deletion in the small-cell lung carcinoma (SCLC) cell line U2020. Genes Chromosomes Cancer. 5:67-74, 1992.

30.   Hosoe S, Ueno K, Shigedo Y, Tachibana I, Osaki T, Kumagai T, Tanio Y, Kawase I, Nakamura Y and Kishimoto T. A frequent deletion of chromosome 5q21 in advanced small cell and non-small cell carcinoma of the lung. Cancer Res. 54:1787-90, 1994.

31.   Murata Y, Tamari M, Takahashi T, Horio Y, Hibi K, Yokoyama S, Inazawa J, Yamakawa K, Ogawa A, et al. Characterization of an 800 kb region at 3p22-p21.3 that was homozygously deleted in a lung cancer cell line. Hum Mol Genet 3:1341-4, 1994.

32.   Todd S, Roche J, Hahner L, Bolin R, Drabkin HA and Gemmill RM. YAC contigs covering an 8-megabase region of 3p deleted in the small- cell lung cancer cell line U2020. Genomics. 25:19-28, 1995.

33.   Yamakawa K, Takahashi T, Horio Y, Murata Y, Takahashi E, Hibi K, Yokoyama S, Ueda R, Takahashi T and Nakamura Y. Frequent homozygous deletions in lung cancer cell lines detected by a DNA marker located at 3p21.3-p22. Oncogene 8:327-30, 1993.

34.   Kishimoto Y, Sugio K, Mitsudomi T, Oyama T, Virmani AK, McIntire DD and Gazdar AF. Frequent loss of the short arm of chromosome 9 in resected non-small-cell lung cancers from Japanese patients and its association with squamous cell carcinoma. Journal of Cancer Research & Clinical Oncology 121:291-6, 1995.

35.   Olopade OI, Buchhagen DL, Malik K, Sherman J, Nobori T, Bader S, Nau MM, Gazdar AF, Minna JD and Diaz MO. Homozygous loss of the interferon genes defines the critical region on 9p that is deleted in lung cancers. Cancer Res. 53 (10 Suppl):2410-5, 1993.

36.   Xiao S, Li D, Corson JM, Vijg J and Fletcher JA. Codeletion of p15 and p16 genes in primary non-small cell lung carcinoma. Cancer Research 55:2968-71, 1995.

37.   Morstyn G, Brown J, Novak U, Gardner J, Bishop J and Garson M. Heterogeneous cytogenetic abnormalities in small cell lung cancer cell lines. Cancer Res. 47:3322-3327, 1987.

38.   D'Amico D, Carbone DP, Johnson BE, Meltzer SJ and Minna JD. Polymorphic sites within the MCC and APC loci reveal very frequent loss of heterozygosity in human small cell lung cancer. Cancer Research 52:1996-1999, 1992.

39. Cannizzaro LA, Skolnik EY, Margolis B, Croce CM, Schlesinger J and Huebner K. The human gene encoding phosphatidylinositol-3 kinase associated p85 alpha is at chromosome region 5q12-13. Cancer Res. 51:3818-20, 1991.

40. Bishop DT and Westbrook C. Report of the committee on the genetic constitution of chromosome 5. Cytogenet Cell Genet 55:111-7, 1990.

41. Escobedo JA, Navankasattusas S, Kavanaugh WM, Milfay D, Fried VA. and Williams LT. cDNA cloning of a novel 85 kd protein that has SH2 domains and regulates binding of PI3-kinase to the PDGF beta-receptor. Cell 65:75-82, 1991.

42. Rasio D, Negrini M, Manenti G, Dragani TA and Croce CM. Loss of heterozygosity at chromosome 11q in lung adenocarcinoma: identification of three independent regions. Cancer Research. 55:3988-91, 1995.

43. Miura I, Graziano SL, Cheng JQ, Doyle LA and Testa JR. Chromosome alterations in human small cell lung cancer: frequent involvement of 5q. Cancer Res 52:1322-8, 1992.

44. Harbour JW, Lai SL, Whang-Peng, J, Gazdar AF, Minna JD and Kaye FJ. Abnormalities in structure and expression of the human retinoblastoma gene in SCLC. Science 241:353-357, 1988.

45. Nigro J, Baker S, Preisinger A, Jessup J, Hostetter R, Cleary K, Bigner S, Davidson N, Baylin S, Devilee P, Glover T, Collins F, Weston A, Modali R, Harris C and Vogelstein B. Mutations in the p53 gene occur in diverse human tumour types. Nature 342:705-708, 1989.

46. Bronner CE, Baker SM, Morrison PT, Warren G, Smith LG, Lescoe MK, Kane M, Earabino C, Lipford J, Lindblom A, et al. Mutation in the DNA mismatch repair gene homologue hMLH1 is associated with hereditary non-polyposis colon cancer. Nature 368:258-61, 1994.

47. Papadopoulos N, Nicolaides NC, Wei YF, Ruben SM, Carter KC, Rosen CA, Haseltine WA, Fleischmann RD, Fraser CM, Adams MD, Venter JC, Hamilton SR, Petersen GM, Watson P, Lynch HT, Peltomäki P, Mecklin J-P, de la Chapelle A, Kinzler KW and Vogelstein B. Mutation of a mutL homolog in hereditary colon cancer. Science 263:1625-9, 1994.

48. Leach FS, Nicolaides NC, Papadopoulos N, Liu B, Jen J, Parsons R, Peltomaki P, Sistonen P, Aaltonen LA, Nystrom-Lahti M, et al. Mutations of a mutS homolog in hereditary nonpolyposis colorectal cancer. Cell 75:1215-25, 1993.

49. Fishel R, Lescoe MK, Rao MR, Copeland NG, Jenkins NA, Garber J, Kane M and Kolodner R. The human mutator gene homolog MSH2 and its association with hereditary nonpolyposis colon cancer. Cell. 75:1027-38, 1993.

50. Ionov Y, Peinado MA, Malkhosyan S, Shibata D and Perucho M. Ubiquitous somatic mutations in simple repeated sequences reveal a new mechanism for colonic carcinogenesis. Nature 363:558-61, 1993.

51. Thibodeau SN, Bren G and Schaid D. Microsatellite instability in cancer of the proximal colon. Science 260:816-9, 1993.

52. Merlo A, Mabry M, Gabrielson E, Vollmer R, Baylin SB and Sidransky D. Frequent microsatellite instability in primary small cell lung cancer. Cancer Res 54:2098-101, 1994.

53. Mitsudomi T, Viallet J, Mulshine JL, Linnoila RI, Minna JD and Gazdar AF. Mutations of *ras* genes distinguish a subset of non-small-cell lung cancer cell lines from small-cell lung cancer cell lines. Oncogene. 6:1353-1362, 1991.

54. Carbone DP, Mitsudomi T, Chiba I, Piantadosi S, Rusch V, Nowak JA, McIntire D, Slamon D, Gazdar A and Minna J. p53 immunostaining positivity is associated with reduced survival and is imperfectly correlated with gene mutations in resected non-small cell lung cancer. A preliminary report of LCSG 871. Chest 106:377S-381S, 1994.

55. Geradts J, Fong KM, Zimmerman PV, Maynard R and Minna JD. Correlation of abnormal RB, p16ink4a, and p53 expression with 3p loss of heterozygosity, other genetic abnormalities, and clinical features in 103 primary non-small cell lung cancers. Clin Cancer Res 5:791-800, 1999.

56. Heighway J, Thatcher N, Cerny T and Hasleton P. Genetic predisposition to human lung cancer. Br J Cancer 53:453-457, 1986.

57. Mitsudomi T, Steinberg SM, Oie HK, Mulshine JL, Phelps R, Viallet J, Pass H, Minna JD and Gazdar AF. *ras* gene mutations in non-small cell lung cancers are associated with shortened survival irrespective of treatment intent. Cancer Research 51:4999-5002, 1991.

58. Nau MM, Brooks BJ, Battey J, Sausville E, Gazdar AF, Kirsch IR, McBride O W, Bertness V, Hollis GF. and Minna J D. L-*myc*, a new *myc*-related gene amplified and expressed in human small cell lung cancer. Nature (London). 318:69-73, 1985.

59. Johnson B, Makuch R, Simmons A, Gazdar A, Burch D and Cashell A. myc family DNA amplification in small cell lung cancer patients' tumors and corresponding cell lines. Cancer Res 48:5163-5166, 1988.

60. Brennan J, O'Connor T, Makuch RW, Simmons AM, Russell E, Linnoila RI, Phelps RM, Gazdar AF, Ihde DC. and Johnson, B. E. myc family DNA amplification in 107 tumors and tumor cell lines from patients with small cell lung cancer treated with different combination chemotherapy regimens. Cancer Research. 51:1708-12, 1991.

61. Takahashi T, Obata Y, Sekido Y, Hida T, Ueda R, Watanabe H, Ariyoshi Y, Sugiura T and Takahashi T. Expression and amplification of myc gene family in small cell lung cancer and its relation to biological characteristics. Cancer Res. 49:2683-2688, 1989.

62. Slebos R, Evers S, Wagenaar S and Rodenhuis, S. Cellular protooncogenes are infrequently amplified in untreated non-small cell lung cancer. Br J Cancer 59: 76-80, 1989.

63. Taguchi T, Cheng GZ, Bell DW, Balsara B, Liu Z, Siegfried JM and Testa JR. Combined chromosome microdissection and comparative genomic hybridization

detect multiple sites of amplification DNA in a human lung carcinoma cell line. Genes Chromosomes Cancer 20:208-12, 1997.

64.   Okazaki T, Takita J, Kohno T, Handa H and Yokota J. Detection of amplified genomic sequences in human small-cell lung carcinoma cells by arbitrarily primed-PCR genomic fingerprinting. Hum Genet 98:253-8, 1996.

65.   Dowdy SF, Hinds PW, Louie K, Reed SI, Arnold A and Weinberg RA. Physical interaction of the retinoblastoma protein with human D cyclins. Cell 73: 499-511, 1993.

66.   Ewen ME, Sluss HK, Whitehouse LL and Livingston DM. TGF beta inhibition of Cdk4 synthesis is linked to cell cycle arrest. Cell 74:1009-20, 1993.

67.   Kato J, Matsushime H, Hiebert SW, Ewen ME and Sherr CJ. Direct binding of cyclin D to the retinoblastoma gene product (pRb) and pRb phosphorylation by the cyclin D-dependent kinase CDK4. Genes Dev 7:331-42, 1993.

68.   Kratzke RA, Greatens TM, Rubins JB, Maddaus MA, Niewoehner DE, Niehans GA and Geradts J. Rb and p16INK4a expression in resected non-small cell lung tumors. Cancer Res 56:3415-20, 1996.

69.   Huang H-J, Yee J-K, Shew J-Y, Chen P-L, Bookstein R, Friedmann T, Lee E-H and Lee W-H. Suppression of the neoplastic phenotype by replacement of the RB gene in human cancer cells. Science 242:1563-6, 1988.

70.   Symonds H, Krall L, Remington L, Saenz-Robles M, Lowe S, Jacks T and Van Dyke T. p53-dependent apoptosis suppresses tumor growth and progression in vivo. Cell 78:703-11, 1994.

71.   Kastan MB, Zhan Q, El DW, Carrier F, Jacks T, Walsh WV, Plunkett BS, Vogelstein B and Fornace AJJ. A mammalian cell cycle checkpoint pathway utilizing p53 and GADD45 is defective in ataxia-telangiectasia. Cell 71:587-97, 1992.

72.   Chiba I, Takahashi T, Nau MM, D'Amico D, Curiel D, Mitsudomi T, Buchhagen D, Carbone D, Koga H, Reissmann PT, Slamon DJ, Holmes EC and Minna JD. Mutations in the p53 gene are frequent in primary, resected non-small cell lung cancer. Oncogene 5:1603-1610, 1990.

73.   D'Amico D, Carbone D, Mitsudomi T, Nau M, Fedorko J, Russell E, Johnson B, Buchhagen D, Bodner S, Phelps R, Gazdar A. and Minna JD. High frequency of somatically acquired p53 mutations in small cell lung cancer cell lines and tumors. Oncogene 7:339-346, 1992.

74.   Bodner SM, Minna J, Jensen SM, D'Amico D, Carbone D, Mitsudomi T, Fedorko J, Nau MM, Gazdar AF and Linnoila RI. Expression of mutant p53 proteins in lung cancer correlates with the class of p53 gene mutation. Oncogene. 7:743-749, 1992.

75.   Sanchez-Cespedes M, Reed AL, Buta M, Wu L, Westra WH, Herman JG, Yang, SC, Jen J and Sidransky D. Inactivation of the INK4A/ARF locus frequently coexists with TP53 mutations in non-small cell lung cancer [In Process Citation]. Oncogene 18:5843-9, 1999.

76. Vonlanthen S, Heighway J, Tschan MP, Borner MM, Altermatt HJ, Kappeler A, Tobler A, Fey MF, Thatcher N, Yarbrough WG and Betticher DC. Expression of p16INK4a/p16alpha and p19ARF/p16beta is frequently altered in non-small cell lung cancer and correlates with p53 overexpression. Oncogene 17:2779-85, 1998.

77. Schneider PM, Hung MC, Chiocca SM, Manning J, Zhao XY, Fang K and Roth JA. Differential expression of the c-erbB-2 gene in human small cell and non-small cell lung cancer. Cancer Res 49:4968-71, 1989.

78. Kern JA, Schwartz DA, Nordberg JE, Weiner DB, Greene MI, Torney L and Robinson, R. A. p185neu expression in human lung adenocarcinomas predicts shortened survival. Cancer Res 50:5184-7, 1990.

79. Yu D, Wang SS, Dulski KM, Tsai CM, Nicolson GL and Hung MC. c-erbB-2/neu overexpression enhances metastatic potential of human lung cancer cells by induction of metastasis-associated properties. Cancer Res 54:3260-6, 1994.

80. Kern JA, Torney L, Weiner D, Gazdar A, Shepard HM and Fendly B. Inhibition of human lung cancer cell line growth by an anti-p185HER2 antibody. Am J Respir Cell Mol Biol 9:448-54, 1993.

81. Cerny T, Barnes D, Hasleton P, Barber P, Healy K, Gullick W and Thatcher N. Expression of epidermal growth factor receptor (EGF-R) in human lung tumours. Br J Cancer 54:265-269, 1986.

82. Garcia de Palazzo IE, Adams GP, Sundareshan P, Wong AJ, Testa JR, Bigner D. D and Weiner LM. Expression of mutated epidermal growth factor receptor by non-small cell lung carcinomas. Cancer Res 53:5217-20, 1993.

83. Baguley BC, Marshall ES, Holdaway KM, Rewcastle GW and Denny WA. Inhibition of growth of primary human tumour cell cultures by a 4-anilinoquinazoline inhibitor of the epidermal growth factor receptor family of tyrosine kinases. Eur J Cancer 34:1086-90, 1998.

84. Suarez Pestana E, Greiser U, Sanchez B, Fernandez LE, Lage A, Perez R and Bohmer FD. Growth inhibition of human lung adenocarcinoma cells by antibodies against epidermal growth factor receptor and by ganglioside GM3: involvement of receptor-directed protein tyrosine phosphatase(s). Br J Cancer 75:213-20, 1997.

85. Griffin C and Baylin S. Expression of the c-*myb* oncogene in human small cell lung carcinoma. Cancer Res 45:272-275, 1985.

86. Graziano SL, Pfeifer AM, Testa JR, Mark GE, Johnson BE, Hallinan EJ, Pettengill OS, Sorenson GD, Tatum AH, Brauch H, et al. Involvement of the RAF1 locus, at band 3p25, in the 3p deletion of small-cell lung cancer. Genes Chromosom Cancer 3:283-93, 1991.

87. Hibi K, Takahashi T, Sekido Y, Ueda R, Hida T, Ariyoshi Y, Takagi H. and Takahashi, T. Coexpression of the stem cell factor and the c-kit genes in small-cell lung cancer. Oncogene 6:2291-6, 1991.

88. Sekido Y, Obata Y, Ueda R, Hida T, Suyama M, Shimokata K, Ariyoshi Y and Takahashi T. Preferential expression of c-kit protooncogene transcripts in small cell lung cancer. Cancer Res. 51:2416-9, 1991.

89. Antoniades HN, Galanopoulos T, Neville GJ and O'Hara CJ. Malignant epithelial cells in primary human lung carcinomas coexpress in vivo platelet-derived growth factor (PDGF) and PDGF receptor mRNAs and their protein products. Proc Natl Acad Sci USA 89:3942-6, 1992.

90. Bravo M, Väsquez R, Rubio H, Salazar M, Pardo A and Selman M. Production of platelet-derived growth factor by human lung cancer. Respir Med 85:479-85, 1991.

91. Plummer HD, Catlett J, Leftwich J, Armstrong B, Carlson P, Huff T and Krystal G. c-myc expression correlates with suppression of c-kit protooncogene expression in small cell lung cancer cell lines. Cancer Res 53:4337-42, 1993.

92. Wistuba II, Lam S, Behrens C, Virmani AK, Fong KM, LeRiche J, Samet JM, Srivastava S, Minna JD and Gazdar AF. Molecular damage in the bronchial epithelium of current and former smokers. J Natl Cancer Inst 89:1366-73, 1997.

93. Mao L, Lee DJ, Tockman MS, Erozan YS, Askin F and Sidransky D. Microsatellite alterations as clonal markers for the detection of human cancer. Proc Natl Acad Sci USA 91:9871-5, 1994.

94. Mao L, Hruban RH, Boyle JO, Tockman M and Sidransky D. Detection of oncogene mutations in sputum precedes diagnosis of lung cancer. Cancer Res 54: 1634-7, 1994.

95. Peck K, Sher YP, Shih JY, Roffler SR, Wu CW and Yang PC. Detection and quantitation of circulating cancer cells in the peripheral blood of lung cancer patients. Cancer Res 58:2761-5, 1998.

96. Giatromanolaki A, Koukourakis MI, Kakolyris S, Turley H, O'Byrne K, Scott PA, Pezzella F, Georgoulias V, Harris AL and Gatter KC. Vascular endothelial growth factor, wild-type p53, and angiogenesis in early operable non-small cell lung cancer. Clin Cancer Res 4:3017-24, 1998.

97. Suzuki M, Iizasa T, Fujisawa T, Baba M, Yamaguchi Y, Kimura H and Suzuki H. Expression of Matrix Metalloproteinases and Tissue Inhibitor of Matrix Metalloproteinases in Non-Small-Cell Lung Cancer. Invasion Metastasis 18: 134-141, 1999.

98. Zucker S, Wieman J, Lysik RM, Imhof B, Nagase H, Ramamurthy N, Liotta LA and Golub LM. Gelatin-degrading type IV collagenase isolated from human small cell lung cancer. Invasion Metastasis 9:167-81, 1989.

99. Iizasa T, Fujisawa T, Suzuki M, Motohashi S, Yasufuku K, Yasukawa T, Baba M and Shiba M. Elevated levels of circulating plasma matrix metalloproteinase 9 in non- small cell lung cancer patients. Clin Cancer Res 5:149-53, 1999.

100. Itoh T, Tanioka M, Yoshida H, Yoshioka T, Nishimoto H and Itohara S. Reduced angiogenesis and tumor progression in gelatinase A-deficient mice. Cancer Res 58:1048-51, 1998.

101. Kitamura H, Oosawa Y, Kawano N, Kameda Y, Hayashi H, Nakatani Y, Udaka N, Ito T and Miyazaki K. Basement membrane patterns, gelatinase A and tissue inhibitor of metalloproteinase-2 expressions, and stromal fibrosis during the development of peripheral lung adenocarcinoma. Hum Pathol 30:331-8, 1999.

102. Fong KM, Kida Y, Zimmerman PV and Smith PJ. TIMP1 and adverse prognosis in non-small cell lung cancer. Clin Cancer Res 2:1369-72, 1996.

103. Lozonschi L, Sunamura, M, Kobari M, Egawa S, Ding L and Matsuno S. Controlling tumor angiogenesis and metastasis of C26 murine colon adenocarcinoma by a new matrix metalloproteinase inhibitor, KB-R7785, in two tumor models. Cancer Res 59:1252-8, 1999.

104. Shalinsky DR, Brekken J, Zou H, McDermott CD, Forsyth P, Edwards D, Margosiak S, Bender S, Truitt G, Wood A, Varki NM and Appelt K. Broad antitumor and antiangiogenic activities of AG3340, a potent and selective MMP inhibitor undergoing advanced oncology clinical trials. Ann NY Acad Sci 878:236-70, 1999.

105. Steward WP. Marimastat (BB2516): current status of development. Cancer Chemother Pharmacol 43:S56-60, 1999.

106. Takahashi, T., Carbone, D., Takahashi, T., Nau, M. M., Hida, T., Linnoila, I., Ueda, R. and Minna, J. D. Wild-type but not mutant p53 suppresses the growth of human lung cancer cells bearing multiple genetic lesions. Cancer Research 52: 2340-2343, 1992.

107. Bookstein R, Shew JY, Chen PL, Scully P and Lee WH. Suppression of tumorigenicity of human prostate carcinoma cells by replacing a mutated RB gene. Science 247:712-5, 1990.

108. Fujiwara T, Grimm EA, Mukhopadhyay T, Cai DW, Owen-Schaub LB and Roth JA. A retroviral wild-type p53 expression vector penetrates human lung cancer spheroids and inhibits growth by inducing apoptosis. Cancer Res 53:4129-33, 1993.

109. Cai DW, Mukhopadhyay T, Liu Y, Fujiwara T and Roth JA. Stable expression of the wild-type p53 gene in human lung cancer cells after retrovirus-mediated gene transfer. Hum Gene Ther 4:617-24, 1993.

110. Fujiwara T, Cai DW, Georges RN, Mukhopadhyay T, Grimm EA and Roth JA. Therapeutic effect of a retroviral wild-type p53 expression vector in an orthotopic lung cancer model. J Natl Cancer Inst 86:1458-62, 1994.

111. Roth JA. Therapy of human lung cancer with a retrovirus carrying wild-type p53. Nature Medicine, In press, 1996.

112. Swisher SG, Roth JA, Nemunaitis J, Lawrence DD, Kemp BL, Carrasco CH, Connors DG, El-Naggar AK, Fossella F, Glisson BS, Hong WK, Khuri FR, Kurie JM, Lee JJ, Lee JS, Mack M, Merritt JA, Nguyen DM, Nesbitt JC, Perez-Soler R, Pisters KM, Putnam JB, Jr., Richli WR, Savin M, Waugh MK, et al. Adenovirus-mediated p53 gene transfer in advanced non-small-cell lung cancer. J Natl Cancer Inst 91:763-71, 1999.

113. Deshane J, Siegal GP, Alvarez RD, Wang MH, Feng M, Cabrera G, Liu T, Kay M and Curiel DT. Targeted tumor killing via an intracellular antibody against erbB-2. J Clin Invest 96:2980-2989, 1995.

114. Slebos RJ, Kibbelaar RE, Dalesio O, Kooistra A, Stam J, Meijer CJ, Wagenaar SS, Vanderschueren RG, van Zandwijk N, Moot WJ, Bos JL and Rodenhuis S. K-ras oncogene activation as a prognostic marker in adenocarcinoma of the lung. N Engl J Med 323:561-5, 1990.

115. Georges RN, Mukhopadhyay T, Zhang Y, Yen N and Roth JA. Prevention of orthotopic human lung cancer growth by intratracheal instillation of a retroviral antisense K-ras construct. Cancer Res 53:1743-6, 1993.

116. Mukhopadhyay T, Tainsky M, Cavender AC and Roth JA. Specific inhibition of K-ras expression and tumorigenicity of lung cancer cells by antisense RNA. Cancer Res 51:1744-8, 1991.

117. Ziegler A, Luedke GH, Fabbro D, Altmann KH, Stahel RA and Zangemeister-Wittke U. Induction of apoptosis in small-cell lung cancer cells by an antisense oligodeoxynucleotide targeting the Bcl-2 coding sequence [see comments]. Journal of the National Cancer Institute 89:1027-36, 1997.

118. Moolten FL. Drug sensitivity ("suicide") genes for selective cancer chemotherapy. Cancer Gene Ther 1:279-87, 1994.

119. Richards CA, Austin EA and Huber BE. Transcriptional regulatory sequences of carcinoembryonic antigen: identification and use with cytosine deaminase for tumor-specific gene therapy. Hum Gene Ther 6: 881-93, 1995.

120. Freeman SM, Abboud CN, Whartenby KA, Packman CH, Koeplin DS, Moolten FL and Abraham GN. The bystander effect: tumor regression when a fraction of the tumor mass is genetically modified. Cancer Res 53:5274-83, 1993.

121. Sharma S, Miller PW, Stolina M, Zhu L, Huang M, Paul RW and Dubinett SM. Multicomponent gene therapy vaccines for lung cancer: effective eradication of established murine tumors in vivo with interleukin- 7/herpes simplex thymidine kinase-transduced autologous tumor and ex vivo activated dendritic cells. Gene Ther 4:1361-70, 1997.

122. Sharma S, Wang J, Huang M, Paul RW, Lee P, McBride WH, Economou JS, Roth MD, Kiertscher SM and Dubinett SM. Interleukin-7 gene transfer in non-small-cell lung cancer decreases tumor proliferation, modifies cell surface molecule expression, and enhances antitumor reactivity. Cancer Gene Ther 3:302-13, 1996.

123. Smythe WR, Hwang HC, Amin KM, Eck SL, Davidson BL, Wilson JM, Kaiser LR and Albelda SM. Use of recombinant adenovirus to transfer the herpes simplex virus thymidine kinase (HSVtk) gene to thoracic neoplasms: an effective in vitro drug sensitization system. Cancer Res 54:2055-9, 1994.

124. Treat J, Kaiser LR, Sterman DH, Litzky L, Davis A, Wilson JM. and Albelda, S. M. Treatment of advanced mesothelioma with the recombinant adenovirus H5.010RSVTK: a phase 1 trial (BB-IND 6274). Hum Gene Ther 7:2047-57, 1996.

125. Chen HL and Carbone DP. p53 as a target for anti-cancer immunotherapy. Molecular Medicine Today 3:160-7, 1997.

126. Vierboom M P M, Nijman HW, Offringa R, van der Voort EIH, van Hall T, van den Broek L, Fleuren GJ, Kenemans P, Kast WM and Melief CJM. Tumor Eradication by Wild-type p53-specific Cytotoxic T Lymphocytes. Journal of Experimental Medicine 186:695-704, 1997.

127. McKneally MF, Maver C, Kausel HW and Alley RD. Regional immunotherapy with intrapleural BCG for lung cancer. Journal of Thoracic & Cardiovascular Surgery 72:333-8, 1976.

128. Holmes EC and Gail M. Surgical adjuvant therapy for stage II and stage III adenocarcinoma and large-cell undifferentiated carcinoma. Journal of Clinical Oncology 4:710-5, 1986.

129. McCracken JD, Chen T, White J, Samson M, Stephens R, Coltman CA, Jr, Saiki J, Lane M, Bonnet J and McGavran, M.   Combination chemotherapy, radiotherapy, and BCG immunotherapy in limited small-cell carcinoma of the lung: a Southwest Oncology Group Study. Cancer 49:2252-8, 1982.

130. Yasumoto K, Yaita H, Ohta M, Azuma I, Nomoto K, Inokuchi K and Yamamura Y. Randomly controlled study of chemotherapy versus chemoimmunotherapy in postoperative lung cancer patients. Cancer Research 45:1413-7, 1985.

131. Hollinshead A, Stewart TH, Takita H, Dalbow M and Concannon J. Adjuvant specific active lung cancer immunotherapy trials. Tumor-associated antigens. Cancer 60:1249-62, 1987.

132. Topalian SL and Rosenberg SA. "Adoptive Cellular Therapy: Basic Principles." Biologic Therapy of Cancer. DeVita, Hellman and Rosenberg ed. 1991 J. B. Lippincott. Philadelphia.

133. Tan Y, Xu M, Wang W, Zhang F, Li D, Xu X, Gu J and Hoffman RM. IL-2 gene therapy of advanced lung cancer patients. Anticancer Research 16:1993-8, 1996.

134. Ratto GB, Zino P, Mirabelli S, Minuti P, Aquilina R, Fantino G, Spessa E, Ponte M, Bruzzi P and Melioli G. A randomized trial of adoptive immunotherapy with tumor-infiltrating lymphocytes and interleukin-2 versus standard therapy in the postoperative treatment of resected nonsmall cell lung carcinoma. Cancer 78: 244-51, 1996.

135. Melief CJM and Kast WM. Potential immunogenicity of oncogene and tumor suppressor gene products. Curr Op Immunol 5:709-713, 1993.

136. Robbins PF and Kawakami Y. Human tumor antigens recognized by T cells. Current Opinion in Immunology 8: 628-36, 1996.

137. Pardoll DM. Cancer vaccines. Nat Med 4:525-31, 1998.

138. Roth J, Dittmer D, Rea D, Tartaglia J, Paoletti E and Levine AJ. p53 as a target for cancer vaccines: recombinant canarypox virus vectors expressing p53 protect mice against lethal tumor cell challenge. Proceedings of the National Academy of Sciences of the United States of America 93:4781-6, 1996.

139. Ishida T, Stipanov M, Chada S, Gabrilovich DI and Carbone DP. Dendritic cells transduced with wild type p53 gene elicit potent antitumor immune responses. Journal of Clinical and Experimental Immunology 117:244-51, 1999.

140. Houbiers JG, Nijman HW, van der Burg SH, Drijfhout JW, Kenemans P, van de Velde CJ, Brand A, Momburg F, Kast WM and Melief CJ. In vitro induction of human cytotoxic T lymphocyte responses against peptides of mutant and wild-type p53. European Journal of Immunology 23:2072-7, 1993.

141. Ciernik IF, Berzofsky JA and Carbone DP. Mutant oncopeptide immunization induces CTL specifically lysing tumor cells endogenously expressing the corresponding intact mutant p53. Hybridoma 14:139-142, 1995.

142. Yanuck M, Carbone DP, Pendleton CD, Tsukui T, Winter SF, Minna JD and Berzofsky JA. A mutant p53 tumor suppressor protein is a target for peptide-induced CD8+ cytotoxic T cells. Cancer Research 53:3257-3261, 1993.

143. Ciernik IF, Berzofsky JA and Carbone DP. Induction of cytotoxic T lymphocytes and anti-tumor immunity with DNA vaccines expressing single T cell epitopes. Journal of Immunology 56:2369-2375, 1996.

144. Ciernik IF, Berzofsky JA and Carbone DP. Human lung cancer cells endogenously expressing mutant p53 process and present the mutant epitope, and are lysed by mutant-specific CTL. Clinical Cancer Research 2:877-882, 1996.

145. Lee CT, Ciernik IF, Wu S, Tang DC, Chen HL, Truelson JM and Carbone DP. Increased immunogenicity of tumors bearing mutant p53 and P1A epitopes after transduction of B7-1 via recombinant adenovirus. Cancer Gene Therapy 3:238-244, 1996.

146. Winter SF, Minna JD, Johnson BE, Takahashi T, Gazdar AF and Carbone DP. Development of antibodies against p53 in lung cancer patients appears to be dependent on the type of p53 mutation. Cancer Research. 52: 4168-4174, 1992.

147. Tilkin AF, Lubin R, Soussi T, Lazar V, Janin N, Mathieu MC, Lefrere I, Carlu C, Roy M, Kayibanda M, et al. Primary proliferative T cell response to wild-type p53 protein in patients with breast cancer. European Journal of Immunology 25: 1765-9, 1995.

148. Gabrilovich DI, Nadaf S, Cunningham T, Rogers P, Kavanagh D, Ciernik IF, Gazdar AF, Kelley MI, Smith MC, Berzofsky JA and Carbone DP. Cytotoxic T-lymphocytes (CTL) specific for mutant p53-peptides in peripheral blood of patients with cancer: support for specifc immune intervention. The 9th International Congress of immunology A3964, 1995.

149. Grant SC, Kris MG, Miller V, Yao TJ, Houghton AN and Chapman PB. Long survival in 15 patients (pts) with small cell lung cancer (SCLC) immunized with BEC2 plus BCG after initial therapy: an update (Meeting abstract). Proc Annu Meet Am Soc Clin Oncol 1997.

150. Itaya T, Yamagiwa S, Okada F, Oikawa T, Kurumaki N, Takeichi N, Hosokawa, M and Kobayashi H. Xenogenization of a mouse lung carcinoma (3LL) by transfection with an allogenic class I Major Histocompatibility Complex gene (H-2Ld). Cancer Res 47:3136-3140, 1987.

151. Plautz GE, Yang ZY, Wu BY, Gao X, Huang L and Nabel G J. Immunotherapy of malignancy by in vivo gene transfer into tumors. Proceedings of the National Academy of Sciences of the United States of America 90:4645-9, 1993.

152. Nabel GJ, Nabel EG, Yang ZY, Fox BA, Plautz GE, Gao X, Huang L, Shu S, Gordon D and Chan AE. Direct gene transfer with DNA-liposome complexes in melanoma: expression, biological activity, and lack of toxicity in humans. Proc Natl Acad Sci, USA 90:11307, 1993.

153. June CH, Bluestone JA, Nadler LM and Thompson CB. The B7 and CD28 receptor families. Immunol Today 15:321-31, 1994.

154. Guinan EC, Gribben JG, Boussiotis VA, Freeman GJ, Nadler LM, June CH, Bluestone JA, Nadler LM and Thompson CB. Pivotal role of the B7:CD28 pathway in transplantation tolerance and tumor immunity. The B7 and CD28 receptor families. Blood 84:3261-82, 1994.

155. Geldhof AB, Raes G, Bakkus M, Devos S, Thielemans K and De Baetselier P Expression of B7-1 by a highly metastatic mouse T lymphoma induces optimal natural killer cell-mediated cytotoxicity. Cancer Res 55:2730-2733, 1995.

156. Porgador A, Gansbacher B, Bannerji R, Tzehoval E, Gilboa E, Feldman M and Eisenbach L. Anti-metastatic vaccination of tumor-bearing mice with IL-2-gene-inserted tumor cells. Int J Cancer 53:471-7, 1993.

157. Porgador A, Bannerji R, Watanabe Y, Feldman M, Gilboa E and Eisenbach L. Antimetastatic vaccination of tumor-bearing mice with two types of IFN-gamma gene-inserted tumor cells. J Immunol 150:1458-70, 1993.

158. Dranoff G, Jaffee E, Lazenby A, Golumbek P, Levitsky H, Brose K, Jackson V, Hamada H, Pardoll D and Mulligan RC. Vaccination with irradiated tumor cells engineered to secrete murine granulocyte-macrophage colony-stimulating factor stimulates potent, specific, and long-lasting anti-tumor immunity. Proc Natl Acad Sci U S A 90:3539-43, 1993.

159. Inaba K, Inaba M, Romani N, Aya H, Deguchi M, Ikehara S, Muramatsu S and Steinman RM. Generation of large numbers of dendritic cells from mouse bone marrow cultures supplemented with granulocyte/macrophage colony-stimulating factor. J Exp Med 176:1693-702, 1992.

160. Lee C-T, Wu S, Ciernik IF, Chen HL, Nadaf-Rahrov S, Gabrilovich D and Carbone DP. Genetic immunotherapy of established tumors with adenovirus-murine granulocyte-macrophage colony-stimulating factor. Human Gene Therapy 8:187-93, 1997.

161. Gabrilovich DI, Nadaf S, Corak J, Berzofsky JA and Carbone DP. Dendritic cells in anti-tumor immune responses. II. Dendritic cells grown from bone marrow precursors, but not mature DC from tumor-bearing mice are effective antigen carriers in the therapy of established tumors. Cellular Immunology 170:111-119, 1996.

162. Gabrilovich DI, Cunningham HT and Carbone DP. IL-12 and mutant p53 peptide-pulsed dendritic cells for the specific immunotherapy of cancer. Journal of Immunotherapy 19:414-418, 1997.

163. Gabrilovich DI, Corak J, Ciernik IF, Kavanaugh D and Carbone DP. Decreased antigen presentation by dendritic cells in patients with breast cancer. Clinical Cancer Research 3:483-490, 1997.

164. Gabrilovich DI, Chen HL, Girgis KR, Cunningham T, Meny GM, Nadaf S, Kavanaugh D and Carbone DP. Production of vascular endothelial growth factor by human tumors inhibits the functional maturation of dendritic cells. Nature Medicine. 2:1096-1103, 1996.

165. Gabrilovich DI, Ishida T, Nadaf S, Ohm JE and Carbone DP. Antibodies to vascular endothelial growth factor enhance the efficacy of cancer immunotherapy by improving endogenous dendritic cell function. Clin Cancer Res 5:963-70, 1999.

THE EPIDEMIOLOGY OF LUNG CANCER

Mark D. Williams M.D.
Indiana University School of Medicine, Indianapolis, IN 46202 USA

Alan B. Sandler M.D.
Vanderbilt University Medical Center, Nashville, TN 37232 USA

INTRODUCTION

Lung cancer continues to lead cancer deaths in men and women from the United States and in men worldwide. Although the incidence in males is slowly decreasing, the incidence in women is increasing worldwide. There is irrefutable evidence that tobacco smoking causes bronchogenic carcinoma in approximately 85-90% of lung cancer victims. There is also evidence that environmental tobacco exposure or second-hand smoke also may cause lung cancer in life-long non-smokers. Other environmental exposures, such as pollution and domestic radon, have been proposed as contributors to lung malignancy. Many occupational agents have been identified as independent or contributing risk factors for bronchogenic carcinoma. Genetic and dietary factors have also been proposed as potential risk factors. Finally, advances in molecular biology have led to growing interest in investigation of biological markers, which may increase predisposition to smoking-related carcinogenesis.

INCIDENCE AND MORTALITY FOR THE UNITED STATES

Background

The incidence and mortality of lung cancer in American men and women has reached epidemic proportions during the 20th century. Among men, lung cancer mortality began rising in the 1950s, but the female epidemic did not begin until the mid 1960s (Figure 1A and 1B) (1). Cancer was the second leading cause of death in males and females in 1995, when all ages are combined together (2). However, for women less than 80 years of age, cancer was the leading cause of death over heart disease (2). Mortality from lung cancer in men peaked in the late 80s and is now stabilizing in women as we end the 20th century. Despite advances in surgical and non-surgical therapy for this devastating disease, the overall 5-yr survival rates have only modestly increased over the last 25 years, remaining at approximately 14% (3).

An estimated 158,900 Americans, 90,900 males and 68,000 females, died in 1999 from lung cancer (1). This represented approximately 31% of male and 25% of female cancer deaths.

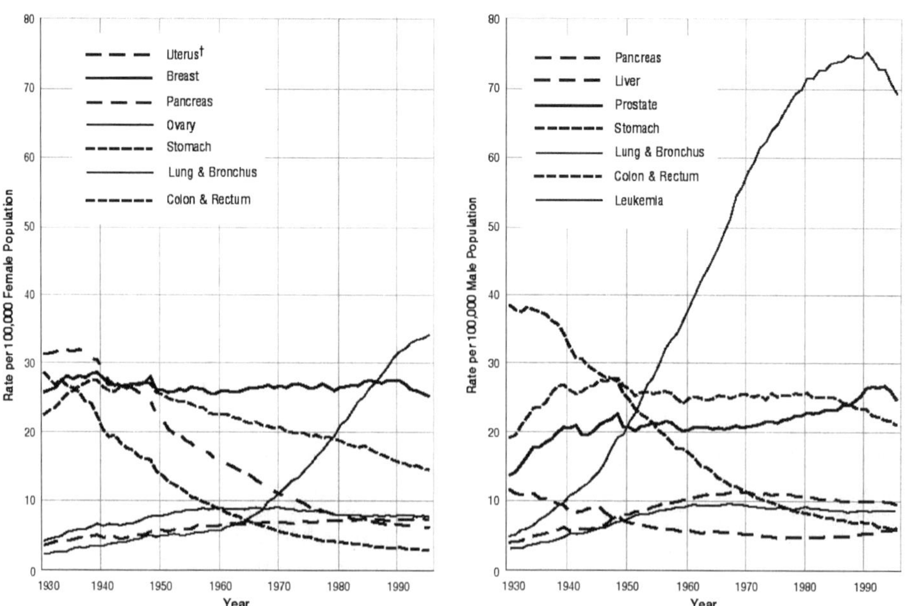

Figures 1A and 1B. Age-adjusted death rates from cancer by site, males and females in the United States, 1930-1995.*

** From Cancer Statistics, 1999, CA Cancer J Clin 49:8-31,1999*

The incidence of lung cancer in men peaked in the late 1980s, and has just now begun to level off in women at the end of the last decade (Figure 2A and 2B) (1). This has been attributed to slowl declining tobacco use in this country. However, this deadly disease remains an incessant reminder of the devastating nature of cancer. An estimated 94,000 men and 77,600 women were newly diagnosed with lung cancer in 1999 (1). The NCI Surveillance, Epidemiology, and End Results (SEER) program has estimated that 1 in 12 males and 1 in 18 females will develop lung cancer during their lifetime (4). The American Cancer Society estimated for 1999 that lung cancer would represent 15% of new cancer diagnoses in males, second only to prostate cancer (29%) (1). In females, it was estimated that lung cancer would represent 13% of new cancer diagnoses, second to breast cancer (29%).

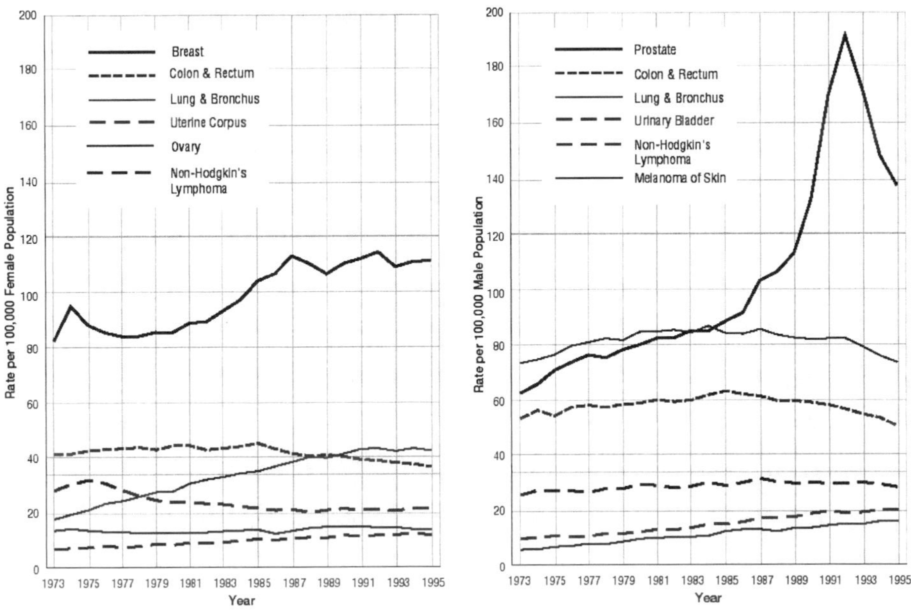

Figures 2A and 2B. Age adjusted incidence rates of cancer by site, males and females in the United States, 1930-1995.*

** From Cancer Statistics, 1999, CA Cancer J Clin 49:8-31,1999*

Ethnicity and Race

Race has been shown to be an important variable in the incidence and mortality of lung carcinoma. From 1990 - 1995, lung cancer incidence rates were 74.3 and 114.4 per 100,000 among white and African-American men, respectively and 43.3 and 46.4 per 100,000 among white and African American women (Table 1). Lung cancer mortality rates for the same time period showed 70.7 and 102 per 100,000 among white and African-American men and 33.6 and 32.7 per 100,000 among white and African-American women (Table 1). These increases in lung cancer incidence and mortality in African-American males have been attributed to lower socioeconomic status, which influences tobacco usage and occupational exposure (5). Many studies have demonstrated that lower socioeconomic status leads to lower education levels, which is a predictor of increased tobacco use (6,7). Investigators have shown higher serum nicotinine levels in blacks, independent of differences in smoking habits, which may suggest a difference in tobacco smoke metabolism (8). Some authors have proposed that American-Americans have higher intake of dietary fats, which may increase carcinogenesis (9). Recently, a study suggested that African- American men have higher lung cancer mortality, in part because they are offered potential curative surgery less frequently than white men (10).

*Table 1. Incidence and Mortality of Lung Cancer by Race**

	White	**African-American**
Incidence		
Male	74.3	114
Female	43.3	46.4
Total	**56.4**	**75**
Mortality		
Male	70.7	102
Female	33.6	32.7
Total	**49.4**	**61**

**Data from Cancer Statistics, CA Cancer J Clin 48:8-31, 1999. Rates are per 100,000 population.*

Incidence and mortality rates have been shown to be less for other American ethnic groups such as Hispanics and Asians (11,12,13). Some studies have shown that these ethnic groups typically smoke less than whites (14,15). Among American ethnic groups, native Americans, Hispanic and Japanese Americans have the lowest lung cancer incidence rates (2). In these groups, men have at least 2.5 times the rate of incidence of lung cancer than women. The differences between white Americans and ethnic Americans are likely multiple, including genetic, dietary and tobacco habit differences.

Gender

Historically, males have had a predominance of lung cancer incidence and mortality, due to gender differences in tobacco use. This has been attributed to the fact it was not acceptable for women to openly smoke, in the first half of the 20th century. Women also have been shown to typically start smoking at a later age than men, and to have less intensity and frequency of smoking (16). There is no consensus whether lung cancer is more common in males or females, when smoking habits are controlled for. Some studies have shown that when adjustments are made for smoking, men still have a higher incidence of lung cancer (17). Many have postulated that this represents increased risk in men due to environmental exposures. In contrast, other studies have suggested that women have a higher incidence, especially for small cell lung cancer and adenocarcinoma (18,19). Some have attributed the increased risk for adenocarcinoma in women to hormonal factors, such as estrogen (20). Non-smokers who develop lung cancer are more frequently female, presumably due to increased environmental tobacco smoke in their household (21).

Age

Lung cancer is typically a disease of older adults, but can occur in younger patients. In 1995, lung cancer represented approximately 10% of cancer deaths in the age group 20-39, 22% in age group 40-59 and 28% in the age group 60-79 years of age (2). There have been downward trends in lung cancer incidence and mortality in whites and African-Americans for many years due to the efforts in tobacco cessation. Unfortunately, tobacco use among teenagers has been increasing over the last decade (22). Lung cancer in younger patients is attributed to smoking more frequently, at an earlier age and smoking cigarettes higher in tar and nicotine. Younger lung cancer victims have been shown to have stronger familial risk for lung cancer (23). Many studies have shown that adenocarcinoma is more prevalent in younger versus older lung cancer groups (24,25). In the past, some have suggested that lung cancer in young patients behaves more aggressively with higher mortality, but recent studies have shown equivalent survival between these two groups (26).

INTERNATIONAL TRENDS

Lung cancer has been the leading cause of cancer death worldwide for several years by surpassing gastric and colon cancer (1). The estimated worldwide incidence rates for 1998 per 100,000 people were 37.5 for men and 10.8 for women (Table 2). Lung cancer mortality in 1998 per 100,000 was estimated at 33.7 and 9.2 for men and women, respectively (Table 2). Recently, it was estimated that lung cancer represents 18% of new cancers in males and 7% of females worldwide, with a total incidence of 12.8 % of all new cancers (1). Regarding cancer deaths, it was estimated that lung cancer causes 23.4 % of male cancer deaths and 10.2 % of female deaths, with a total mortality of 17.8 % (1). Lung cancer is most prevalent in North America and Europe. Other countries with significant incidence and mortality include China, Japan, Australia, New Zealand, Asia and temperate South America (1). The incidence of lung cancer is strongly associated with tobacco consumption within each country. Although the incidence has peaked in the USA and most of Europe, many developed and developing countries are having increasing incidence and mortality from bronchogenic carcinoma. Incidence and mortality continues to climb for women in most countries, as predicted by later onset tobacco abuse, worldwide. Women in China have a particularly high incidence of lung cancer, despite many being non-smokers. This has been attributed to environmental exposures to cooking oils and fossil fuel combustion products (27). The Japanese have lower incidence of lung cancer compared to Europe or the United States, which has been attributed to charcoal filtered cigarettes and possible protective effect of green tea (28). Lung cancer will continue to remain a worldwide plague due to relentless, international cigarette smoking.

*Table 2. International Incidence and Mortality of Lung Cancer**

	<u>Men</u>	<u>Women</u>
<u>Incidence</u>		
	37.5	10.8
<u>Morality</u>		
	33.7	9.2

**Data from Cancer Statistics, CA Cancer J Clin 48:8-31, 1999. Rates are per 100,000 population.*

ETIOLOGY

Tobacco

It has been written that Christopher Columbus became a tobacco smoker within 24 hours of his arrival on this continent. Certainly, the increasing habit of cigarette smoking during this century represents one of the greatest man-made plagues to ever afflict the western world. At the start of the 20th century, lung cancer was a very rare disease with a death rate of much less than 10 per 100,000 population each year. During the civil war smoking significantly increased in men, since there was a levy placed on cigarettes which benefitted the costs of war (29). Therefore, tobacco smoking was even seen as patriotic at that time. After World War I, cigarette smoking significantly increased for many reasons including advances in cigarette production and glamorization in the media (6). In the 1930s researchers began to suspect tobacco smoking was linked to lung cancer. In 1950, Wynder and Graham published a landmark study in JAMA, which detailed 684 lung cancer victims and a similar number of controls, with respect to their smoking habits (30). Doll and Hill, also in 1950, published a critical article in the British Medical Journal, which confirmed the strong association between tobacco habits and lung cancer (31). In 1957, Hoffmann was the first scientist to identify the presence of the carcinogen benzo(a)pyrene in tobacco smoke (32). Since that time over 40 carcinogens have been identified in cigarette smoke (33). There is irrefutable evidence that tobacco smoking causes lung cancer, as reported in numerous reports from the US Surgeon General and others (34-37).

As mentioned above, the smoking population increased exponentially in the 20th century with a peak cigarette consumption in the United States occurring in the 1960s of over 4000 cigarettes per adult per year, or over 200 packs per year (38). Efforts in tobacco cessation have significantly decreased smoking rates in this country and Europe, but unfortunately smoking prevalence is increasing in developing countries. The risk of lung cancer due to tobacco use is related to the number of cigarettes smoked daily, duration of smoking in years, and age of initiation (39). Table 3 illustrates the relative risk of death from lung cancer, according to the number of pack-years of smoking. In the past, studies have claimed that smoking filtered, lower tar cigarettes decreased a smoker`1s risk for lung cancer (40,41). However, more recent studies suggest that these smokers tend to inhale the smoke more intensely, thereby increasing potential carcinogenesis (42). It has been proposed that African-Americans tend to smoke less than whites, but smoke cigarettes with higher percentage of tar and nicotine (43). African-Americans may smoke mentholated cigarettes more than white smokers, but this has not been shown to be an independent risk factor for lung cancer (44). Unfortunately, tobacco use among teenagers has been increasing over the last decade, despite aggressive anti-smoking campaigns (45). Finally, during the last half of the 20th century, women began smoking at an earlier age and therefore their pack-years increased significantly, which has led to equivalent lung cancer risk in females (1).

*Table 3. Relative Risk for Lung Cancer**

Smoking History	Risk Ratio
Lifelong non-smoker	1
Cigarette smoker	
< ½ pack/day	15
½ - 1 pack/day	17
1-2 pack/day	42
> 2 pack/day	64
Ex-smoker	1.5 - 2.0

Other forms of tobacco have also been implicated in causing lung cancer. Although the risk is less than cigarette smoking, pipe and cigar smoking have been shown to cause lung cancer (46). The risk may increase with the number of pipes or cigars smoked daily, and with the intensity of inhalation. Recently, the Surgeon General, reported on the significant dangers associated with cigar smoking (47). Chewing tobacco is associated with oral malignancy, but has not been shown to cause lung cancer. Recently, smokers of marijuana and crack cocaine were shown to have abnormalities in bronchial epithelium analogous to cigarette smokers (48).

Tobacco cessation is an essential focus for preventative medicine in all patients. Smoking cessation does significantly reduce lung cancer risk, but the relative risk remains 1.5 to 2 times the risk of a life-long non-smoker (49). Some have shown that in the initial few years of quitting smoking, the lung cancer risk may actually increase since many patients quit smoking due to symptoms, which may be caused by a lung cancer. The risk of lung cancer does decrease with duration of cessation and typically plateaus at 20 years (50). Some studies have shown that the risk for adenocarcinoma in former smokers, remains higher than other lung cancers (51).

Environmental smoke

Environmental tobacco smoke has been shown to adversely affect the health of non-smokers, especially children. Investigators have theorized for years that environmental smoke causes a majority of lung cancers in non-smokers. Most studies have examined the effect of household environmental smoke on lung cancer incidence in life-long non-smokers. In 1986 the Surgeon General issued a report stating that environmental smoke was a cause of lung cancer in non-smokers (52). Also in 1986, the National Research

Council performed a meta-analysis of 13 published studies on this subject, and concluded that there was an association between environmental smoke and lung cancer. This study concluded that the relative risk of lung cancer in non-smokers exposed to home environmental smoke was 1.34 or 34% (53). Subsequently, the Environmental Protection Agency published a report, which classified environmental smoke as a group A carcinogen and estimated that 3000-4000 of lung cancer deaths were attributable to passive smoke each year (54).

Breathing environmental smoke is certainly less than active inhalation, but side-stream smoke has a different constitution. Sidestream smoke has twice as much nicotine, and may have increased concentrations of carcinogens, such as 4-aminobiphenyl (21). Studies have shown that non-smokers who breathe environmental smoke, inhale the smoke and metabolize its carcinogens (53). Many studies have shown the significant exposure to environmental smoke in the work-place (55). The Occupational Safety and Health Administration (OSHA) has regulated indoor air quality in an effort to reduce the significant exposure to passive smoking (56). A recent large multi-center case control study of environmental smoke exposure and lung cancer risk performed in Europe, demonstrated that if exposure ended more that 15 years ago, there was no increased risk (57). This finding supports tobacco cessation as a critical preventative medicine measure for smokers and non-smokers exposed to their sidestream smoke. Stricter smoking regulations within the workplace have also been shown to significantly decrease the amount of cigarette consumption within a population (58).

Environmental factors

Radon gas is formed by the natural decay of uranium and radium from the earth. Radon gas decay products are carcinogens and have been shown to cause lung cancer in smoking and non-smoking underground miners (59). This colorless and odorless gas may be found in high concentrations within homes and other buildings. The indoor radon level depends on the soil concentration and ventilation rate. Decay products typically enter the home through defects in the foundation or pipes (60). Groundwater contamination has also been shown as a potential source. There is concern that exposure to radon gas is a significant cause of lung cancer in non-smokers, but the literature is inconsistent. A review of domestic radon and lung cancer risk did not show convincing evidence for causation, but concluded that an increased risk should be presumed (61). Smoking has been definitively shown to markedly increase the risk of lung cancer caused from radon exposure (62).

The concentration of radon within homes ranges from 0 to 100 pCi/L, with a mean concentration of 1.25 pCi/L (63). Generally, homes with a concentration of greater than 4 pCi/L are considered unsafe and reductive measures are recommended (64). Authors have estimated that approximately 5-10% of lung cancers may be caused by radon, however clinical studies have not conclusively characterized the risk of home radon exposure.

Air pollution has been implicated in causing lung cancer due to the larger number of carcinogens in ambient air. However, studies have demonstrated that air pollution causes less than 1% of lung cancers (65). Major air pollutants include carbon monoxide, hydrocarbons, sulfur oxides, nitrogen oxide and particulate matter (66). Automobiles and industry are the major causes of air pollution. Heavy exposure to electromagnetic fields has been proposed as an independent risk factor for lung cancer, but published studies are inconclusive (67,68). Diesel fuel exhaust contains many carcinogens and studies have shown that truck drivers have an increased risk of lung cancer, even after correction for smoking (69). The federal Environmental Protection Agency (EPA) has been examining the effects of diesel exhaust for many years. Recently, the California EPA published a meta-analysis of occupation exposure to diesel exhaust and concluded that the pooled smoking-adjusted relative risk was 1.47 (70). Thus, active measures are being followed to reduce this dangerous exposure to certain workers.

Occupational agents

It has been estimated that approximately 10-15% of lung cancer may be attributed to occupational exposures (71). The exact contribution of occupational agents can be difficult to conclusively determine, since smoking is more prevalent in blue collar workers (72). In addition, smoking histories in lung cancer victims may be inaccurate due to potential litigation. There is definitive proof that smoking and exposure to certain occupational agents, such as asbestosis, results in multiplicative risk (73). Occupational agents can cause lung cancer, but most lung cancer in high risk workers is preventable with tobacco cessation. Occupational carcinogens are classified according to the International Agency for Research on Cancer (IARC) as follows: Group 1 (known carcinogen), Group 2A (probable carcinogen) and Group 2B (possible carcinogen) (74).

Group 1 carcinogens for lung cancer include asbestos, arsenic, bis(chloromethyl) ether, chromium, nickel, vinyl chloride and polycyclic aromatic hydrocarbons. Group 2A carcinogens include beryllium, cadmium, acrylonitrile and formaldehyde. Group 2B carcinogens include acetaldehyde, welding fumes, crystalline silica and man-made mineral fibers.

Asbestos is a group of naturally occurring silicates that has been used commercially for over 100 years. It has been estimated that over 8 million workers have been exposed to asbestos in the United States. Common exposures occurred in mines, textile plants, cement plants, shipyards, automobile shops, construction and insulation work. Asbestos fibers are classified as either chrysotile or amphibole, and chrysotile fibers represent 90% of the asbestos used in the United States. All types of asbestos fibers have been shown to cause lung cancer, but generally long-term exposure to crocidolite or amosite carries a higher risk for developing lung cancer (75). Asbestos-related lung cancers tend to be peripheral and in the lower lung fields (76). Asbestos has been shown to be the most common occupational cause of cancer (77). Studies have shown that workers with asbestosis, rather that asbestos exposure, have an increased lung cancer risk (78). The risk of lung cancer in a patient with asbestosis who smokes is multiplicative, with an estimated risk of greater than 50-fold that of a lifelong non-smoker (79). The risk is dependent on cumulative exposure to the asbestos fibers (80). There is a latency period for the development of lung cancer in asbestos workers estimated at 25-40 years (81). Given the current low levels of occupational exposure to asbestos, the excess risk for lung cancer in the work place will continue to decrease.

Arsenic is a naturally occurring metal that is produced as a by-product of copper, lead, zinc and tin ore smelting and combustion of fossil fuels and wood (77). It is also present in agricultural pesticides and in marine organisms. Exposures to arsenic occur via air, water, soil and foods. An individuals concentration of arsenic is influenced by the quantity of seafood in their diet. Cumulative exposure to arsenic has been shown to be an independent risk factor for lung cancer (82). The interaction between smoking and arsenic exposure is generally considered less multiplicative than smoking and asbestos exposure (83). There is a latency period between exposure initiation and cancer occurrence of approximately 20-30 years (84). Unlike smoking, there is no decline in risk after exposure to arsenic has stopped (85).

Bis(chloromethyl) ether (BCME) is a product of chloromethylation processes performed in paint, textile and insulation industries (77). Studies have shown a dose-dependent relationship between exposure and lung cancer risk. After controlling for smoking, the relative risk for lung cancer is up to 10-fold for BCME (86). The majority of lung cancer caused by BCME is small-cell carcinoma (87). This carcinogen has been strictly regulated by OSHA and occupational risks have almost been completely eliminated.

Chromium has been a commonly used agent for metal alloys, paint pigments, rubber, cement, stainless steel, chrome plating, wood preservation and chemical manufacturing (77). Typically, workers are exposed in jobs such as: electroplating, arc welding, chromate-pigment manufacturing, mining and cutting/grinding of chromium alloys. Chromium exposure alone is felt to increase lung cancer risk by 2 to 3-fold (88).

Nickel has also been a popular component of metal alloys because of its strength. This metal has been used in stainless steel, plumbing, pumps, welding electrodes, coins, paint pigments, ceramics and batteries (77). Nickel sulfides and oxides have been shown to be carcinogens, with a dose-dependent causation of lung cancer (89). The relative risk of nickel exposure has been estimated at 1.56 (90). Frequently, workers exposed to nickel are also exposed to many other carcinogens. Finally, the relationship between cigarette smoking and nickel exposure is less clear.

Vinyl chloride is a colorless chemical used to make a type of plastic. The result is polyvinyl chloride (PVC), for example a PVC pipe. Vinyl chloride is also used in cosmetic products as a propellant. Exposures occur via hazardous waste sites, plastic factories or contaminated drinking water. It is a known cause of liver angiosarcoma, but its role in causing lung cancer is much less clear. Some studies have shown increases in lung cancer risk, but dose-dependence has not been documented (91). However, generally vinyl chloride is considered a small risk factor for lung cancer.

Polycyclic aromatic hydrocarbons (PAHs) are formed from incomplete combustion of organic material. The chemicals are ubiquitous and exposures occur in food intake, cigarette smoke, wood burning, diesel exhaust, coal tar, roofing tar and iron and steel founding (77). Many studies have demonstrated the excess risk of lung cancer in foundry workers (92). The relative risk of PAHs causing lung cancer ranges from 1.5 to 2.5, when controlled for smoking (93). Coke oven workers are at high risk and OSHA has enforced strict regulations for proper monitoring of these workers.

Group 2A carcinogens have been proven in experimental animals, but the evidence for humans is limited. Beryllium is a popular metal for alloys because of its high heat absorption and hardness. Exposures have occurred in mining, metal alloy manufacturing, ceramics and the electronic industry. During World War II, acute berylliosis was identified in miners with intense exposure. Many of these individuals also developed lung cancer (94). Animal studies have definitively proven beryllium as a pulmonary carcinogen, but human studies are inconsistent (95). Regardless, current strict exposure limits have likely minimized any relative risk. Cadmium is another metal that has been classified as a probable pulmonary carcinogen. Typically, it has been used for electroplating metals, pigments, batteries and plastic stabilization. Attributing relative risk for lung cancer from cadmium is difficult because of concomitant exposure to nickel or arsenic (96). Many studies have shown increased relative risk due to cadmium, but smoking is not controlled for reliably in these studies (97). Acrylonitrile is a flammable liquid used for acrylic fibers in textiles, plastics, rubbers and pipes. Small studies have reported a small increase in relative risk for lung cancer, but other carcinogens and smoking habits were not reliably controlled for (77). Therefore, the data is inconclusive, but regulations have been recommended. Formaldehyde is a reactive molecule used for adhesives, insulating materials, photographic film, cosmetics, embalming, rubbers and clothing. Naso-pharyngeal carcinomas in animals have been caused by formaldehyde exposure. There is little evidence that prolonged formaldehyde exposure is a significant risk factor for lung cancer. A very large study of 26,561 formaldehyde workers showed no causal relationship (98).

Group 2B carcinogens include agents with limited human data and no evidence for in experimental animals or no evidence in humans with sufficient animal data. Acetaldehyde, like formaldehyde, has been used for plastics, rubbers, resins and dyes. Animal studies have documented it as a cause of pulmonary cancer, but human studies are very limited (99). Welding fumes are composed of particulates, vapors and gases. Fumes consisting of nickel and chromium are well described in welding, but the relative risk in humans has not been clearly determined due to concomitant smoking and asbestos exposure (100). Man-made fibers are produced by the melting of raw materials and molding of the molten liquid. These are classified as mineral wools, fibrous glass and ceramic fibers. Commonly these fibers are produced by spinning or blowing molten glass or ceramic material. Animal studies have shown pulmonary carcinogenesis, but human studies show very weak association with lung cancer (101). Finally, silica is a very common component in commercial sands. Exposures typically have occurred in mining, metal foundry industry, sandblasting, ceramics, glass manufacturing, agricultural operations and rock processing. Many animal studies have proven that crystalline silica caused lung cancer, usually in the presence of fibrosis (102). Human studies have shown increased relative risk, especially in the setting of silicosis, which demonstrates a dose-responsive causal relationship (103). However, some autopsy studies of silicosis patients have not shown an increased rate of lung cancer. Given the decrease in silicosis, the risk for lung cancer from crystalline silica is likely to be low.

Preexisting lung disease

As mentioned above, lung cancer occurs in patients with pulmonary fibrosis from asbestos or silica. Other chronic lung diseases such as asthma, emphysema, idiopathic pulmonary fibrosis, tuberculosis, chronic bronchitis and pneumonia have been associated with increased lung cancer incidence in non-smokers. A large multicenter, retrospective study showed that any history of chronic lung disease yielded an elevated risk ratio of 1.56 (104). Tuberculosis has been shown to be a significant risk factor for the formation of adenocarcinoma from granulomatous lesions (105). Many studies have proven that heavy smokers who have airflow obstruction (COPD) have significantly higher risk for lung cancer. In fact a recent study proposed that these particular patients receive lung cancer screening using spiral chest CT scans (106). Finally, idiopathic pulmonary fibrosis patients have been shown to have a higher incidence of lung cancer, even after controlling for smoking habits (107).

Genetic

It is universally accepted that tobacco is responsible for the majority of lung cancers, however only approximately 1 out of 8 to 10 heavy smokers develop the deadly disease. Therefore, it is intuitive that there are genetic variables regarding the susceptibility of tobacco smoke carcinogens. Many studies have shown genetic predispostion for lung cancer (108,109). Studies have shown a smoking-adjusted 2 to 4-fold increase of lung cancer among individuals with a strong family history of lung cancer (110). Non-smokers with a family history of lung cancer have an estimated 2 to 3-fold increased relative risk (111). Familial aggregation of lung cancer has been attributed to genetics and also to similar smoking habits and environmental exposures. Some have hypothesized that familial aggregation of lung cancer may be due to inheritance of an autosomal gene that directly influences the risk of cigarette smoke (112).

Biomarkers are genetic markers that can be identified as associated with increased susceptibility to carcinogens. Many studies have examined the role of specific biomarkers for lung cancer (113). Studies of smoke carcinogen metabolism have shown individual differences in detoxification of carcinogens (114). The ability of carcinogens to cause covalent modification of DNA within bronchial tissue is measured by the degree of DNA adduct formation (115). Polycyclic aromatic hydrocarbons (PAHs) induce DNA adduct formation in the lung in a dose-dependent relationship with cigarette smoking (116). PAHs induce the cytochrome P450 enzyme, aryl hydrocarbon hydroxylase (CYP1A1), to form potent carcinogens. Genetic studies have demonstrated individual variability with this enzyme, which helps explain individual smoker differences in lung cancer risk (117). One study demonstrated that smokers with a rare homozygous allele for CYP1A1 had an increased relative risk of 7.3 for developing lung cancer (118).

Another cytochrome P450 gene associated with lung cancer is CYP2D6, which is involved in metabolism of certain anti-hypertensive drugs (119). Many studies have shown that increased activity of this gene is associated with an increased lung cancer risk (120). Tobacco smoke nitrosamines are probable substrates for this enzyme (121). After adjusting for smoking, age and sex, individuals with excess CYP2D6 activity have been shown to have a relative risk of 4 to 6 for developing lung cancer (122). A similar enzyme, CYP2A6, has been reported to effect the metabolism of nicotine. One study concluded that deficiency in this particular enzyme reduced smoking in individuals and therefore may lessen lung cancer risk (123). However, a recent study found no evidence that a deficiency of this enzyme led to decreased smoking or lung cancer risk (124). Another class of genes, glutathione-S-transferases (GSTs), have been studied for their effect on lung cancer risk (125). These enzymes are involved in detoxification of carcinogens (126). Microbiologic studies have demonstrated that cells deficient in such enzymes are susceptible to mutagens (127). A recent meta-analysis regarding deficiency of GST showed a relative risk of 1.4 (21). Recently, investigators demonstrated that non-smoking women with the homozygous null genotype for GST-M1 have a greater risk of lung cancer due to environmental tobacco smoke (128).

Advances in genetics have led to increased recognition of gene mutations or over-expression in lung cancer. Many studies have examined the role of oncogenes in the epidemiology of lung cancer. The most important oncogenes for lung cancer are the *ras* and *myc* oncogene families. The *ras* genes are frequently abnormal in lung cancer victims. These genes can induce a p21 protein to transform normal cells into cancerous cells (129). K-*ras* oncogene activation has been associated with a poorer long-term prognosis in non-small cell lung cancer. A recent study showed that the K-*ras* codon 12 mutation is a marker of aggressive non-small cell lung cancer with increased mortality (130). The *myc* genes have been shown to be involved in cell transcriptional regulation (131). Most studies have demonstrated that c-*myc* oncogene expression is associated with an increased risk of small cell lung cancer and a worse prognosis (132). For example, patients treated for relapsed small cell lung cancer who had excess c-*myc* levels have been shown to have decreased survival (133).

Other studies have focused on another oncogene, c-*erb*B-1, which is involved in epidermal growth factor receptor regulation. Over-expression of this gene has been demonstrated in both cancerous lung tissue and premalignant lesions (134). The effect of this gene on lung cancer prognosis is controversial. A similar oncogene, c-*erb*B-2 or HER2, has been shown to be expressed in certain non-small cell lung cancers (135). In adenocarcinoma, this oncogene has been associated with shorter survival (136). Recently, immunotherapy trials using anti-HER2 have begun in breast cancer, and it is likely that such trials will also be done for non-small cell lung cancer. Finally, tumor suppressor genes have been extensively studied regarding their role in the etiology of lung cancer. The two tumor suppressor genes most studied are the p53 and Rb anti-oncogenes. Abnormalities in the p53 gene are well-described in the literature and have been shown to occur in approximately 20-40% of non-small cell lung cancers and 80% of small cell lung cancers (137). Defects in the p53 gene have been associated with increased incidence of lung cancer. The Rb gene was the first tumor suppressor gene identified and is involved in regulation of cell cycle. Its deficiency or absence occurs in approximately all small cell lung cancer patients and approximately 20% of non-small cell patients (138). Despite the advances in molecular biology, there remains no serologic or genetic test widely available to define those smokers with particularly high risk for developing lung cancer.

Dietary

Multiple studies have investigated the role of dietary factors in the epidemiology of lung cancer. Generally, it is accepted that a diet rich in fruits and vegetables leads to lower incidence of lung cancer. Many studies have attributed most of this protective effect to beta-carotene. Beta-carotene is a precursor to vitamin A, which has been shown to have a protective effect on malignant cell differentiation and growth (139). This compound has also been shown to be a free radical scavenger. One large prospective study reported that beta-carotene had a significant protective effect against lung cancer, especially in patients with prolonged number of pack-years (140). Many retrospective studies have demonstrated the inverse relationship between beta-carotene intake and lung cancer incidence, with relative risk ranging from 0.37 to 0.67 (141). Beta-carotene serum levels in smokers are lower than non-smokers, but it is unclear whether this is simply due to differences in dietary intake (142).

Vitamin E has antioxidant properties that can inhibit bronchial carcinogenesis (143). The dietary intake of this fat-soluble vitamin is difficult to assess because it is ubiquitous in a standard diet. Serum vitamin E levels have been shown to be inversely proportional to lung cancer risk in some studies, but other investigation have shown no such relationship (144,145). The National Health and Nutrition Examination Survey (NHANES I) epidemiologic followup study demonstrated that higher vitamin E intake was associated with a lower lung cancer risk (relative risk of 0.36) (146). Vitamin C has been proposed as a protective agent because of its free radical scavenger properties. The NHANES I study reported that vitamin C intake reduced lung cancer incidence, with a relative risk of 0.66 (146). These studies of vitamin intake and lung cancer risk prompted chemoprevention trials in lung cancer. The Beta-Carotene and Retinol Efficacy trial unexpectantly showed an increased incidence of lung cancer in the group using beta-carotene (147). Therefore, some have postulated that the apparent protective effect of fruits and vegetables may be due to other compounds. One large study from Finland showed that flavonoid intake was independently associated with decreased lung cancer incidence (148).

Other dietary factors have been studied with respect to lung cancer incidence. Several studies have purported that a diet high in fat and cholesterol may increase lung cancer risk. One large study of approximately 25,000 men and 25,000 women in Norway, showed that cod liver oil supplement and skim milk intake was associated with relative risks of lung cancer of 0.5 (149). Cod liver oil has been shown to contain both vitamin A and omega-3 fatty acids, which are known to inhibit carcinogenesis. This study showed no association between lung cancer risk and dietary cholesterol and saturated fat. However, other studies have concluded that increased cholesterol is independently associated with a higher lung cancer incidence (150). Finally, a high concentrations of selenium, a mineral involved in the protection of cellular membranes, has been shown to be associated with lower cancer risk (151). Although dietary factors are important considerations for lung cancer risk, certainly smoking cessation remains our greatest hope in lung cancer prevention.

Summary

Lung cancer continues to be the leader in cancer deaths in the United States. The incidence of lung cancer in men has slowly decreased since the late 1980s, but has just now begun to plateau in women at the end of this decade. Despite modest advances in chemotherapy for treating lung cancer, it remains a deadly disease with overall 5-yr survival rates having not increased significantly over the last 25 years, remaining at approximately 14%. Tobacco smoking causes approximately 85-90% of bronchogenic carcinoma. Environmental tobacco exposure or a second-hand smoke also may cause lung cancer in life-long non-smokers. Certain occupational agents such as arsenic, asbestos, chromium, nickel and vinyl chloride increase the relative risk for lung cancer. Smoking has an additive or multiplicative effect with some of these agents. Familial predisposition for lung cancer is an area with advancing research. Developments in molecular biology have led to growing interest in investigation of biological markers, which may increase predisposition to smoking-related carcinogenesis. Hopefully, in the future we will be able to screen for lung cancer by using specific biomarkers. Finally, dietary factors have also been proposed as potential risk modulators, with vitamins A, C and E proposed as having a protective effect. Despite the slow decline of smoking in the United States, lung cancer will likely continue its devastation for years to come.

REFERENCES

1.   Landis S, Murray T, Bolden S and Wingo P. Cancer statistics, 1999. CA Cancer J Clin 49:8-31, 1999.
2.   National Center for Health Statistics: Public use data file documentation: Mortality data from ICD-9, 1995. Hyattsville, MD, Public Health Service, 1997.
3.   Wingo P, Ries L, Rosenberg H, et al. Cancer incidence and mortality, 1973-1995: A report card for the US. Cancer 82:1197-1207, 1998.
4.   National Cancer Institute: SEER Cancer Incidence Public-Use Database CD-ROM, 1973-1995, Bethesda MD, US Department of Health and Human Services, Public Health Service, 1998.
5.   Baquet C, Horm J, Gibbs T et al. Socioeconomic factors and cancer incidence among blacks and whites. J NCI 83:551-557, 1991.

6.   Wynder E. The past, present and future of the prevention of lung cancer. Cancer Epidemiology, Biomarkers and Prevention 7:735-48, 1998.

7.   American Cancer Society. Tobacco Use. Trends in smoking, p.24, Cancer Facts and Figures, 1996. Atlanta: American Cancer Society, Inc. 1996.

8.   Wagenknecht L, Cutter G, Haley N et al. Racial differences in serum cotinine levels among smokers in the coronary artery risk development in young adults study. Am J Public Health 80:1053, 1990.

9.   Richie J, Carlemma S, Muscat J, et al. Differences in the urinary metabolites of the tobacco-specific lung carcinogen 4-(methylnitrosamino)-1-(3-pyridyl)-1-butanone (NNK) in black and white smokers. Cancer Epidemiol Biomark Prev 6:783-90, 1997.

10. Bach P, Cramer L, Warren J and Begg C. Racial differences in the treatment of early-stage lung cancer. New Engl J Med 341:1198-205, 1999.

11. Mahoney M and Michalek A. A meta-analysis of cancer incidence in United States and Canadian native populations. Int J Epidemiol 20:323-327, 1991.

12. Samet J, Wiggins C, Key C et al. Mortality from lung cancer and chronic obstructive pulmonary disease in New Mexico, 1958-82. Am J Public Health 78:1182-86, 1988.

13. American Cancer Society: Cancer facts and figures, California 1993. Oakland, CA, American Cancer Society, California Division, Inc., 1993.

14. Markides K, Coreil J and Ray L. Smoking among Mexican-Americans: a three generation study. Am J Public Health 77:708, 1987.

15. Marin G, Perez-Stable E, Marin B. Cigarette smoking among San Francisco Hispanics: the role of acculturation and gender. Am J Public Health 79:196, 1989.

16. U.S. Department of Health and Human Services (DHHS). The health consequences of smoking for women. Washington, DC: DHHS. Public Health Service, Office of the Assistant Secretary for Health, Office on Smoking and Health, 1980.

17. Samet J, Skipper B, Humble C, et al. Lung cancer risk and vitamin A consumption in New Mexico. Am Rev Respir Dis 131:198-202, 1985.

18. Garfinkel L and Stellman S. Smoking and lung cancer in women: Findings in a prospective study. Cancer Res 48:6951, 1988.

19. Samet J, Wiggins C, Humble C et al. Cigarette smoking and lung cancer in New Mexico. Am Rev Respir Dis 137:1110-1113, 1998.

20. Kubat G. Aspects of the epidemiology of lung cancer in smokers and nonsmokers in the United States. Lung Cancer 15:1-20, 1996.

21. Brownson R, Alavanja M, Caporaso N et al. Epidemiology and prevention of lung cancer in nonsmokers. Epidemiologic Reviews 20:218-236, 1998.

22. Redmond W. Trends in adolescent cigarette use: The diffusion of daily smoking. J of Behavioral Medicine 22(4):379-95, 1999.

23. Kreuzer M, Kreienbroch L, Gerken M et al. Risk factors for lung cancer in young adults. Am J of Epidemiol 147:1028-1037, 1998.

24. Bourke W, Milstein D, Giura R et al. Lung cancer in young adults. Chest 102:1723-9, 1992.

25. Rocha M, Fraire A, Guntupalli K et al. Lung cancer in the young. Cancer Detect Prev 18:349-55, 1994.

26. Sekine I, Nishiwaki Y, Yokose T et al. Young lung cancer patients in Japan: Different characteristics between the sexes. Ann Thorac Surg 67:1451-55, 1999.

27. Wu-Williams A, Dai X, Blot W et al. Lung cancer among women in north-east China. Br J Cancer 1990;62:982-7, 1990.

28. Hirayama T. Life-style and mortality. A large-scale census-based cohort study in Japan. In: J. Wahrendorf (ed.), Contributions to Epidemiology and Biostatistics. Vol. 1, 1-133. Basel: S. Karger AG, 1993.

29. The female smoker: From addiction to recovery. Christen J and Christen A. Creative Services, Indiana University School of Medicine, Indianapolis, IN, 1998.

30. Wynder E and Graham E. Tobacco smoking as a possible etiologic factor in bronchiogenic carcinoma. A study of six hundred and eighty-four proved cases. JAMA 143:329-336, 1950.

31. Doll R and Hill A. Smoking and carcinoma of the lung. Preliminary report. Br Med J 2:739-748, 1950.

32. Wynder E and Hoffman D. A study in tobacco carcinogenesis. VII. The role of higher polycyclic hydrocarbons. Cancer (Phila.) 12:1079-86, 1959.

33. Wynder E, Hoffman D. Tobacco and tobacco smoke: studies in experimental carcinogenesis. New York, Academic Press, 1967.

34. US Public Health Service: Smoking and Health. A Report on the Advisory Committee to the Surgeon General of the Public Health Service. US Department of Health, Education and Welfare, Center for Disease Control, 1964.

35. US Public Health Service: Smoking and Health. A Report of the Surgeon General. Rockville, Maryland, US Department of Health, Education, and Welfare, Public Health Service, Office on Smoking and Health, 1979.

36. Doll R and Peto R. Mortality in relation to smoking: 20 years= observations on male British doctors. Br Med J 2:1525, 1976.

37. Rogot E and Murray J. Smoking and causes of death among US veterans: 16 years of observation. Public Health Rep 15:213, 1980.

38. US Department of Health and Human Services: Smoking and health in the Americas. Atlanta, US Department of Health and Human Services, Public Health Service, Centers for Disease Control, National Center for Chronic Disease Prevention and Health Promotion, Office on Smoking and Health, 1992; DHHS Publication No. [CDC] 92-8419.

39. Doll R and Peto R. Cigarette smoking and bronchial carcinoma: Dose and time relationships among regular smokers and lifelong non-smokers. J Epidemiol Community Health 32:303-313, 1978.

40. Stellman S and Garfinkel L. Lung cancer risk is proportional to cigarette tar yield: evidence from a prospective study. Prev Med 18:518, 1989.

41. Lubin J, Blot W, Berrino F et al. Patterns of lung cancer risk according to type of cigarette smoked. Int J Cancer 33:569-576, 1984.

42. United States Department of Health and Human Services. Strategies to control tobacco use in the United States. Smoking Tobacco Control Monogr (NIH) 1:1-307, 1991.

43. Cummings K, Giovino G and Mendicino A. Cigarette advertising and black-white differences in brand preference. Public Health Rep 102:698-701, 1987.

44. Kabat G and Hebert J. Use of mentholated cigarettes and lung cancer risk. Cancer Res 51:6510-6513, 1991.

45. Redmond W. Trends in adolescent cigarette use: The diffusion of daily smoking. J of Behavioral Med 22(4):379-95, 1999.

46. Damber L and Larsson L. Smoking and lung cancer with special regard to type of smoking and type of cancer: a case-control study in north Sweden. Br J Cancer 53:673, 1986.

47. Satcher D. Cigars and public health. NEJM 340(23):1829-31, 1999.

48. Barsky S, Roth M, Kleerup E et al. Histopathologic and molecular alterations in bronchial epithelium in habitual smokers of marijuana, cocaine and/or tobacco.

J of the Natl Cancer Inst 90:1198-1205, 1998.

49. Becher H, Jockel K, Timm J et al. Smoking cessation and nonsmoking intervals: Effect of different smoking patterns on lung cancer risk. Cancer Causes and Control 2:381-87, 1991.

50. US Department of Health and Human Services: The Health Benefits of Smoking Cessation: US Department of Health and Human Services, Public Health Service, Centers for Disease Control, Center for Chronic Disease Prevention and Health Promotion, Office on Smoking and Health. DHHS Publication No. (CDC) 90-8416, 1990.

51. Higgins I and Wynder E. Reduction in risk of lung cancer among ex-smokers with particular reference to histologic type. Cancer 62:2397-2401, 1988.

52. US Surgeon General. The health consequences of involuntary smoking. Washington, DC, United States Department of Health and Human Services, Centers for Disease Control, Publication No. 87-8398,1986.

53. Committee on Passive Smoking, Board on Environmental Studies and Toxicology, National Research Council: Environmental Tobacco Smoke: Measuring Exposures and Assessing Health Effects. Washington, DC, National Academy Press, 1986.

54. US Environmental Protection Agency: Health Effects of Passive Smoking: Assessment of Lung Cancer in Adults and Respiratory Disorders in Children. EPA Publication No. 600/6-90/006A.

55. Hammond S. Exposure of US workers to environmental tobacco smoke. Environ Health Perspect 107(Suppl 2):329-340, 1999.

56. NIOSH: Current Intelligence bulletin 54. Environmental tobacco smoke in the workplace. Lung cancer and other health effects. US Department of Health and Human Services, Public Health Service, Centers for Disease Control, National Institute for Occupational Safety and Health, Cincinnati, 1991.

57. Boffetta P, Agudo A, Ahrens W et al. Multicenter case-control study of exposure to enviromental tobacco smoke and lung cancer in Europe. J of the Natl Cancer Inst 90:1440-50, 1998.

58. Chapman S, Borland R, Scollo M et al. The impact of smoke-free workplaces on declining cigarette consumption in Australia and the United States. Am J of Public Health 89:1018-1023, 1999.

59. Saccomanno G, Huth G, Auerbach O et al. Relationship of radioactive radon daughters and cigarette smoking in the genesis of lung cancer in uranium miners. Cancer 62:1402-1408, 1988.

60. Oge, M. Radon risk in the home. Science 255:1194, 1992.

61. Samet J. Radon and lung cancer. J Natl Cancer Inst 81:745-757, 1989.

62. American Medical Association Council of Scientific Affairs: Health Effects of radon exposure. Arch Intern Med 151:674-77, 1991.

63. Samet J, Stolwijk J, Rose S. Summary: International Workshop on Residential Radon Epidemiology. Health Physics 60:223-227, 1991.

64. Samet J and Hornung R. Review of radon and lung cancer risk. Risk Analysis 10:65-75, 1990.

65. U.S. Environmental Protection Agency. Cancer risk from outdoor exposure to air toxins, Vol. 1, final report. Research Triangle Park, NC: Environmental Criteria and Assessment Office, EPA/450/1-90/004A, 1990.

66. Natusch D. Potentially carcinogenic species emitted to the atmosphere by fossil-fueled power plants. Environ Health Perspect 22:79-90, 1978.

67. Robinette C, Silverman C and Jablon S. Effects upon health of occupational exposure to microwave radiation (radar). Am J Epidemiol 112:39-53, 1980.

68. Vogero D, Ahlbom A, Olin R et al. Cancer morbidity among workers in the telecommunications industry. Br J of Ind Med 42:191-195, 1985.

69. Steenland K. Lung cancer and diesel exhaust: A review. Am J Ind Med 10:177-189, 1986.

70. Lipsett M and Campleman S. Occupational exposure to diesel exhaust and lung cancer: A meta-analysis. Am J Public Health 89:1009-17, 1999.

71. Samet J and Lerchen M. Proportion of lung cancer caused by occupation: a critical review. In: Gee J, Morgan W and Brooks S, eds. Occupational lung disease. New York, Raven Press: 55, 1984.

72. Nelson D Emont S, Brackbill R et al. Cigarette smoking prevalence by occupation in the United States: a comparison between 1978 to 1980 and 1987 to 1990. J Occup Med 36:516-525, 1994.

73. Selikoff I, Hammond E and Churg J. Asbestos exposure, smoking andneoplasia. JAMA 204:104, 1968.

74. International Agency for Research on Cancer (IARC). IARC monographs on the evaluation of carcinogenic risks to humans. Overall evaluations of carcino- genicity: an updating of IARC monographs volumes 1 to 42 (Suppl 7). Lyon: IARC, 1987.

75. Health and Safety Commission: Asbestos. Vol. 2: Papers Prepared for the Advisory Committee. London, Her Majesty's Stationery Office, pp. 8-55, 1979.

76. Weiss W. Lobe of origin in the attribution of lung cancer to asbestos. Br J of Ind Med 45:544-547, 1986.

77. Steenland K, Loomis D, Shy C and Simonsen N. Review of occupational lung carcinogens. Am J of Ind Med 29:474-490, 1996.

78. Weiss W. Asbestosis: A marker for the increased risk of lung cancer among workers exposed to asbestos. Chest 115:536-549, 1999.

79. Hammond E, Selikoff I and Seidman H. Asbestos exposure, cigarette smoking and death rates. Ann NY Acad Sci 330:473-90, 1979.

80. Browne K. A threshold for asbestos related lung cancer. Br J Ind Med 43:556-58, 1986.

81. Liddell F. Latent periods in lung cancer mortality in relation to asbestos dose and smoking. In: Wagner J and Davis W, eds, Biological Effects of Mineral Fibres, Lyon, IARC, pp. 661-665, 1980.

82. Enterline P, Marsh G, Esmen N et al. Some effects of cigarette smoking, arsenic and SO_2 on mortality among US copper smelter workers. J Occup Med 29:831-38, 1987.

83. Pershagen G, Wall S, Taube A et al. On the interaction between occupational arsenic exposure and smoking and its relationship to lung cancer. Scand J Work Environ Health 7:302-09, 1981.

84. Brown C and Chu K. Implications of the multistage theory of carcinogenesis applied to occupational arsenic exposure. J Natl Cancer Inst 70:455-63, 1983.

85. Sobel W, Bond G, Baldwin C et al. An update of respiratory cancer and occupational exposure to arsenicals. Am J Ind Med 13:263-70, 1988.

86. McCallum R, Woolley V and Petrie A. Lung cancer associated with chloromethyl methyl ether manufacture: An investigation at two factories in the United Kingdom. Br J Ind Med 40:384-89, 1983.

87. Weiss W, Moser R and Auerbach O. Lung cancer in chloromethyl ether workers. Am Rev Respir Dis 120:1031-37, 1979.

88. Hayes R, Sheffet A and Spirtas R. Cancer mortality among a cohort of chromium pigment workers. Am J Ind Med 16:127-33, 1989.

89.   Doll R, Mathews J, and Morgan L. Cancers of the lung and nasal sinuses in nickel workers: A reassessment of the period of risk. Br J Ind Med 34:102-05, 1977.

90.   International Committee on Nickel Carcinogenesis in Man. Report of the International Committee on Nickel Carcinogenesis in Man. Scand J Work   Environ Health 16:1-82, 1990.

91.   Simonato L, L'Abbe K, Andersen A et al. A collaborative study of cancer incidence and mortality among vinyl chloride workers. Scand J Work Environ Health 17:159-69, 1991.

92.. International Agency for Research on Cancer (IARC). IARC monographs on the evaluation of carcinogenic risk of chemicals to humans. Polynuclear aromatic hydrocarbons, part 1, chemical, environmental and experimental data. Lyon: IARC, 32, 1983.

93.   Lloyd J. Long-term mortality study of steelworkers. Respiratory cancer in coke plant workers. J Occup Med 13:53-68, 1971.

94.   Steenland K and Ward E. Lung cancer incidence among patients with beryllium disease: a cohort mortality study. J Natl Cancer Inst 83:1380-85, 1991.

95.   MacMahon B. The epidemiological evidence on the carcinogenicity of beryllium in humans. J Occup Med 36:15-26, 1994.

96.   Lamm S, Parkinson M, Anderson M and Taylor W. Determinants of lung cancer risk among cadmium-exposed workers. Ann Epidemiol 2:195-211, 1992.

97.   Thun M, Schnorr T, Smith A et al. Mortality among a cohort of US cadmium production workers B An update. J Natl Cancer Inst 74:235-33, 1985.

98.   Marsh G, Stone R and Henderson V. A reanalysis of the National Cancer Institute study on lung cancer mortality among industrial worker exposed to formaldehyde. J Occup Med 34:42-44, 1992.

99.   U.S. Environmental Protection Agency. Health assessment document for acetaldehyde. Research Triangle Park, NC: Office of Health and Environmental Assessment. 1987:EPA/600/8-86/015A.

100. International Agency for Research on Cancer (IARC). IARC monographs on the evaluation of carcinogenic risks to humans. Chromium, nickel and welding fumes. Lyon: IARC 49:447-525, 1990.

101. Miettinen O and Rossiter C. Man-made mineral fibers and lung cancer: epidemiologic evidence regarding the causal hypothesis. Scand J Work Environ Health 16:221-231, 1990.

102. Saffiotti U. Lung cancer induction by crystalline silica. Prog Clin Biol Res 374:51-69, 1992.

103. Simonato L, Fletcher A, Saracci R and Thomas T. Occupational exposure to silica and cancer risk. IARC Sci Publ 97:55-64, 1990.

104. Wu A, Fontham E, Reynolds P et al. Previous lung disease and risk of lung cancer among lifetime nonsmoking women in the United States. Am J Epidemiol 141:1023-32, 1995.

105. Zheng W, Blot W, Liao M et al. Lung cancer and prior tuberculosis infection in Shanghai. Br J Cancer 56:501, 1987.

106. Henschke C, McCauley D, Yankelevitz D et al. Early lung cancer action project: overall design and findings from baseline screening. Lancet 354:99-105, 1999.

107. Turner-Warwich M, Lebowitz M, Burrows B and Johnson A. Cryptogenic fibrosing alveolitis and lung cancer. Thorax 35:496-99, 1980.

108. Sellers T, Bailey-Wilson J, Elston R et al. Evidence for Mendelian inheritance in the pathogenesis of lung cancer. J Natl Cancer Inst 82:1272, 1990.

109. Samet J, Humble C and Pathak D. Personal and family history of respiratory disease and lung cancer risk. Am Rev Resp Dis 134:466, 1986.

110. Osann K. Lung cancer in women: The importance of smoking, family history of cancer and medical history of respiratory disease. Cancer Res 51:4893-97, 1989.

111. Tokuhata G and Lilienfeld A. Familial aggregation of lung cancer in humans. J Natl Cancer Inst 30:289-312, 1963.
112. Fain P, Lynch H, Albano et al. Sex differences in lung cancer incidence: A genetic model. Med Hypoth 7:1109-1112, 1981.
113. Perera F and Weinstein I. Molecular epidemiology and carcinogen DNA adduct detection: New approaches to studies of human cancer causation. J Chron Dis 35:581-600, 1982.
114. Harris C. Interindividual variation among humans in carcinogen metabolism, DNA adduct formation and DNA repair. Carcinogenesis 10:1563-66, 1989.
115. Glickman B. DNA repair and its relationship to the origins of human cancer. In: Cleton F and Simons J (eds), Genetic origin of tumor cells. Nijhoff, The Hague, 25-51, 1980.
116. Phillips D, Hewer A, Matin C et al. Correlation of DNA adduct levels in human lung with cigarette smoking. Nature 336:790-92, 1982.
117. Strong L and Amos C. Inherited susceptibility. In: Schottenfeld D and Fraumeni J (eds). Cancer epidemiology and prevention. Oxford University Press, New York, 559-583,1996.
118. Nakachi K, Imai K, Hayashi S et al. Genetic susceptibility to squamous cell carcinoma of the lung in relation to cigarette smoking dose. Cancer Res 51:5177-80, 1991.
119. Meyer U, Zanger U, Zanger D et al. Genetic polymorphisms of drug metabolism. Adv Drug Res 19:197-241, 1990.
120. Caporaso N, Tucker M, Hoover R et al. Lung cancer and the debrisoquine metabolic phenotype. J Natl Cancer Inst 82:1264-72, 1990.
121. Crespi C, Penman B, Gelboin H et al. A tobacco smoke-derived nitrosamine, 4-(methylnitrosamino)-1-(3-pyridyl)-1-butanone, is activated by multiple human cytochrome P450=s including the polymorphic human cytochrome P4502D6. Carcinogenesis 11:1293-1300, 1990.
122. Caporaso N, Tucker M, Hoover R et al. Lung cancer and the debrisoquine metabolic phenotype. J Natl Cancer Inst 82:1264-72, 1990.
123. Pianezza M, Sellers E and Tyndale R. Nicotine metabolism defect reduces smoking. Nature 393:750, 1998.
124. London S, Idle J, Daly A and Coetzee G. Genetic variation of CYP2A6, smoking, and risk of cancer. Lancet 353:898-899, 1999.
125. Seidegard J, Pero R, Miller D et al. Glutathione transferase in human leukocytes as a marker for the susceptibility to lung cancer. Carcinogenesis 751-53, 1986.
126. Nazar-Stewart V, Motulsky A, Eaton D et al. The glutathione S-transferase polymorphism as a marker for susceptibility to lung carcinoma. Cancer Res 53:2313, 1993.
127. Wiencke J, Kelsey K, Lamela R et al. Human glutathione-S-transferase deficiency as a marker of susceptibility to epoxide-induced cytogenetic damage. Cancer Res 50:1585-90, 1990.
128. Bennett W, Alavanja M, Blomeke B et al. Environmental tobacco smoke, genetic susceptibility, and risk of lung cancer in never-smoking women. J Natl Cancer Inst 91:2009-14, 1999.
129. Rodenhuis S and Slebus R. The RAS oncogene in human lung cancer. Am Rev Resp Dis 142:527-30, 1990.
130. Nelson H, Christiani D, Mark E et al. Implications and prognostic value of K-ras mutation for early-stage lung cancer in women. J Natl Cancer Inst 91:2032-38, 1999.
131. Minna J, Battey J, Brooks B et al. Molecular genetic analysis reveals chromosomal deletion, gene amplification, and autocrine growth factor production in the pathogenesis of human lung cancer. Cold Spring Harbor Symp Quant Biol 51: 843-53, 1986.

132. Funa K, Steinholz L, Nou et al. Increased expression of N-*myc* in human small cell lung cancer biopsies predicts lack of response to chemotherapy and poor prognosis. Am J Clin Pathol 88:216-20, 1987.

133. Johnson B, Ihde D, Makuch R et al. *myc* family oncogene amplification in tumor cell lines established from small cell lung cancer patients and its relationship to clinical course. J Clin Invest 79:1629-34, 1987.

134. Hendler F and Ozanne B. Human squamous cell lung cancers express increased epidermal growth factor receptor. J Clin Invest 74:647-51, 1984.

135. Schneider P, Hung M, Chiocca S, et al. Differential expression of the c-*erb*B-2 gene in human small cell and non-small lung cancer. Cancer Res 49:4968-71, 1989.

136. Kern F, Schwartz D, Nordberg J, et al. p185 ^{neu} expression in human lung adenocarcinomas predicts shortened survival. Cancer Res 50:5184-91, 1990.

137. Takashi T, Nau M, and Chiba I. p53: A frequent target for genetic abnormalities in lung cancer. Science 246:491-94, 1989.

138. Harbor J, Sali S, Whang-Peng J, et al. Abnormalities in structure and expression of the human retinoblastoma gene in SCLC. Science 241:353-57, 1988.

139. Peto R, Doll R, Buckley J et al. Can dietary beta-carotene materially reduce human cancer rates? Nature 290:201-208, 1981.

140. Shekelle R, Liu S, Raynor W, et al. Dietary vitamin A and risk of cancer in the Western Electric Study. Lancet 2:1185-90, 1981.

141. Byers T, Graham S, Haughey B et al. Diet and lung cancer risk: Findings from the western New York diet study. Am J Epidemiol 125:351-63, 1987.

142. Stryker W, Kaplan L, Stein E, et al. The relation of diet, cigarette smoking and alcohol consumption to beta-carotene and alpha-tocopherol levels. Am J Epidemiol 127:283-96, 1988.

143. Chow C. Dietary vitamin E and cellular susceptibility to cigarette smoke. Ann NY Acad Sci 393:426-36, 1982.

144. Menkes M, Comstock G, Vuilleumeir J et al. Serum beta-carotene, vitamins A and E, selenium, and the risk of lung cancer. N Engl J of Med 315:1250-54, 1986.

145. Willett W, Polk B, Underwood B et al. Relation of serum vitamins A and E and carotenoids to the risk of cancer. N Engl J Med 310:430-34, 1984.

146. Yong L, Brown C, Schatzkin A, et al. Intake of vitamins E, C and A and risk of lung cancer. The NHANES I epidemiologic followup study. Am J of Epidemiol 146:231-43, 1997.

147. Omenn G, Goodman G, Thonquist et al. Effects of a combination of beta-carotene and vitamin A on lung cancer and cardiovascular disease. N Engl J Med 334:1150-5, 1996.

148. Knekt P, Jarvinen R, Seppanen R, et al. Dietary flavonoids and the risk of lung cancer and other malignant neoplasms. Am J of Epidemiol 146:223-30, 1997.

149. Vierod M, Laake P and Thelle D. Dietary fat intake and risk of lung cancer: a prospective study of 51,452 Norwegian men and women. Eur J of Cancer Prevention 6:540-49, 1997.

150. Knekt P, Seppanen R, Jarvinen R et al. Dietary cholesterol, fatty acids and the risk of lung cancer among men. Nutr Cancer 16:267-75, 1991.

151. Salonen J, Alfthan G, Huttenen J et al. Association between serum selenium and risk of cancer. Am J Epidemiol 120:342-49, 1984.

STAGING AND PROGNOSIS IN LUNG CANCER: MAKING THE COMPLEX ACCESSIBLE

Corey J. Langer, M.D.
Fox Chase Cancer Center Philadelphia, PA 19111 USA

INTRODUCTION

Long-term survival in lung cancer remains relatively dismal (1). With the exception of resectable patients with either minimal or no node involvement, selected locally advanced patients with NSCLC, and selected limited disease patients with SCLC, cure remains elusive (2,3). As we tease out those who may benefit from aggressive therapy, the intricacies of the staging system appear to grow inversely proportional to the prospect of cure using conventional therapeutic maneuvers. Therapeutic nihilists would argue that staging, in such a setting, is largely irrelevant or useless. However, the nuances of treatment hinge directly on appropriate staging. In addition, carefully defined staging constitutes a common language for clinicians, particularly in the interdisciplinary setting which ideally is required for the optimal treatment of lung cancer. For staging to be meaningful, it must be methodical, comprehensive and reproducible. Otherwise, the putative stage assignment is meaningless.

Within this paradigm, prognosis and treatment decisions are further informed by basic prognostic factors, including performance status, pre-existing weight loss, and, to a lesser extent, gender (4,5). These factors, however, have not yet been routinely incorporated into current lung cancer staging criteria.

The Evolution of NSCLC Staging: *1973 AJCC Criteria (6)*

Initial staging guidelines promulgated in the early 70s attempted to impose consistency in treatment decision making, but quickly proved outmoded. At that time, tumor extent was defined as stages I, II, or III. Stage I (operable) NSCLC included patients with T_1 N_{0-1} and T_2 N_0 disease, while Stage II (also operable), consisted of a relatively small cohort: T_2 N_1 M_0 disease. All other tumors, including T_3, N_2 and M_1 lesions were lumped into Stage III; by the standards of more than a quarter of a century ago, these patients were considered unresectable and therefore incurable. Given the limited treatment options available at that time, this surgically driven staging system was probably appropriate (Table I). It quickly became apparent that this system was based, in large part, on limited, relatively inadequate staging tools available at that time, and that the diverse T_3 category included groups who were potentially curable, as well as those who could not be cured. With the exception of $T_3 N_0$ disease, virtually all stage III patients had a poor prognosis. In addition, there was no attempt, at that time, to tease out locally advanced N_2 or N_3 disease, where aggressive local radiotherapy might benefit patients, and M_1 (extrathoracic) disease where prognosis was uniformly fatal and local irradiation had no curative role.

Table 1. Stage Grouping (TNM combinations)

1974		1986		1997	
Occult	$T_x N_0 M_0$	Occult	$T_x N_0 M_0$	Occult	$T_{xs} N_0 M_0$
Stage 0	$T_{is} N_0 M_0$	Stage 0	$T_{is} N_0 M_0$	Stage 0	$T_{is} N_0 M_0$
Stage I	$T_1 N_0 M_0$ $T_2 N_0 M_0$ $T_1 N_1 M_0$	Stage I	$T_1 N_0 M_0$ $T_2 N_0 M_0$	Stage IA Stage IB	$T_1 N_0 M_0$ $T_2 N_0 M_0$
Stage II	$T_2 N_1 M_0$	Stage II	$T_1 N_1 M_0$ $T_2 N_1 M_0$	Stage IIA Stage IIB	$T_1 N_1 M_0$ $T_2 N_1 M_0$ $T_3 N_0 M_0$
Stage III M M M	T_3, any N, any Any T, N_2 any Any T, any N,	Stage IIIA	$T_3 N_0 M_0$ $T_3 N_1 M_0$ $T_1 N_2 M_0$ $T_2 N_2 M_0$ $T_3 N_2 M_0$	Stage IIIA	$T_3 N_1 M_0$ $T_1 N_2 M_0$ $T_2 N_2 M_0$ $T_3 N_2 M_0$
		Stage IIIB	T_4 any N, M_0 AnyT,N_3,M_0	Stage IIIB	T_4,any N, M_0 Any T, N_3, M_0
		Stage IV	Any T, any N, M	Stage IV	Any T, any N, M

1986 TNM Update (7)

A comprehensive overhaul of the staging system occurred in the mid 80s based in part on improved imaging techniques, and in part on the recognition that refined treatment approaches, including combined modality therapy, could lead to improved prognosis particularly for locally advanced, resectable or potentially resectable disease (Table I). This collaborative effort of the AJCC, UICC and Japanese and German representatives evaluated databases comprised of records of 3753 lung cancer patients from the now-defunct North American Lung Cancer Study Group and reference data from M.D. Anderson Cancer Center in Houston. The revised International Staging System was published in 1986, and represented a major leap forward in refining prognostic subgroups, and establishing meaningful treatment guidelines. Tumors invading vital mediastinal structures, e.g., superior vena cava, esophagus, trachea, and vertebral body invasion as well as tumors associated with malignant pleural effusions, were moved from the T_3 category into a new T_4 category. In addition, malignant effusion was specifically defined to exclude cytologically negative, non-bloody, non-exudative effusions. The T_3 category now specifically referred to patients with limited, circumscribed extrapulmonary extension (e.g. chest wall, including superior sulcus, pericardium, diaphragm, mediastinal pleura). The T_3 category also included tumors within 2 cm of the carina, with no evidence of carinal involvement.

In addition, mediastinal nodes were divided into two separate categories. N_2 designated ipsilateral, mediastinal and subcarinal nodal involvement, a group in whom resection was potentially feasible, while a new category (N_3), encompassed supraclavicular and contralateral hilar and contralateral mediastinal nodes. Although N_3 disease, was recognized as a poor prognostic sign, this accommodation recognized the regional nature of N_3 involvement, and the capacity of modern radiation techniques to encompass this type of disease. The N_1 category specifically referred to intrapulmonary or ipsilateral hilar nodal involvement, which by definition, was resectable upfront.

In addition to revisions in TNM staging, the staging subgroups were also revised. Patients with T_1 and T_2N_0 disease, recognized as a particularly favorable subgroup, were designated stage I, while T_1 N_1 disease, with poorer prognosis based on nodal involvement and the attendant risk of occult extra-thoracic spread, was combined with T_2 N_1 disease and considered stage II. The hitherto, highly heterogeneous stage III category of the first AJCC system was divided into two major subgroups: stage III indicative of locally advanced disease, and stage IV (M_1) indicative of extrathoracic disseminated spread. In recognition of the complex nature of stage III patients, this category was further subdivided into III-A (T_3 and/or N_2) where complete resection might be feasible upfront or reasonable after appropriate induction therapy, and III-B (T_4 and/or N_3), where resection rarely, if ever, was feasible, but where local irradiation might have a definitive role. Unfortunately the T_4 category did not discriminate between lesions invading vital mediastinal structures (e.g. trachea, vertebral body, heart, etc.) where irradiation could potentially have a definitive role and malignant pleural effusions or multifocal ipsilateral pulmonary or pleural disease, where irradiation would not likely provide any long-term benefit. Overall, the 1987 revision was fairly radical, and represented a major improvement in tailoring staging to prognostic subgroups.

1997 AJCC Revision (8)

After more than a decade of familiarity with the 1986 system, the staging criteria were again revised, based on outcomes for over over 5000 patients treated at M.D. Anderson Cancer Center (1975-1988), and by the North American Lung Cancer Study Group (1977-1982). Compared to the 1986 revision, the staging modifications introduced in the late 90s were relatively minor, and were based on the recognition of varying prognoses for additional subgroups. Stage I was subdivided into I-A and I-B, based on tumor size (3 cm or less (T_1) vs. more than 3 cm (T_2)), the absence (T_1) or presence of visceral pleural invasion (T_2) or extension into the mainstem bronchus (T_2) (9,10,11). Stage II (N_1) disease was subdivided into II-A and II-B based on identical criteria. In addition, $T_3 N_0 M_0$ patients were downstaged from III-A to II-B based on the observation

Table 2. Anatomical Staging for Lung Cancer. TNM Categories Definitions

Primary Tumor (T)

Tx	Primary tumor cannot be assessed, or tumor proven by presence of malignant cells in sputum or bronchial washings but not visualized by imaging or bronchoscopy
T0	No evidence of primary tumor
Tis	Carcinoma *in situ*
T1	Tumor 3 cm or less in greatest dimension, surrounded by lung or visceral pleura, without bronchoscopic evidence of invasion more proximal than the lobar bronchus* (i.e., not in main bronchus)
T2	Tumor with *any* of the following features of size or extent: More than 3 cm in greatest dimension Involves main bronchus, 2 cm of more distal to the carina Invades the visceral pleura Associated with atelectasis or obstructive pneumonitis that extends to the hilar region but does not involve the entire lung
T3	Tumor of any size that directly invades any of the following: chest wall (including superior sulcus tumor), diaphragm, mediastinal pleura, parietal pericardium; or tumor in the main bronchus less than 2 cm distal to the carina but without involvement of the carina; or associated atelectasis or obstructive pneumonitis of the entire lung
T4	Tumor of any size that invades any of the following: mediastinum, heart, great vessels, trachea, esophagus, vertebral body, carina; separate tumor nodule(s) in the same lobe; or tumor with a malignant pleural effusion**

*The uncommon superficial tumor of any size with its invasive component limited to the bronchial wall, which may extend proximal to the main bronchus, is also classified T1.

**Most pleural effusions associated with lung cancer are due to tumor. However, there are a few patients in whom multiple cytopathologic examinations of pleural fluid are negative for tumor. In these cases, fluid is nonbloody and is not an exudate. When these elements and clinical judgement dictate that the effusion is not related to the tumor, the effusion should be excluded as a staging element and the patient should be staged T1, T2, or T3.

Regional Lymph Nodes (N)

NX	Regional lymph nodes cannot be assessed
N0	No regional lymph node metastasis
N1	Metastasis to ipsilateral peribronchial and/or ipsilateral hilar lymph nodes and intrapulmonary nodes involved by direct extension of the primary tumor
N2	Metastasis to ipsilateral mediastinal and/or subcarinal lymph node(s)
N3	Metastasis in contralateral mediastinal, contralateral hilar, ipsilateral or contralateral scalene or supraclavicular lymph node(s)
MX	Distant metastasis cannot be assessed
MO	No distant metastasis
M1	Distant metastasis present (includes synchronous separate nodule(s) in a different lobe)

Stage Grouping

Occult	TX	N0	M0
Stage 0	Tis	N0	M0
Stage IA	T1	N0	M0
Stage IB	T2	N0	M0
Stage IIA	T1	N1	M0
Stage IIB	T2	N1	M0
	T3	N0	M0
Stage IIIA	T3	N1	M0
	T1	N2	M0
	T2	N2	M0
	T3	N2	M0
Stage IIIB	Any T	N3	M0
	T4	Any N	M0
Stave IV	Any T	Any N	M1

Anatomical Staging for Lung Cancer, (IUCC-AJCC, 1997), Chest 111; 1710-17, Mountain CF that this group was potentially curable with surgery alone, and that the cure rate with surgery alone in this group far exceeded that of other stage III patients (12,13,14). In a controversial move, which many clinicians considered regressive, tumors with satellite nodules in the same lobe were upstaged from T_2 to T_3 or T_3 to T_4 (stage III-B); and synchronous lesions in a different ipsilateral lobe, were considered M_1. This bow to pathology, the recognition that multifocal intrathoracic disease is, in fact, metastatic defies clinical reality; many of these patients can benefit from resection.

Nevertheless, the 1997 revision represents the current state of the art. Studies initiated in the late 90s have based eligibility on this revision. For example, an intergroup trial evaluating the chemopreventive role of selenium specifically targets I-A and I-B disease, while other trials evaluating adjuvant chemotherapy target stage I-B and +/- stage II patients.]

ONGOING CONTROVERSIES

The 1997 staging revision is more complicated and more comprehensive than previous staging criteria. Despite this level of complexity, several compelling issues have been side-stepped.

Satellite Nodules and Other Orbits (Lobes)

In a footnote to the Fourth Edition of the AJCC Staging Manual published in 1993, satellite lesions in the same lobe upstaged the primary by one T category and the presence of the synchronous ipsilateral lesion in a separate lobe was considered T_4. Several investigators have questioned the latter designation, citing hematogenous and therefore metastatic spread to other lobes as a reason to consider such lesions M_1.

Deslauriers retrospectively evaluated 84 patients with primary lung tumors, accompanied by one or more satellite nodules, and over 1000 patients with primary lung tumor but no satellite nodules, all of whom had undergone resection between 1969 and 1986 (15). In the majority of patients, satellite nodules were observed in the same lobe as the primary (68/84). Survival, based on 1974 guidelines, was compared stage-for-stage between patients with satellite nodules and those without. The five-year survival rates respectively for those without satellite nodules and for those with satellite nodules were 54.4% vs. 32% for stage I; 40.4% vs. 12.5% for stage II, and 20.3% vs. 5.6% for stage III. Because so few patients had satellite nodules in different, ipsilateral lobe(s), further subset analysis was not conducted. The work of Deslauriers clearly showed that the presence of satellite nodules impaired prognosis, but it also demonstrated that satellite lesions, in and of themselves, did not automatically constitute a fatal prognosis.

Shimizu noted a two-year survival rate of 41.5% in patients with satellite lesions in the same lobe as the primary tumor, compared to 20% in patients in whom satellite nodules occurred in a different, ipsilateral lobe (16). Again, the presence of satellite nodules did not preclude long-term survival after surgery. In a series of 49 patients, Watanabe observed that the survival rate in patients with satellite lesions was similar to other stage III-A patients without satellite lesions and superior to stage III-B patients without satellite lesions (12). Survival following surgery, even for those with involvement in different, ipsilateral lobes, was clearly better than expected for M_1 disease. Nevertheless, synchronous lesions outside the primary tumor lobe, but in the same lung, by 1997 criteria are now considered M_1, a distinction based on putative biology, rather than clinical reality. Lesions in the same lobe are generally thought to represent tumor emboli, while those in different lobes are felt to represent hematogenous spread. Unfortunately the T_4 designation for satellite lesions in the same lobe denotes a prognosis poorer than established; likewise, available data would suggest that an M_1 designation for spread to a different ipsilateral lobe conveys a false impression. Many therefore contend that the staging system, at least in this regard, should return to the previous format.

Pleural Effusions

Malignant pleural effusions containing malignant cells and/or either bloody or exudative effusions were, by definition, in the 1986 criteria, considered malignant. It has been long recognized that pleural effusions are associated with poor prognosis (17). Including malignant pleural effusions in the T_4 category was based in part on data from Naruke (9): The five-year survival rate in 48 patients with malignant pleural involvement at surgery was 10.7%, similar to that of other operated patients with T_4 disease (8.4%), using the database from the 1986 staging system. Others have failed to demonstrate similar survival rates, and more recent data strongly suggest that the survival of patients with malignant pleural effusion more closely approximates that observed for other patients with stage IV disease. Sugiura and colleagues investigated the impact of pleural effusion in patients with advanced stage III or stage IV-B NSCLC (18). Median survival for patients with stage III-B disease with no pleural effusion was 15.3 months, compared to 7.5 months for patients with stage III-B disease and pleural effusion. Median survival for stage IV disease was not significantly different at 5.5 months. Moreover, there was no significant difference in survival between patients with cytologically positive and cytologically negative pleural effusions.

As treatment techniques become better defined, the vast majority of fit patients with stage III-B disease, exclusive of malignant pleural effusions, receive combined modality therapy, which is generally not appropriate in the face of diffuse pleural involvement.

To reflect the generally palliative nature of treatment for this category, many investigators feel strongly that malignant pleural effusions deserve a stage IV designation, even though they do not necessarily denote hematogenous spread. On the other hand, work at FCCC evaluating systemic therapy with carboplatin and paclitaxel has demonstrated superior survival for patients with malignant pleural effusion (77 wks) vs. those with metastatic disease (50 wks), with one and two-year survival rates 67% and 27% vs. 47% and 12%, respectively (19). For this category of patients, some investigators would favor a stage IV-A designation, to distinguish it from those with frank metastatic, extra-thoracic disease (stage IV-B).

Pleural Nodules in the Absence of Pleural Effusion

In the absence of pleural effusion, multifocal pleural nodules are considered T_4 based on the footnote to the 1986 staging classification, but the data are scarce. Akaogi assessed 23 patients with pleural involvement, but no distant metastases, all of whom underwent pleural pneumonectomy (20). Thirteen had small pleural nodules, and either no effusion or minimal effusion; ten of the thirteen had involvement of the parietal pleura. In six of ten, parietal involvement was considered extensive. By and large, those with pleural involvement, particularly those with N_2 spread, did poorly. Shimizu cited a 19.4% five-year survival rate in 38 patients with pleural dissemination, without pleural effusion, a rate generally better than expected for patients with pleural dissemination (21).

THE INFLUENCE OF BASIC PROGNOSTIC FACTORS, HISTOLOGY, AND TUMOR MARKERS: HOW ARE THEY WOVEN IN?

Histology: Should we lump or split

The three major histologic NSCLC subtypes, adenocarcinoma, squamous cell, large cell are grouped together under the same rubric. Yet, stage-for-stage, particularly in patients who undergo definitive curative treatment, patients with squamous cell carcinoma tend to do better than those with adenocarcinoma. In addition, squamous cell histology is the most likely of all pulmonary neoplasms to remain localized. In autopsy series, 15-30% of patients with squamous cell cancer expired from local disease, with absolutely no evidence of systemic spread (22). The recurrence rates per person per year in a study by Gail and colleagues was 0.105 in squamous cell histology, compared to 0.207 for non-squamous patients, suggesting a favorable impact of squamous histology on prognosis (23). Conversely, large cell tumors, though relatively rare (10-15% of all NSCLC), tend to be more aggressive, with generally higher propensity to metastasize to regional lymph nodes and distant sites and poorer survival (24). A separate histologic subgroup, large cell neuroendocrine carcinomas, do even worse; Dresler et al. has cited a median survival in resected patients of only 14 months (25).

To date, however, histology in the NSCLC category has not typically influenced treatment approaches. Until these are cogent evidence that NSCLC patients with identical stage, but different histology, benefit from alternative treatment approaches, histologic data will very likely not be included in the staging system.

The Influence of Weight Loss on Performance Status

Within given stages, particularly advanced stages, the most important prognostic factor remains performance status. The Karnofsky and ECOG/Zubrod scales define performance status readily, discriminating between patients who are ambulatory and asymptomatic, those who have symptoms, and those whose mobility and activity during the day are compromised (26, 27). Likewise, patients who have lost more than 5% of their baseline body weight during the 3-6 month period preceding diagnosis, consistently have a worse prognosis than those who have not lost significant amounts of weight. These distinctions are not trivial. Although they are not integrated into the current staging system, they do discriminate between treatment approaches, particularly in patients with locally advanced NSCLC, who may benefit from combined modality treatment.   To date, consistent benefit has not been demonstrated for this approach in patients who have poor prognostic criteria (> 5% weight loss or KPS <70). Aside from stage, performance status is the most important prognostic variable. Out of 15 studies, 14 demonstrated critical importance of performance status in determining prognosis. Other suggestive factors that have been less well evaluated, or whose impact is occasionally ambiguous, include gender, age, LDH, plasma albumin, and baseline hemoglobin (4,5; 28-44).

In stage IV disease, the role of various, readily identifiable, clinical prognostic factors have been explored in detail.   In several retrospective analyses of the Eastern Cooperative Oncology Group database, performance status and anorexia/weight loss are two of the most important factors (4,5,31).   Other important factors included the presence or absence of bone, liver, subcutaneous metastases and gender, with men generally doing more poorly than women (31). A landmark report by Stanley evaluating more than 70 prognostic factors in over 5000 patients with advanced NSCLC identified the critical importance of Karnofsky performance status, extent of disease and weight loss (43). Jiroutek and colleagues in an analysis of randomized phase III studies of the ECOG demonstrated the importance of performance status, age, and appetite (weight loss) in determining outcome (Table 3) (44). O'Connell et al in a much smaller study of 378 advanced patients receiving platinum based combination chemotherapy, also identified Karnofsky performance status, as well as the presence of bone metastases, elevated serum LDH, male gender, and two or more extra-thoracic metastatic sites as important adverse prognostic factors (42). Performance status, in and of itself, will generally indicate whether the use of aggressive systemic therapy in advanced disease is reasonable or futile.

Table 3. Recursive Partitioning Analysis Terminal Nodes

	Appetite Intact (No. of Patients)	Appetite Diminished (No. of Patients)
PS-0		
Female	12.58 (111)	8.54 (15)
Male	9.86 (219)	6.74 (50)
PS-1		
Female	7.77 (214)	6.95 (102)
Male	6.70 (421)	5.08 (224)
PS-2		
Female	5.31 (24)	2.30 (27)
Male	4.30 (64)	3.43 (100)

… Jiroutek, et al.

Serum and Tumor Markers

Readily measurable chemistries can be highly predictive. Multiple studies have shown a strong association between elevated serum lactate dehydrogenate level, metastatic spread, either occult or clinical, and poor prognosis. Similarly, elevations of white counts have been associated with reduced prognosis. Tumor markers, including CEA, may also be predictive (48).

Histopathologic Findings

Tumor necrosis appears to be an adverse predictor of survival. Ellson and colleagues showed a statistically significant association between extent of tumor necrosis on survival in 47 surgically resected patients (45). Shahab objectively evaluated the extent of tumor necrosis by computer assisted morphometry in 28 patients, and corroborated Ellson's findings (46). The increased deposition of basement membrane by tumor cells has also been suggested to represent a sign of improved prognosis, independent of tumor stage. Ten Velde and colleagues used polyclonal antibodies against type II human collagen in 68 patients with squamous cell malignancy to assess basement membrane substance (47). 27 of 62 patients had extensive basement membrane depositions and significantly improved prognosis compared to those without heightened base membrane deposition. Other negative prognostic determinants (49-57) have included lack of tumor differentiation, lymphatic vessel invasion in node (-) disease, blood vessel permeation, increased mitotic index, loss or alteration of blood group antigens and other tumor associated carbohydrate antigens (e.g., H/LE) (Y) (LE) (B), sialyl Lewis (X) and sialyl Lewis (a)). Studies evaluating flow cytometric analysis of DNA content and ploidy have yielded conflicting results: some studies have demonstrated that patients with diploid tumors do better than those with aneuploid tumors; other studies have shown no difference (58-62).

Molecular Genetics

The field of molecular genetics and its potential role in predicting prognosis is just emerging. Mutations in K^{ras} have repeatedly demonstrated an adverse effect on survival, particularly in adenocarcinoma and in other cell types (63-71). Overexpression of the erb/B2 protein has also been associated with shorter survival, though these findings are largely limited to resected adenocarcinoma (72-77). In addition, in one study, the combination of K^{ras} mutations and erb/B2 overexpression have had an additive negative impact on survival (76). Alterations in p53 gene have been associated with conflicting results. Several studies have demonstrated decreased survival in patients with p53 overexpression; however, three studies failed to demonstrate a difference in survival between those with p53+ and p53- tumors; and two studies demonstrated that p53 expression had a positive impact (78-83). Other studies have proven inconclusive (84-89).

Inappropriately high levels of chromosomal telomerase have been associated with long repeat DNA sequences, and may contribute to the lack of growth control exhibited by cancer cells (90). There is emerging evidence that this phenomenon in lung cancer is associated with worse prognosis, although confirmatory studies are needed. Loss of p21 is also associated with poor prognosis in two separate studies of NSCLC by immunohistochemical staining (91).

Two recent large molecular-clinical correlative studies of NSCLC have enhanced our understanding of prognosis in NSCLC, and its relationship to molecular biology. In one study of 180 patients undergoing definitive surgery, p53 expression, K^{ras} exon 12 mutations, and loss of p21 H-^{ras} expression were associated with poorer prognosis (92). In addition, patients with lymphatic invasion, tumor size >4 cm, and solid tumor with mucin expression did poorly. The five-year cancer-free survival rate of resected patients with two or fewer factors was 87%, but only 21% in those with four or more adverse factors. In the same study, Bcl-2 overexpression predicted an improved five-year cancer free survival rate in patients who underwent lobectomy or pneumonectomy, a somewhat unexpected result. A second study by Kim and colleagues evaluated the separate and combined value of Ras, HER-2/neu, p53 and Bcl-2 expression as determined by IHC staining in 238 Korean NSCLC patients (93). Univariate analysis demonstrated that Bcl-2 overexpression was associated with significantly poorer prognosis, as were the combinations of; Bcl-2, HER-2/neu, p53, and Bcl-2/Her-2/neu; p53 and K^{ras}, with rising hazard ratios for each grouping. By multivariate analysis, only the combination of Bcl-2 and HER-2/neu were independent markers of poor survival (p=0.003).

STAGING WORKUP

Staging workup includes history and physical exam, chest film, blood counts, chemistry panel, and, in most instances, chest and upper abdominal CT scan imaging. Further workup, including bone scan, brain CT or MRI, depend on clinical circumstances. Invasive staging procedures are generally directed toward those patients being considered for surgical resection.

History and Physical Exam

Early stage lung cancers are generally asymptomatic, whereas symptoms of local or systemic involvement frequently herald locally advanced stage III or stage IV disease. Changes in cough, hemoptysis, and history of repeated respiratory infections are often associated with local disease involving the airway. Similarly, dyspnea, wheezing and hemoptysis may be due to intrinsic airway obstruction. Progressive dyspnea may also be due to increasing pleural effusion. Symptoms of pneumonia may herald partial or complete bronchial obstruction. Chest pain is often due to invasion of the chest wall or extensive mediastinal involvement. Shoulder and arm pain may be due to infiltration by apical tumor into the brachial plexus, with secondary radiculopathy. These tumors are often difficult to see on routine CXR. The relatively rare triad of ptosis, meiosis, and ipsilateral anhidrosis, also known as Horner's syndrome, is typically due to apical tumors invading sympathetic nerve root ganglia. Hoarseness may be due to recurrent laryngeal nerve compression by nodal involvement or local invasion of a left sided T3 or T4 tumor. In addition, symptoms consistent with local regional spread, including chest pain, neck or facial fullness, or facial nerve paresis or pleurisy usually signal unresectable disease. Patients should also be queried about the presence of palpable lesions, bone pain, headache, change in vision, or other neurologic complaints. Establishment of baseline weight and recent weight loss is absolutely essential.

Physical exam should focus on signs of airway obstruction, including consolidation, and/or wheezing; pleural effusions (dullness to percussion); chest wall involvement (palpable bony deformity), and evidence of supraclavicular spread. Not only does supraclavicular nodal involvement instantly upstage tumor to N_3 (IIIB), these nodes are readily accessible, and can frequently establish diagnosis by fine needle aspiration (FNA), avoiding more invasive and more costly procedures. Finally, enlargement of the liver, though rare on initial evaluation, frequently heralds hepatic metastases. Newly diagnosed patients should be screened for signs of cardiac tamponade. In addition, evidence of paraneoplastic syndromes is often evinced on physical exam. New onset clubbing may herald pulmonary malignancy. Local swelling or pain over the distal tibia and ankle region may indicate hypertrophic pulmonary osteoarthropathy.

Laboratory Workup

CBC, differential, and platelet count, and full chemistry screen, including alkaline phosphatase, lactic dehydrogenase, and calcium are important. Abnormalities in these findings often predict metastatic disease, and are associated with poor prognosis. In addition, they are readily available on routine chemistry screening, and will often direct further investigation for suspected metastases. Tumor markers, including CEA, have not yet been included as part of the standard initial workup, though once diagnosis is established, they may enhance our ability to gauge treatment response, particularly in the absence of readily measurable tumor.

Imaging Studies

Routine chest films (AP and lateral), by themselves, can help elucidate stage. Bulky mediastinal adenopathy generally indicates N_2 or N_3 disease at the outset. Local invasion into the chest wall structures like the ribs similarly indicates T_3 disease. Visible effusions on chest film are usually indicative of T_4 disease. The presence of synchronous pulmonary nodules are often detected by this technique. However, chest films alone are suboptimal, particularly in the assessment of patients being considered for resection.

Virtually all newly diagnosed NSCLC patients in North America who are not automatically consigned to hospice undergo computerized tomographic (CT) scans. Ideally, chest CTs are carried through the level of the liver and adrenals to accommodate the inferior dip in pleural sulci posteriorly. Chest CTs should include 2-5 mm cuts through the suspicious lesion, especially if it is smaller than 3 cm in diameter. This method best gauges size, extent, and local invasion. CT imaging with intravenous contrast often helps to evaluate more central lesions, defining potential vascular invasion, and delineating nodal tissue from vascular structures. In addition, CT imaging can help differentiate atelectasis and adjacent consolidation from the primary tumor process. It may also delineate satellite lesions or intrathoracic metastases (94). Short of mediastinoscopy or resection, CT scans are the best approach to elucidate clinical TNM stage.

Multiple controversies exist. The mere presence of nodes on CT scan does not necessarily indicate pathologic involvement. Nodes less than 1 cm in greatest diameter unless clustered or coalescent are, more often than not, pathologically benign, with metastatic involvement found in less than 10% of cases (95). Those between 1-2 cm in greatest diameter are pathologically involved 30% of the time, while pathologic involvement is found in 60% of those nodes greater than 2 cm (96, 98). Moreover, benign etiologies for mediastinal nodal enlargement are not uncommon in patients with post obstructive infection (97-99). Mediastinoscopy remains the definitive diagnostic procedure regarding nodal involvement (100-102). Overall, CT scans are roughly 80% sensitive in identifying pathologic mediastinal adenopathy. Their specificity is generally lower, approximately 65%, compared to surgical staging. The predictive index improves to 85% or higher when nodes are larger than 1.5 cm in size. Others have discovered a higher percentage of false positive CT results. Gallardo et al. in a series of 167 patients noted pathologic involvement in only 23% of those whose nodes were enlarged on CT scan (99). Such high false positive rates mandate the use of surgical staging or other procedures to definitively define nodal involvement (96, 103-105).

CT imaging of the liver can help delineate benign cyst-like structures from less well defined metastatic sites. MRI may help to elucidate equivocal lesions. CT scan also remains the most sensitive method of detecting adrenal metastases (106-108). Most of these are asymptomatic, and discovered incidentally during CT evaluation of the chest. In autopsy series, 40% or more of NSCLC patients had adrenal involvement (109). Enlarged lesions on CT scan should be evaluated either by MRI or by fine needle aspirate under CT guidance (110-112).

The routine use of bone scan and/or either CT scan or MRI imaging of the brain in the absence of symptoms or signs is not generally advocated outside a protocol setting. Nevertheless, asymptomatic bone and/or brain metastases are reported in up to 10-15% of patients undergoing noninvasive clinical staging (113-118). While these numbers are not high overall, it is not unreasonable to include these imaging approaches in otherwise asymptomatic patients to avoid the morbidity of unnecessary surgical resection.

Bronchoscopy and Mediastinoscopy

In any patient diagnosed with pulmonary malignancy, bronchoscopy is absolutely essential. Flexible fiberoptic instruments are safe, allow fairly rapid, relatively meticulous inspection of the proximal tracheal bronchial tree up to the second and third subsegmental divisions, and readily assess the intraluminal extent of proximal lesions; they also rule out the potential presence of synchronous lesions. The diagnostic yield for visible lesions is greater than 85-90% (119). In addition, in undiagnosed patients, post bronchoscopy sputum cytology as opposed to induction cytology, has far greater yield (120). Bronchoscopy is crucial in the assessment of proximal lesions; it is superior to CT scans in determining local extent, including proximity to carina, and carinal involvement.

In assessing the mediastinum, mediastinoscopy or mediastinotomy remains the standard of comparison. Mediastinoscopy is 89% sensitive and nearly 100% specific in nodal staging of NSCLC patients (101,121). Investigators have contrasted this to CT scan, where sensitivity and specificity are 63% and 57%, respectively (122,123). Patients with peripheral T_1 lesions, and no visible nodal enlargement on CT scan can probably forego mediastinoscopy, as long as nodal sampling or dissection is performed at the time of thoracotomy. Virtually all other patients require mediastinoscopy. In a series of 681 patients of whom over 500 had normal size mediastinal nodes, only 37 (7.4%) were found to have positive nodes at mediastinoscopy or thoracotomy (121,122). Regardless, the majority underwent definitive resection, and in this group, five-year survival rates were 31%. Under these circumstances, if full mediastinal node dissection is planned, and nodes appear normal size on CT scan, mediastinoscopy *may be* bypassed. The same recommendations do not hold for central tumors or for those with visible nodal enlargement on CT scan or chest film.

Finally, mediastinoscopy is crucial in delineating N_2 disease, for which induction therapy followed by surgery may be reasonable, from N_3 disease, in which a combined modality non-surgical approach is most likely preferable. For those patients with left upper lobe tumors, extended mediastinoscopy or anterior mediastinotomy (Chamberlain procedure) are the preferred diagnostic approaches (124,125). This affords evaluation of level V and level VI mediastinal nodes, not readily assessable by conventional mediastinoscopy.

Endoscopic Ultrasound (EUS)

Several centers have begun to evaluate EUS in improving staging accuracy. EUS enables investigators to assess nodes based on thickness, contour, and internal architecture, rather than size alone. Kondo and colleagues evaluated EUS in 101 Japanese patients with lung cancer: sensitivity was 73.6%; specificity 97.5% (126). In addition, EUS affords accessibility for FNA of abnormal nodes or those nodes inaccessible to conventional mediastinoscopy (127). The main drawback of EUS is that it can only be used to evaluate nodes adjacent to the esophagus. As such, it complements, but does not replace, chest CT and mediastinoscopy.

Positron Emission Tomography (PET) (128-148)

Far more popular, in may quarters, is the routine use of PET imaging as part of the metastatic workup. Although multiple studies have extolled its potential virtues, this technology remains investigational. PET scan imaging relies on enhanced glucose uptake by malignant tissue, compared to adjacent normal or non-malignant tissue. When PET scans are done in conjunction with CT imaging, computerized technology permits three-dimensional reconstruction of images, honing in on "hot" areas in which uptake of 18-fluoro-deoxyglucose (FDG) is increased. One study documented a 94% sensitivity and 80% specificity in the diagnosis of lung nodules. In another group of 76 patients studied prospectively with both PET imaging and CT scans (131), sensitivity was 83%, and specificity 94% in the diagnosis of N_2 nodal involvement. In addition, PET scans demonstrated unsuspected distant metastases in 11% of patients (131).

Ultimately, PET imaging has much stronger negative, compared to positive, predictive value, because non-malignant, metabolically active, processes may also yield increased FDG uptake. Anecdotally, false (+) results have been observed in patients with granulomatous disease or other benign inflammatory lesions. Conversely, smaller parenchymal lesions (< 10 mm) or those that are better differentiated, may prove falsely (-). Sazon and colleagues reported 100% sensitivity and 52% specificity in predicting malignant nature of radiographic abnormalities (129). Others have observed less impressive findings, but a general sensitivity rate on the order of 90% has been observed consistently in multiple studies (138-140). PET has proven superior to CT scan in both sensitivity and specificity of mediastinal node stage, 93% and 97%, respectively (141).

Its ultimate utility in defining stage and potentially replacing other imaging modalities remains to be determined. Ideally, PET imaging should be used in conjunction with CT imaging. Fusion images of CT and FDG PET may prove superior to either modality alone and can yield precise anatomic correlation (142). In a controversial move, the United States Healthcare Financing Administration (HCFA) has authorized Medicare to pay for PET scans in the routine staging of patients with NSCLC (128,130).

Semi-quantitative measurements of FDG uptake on PET scan may have prognostic importance (134,135). PET scans may also have a role in guiding management and follow-up. PET scan imaging may help delineate whether viable tumor remains after induction chemotherapy or chemoradiation. Multiple investigators are assessing whether PET scan imaging can be used, in lieu of mediastinoscopy, to guide management of patients who have received induction therapy (132-135). Others are investigating the use of this technique to detect recurrence (143-147).

Intraoperative Staging (Figure 1) (149-154)

Intraoperative staging at this time remains the ultimate gold standard for determining the presence of a nodal metastasis. During right-sided thoracotomy, at the very least, levels IV, VII and X nodes should be sampled, if not dissected; at the time of left thoracotomy, levels V and/or VI as well as VII are accessible and should be removed. Visual inspection alone or manual palpation is insufficient. Unfortunately, node sampling and/or dissection is rarely performed in the community outside an academic center. Such patients are inadequately staged. In such circumstances, when conclusive pathologic material is unavailable, treatment recommendations are difficult, if not impossible, to make. Proper mediastinal node dissection is associated with minimal morbidity, and ultimately increases the length of operative procedure only marginally.

STAGE DIRECTED GUIDELINES: DOES TREATMENT INFLUENCE OUTCOME

Stage I

Pathologically proven stage I lesions remain in the province of surgery. Five-year survival rates are 65 to 75% (155) Preoperative or postoperative radiation has yet to change prognosis. The recent Port analysis suggested a decrement in survival in stage I patients who underwent postoperative radiation (156). Adjuvant cytotoxic studies examining single agents or a combination chemotherapy have been consistently negative with two prominent exceptions: a Finnish study (157) which demonstrated the superiority of CAP chemotherapy to observation with improvement in five-year survival from 48 to 60%; and a Japanese study (158) evaluating the utility of UFT, an oral fluoro-pyridimine, either alone or in combination with cisplatin and vindesine vs. observation, in which virtually identical survival data were observed for both groups of patients receiving UFT. Wedge resections or segmental resections have proven inferior to anatomic lobe resections, i.e., lobectomy (159). Patients who undergo limited surgery, in the absence of compelling physiologic reasons (160), have higher local recurrence rates, higher incidence of CNS metastasis, and poorer survival. Ongoing intergroup trials are evaluating the role of newer chemotherapy regimens such as paclitaxel-carboplatin and vinorelbine-cisplatin in the adjuvant setting in patients with IB disease.

Stage II NSCLC

Patients with N_1 (peribronchial or hilar node) involvement, have a substantially reduced prognosis compared to patients with stage I disease; five-year survival rates are in the range of 30 to 40% at best. Hilar node involvement signals increased risk of occult systemic spread (161-165). Surgery, as in stage I disease, remains the cornerstone of treatment. Postoperative radiation, particularly in squamous cell malignancy, has reduced the risk of local relapse, but has not affected long-term survival (166). Adjuvant cytotoxics (e.g., CAP) have prolonged disease-free survival and median survival, but, with the exception of the UFT trial, have not improved long-term survival (167,168). A recent study conducted by ECOG/RTOG comparing postoperative radiation alone to concurrent chemoradiotherapy with etoposide and cisplatin demonstrated absolutely no difference in median survival, two-year survival, and three-year survival rates, though it should be noted that both groups, in whom proper surgical staging was performed, enjoyed substantially better survival compared to historic controls (169).

For those with chest wall disease (T_3N_{0-1}), in the absence of obvious mediastinal node involvement, surgical resection remains the cornerstone of treatment (170,171). There is no evidence that adjuvant therapy of any sort, in this situation, yields additional benefit.

Stage IIIA NSCLC

Ultimately, from a practical standpoint, stage IIIA NSCLC, an innately heterogeneous grouping, is divided into three subcategories : incidental N_2 involvement appreciated only at the time of mediastinal node dissection, after (-) preoperative assessment; non-bulky, potentially resectable, N_2 (mediastinal) involvement with nodes appreciated only on CT scan, but not on chest x-ray or at bronchoscopy; or single station nodes on mediastinoscopy; bulky N_2 disease with paratracheal nodes clearly visible on chest film, or splaying of the carina at bronchoscopy, indicating fairly bulky disease, not readily amenable to resection.

Heretofore, conventional adjuvant therapy has failed to improve outcome. However, two randomized controlled phase III trials evaluating the role of induction chemotherapy followed by surgery, compared to surgery alone, have proven positive. One study from Spain (172) , employing a mitomycin-ifosfamide-cisplatin regimen, demonstrated a marked improvement in median and two-year survival rates, though it should be noted the surgery only group did more poorly than historic controls. Another study from the United States using an etoposide-cisplatin based chemotherapy regimen demonstrated similar results (173), with three-year survival rates in the combined modality arm exceeding 50%. Finally, a much larger study from France (174) evaluating induction therapy with mitomycin, ifosfamide, and cisplatin followed by surgery vs. surgery alone in stage IIIA patients (as well as earlier stage patients) demonstrated a compelling trend toward improved median survival (36 vs. 26 months), and three-year survival rate (52% vs. 41%, p=0.09). Taken together, these studies strongly suggest a benefit for neoadjuvant or induction chemotherapy, and also indicate that induction therapy may ultimately perturb the natural history of locally advanced, resectable NSCLC.

For patients with bulky IIIA disease, who are not candidates for resection, but who have experienced minimal weight loss and have intact functional status, eight separate randomized controlled phase III trials have demonstrated the superiority of chemo/radiation to radiation alone (175-184). Four trials have shown superiority of induction chemotherapy followed by radiation vs. radiation alone (175-180). Each of these used cisplatin-based regimens. Three other trials, one using cisplatin and two employing carboplatin-based therapy, have demonstrated a radiosensitizing effect for systemic agents given concurrently with radiation, with improved local control and ultimately improved long-term survival (181-184). Finally, a Japanese study demonstrated the superiority of concurrent high dose chemo-radiation to sequential chemotherapy followed by RT (184). Survival rates in some of these efforts at 4-5 years have exceeded 20%, as opposed to 5-7% in the control groups (182,183).

In addition, altered radiation fractionation schedules, in particular CHART (continuous hyperfractionated accelerated radiation) to a total dose of 54 Gy over 12 consecutive days has proven superior to standard RT (60 Gy over six weeks), with nearly 50% improvement in two-year survival rates (185,186).

Preoperative chemotherapy either alone or combined with radiation can render 40 to 70% of bulky N_2 patients resectable, with pathologic complete remissions observed in 10-25% and three to five-year survival rates ranging from 15-25% (187-191). Unfortunately, this approach has not yet been successfully tested in a randomized phase III setting. An ongoing intergroup study assessing definitive chemoradiation vs. chemoradiation followed by surgery will determine whether tri-modality therapy is, in fact, superior to bi-modality therapy, or whether surgery merely selects out those patients destined to do well, while exacerbating morbidity.

Stage IIIB NSCLC

With the exception of patients who have malignant pleural or pericardial effusions, IIIB patients are treated similarly to those with bulky IIIA disease. For those receiving RT alone, survival rates at five years are generally less than 5%. On the other hand, chemoradiation in fit patients has yielded benefits similar to those observed in unresectable IIIA patients (192).

Stage IV NSCLC

Median survival for best supportive care alone is poor, 3 to 6 months at best, and is substantially worse in those with impaired performance status; declining appetite or weight; or metastasis to bone, brain, liver, or subcutaneous tissue (4,5,31). In addition, gender makes a difference: men do more poorly than women. In specific studies (36,193) and in a large meta-analysis, the advent of cisplatin-based therapies has yielded a three-four month improvement in median survival, and 10% improvement in one-year survival rates from 10-15% to 20-25% (194). However, improvements in response rate to systemic therapy do not necessarily translate into improved survival (195,196); and higher doses of cisplatin have yielded more toxicity, but no survival advantage (197-199). In the era of modern chemotherapy, three separate trials employing gemcitabine, vinorelbine, and tirapazamine in combination with cisplatin, have proven superior to cisplatin alone, not merely in response rate, but in time to progression and survival (200-202). Only two regimens (vinorelbine-cisplatin and paclitaxel-cisplatin) have proven superior to older cisplatin combinations (203,204). Recently completed trials have also demonstrated the therapeutic equivalence of single agent, relatively non-toxic, monotherapy (gemcitabine) to cisplatin-etoposide and single agent vinorelbine to cisplatin-vindesine (205,206). In the elderly (greater than 70 years of age, performance status 0-2), vinorelbine monotherapy has improved six-month and one-year survival rates substantially, compared to best supportive care (207). The 50% one-year survival bar, however, has not been consistently hurdled; and it seems unlikely that novel permutations and combinations of new agents will provide substantial additional benefit.

SMALL CELL CARCINOMA OF THE LUNG

Basic Staging

In small cell carcinoma, the AJCC staging criteria, though often imposed by tumor registries, are irrelevant. From a practical standpoint, small cell carcinoma is divided simply and cleanly into limited and extensive categories. By definition, limited disease is confined to a single radiation portal, and in the era of modern treatment, concurrent chemoradiation offers a real chance of cure (208-212). Extensive disease, on the other hand, denotes involvement beyond a single radiation portal and, by definition, is incurable. There are, however, patients with extensive disease confined to a single, often otherwise asymptomatic site, whose prognosis is intermediate between that typically observed for limited and extensive disease (212-214).

Hence, the major thrust of staging is to rule out the presence of disease beyond a single radiation portal. Once that presence is established, further exhaustive workup to document other sites of metastases, outside of a protocol setting, is probably unnecessary. By and large, micro-dissemination is present even in SCLC patients ultimately thought to be cured of their original tumor. In one series of patients who had undergone surgical resection and had died of other causes, 69% had persistent tumor and in the vast majority (63%), tumor had spread beyond the chest (215). This rate is far higher than that observed in similar series of squamous cell carcinoma, adenocarcinoma, and large cell carcinoma.

With the rare exception of clinical stage I or II patients, who may potentially benefit from surgical resection (216-219), the vast majority of those diagnosed with limited SCLC have evidence of hilar or mediastinal node involvement. By convention, the presence of supraclavicular nodal involvement and/or ipsilateral pleural effusion indicates disease beyond an easily managed radiation portal.

Presentation

By and large, patients with small cell carcinoma of the lung have very short interval from initial onset of symptoms to diagnosis. Signs and symptoms correlate with the size and location of the primary tumor, and the presence or absence of regional and distant metastases. Almost invariably, patients present with cough and some combination of the following symptoms: dyspnea, wheezing, hemoptysis, and/or chest pain. On plain chest x-ray, disease is rarely peripheral. For the most part, patients have evidence of central involvement, with clearly evident widening of the mediastinum, and frequent evidence of atelectasis and post obstructive pneumonitis. Pleural effusions are common; cavitation is not. In addition, a significant percentage of patients will present with superior vena cava syndrome at diagnosis; a relatively smaller percentage have symptoms due to paraneoplastic syndromes, including SIADH or Eaton-Lambert syndrome.

Diagnostic Workup

In general, diagnosis is readily secured by either sputum cytology, fiberoptic bronchoscopy (FOB), or fine needle aspirate. FOB, will confirm cancer in more than 90% of patients, including 8-10% of those whose tumors are not readily apparent on chest film; it will also help define the extent of disease (220). CT of the thorax is superior to chest film alone in defining the extent of parenchymal, mediastinal, and pleural involvement. The routine use of chest MRI adds little.

Basic Staging Evaluation

At a minimum, patients with limited small cell carcinoma require a thorough history and physical; pathologic review to exclude non-small cell histology; chest film; routine blood work including CBC, differential, platelets, electrolytes and LFTs (including LDH and alkaline phosphatase). In addition, the basic workup includes a CT of the chest, with full cuts of the liver and adrenal, and brain scan, either CT or MRI. Most practitioners will also obtain bone scan. These studies will almost always delineate limited from extensive disease and are appropriate in patients destined to receive aggressive therapy, i.e., performance status 0-2 patients with adequate physiologic indices, including reasonable cardiopulmonary, renal, and hepatic function. Further workup beyond this initial evaluation, outside of protocol setting, is usually unnecessary, though many practitioners will still obtain unilateral or bilateral bone marrow biopsies and aspirates in patients who otherwise have limited disease, especially if there are derangements in LDH (221).

Basic staging will confirm limited disease in 30-40% of patients, and extensive disease in 60-70% (209,212,222). The most common sites of extra-thoracic involvement are listed in Table III (212,222,229):

	Clinical	Autopsy (223,224)
Bone	20-40%	38%
Liver	15-35%	62%
Bone Marrow	15-25%	N/A
Brain	0-20%	31%
Lymph Nodes	7-25%	57%
Soft Tissue	2-11%	N/A

Bone scans are generally reliable, clearly more sensitive than conventional radiographs, but prone to false positive interpretations. Hence, bone scans by themselves, should not be the sole determinate for making life and death therapeutic decisions. Abnormalities that are not clearly degenerative in etiology warrant further evaluation: either conventional x-rays and/or MRI.

Bilateral bone marrow biopsies will detect disease in up to 25% of patients, but fewer than 5% of patients will have bone marrow involvement as the only site of extensive disease (225-228). Not all patients with positive bone marrow have abnormalities on bone scan.

Liver involvement is generally heralded by LFT abnormalities. CT scans of the liver, generally included in the initial diagnostic workup, are usually sufficient to detect or exclude hepatic involvement and will reveal involvement in over one-third of patients (230). CT guided FNAs will usually confirm involvement if there are no other sites of metastases, but very rarely reveal metastatic dissemination not readily identifiable by other means.

Brain metastases are extraordinarily common, occurring in at least 30% of patients, either at diagnosis or during treatment course. Nuclear brain scans are outmoded; CT scans of the brain, at the very least, are usually recommended as part of staging. In the absence of symptoms, CT scan will reveal involvement of 5-10% of patients (231-235). Magnetic resonance imaging studies are relatively more sensitive, and will frequently resolve diagnostic dilemmas raised on CT scan. To date, though not well studied, there is no evidence that detection of brain metastases in patients without symptoms alters survival, compared to patients whose metastases are indicated by neurologic symptoms or signs. Median survival in patients with brain metastasis-only disease are similar to those with limited disease, but long-term survival is rare (214).

To date, there is no indication for PET scan imaging. Radiolabelled octreotide, based on its detection of neuroendocrine tumors, is undergoing active investigation as a staging tool. Similarly, tumor markers have added little to routine radiographic screening and follow-up. Murine specific amylase, creatine kinase-BB, neuron-specific enolase, and CEA all correlate with tumor burden, but their routine use outside of a research setting is not advocated (236-242). Routine laboratory tests, including LDH and alkaline phosphatase are more useful (251). Elevations of either strongly suggest that additional workup to exclude metastatic disease is warranted.

Recent studies have suggested that metalloproteinase levels correlate with survival. MMPs and their tissue inhibitors (TIMPs) are widely expressed in SCLC (243,244). Increased tumoral expression of MMP-3, 11, and 14 are independent negative prognostic factors.

Histology as Predictor of Prognosis

Conflicting data exist regarding the influence of histology. There is no apparent difference between classical and intermediate small cell subtype. However, mixed small cell/large cell variant, which occurs in 4% or more of patients, in some series has been associated with decreased response to combination chemotherapy and inferior survival (245). Other series have not observed similar decrements in survival (246). In addition, in one autopsy series, 13% of small cell patients with non-small cell components at autopsy, had significantly shorter survival compared to patients with pure SCLC (247). Heightened microvascular density has also correlated with decreased survival.

Basic Prognostic Breakdown

How well or poorly patients do can be predicted readily by initial evaluation (248-252).

Tumor factors

stage of disease (limited vs. extensive);
single organ vs. multi-organ extensive involvement;
absence or presence of hepatic or CNS involvement;
elevations in LDH +/- alkaline phosphatase c/w increased tumor burden;
low sodium c/w SAIDH, correlated with poor outcome.

Host Factors

Performance Status (0-1 vs. 2 or worse)
Gender (women have more favorable prognosis)
Weight loss
Age: (younger patients tolerate treatment better and consequently have better prognosis).

STAGE DIRECTED TREATMENT GUIDELINES IN SCLC: DOES TREATMENT INFLUENCE OUTCOME?

In the era of modern chemotherapy, the prognosis for small cell carcinoma of the lung has improved 5 to 6-fold (253,254). Well staged patients with limited disease, who previously lived 3-4 months on average, have consistent median survivals in the 18-24 month range; and five-year survival rates, generally tantamount to cure, now approach 15-25% (255-259). Extensive disease patients who, without treatment, lived 6-8 weeks at best, now have median survivals of 7-11 months, and two-year survival rates of 5 to 10%. Over the past 20 years, however, the improvement in median survival has been quite modest, roughly two months (260).

Limited Disease

A landmark meta-analysis by Pignon and colleagues confirmed the importance of combined modality therapy vs. chemotherapy alone. Chemotherapy and radiation together resulted in an absolute 5% improvement in survival at two years (261). These results, however, were not demonstrated in the elderly (> 70 yrs), and have therefore been interpreted by many investigators, particularly those in Europe, as evidence that the elderly do not benefit from aggressive combined modality treatment.

The timing of chemotherapy and radiation has also altered prognosis. The Japanese have demonstrated a significant improvement in survival for concurrent upfront chemoradiation compared to sequential chemotherapy followed by radiation (262). In a similar vein, the NCI-Canada demonstrated superior survival at five years (20% vs. 10%) for early concurrent chemoradiation compared to delayed concurrent chemoradiation (263). Finally, an intergroup study mounted by the Eastern Cooperative Oncology Group and the Radiation Therapy Oncology Group demonstrated the best survival data to-date in this disease: hyperfractionated (bid) radiation, given concurrently with chemotherapy, yielded a five-year survival rate of 26%, compared to 16% for single daily fractionated RT and concurrent chemotherapy (258). This approach in reasonably good performance status patients represents state-of-the-art therapy and remains the "standard of comparison."

A recent meta-analysis also puts into perspective the potential role of PCI: an absolute improvement of 5% in three-year survival rates was observed in patients receiving PCI, in the presence of either CR or good PR, and in the absence of extensive disease (264). This "advantage" was virtually identical to the advantage for chemoradiation, compared to radiation alone, identified by Pignon and his collaborators. The appropriate dose and timing of PCI remains an open question (265-267).

The best prognoses with long-term survival rates of 30-40% are observed in the rare patients with limited stage I or stage II small cell carcinoma of the lung, in whom surgical resection is feasible (268). By and large, these results are observed only when chemotherapy +/- radiation are given as part of the basic treatment.

Long-term survivors have almost invariably been treated with chemoradiation, and in those patients who reach a 30 month survival, three independent factors (269) have predicted survival beyond five years: age ≤ 60 at time of diagnosis; the use of radiotherapy; absence of relapse.

In addition, at 30 months, the risk of second primary tumors due to tobacco exposure exceeds the risk of small cell relapse; and this risk closely correlates with patients smoking status at the time of diagnosis (270,271). Those who continue to smoke through treatment have a 60-fold increase in second primary tumors, compared to the general population. Those who stop at diagnosis have a 20-fold increase, and those who previously quit have a 10-fold increase risk (272-274). In this light, smoking status, in and of itself, has a potential impact on prognosis.

Extensive Disease

Unlike limited small cell; we have made little headway in the past 20 years in the treatment of extensive disease (262,264,270,283). Earlier studies using alkylator based treatments, either single agent or combination, yielded consistent response rates of 30% or greater, and median survival of 5-7 months (275). More modern combination chemotherapy reliably produces response rates in the 50-60% range, and median survival time of 7-11 months (252,254). A recent analysis by Chute and colleagues of twenty years of phase III trials for patients with extensive disease is rather disturbing (252,260). Improvement in median survival time has been modest at best, from seven months between 1972 and 1981 to nine months between 1982 and 1990. An analysis of the Seer database of patients with extensive stage SCLC over the same time course reveals a virtually identical two month prolongation in median survival time. Countless studies, evaluating the role of maintenance treatment, alternating non-cross resisting chemotherapy and dose intensification, have proven disappointing (275-291). Unfortunately, the fundamental assumption that a systemic disorder like SCLC will respond better to more aggressive systemic therapy has been flawed.

The modest increase in survival time, such as it exists, has been attributed to at least three factors: transition to etoposide/cisplatin chemotherapy, the standard treatment since the mid-1980's; improved supportive care over the past two decades; stage migration.

Current studies are evaluating the role of non-cross resistant consolidation, both cytotoxic and biologic. The Eastern Cooperative Oncology Group recently completed a trial assessing whether topotecan, as consolidation, could improve outcome in patients who had previously responded to or stabilized on etoposide/cisplatin. A number of ongoing studies, capitalizing on the observation that elevated metalloproteinase levels correlate with poor prognosis, are assessing the role of metalloproteinase inhibitors in extensive disease. Can these agents prolong time to progression and thereby enhance median and long-term survival? To-date, in extensive SCLC, the twelve month median survival barrier has seldom, if ever, been penetrated by conventional cytotoxics; most modern regimens fall short. In this era of new biologic inhibitors of signal transduction, farnesyl transferase, angiogenesis, etc., it remains to be seen if this barrier in extensive stage SCLC will ever prove surmountable.

REFERENCES

1. Denoix PF. Enquete permanent dans les centres anticancereux. Bull Inst Nat Hyg 1: 70-75, 1946.
2. Wingo PA, Tong T, Bolden S. Cancer statistics. CA Cancer J Clin 45: 8-30, 1995.
3. Martini N. Operable lung cancer. CA Cancer J Clin 43: 210-214, 1993.
4. Albain KS, Crowley JJ, LeBlanc M, Livingston RB. Survival determinants in extensive-stage non-small cell lung cancer: the Southwest Oncology Group experience. J Clin Oncol 9: 1618-1626, 1991.

5. Paesmans M, Sculier JP, Libert P, et al. Prognostic factors for survival in advanced non-small cell lung cancer: univariate and multivariate analysis including recursive partitioning and amalgamation algorithms in 1,052 patients. J Clin Oncol 13: 1221-1230, 1995.

6. Mountain CF, Carr DT, Anderson WAD. A system for the clinical staging of lung cancer. AJR 120: 130-138, 1974.

7. Mountain CF. A new international staging system for lung cancer. Chest 89: 255s-s335, 1986 (supplement).

8. Mountain CF. Revision in the international staging system for staging lung cancer. Chest 111: 1710-1717, 1997.

9. Naruke T, Goya T, Tsuchiya R, Suemasu K. Prognosis and survival in resected lung carcinoma based on the new international staging system. J Thorac Cardiovasc Surg 96: 440-447, 1988.

10. Harpole DH, Herndon JE, Wolfe WG, Iglehart JD, Marks JR. A prognostic model of recurrence and death in stage I non-small cell lung cancer utilizing presentation, histopathology, and oncoprotein expression. Cancer Res 55: 51-56, 1995.

11. Treasure T, Belcher JR. Prognosis of peripheral lung tumours related to size of the primary. Thorax 36: 5-8, 1981.

12. Watanabe Y, Shimizu J, Oda M, Hayashi Y, Iwa T, Nonomura A, Kamimura R, Takashima T. Proposals regarding some deficiencies in the new international staging system for non-small cell lung cancer. Jpn J Clin Oncol 21: 160-168, 1991.

13. Mountain CF. Expanded possibilities for surgical treatment of lung cancer. Survival in Stage IIIA disease. Results of surgical treatment in patients with Stage IIIA non-small cell lung cancer. Chest 97: 1045-1051, 1990.

14. Watanabe Y, Shimizu J, Oda M, et al. Results of surgical treatment in patients with stage IIIA non-small cell lung cancer. Thorac Cardiovasc Surgeon 39: 44-49, 1991.

15. Deslauriers J, Brisson J, Cartier R, Marcien F, Gagnon D, Piraux M, Beaulieu M. Carcinoma of the lung: Evaluation of satellite nodules as a factor influencing prognosis after resection. J Thorac Cardiovasc Surg 97: 504-512, 1989.

16. Shimizu N, Ando A, Date H, Teramoto S. Prognosis of undetected intrapulmonary metastases in resected lung cancer. Cancer 71(12): 3868-3872, 1993.

17. Mountain CF. Prognostic implications of the international staging system for lung cancer. Semin Oncol 15(3): 236-245, 1988.

18. Sugiura S, Ando Y, Minami H, Ando M, Sakai S, Shimokata K. Prognostic value of pleural effusion in patients with non-small cell lung cancer. Clin Cancer Res 3: 47-50, 1997.

19. Rosvold E, Langer CJ, McAleer C, Zipin H, Bonjo C, Ozols R. Advancing age does not exacerbate toxicity or compromise outcome in non-small cell lung cancer patients receiving paclitaxel-carboplatin. Proc Am Soc Clin Oncol 18: 478a, 1999 (abstract A-1846).

20. Akaogi E, Mitsui K, Onizuka M, Ishikawa S, Tsukada H, Mitsui T. Pleural dissemination in non-small cell lung cancer: Results of radiological evaluation and surgical treatment. J Surg Oncol 57: 33-39, 1994.

21. Shimizu J, Oda M, Morita K, Hayashi Y, Arano Y, Matsumoto I, Kobayashi K, Nonomura A, Watanabe Y. Comparison of pleuropneumonectomy and limited surgery for lung cancer with pleural dissemination. J Surg Oncol 61: 1-6, 1996.

22. Thomas PA, Piantadosi S. Postoperative T1N0 non-small cell lung cancer: squamous versus nonsquamous recurrences. J Thorac Cardiovasc Surg 94: 349-354, 1987.

23. Gail MH, Eagan RT, Feld R, Ginsberg R, Goodell B, Hill L, Holmes EC, Lukeman JM, Mountain CF, Oldham RK, Pearson RG, Wright PW, Lake WH, Lung Cancer Study Group. Prognostic factors in patients with resected stage I non-small cell lung cancer. A report from the Lung Cancer Study Group. Cancer 54: 1802-1813, 1984.

24. Williams DE, Pairolero PC, Davis CS, Bernatz PE, Payne WS, Taylor WF, Uhlenhopp MA, Fontana RS. Survival of patients surgically treated for stage I lung cancer. J Thorac Cardiovasc Surg 82: 70-76, 1981.

25. Dresler C, Ritter J, Wick M. Clinical and pathological findings in large cell lung carcinoma with neuroendocrine differentiation. Proc Am Soc Clin Oncol 14: A-1096, 1996.

26. Lipford HH, Scacs DL, Eggleston JC, More CW, Littlemore KD, Baker RR. Prognostic factors in surgically resected limited stage, non-small cell lung cancer. Am J Surg Pathol 8: 357-365, 1984.

27. Soorensen JB, Badsberg JH. Prognostic factors in resected stage I and II adenocarcinoma of the lung: A multivariate analysis of 137 consecutive patients. J Thorac Cardiovasc Surg 99: 218-226, 1990.

28. Green N, Kurohara SS, George FW. Cancer of the lung: an in-depth analysis of prognostic factors. Cancer 28: 1229, 1971.

29. Lanzotti VJ, Thomas DR, Boyle LE, et al. Survival with inoperable lung cancer: an integration of prognostic variables based on simple clinical criteria. Cancer 39: 303, 1977.

30. Miller TP, Chen TT, Coltman CA, et al. Effect of alternating combination chemotherapy on survival of ambulatory patients with metastatic large-cell and adenocarcinoma of the lung. A Southwest Oncology Group study. J Clin Oncol 4: 502-508, 1986.

31. Finkelstein DM, Ettinger DS, Ruckdeschel JC. Long-term survivors in metastatic non-small cell l ung cancer: an Eastern Cooperative Oncology Group study. J Clin Oncol 4: 702-709, 1986.

32. Einhorn LE, Loehrer PJ, Williams SD, et al. Random prospective study of vindesine versus vindesine plus high-dose cisplatin versus vindesine plus cisplatin plus mitomycin C in advanced non-small cell lung cancer. J Clin Oncol 4: 1037-1043, 1986.

33. Evans WK, Nixon DW, Daly JM, et al. A randomized study of oral nutritional support versus ad lib nutritional intake during chemotherapy for advanced colorectal and non-small cell lung cancer. J Clin Oncol 5: 113-124, 1987.

34. O'Connell JP, Kris MG, Gralla RJ, et al. Frequency and prognostic importance of pretreatment clinical characteristics in patients with advanced non-small cell lung cancer treated with combination chemotherapy. J Clin Oncol 4: 1604-1614, 1986.

35. Rapp E, Pater JL, Willan A, et al. Chemotherapy can prolong survival in patients with advanced non-small cell lung cancer: report of a Canadian multicenter randomized trial. J Clin Oncol 6: 633-641, 1988.

36. Sukurai M, Shinkai T, Eguchi K, et al. Prognostic factors in non-small cell lung cancer; multiregression analysis in the National Cancer Center Hospital(Japan). J Cancer Res Clin Oncol 115: 563-566, 1987.

37. Soorensen JB, Badsberg JH, Olsen J. Prognostic factors in inoperable adenocarcinoma of the lung: a mulivariate regression analysis of 259 patients. Cancer Res 49: 5748-5754, 1989.

38. Shinkai T, Eguchi K, Sasaki Y, et al. A prognostic factor risk index in advanced non-small cell lung cancer treated with cisplatin-containing combination chemotherapy. Cancer Chemother Pharmacol 30: 1-6, 1992.

39. Kojima A, Shinkai T, Eguchi K, et al. Analysis of three-year survivors among patients with advanced inoperable non-small cell lung cancer. Jpn J Clin Oncol 21: 276-281, 1991.

40. Kawahara M, Furuse K, Kodama N, et al. A randomized study of cisplatin versus cisplatin plus vindesine for non-small cell lung carcinoma. Cancer 68: 714-719, 1991.

41. Bonomi P, Gale M, Rowland K, et al. Pre-treatment prognostic factors in stage III non-small cell lung cancer patients receiving combined modality treatment. Int J Radiat Oncol Biol Phys 20: 247-252, 1991.

42. O'Connell JP, Kris MG, Gralla RJ, et al. Frequency and prognostic importance of pre-treatment clinical characteristics in patients with advanced non-small-cell lung cancer treated with combination chemotherapy. J Clin Oncol 4: 1604-1614, 1986.

43. Stanley KE. Prognostic factors for survival in patients with inoperable lung cancer. J Natl Cancer Inst. 65: 25, 1980.

44. Jiroutek M, Johnson D, Blum R, et al. Prognostic factors in advanced non-small cell lung cancer (NSCLC): analysis of Eastern Cooperative Oncology Group (ECOG) trials from 1981-1992. Proc Am Soc Clin Oncol 17: 461A, 1998.

45. Elson CE, Roggli VL, Vollmer RT, et al. Prognostic indicators for survival in stage I carcinoma of lung. A histologic study of 47 cases. Mod Pathol 1: 288-291, 1988.

46. Shahab I, Fraire AE, Greenberg SD, et al. Morphometric quantitation of tumor necrosis in stage I non-small cell carcinoma of lung: prognostic implications. Mod Pathol 5: 521-524, 1992.

47. Ten Velde GP, Havenith MG, Volovics A, Bosman FT. Prognostic significance of basement membrane deposition in operable squamous cell carcinomas of the lung. Cancer 67: 3001-3005, 1991.

48. Buccheri G, Ferrigno D, Vola F. Carcinoembryonic antigen (CEA), tissue polypeptide antigen (TPA) and other prognostic indicators in squamous cell lung cancer. Lung Cancer 10: 21-33, 1993.

49. Rice TW, Tubbs RR, Hoeltge GA, Kirby TJ, Meeker DP, Medendorp SV, Bukowski RM. Expression of blood group antigen A by stage I non-small cell lung carcinomas. Ann Thorac Surg 59: 568-572, 1995.

50. Dresler CN, Ritter JH, Wick MR, Roper CL, Patterson GA, Cooper JD. Immunostains for blood group antigens lack prognostic significance in T1 lung carcinoma. Ann Thorac Surg 59: 1069-1073, 1995.
51. Orntoft TF, Wolf H, Clausen H, Dabelsteen E, Hakomori SI. Blood group ANH-related antigens in normal and malignant bladder urothelium: possible structural basis for the deletion of type-2 chain ABH antigens in invasive carcinomas. Int J Cancer 43: 774-780, 1989.
52. Miyake M, Taki T, Hitomi S, Hakomori S. Correlation of expression of H/Le^y/Le^b antigens with survival in patients with carcinoma of the lung. N Engl J Med 327: 14-18, 1992.
53. Pantel K, Passlick B, Izbicki JR, Liewald R, Karg O, Riethmuller G. Expression of Lewis Y blood group precursor antigens on non-small cell lung carcinomas is associated with an unfavorable prognosis. Proc Am Soc Clin Oncol 12: 290, 1993.
54. Ogawa J, Sano A, Inoue H, Kolde S. Expression of Lewis-related antigen and prognosis in stage 1 non-small cell lung cancer. Ann Thorac Surg 59: 412-415, 1995.
55. Lee JS, Hong WK. Prognostic factors in lung cancer. N Engl J Med 327: 47-48, 1992.
56. Lee JS, Ro JY, Sabin AA, et al. Expression of blood group antigen A: a favorable prognostic factor in non-small cell lung cancer. N Engl J Med 324: 1084-1090, 1991.
57. Matsumoto H, Muramatsu H, Shimotakahara T, et al. Correlation of expression of ABH blood group carbohydrate antigens with metastatic potential in human lung carcinomas. Cancer 72: 75-81, 1993.
58. Volm M, Hahn EW, Mattern J, et al. Five year follow up study of independent clinical and flow cytometric prognostic factors for the survival of patients with non-small cell carcinoma. Cancer Res 48: 2923-2928, 1988.
59. Miyamoto H, Harada M, Isobe A, et al. Prognostic value of nuclear DNA content and expression of the *ras* oncogene product in lung cancer. Cancer Res 51: 6346-6350, 1991.
60. Zimmerman PV, Hawson GAT, Bint MH, Parsons PG. Ploidy as a prognostic determinant in surgically treated lung cancer. Lancet 2: 530-533, 1987.
61. Zimmerman PV, Bint MH, Hawson GAT, et al. Ploidy as a prognostic determinant in surgically treated lung cancer. Lancet 530, 1987.
62. Sahin A, Lee JS, Ro JY, et al. DNA flow cytometric (FCM) analysis of non-small cell lung cancer (NSCLC). Proc Am Soc Clin Oncol 8: 226, 1989.
63. Rodenhuis S, Van De Wetering MLM, Mooi WJ, Evers SG, van Zandwiijk N, Bos JL. Mutational activation of the K-*ras* oncogene: a possible pathogenetic factor in adenocarcinoma of the lung. N Engl J Med 317: 929-935, 1989.
64. Rodenhuis S, Slebos RJC, Boot AJM, Evers SG, Mooi WJ, Wagenaar SSC, van Bodegom PC, Bos JL. Incidence and possible clinical significance of K-*ras* oncogene activation in adenocarcinoma of the human lung. Cancer Res 48: 5738-5741, 1988.
65. Sugio K, Ishida T, Yokoyama H, Inoue T, Sugimachi K, Sasazuki T. *ras* gene mutations as a prognostic marker in adenocarcinoma of the human lung without lymph node metastasis. Cancer Res 52: 2903-2906, 1992.

66. Mitsudomi T, Steinberg SM, Oie HK, Mulshine J, Phelps R, Viallet J, Pass H, Minna JD, Gazdar AF. *Ras* gene mutations in non-small cell lung cancers are associated with shortened survival irrespective of treatment intent. Cancer Res 51: 4999-5002, 1991.

67. Mitsudomi T, Viallet J, Mulshine JL, Linnoila RI, Minna JD, Gazdar AF. Mutations of *ras* genes distinguish a subset of non-small cell lung cancer cell lines from small-cell lung cancer cell lines. Oncogene 6: 1353-1362, 1991.

68. Rosell R, Molina F, Moreno I, Martinez E, Pifarre A, Font A, Li S, Skacel Z, Gomez-Codina J, Camps C, Monzo M, de Anta JM. Mutated K-*ras* gene analysis in a randomized trial of preoperative chemotherapy plus surgery versus surgery in stage IIIA non-small cell lung cancer. Lung Cancer 12: S59-S70, 1995.

69. Keohavong P, De Michele MAA, Melacrinos AC, Landreneau RJ, Weyant RJ, Sigfried JM. Detection of K-*ras* mutations in lung carcinomas: relationship to prognosis. Clin Cancer Res 2: 411-418, 1996.

70. Martinez E, Vadell C. Clinical implications of genotypic characterization of non-small cell lung cancer based on K-*ras* mutants. Proc Am Soc Clin Oncol 13: 325, 1994.

71. Rodenhuis S, Slebos RJC. Clinical significance of *ras* oncogene activation in human lung cancer. Cancer Res 52: 2665S-2669S, 1992 (suppl).

72. Weiner DB, Norberg J, Robinson R, Nowell PC, Gazdar A, Greene MI, Williams WV, Cohen JA, Kern JA. Expression of the neu gene encoded protein (p185^{neu}) in human non-small cell carcinomas of the lung. Cancer Res 50: 421-425, 1990.

73. Noguchi M, Murakami M, Bennett W, Lupu R, Hui F, Harris CC, Gerwin BI. Biological consequences of overexpression of a transfected c-*erb* B-2 gene in immortalized human bronchial epithelial cells. Cancer Res 53: 2035-2043, 1993.

74. Tateishi M, Ishida T, Mitsudomi T, Kaneko S, Sugimachi K. Prognostic value of c-*erb* B-2 protein expression in human lung adenocarcinoma and squamous cell carcinoma. Eur J Cancer 27: 1372-1375, 1991.

75. Scagliotti GV, Leonardo E, Cappia S, Masiero P, Micela M, Gubetta L, Pozzi E. Epidermal growth factor receptor and *neu*-oncogene expression in lung cancer. Proc Am Soc Clin Oncol 12: 328, 1993.

76. Kern J, Slebos R, Top B, Rodenhuis S, Lager D, Robinson R, Weiner D, Schwartz DA. C-*erb* B-2 expression and codon 12 K-*ras* mutations both predict shortened survival for patients with pulmonary adenocarcinomas. J Clin Invest 93: 516-520, 1994.

77. Volm M, Drings P, Wodrich W. Prognostic significance of the expression of c-*fos*, c-*jun*, and c-*erb* B-1 oncogene products in human squamous cell lung carcinomas. J Cancer Res Clin Oncol 119: 507-510, 1993.

78. Chang F, Syrjanen S, Syrjanen K. Implications of the p53 tumor-suppressor gene in clinical oncology. J Clin Oncol 13: 1009-1022, 1995.

79. Fung CY, Fisher DE. p53: from molecular mechanisms to prognosis in cancer. J Clin Oncol 13: 808-811, 1995.

80. Iggo R, Gatter K, Bartek J, Lane D, Harris AL. Increased expression of mutant forms of p53 oncogene in primary lung cancer. Lancet 335: 675-679, 1990.

81. Chiba I, Takahashi T, Nau MM, D'Amico D, Curiel DT, Mitsudomi T, Buchhagen DL, Carbone D, Piantadosi S, Koga H, Reissman PT, Slamon W, Holmes EC,

Ninna JD. Mutations in the p53 gene are frequent in primary, resected non-small cell lung cancer. Oncogene 5: 1603-1610, 1990.

82. Mitsudomi T, Lyama T, Kusano T, Ohsaki T, Nakanishi R, Shirakusa T. Mutations of the p53 gene as a predictor of poor prognosis in patients with non-small cell lung cancer. Proc Am Assoc Cancer Res 34: 516, 1993 (abstract).

83. Carbone DP, Mitsudomi T, Chiba I, Piantadosi S, Rusch V, Nowak JA, McIntire D, Slamon D, Gazdar A, Minna J. p53 immunostaining positivity is associated with reduced survival and is imperfectly correlated with gene mutations in resected non-small cell lung cancer. Chest 106: 377S-381S, 1994.

84. Hiyoshi H, Matsuno Y, Kato H, Shimosato Y, Hirohashi S. Clinicopathological significance of nuclear accumulation of tumor suppressor gene p53 product in primary lung cancer. Jpn J Cancer Res 83: 101-106, 1992.

85. Quinlan DC, Davidson AG, Summers CL, Warden HE, Doshi HM. Accumulation of p53 protein correlates with a poor prognosis in human lung cancer. Cancer Res 52: 4828-4831, 1992.

86. McLaren R, Kuzu I, Dunnill M, Harris A, Lane D, Gatter KC. The relationship of p53 immunostaining to survival in carcinoma of the lung. Br J Cancer 66: 735-738, 1992.

87. Passlick B, Izbicki JR, Haussinger K, Thetter O, Pantel K. Immunohistochemical detection of p53 protein is not associated with a poor prognosis in non-small cell lung cancer. J Thorac Caradiovasc Surg 109: 1205-1211, 1995.

88. Lee JS, Yoon A, Kalapurakal SK, Ro JY, Lee JJ, Tu N, Hittelman WN, Hong KH. Expression of p53 oncoprotein in non-small cell lung cancer: a favorable prognostic factor. J Clin Oncol 13: 1893-1903, 1995.

89. Top B, Mooi WJ, Klaver SG, Boerrigter L, Wisman P, Elbers HRJ, Visser S, Rodenhuis S. Comparative analysis of p53 gene mutations and protein accumulation in human non-small cell lung cancer. Int J Cancer 64: 83-91, 1995.

90. Shirotani Y, Hiyama K, Ishioka S, et al. Alteration in length of telomeric repeats in lung cancer. Lung Cancer 11: 29-41, 1994.

91. Komiya T, Hosono Y, Hirashima T, Masuda N, Yasumitsu T, Nakagawa K, et al. P21 expression as a predictor for favorable prognosis in squamous cell carcinoma of the lung. Clin Cancer Res 3(10): 1831-1835, 1997.

92. Kwiatkowski DJ, Harpole PH, Jr; Godleski J, Herndon JE, 2nd; Shieh DB, Richards W, Blanco R, Xu HJ, Strauss GM, Sugarbaker DJ. Molecular pathologic substaging in 244 stage I NSCLC patients: clinical implications. J Clin Oncol 7: 16(7): 2468-2477, 1998.

93. Kim Y-C, Kyung J, Park O, Kern JA, Park C-S, Lim S-C, Jang A-S, Yang J-B. The interactive effect of ras, her-2, p53, and BCL-2 expression in predicting survival of non-small cell lung cancer patients. Lung Cancer 22: 181-190, 1998.

94. Keogan MT, Tung KT, Kaplan DK, Goldstraw PJ, Hansell DM. The significance of pulmonary nodules detected on CT staging for lung cancer. Clin Radiology 48: 94-96, 1993.

95. Arita T, Kurainitsu T, Kawamura M, Matsumoto T, Matsunaga N, Sugi K, Esato K. Bronchogenic carcinoma: incidence of metastases to normal sized lymph nodes. Thorax 50: 1267-1269, 1995.

96. Patterson GA, Ginsberg RJ, Poon Y, et al. A prospective evaluation of magnetic resonance imaging, computed tomography and mediastinoscopy in the preoperative assessment of mediastinal node status in bronchogenic carcinoma. J Thorac Cardiovasc Surg 94: 679-684, 1987.

97. Seely JM, Mayo JR, Miller RR, et al. T1 lung cancer: Prevalence of mediastinal nodal metastases and diagnostic accuracy of CT. Radiology 186: 129-132, 1993.

98. McLoud TC, Bourgouin PM, Greenberg RW, Kosiuk JP, Templeton PA, Shepard JO, Moore EH, Wain JC, Mathisen DJ, Grillo HC. Bronchogenic carcinoma: Analysis of staging in the mediastinum with CT by correlative lymph node mapping and sampling. Radiology 182: 319-323, 1992.

99. Gallardo JFM, Naranjo FB, Cansino MT, Rodriguez-Panadero F. Validity of enlarged mediastinal nodes as markers of involvement by non-small cell lung cancer. Am Rev Respir Dis 146: 1210-1212, 1992.

100. Gdeede A, Van Schil P, Corthouts B, Van Mieghem F, Van Meerbeeck J, Van Marck E. Prospective evaluation of computed tomography and mediastinoscopy in mediastinal lymph node staging. Eur Respir J 10: 1547-1551, 1997.

101. Dillemans B, Deneffe G, Verschakelen J, et al. Value of computed tomography and mediastinoscopy in preoperative evaluation of mediastinal nodes in non-small cell lung cancer. Eur J Cardio Thorac Surg 8: 37-42, 1994.

102. Arita T, Kuramitsu T, Kawamura M, et al. Bronchogenic carcinoma: incidence of metastases to normal sized lymph nodes. Thorax 50: 1267-1269, 1995.

103. Pearson FG. Staging of the mediastinum: role of mediastinoscopy and computed tomography. Chest 103(4): 346S-348S, 1993.

104. Libshitz HI, McKenna RJ Jr, Haynie TP, et al. Mediastinal evaluation in lung cancer. Radiology 151: 295-299, 1984.

105. Staples CA, Muller NL, Miller RR, et al. Mediastinal nodes in bronchogenic carcinoma: comparison between CT and mediastinoscopy. Radiology 167: 367-372, 1988.

106. Oliver TW, Bernardino ME, Miller JI, et al. Isolated adrenal masses in non-small cell bronchogenic carcinoma. Radiology 153: 217-218, 1984.

107. Ettinghausen SE, Burt ME. Prospective evaluation of unilateral adrenal masses in patients with operable non-small cell lung cancer. J Clin Oncol 9: 1462-1466, 1991.

108. Sandler MA, Pearlberg JL, Madrazo BL, Gitschlag KF, Gross SC. Computed tomographic evaluation of the adrenal gland in the preoperative assessment of bronchogenic carcinoma. Radiology 145: 733-736, 1982.

109. Allard P, Yankaskas BC, Fletcher RH, et al. Sensitivity and specificity of computed tomography for the detection of adrenal metastatic lesions among 91 autopsied lung cancer patients. Cancer 66: 457-462, 1990.

110. Silverman SG, Mueller PR, Pinkney LP, et al. Predictive value of image-guided adrenal biopsy: analysis of results of 101 biopsies. Radiology 187: 715-718, 1993.

111. Pagani JJ. Non-small cell lung carcinoma adrenal metastases computed tomography and percutaneous cancer. Cancer 53: 1058-1060, 1984.

112. Bernardino M, Walther M, Phillips V, et al. CT-guided adrenal biopsy: accuracy, safety, and indications. AJR 144: 67-69, 1985.

113. Michel F, Soler M, Imhof E, et al. Initial staging of non-small cell lung cancer: value of routine radioisotope bone scanning. Thorax 46: 469-473, 1991.

114. Tarver RD, Richmond BD, Kratte EC. Cerebral metastases from lung carcinomas: neurological and CT correlation. Radiology 153: 689-692, 1984.

115. Merchut MP. Brain metastases from undiagnosed systemic neoplasms. Arch Intern Med 149: 1076-1080, 1989.

116. Newman SJ, Hansen HH. Frequency, diagnosis, and treatment of brain metastases in 247 consecutive patients with bronchogenic carcinoma. Cancer 33: 492-496, 1974.

117. Hooper R, Tenholder M, Underwood G, et al. Computed tomographic scanning of the brain in initial staging of bronchogenic carcinoma. Chest 85: 774-776, 1984.

118. Mintz BJ, Tuhrim S, Alexander S, et al. Intracranial metastases in the initial staging of bronchogenic carcinoma. Chest 86: 850-853, 1984.

119. Warren WH, Faber LP. Bronchoscopic evaluation of the lungs and tracheobronchial tree, in Shields TW (ed): General Thoracic Surgery 250-262, Williams & Wilkins & Wilkins, Baltimore, 1994.

120. Stanley JH, Fish GD, Andriole JG, Gobien RP, Betsill WL, Laden SA, et al. Lung lesions: cytologic diagnosis by fine-needle biopsy. Radiology 162: 389-391, 1987.

121. The Canadian Lung Group: Investigation for mediastinal disease in patients with apparently operable lung cancer. Ann Thorac Surg 60: 1382-1389, 1995.

122. Daly BDT, Mueller JD, Faling LJ, Diehl JT, Bankoff MS, Karp DD, Rand WM. N2 lung cancer: Outcome in patients with false-negative computed tomographic scans of the chest. J Thorac Cardiovasc Surg 105(5): 904-911, 1993.

123. Gdeddo A, Van Schil P, Corthouts B, et al. Prospective evaluation of computed tomography and mediastinoscopy in mediastinal lymph node staging. Eur Respir J 10(7): 1552-1558, 1997.

124. Ginsberg RJ, Rice TW, Goldberg M, et al. Extended mediastinoscopy. J Thorac Cardiovasc Surg 94: 673-678, 1987.

125. McNeil TM, Chamberlain JM. Diagnostic anterior mediastinotomy. Ann Thorac Surg 2: 532, 1966.

126. Kondo D, Imaizumi M, Abe T, Naruke T, Suemasu K. Endoscopic ultrasound examination for mediastinal lymph node metastases of lung cancer. Chest 98: 586-593, 1990.

127. Silvestri GA, Hoffman BJ, Bhutani MS, Hawes RH, Coppage L, Sanders-Cliette A, Reed CE. Endoscopic ultrasound with fine-needle aspiration in the diagnosis and staging of lung cancer. Ann Thorac Surg 61: 1441-1446, 1996.

128. McCann J. PET scans approved for detecting metastatic non-small cell lung cancer. J Natl Cancer Inst 90(2): 94-96, 1998.

129. Sazon DA, Santiago SM, Soo Hoo GW, Khonsary A, Brown C, Mandelkern M, Blahd W, Williams AJ. Fluorodeoxyglucose-positron emission tomography in the detection and staging of lung cancer. Am J Respir Crit Care Med 153: 417-421, 1996.

130. Kutlu C, Pastorino U, Maisey M, et al. Selective use of PET scan in the preoperative staging of NSCLC. Lung Cancer 21: 177-184, 1998.

131. Valk PE, Parnds TR, Hopkins DM, Haseman MK, Hoeb GA, Greiss HB, et al. Staging non-small cell lung cancer by whole-body position emission tomographic imaging. Ann Thorac Surg 60: 1573-1582, 1995.

132. Eberhadt W, Wilke H, Stamatis G, Stuschke M, Harstrick A, Menker H, Krause B, Mueller MR, Stahl M, Flasshove M, Udach V, Greschuchna D, Konietzko N, Sack H, Seeber S. Preoperative chemotherapy followed by concurrent chemoradiation therapy based on hyperfractionated accelerated radiotherapy and definitive surgery in locally advanced non-small cell lung cancer: Mature results of a Phase II trial. J Clin Oncol 16(2): 622-634, 1998.

133. Venugopal P, Bonomi P, Ali A, Patel S, Faber LP, Lincoln S, LaFollette S, Priesler H. Correlation of positron emission tomography (PET) scan, computerized tomographic (CT) scan and histologic response to combined modality chemo-radiotherapy (CT/RT) in Stage III non-small cell lung cancer.

134. Vansteenkoste JF, Stroobants SG, DuPont J, DeLeyn PR, Verbeken EK, Deneffe GJ, Mortelmans LA, Demedts MG. Prognostic importance of the standardized uptake value on 18F-fluoro-2-deoxy-glucose-position Emission Tomography Scan in non-small cell lung cancer: an analysis of 125 cases. J Clin Oncol 17: 3201-3206, 1999.

135. Vansteenkiste JF, Stroobants SG, De Leyn PR, Dupont PJ, Verschakelen JA, Nacckaerts KL, Mortelmans LA, Leuven Lung Cancer Group. Mediastinal lymph node staging with FDG-PET scan in patients with potentially operable non-small cell lung cancer: A prospective analysis of 50 cases. Chest 112: 1480-1486, 1997.

136. Mentzer SJ. Mediastinoscopy, thoracoscopy, and video-assisted thoracic surgery in the diagnosis and staging of lung cancer. Hematol Oncol Clin North Am 11(3): 435-447, 1997.

137. Nabi HA, Steinbrenner L, Lamonica D, Spaulding M. The use of positron emission tomography. Proc Am Soc Clin Oncol 15: A-1204, 1996 (abstract).

138. Dewan N, Shehan C, Reeb S, et al. Likelihood of malignancy in a solitary pulmonary nodule comparison of bayesian analysis and results of FDG PET scan. Chest 112: 416-422, 1997.

139. Patz E Jr, Lowe V, Goodman P, et al. Thoracic nodal staging with positron emission tomography (PET) and 18-F-2-fluoro-2-deoxy-D-glucose in patients with bronchogenic carcinoma. Chest 108: 1617-1621, 1995.

140. Gupta N, Gill H, Graeber G, et al. Dynamic positron emission tomography with F-18-fluorodeoxyglucose imaging in differentiation of benign from malignant lung/mediastinal lesions. Chest 114: 1105-1111, 1998.

141. Steinert H, Hauser M, Allemann F, et al. Non-small cell lung cancer: nodal staging with FDG PET versus CT with correlative lymph node mapping and sampling. Radiol 202: 441-446, 1997.

142. Wahl R, Quint L, Greenough R, et al. Staging of mediastinal non-small cell lung cancer with FDG PET, CT, and fusion images: preliminary prospective evaluation. Radiol 191: 371-377, 1994.

143. Ichiya Y, Kuwabara Y, Otsuka M. Assessment of response to cancer therapy using fluorine-18-fluorodeoxyglucose and positron emission tomography. J Nucl Med 32: 1655-1660, 1991.

144. Frank A, Letkowitz D, Jaeger S, et al. Decision logic for retreatment of asymptomatic lung cancer recurrence based on positron emission tomography findings. Int J Radiat Oncol Biol Phys 32: 1495-1512, 1995.

145. Kubota K, Yamada S, Ishiwata K, et al. Positron emission tomography for treatment evaluation and recurrence detection compared with CT in long-term follow-up cases of lung cancer. Clin Nucl Med 17: 877-881, 1992.

146. Kim E, Chung S, Haynie TP. Differentiation of residual or recurrent tumors from post-treatment changes with F-18-FDG PET. RadioGraphic 12: 269-279, 1992.

147. Patz E, Lowe V, Hoffman J, et al. Persistent or recurrent bronchogenic carcinoma: detection with PET and 2-[F-18]-2-deoxy-D-glucose. Radiol 191: 379-382, 1994.

148. Kerstine KH, Trapp JF, Croft DR, et al. Comparison of positron emission tomography (PET) and computed tomography (CT) to identify N2 and N3 disease in non-small cell lung cancer (NSCLC). Proc Am Soc Clin Oncol 17: 458, 1998 (abstract 1762).

149. Shields TW. The significance of ipsilateral mediastinal lymph node metastases (N2 disease) in non-small cell carcinoma of the lung. J Thorac Cardiovasc Surg 99: 48-53, 1990.

150. Goldstraw P, Mannam GC, Kaplan DK, Mitchail P. Surgical management of non-small cell lung cancer with ipsilateral mediastinal node metastases (N2 disease). J Thorac Cardiovasc Surg 107: 19-28, 1994.

151. Martini N, Flehinger BJ. The role of surgery in N2 lung cancer. Surg Clin North Am 67: 1037-1049, 1987.

152. Mitsukuoka M, Hayashi A, Takamori S, Nagamatsu Y, Matsuo T, Kakegawa T. The significance of lymph nodes (LN) dissection through median sternotomy for left lung cancer. Lung Cancer 11(suppl 1): 149, 1994.

153. Levasseur PH, Regnard JF. Long term results after surgery for N2 non-small cell lung cancer. Presented at the International Association for the Study of Lung Cancer (IASCC) Workshop, Burges, Belgium, June 17-21, 1990.

154. Naruke T, Goya T, Tsuchiya R, Suemasu K. The importance of surgery to non-small cell carcinoma of lung with mediastinal lymph node metastases. Ann Thorac Surg 46: 603-610, 1988.

155. Moores DW, McKneally MF. Treatment of stage I lung cancer (T1N0M0, T2N0M0). Surg Clin North Am 67: 937-943, 1987.

156. PORT Meta-analysis Trialists Group: Postoperative radiotherapy in non-small cell lung cancer: Systemic review and meta-analysis of individual patient data from nine randomized controlled trials. Lancet 352: 257-263, 1998.

157. Niiranen A, Witamo-Korhonen S, Kouri M, Assendelft A, Mattson K, Pyrhonen S. Adjuvant chemotherapy after radical surgery for non-small cell lung cancer: A randomized study. J Clin Oncol 10: 1927-1932, 1992.

158. Wada H, Hitomi S, Teramatsu T, et al. Adjuvant chemotherapy after complete resection in non-small cell lung cancer. J Clin Oncol 114: 1048-1054, 1996.

159. Warren WH, Faber LP. Segmentectomy versus lobectomy in patients with stage I pulmonary carcinoma. J Thorac Cardiovasc Surg 107: 1087-1094, 1994.

160. Yano T, Yokoyama H, Yoshino I, Tayama K, Asoh H, Hata K, et al. Results of a limited resection for compromised or poor-risk patients with clinical stage I non-small cell carcinoma of the lung. J Am Coll Surg 181: 33-37, 1995.

161. Ayoub J, Vigneault J, Hanley A, et al. The Montreal multi-center trial in operable non-small cell lung cancer (NSCLC): a multivariate analysis of the predictors of relapse. Proc Am Soc Clin Oncol 10: 247, 1991 (abstract).

162. Mountain CF. New prognostic factors in lung cancer: biologic prophets of cancer cell aggression. Chest 108: 246-254, 1995.

163. Martini N, Flehinger BJ, Nagasaki F, Hart B. Prognostic significance of N1 disease in carcinoma of the lung. J Thorac Cadiovasc Surg 86: 646-653, 1983.

164. Holmes EC. Treatment of stage II lung cancer (T1N1, T2N1). Surg Clin North Am 67: 945-949, 1987.

165. Yano T, Yokoyama H, Inoue T, Asoh H, Tayama K, Ichinose Y. Surgical results and prognostic factors of pathologic N1 disease in non-small cell carcinoma of the lung. J Thorac Cardiovasc Surg 107: 1398-1402, 1994.

166. Weisenberger TH, Gail M, Lung Cancer Study Group. Effects of postoperative mediastinal radiation on completely resected stage II and stage III epidermoid cancer of the lung. N Engl J Med 315: 1377-1381, 1986.

167. Holmes EC, Gail M, Lung Cancer Study Group. Surgical adjuvant therapy for stage II and III adenocarcinoma and large cell undifferentiated carcinoma. J Clin Oncol 4: 710-715, 1986.

168. Lad T, Rubinstein A, Sadeghi A, et al. The benefit of adjuvant treatment for resected locally advanced non-small cell lung cancer. J Clin Oncol 6: 9-17, 1988.

169. Keller S, Adak S, Wagner H, Herskovic A, Brooks B, Perry M, Livingston R. Prospective randomized trial of postoperative adjuvant therapy in patients with completely resected stage I and stage IIIA non-small cell lung cancer. Proc Am Soc Clin Oncol 18: 465a, 1999 (abstract A-1793).

170. Pichler JM, Pairolero PC, Weiland LH, et al. Bronchogenic carcinoma with chest wall invasion: factors affecting survival following en bloc resection. Ann Thorac Surg 34: 684-691, 1982.

171. Patterson GA, Ilves R, Ginsberg PJ, et al. The value of adjuvant radiotherapy in pulmonary and chest wall resection for bronchogenic carcinoma. Ann Thorac Surg 34: 692-697, 1982.

172. Rosell R, Goméz-Codina J, Camps C, Maestre J, Padille J, Cantró A, et al. A randomized trial comparing preoperative chemotherapy plus surgery with surgery alone in patients with non-small cell lung cancer. N Engl J Med 330: 153-158, 1994.

173. Roth JA, Fossella F, Komaki R, et al. A randomized trial comparing perioperative chemotherapy and surgery with surgery alone in resectable stage IIIA non-small cell lung cancer. J Natl Cancer Inst 86: 673-680, 1994.

174. DePierre A, Milleron B, Moro D, Chaveb S, Braun D, Quoix E, et al. Phase III trial of neo-adjuvant chemotherapy in resectable stage I (except T1N0) II, IIIA non-small cell lung cancer: French experience. Proc Am Soc Clin Oncol 18: 465a, 1999 (abstract A-1792).

175. Dillman RO, Seagren SL, Propert KJ, et al. A randomized trial of induction chemotherapy plus high-dose radiation versus radiation alone in stage III non-small cell lung cancer. N Engl J Med 323: 940-945, 1990.

176. Dillman RO, Seagren SL, Herndon J, Green MR, et al. Randomized trial of induction chemotherapy plus radiation therapy (RT) vs RT alone in stage III non-

small cell lung cancer: five-year follow up of CALGB 84-33. Proc Am Soc Clin Oncol 12: 329, 1993 (abstract).

177. Sause WT, Scott C, Taylor S, et al. Radiation Therapy Oncology Group (RTOG) 88-08 and Eastern Cooperative Oncology Group (ECOG) 4588: preliminary advanced results of a phase III trial of regionally unresectable non-small cell lung cancer. J Natl Cancer Inst 87: 198-205, 1995.

178. LeChevalier T, Arriagada R, Quoix E, et al. Radiotherapy alone versus combined chemotherapy and radiotherapy in nonresectable non-small cell lung cancer: first analysis of a randomized trial in 353 patients. J Natl Cancer Inst 83: 417-423, 1990.

179. LeChevalier T, Arriagada R, Quoix E, et al. Significant effect of adjuvant chemotherapy on survival in locally advanced non-small cell lung carcinoma. J Natl Cancer Inst 84: 58, 1992 (letter).

180. Cullen MA, Billingham LJ, Woodroffe CM, et al. Mitomycin, ifosfamide, and cisplatin in unresectable non-small cell lung cancer: effects on survival and quality of life. J Clin Oncol 17: 3188-3194, 1999.

181. Schaake-Koning C, van den Bogaert W, Dalesio O, et al. Effects of concomitant cisplatin and radiotherapy on inoperable non-small cell lung cancer. N Engl J Med 326: 524-530, 1992.

182. Jeremic B, Shibamoto Y, Acimovic L, Djuric L. Randomized trial of hyperfractionated radiation therapy with or without concurrent chemotherapy for stage III non-small cell lung cancer. J Clin Oncol 13: 452-458, 1995.

183. Jeremic B, Shibamoto Y, Acimovic L, Milisarljenic S. Hyperfractionated radiation therapy with or without concurrent low-dose daily carboplatin-etoposide for stage III non-small cell lung cancer. J Clin Oncol 14: 1065-1070, 1996.

184. Furuse K, Fukuoka F, Takada Y, et al. Phase III study of concurrent vs sequential thoracic radiotherapy in combination with mitomycin, vindesine, and cisplatin in unresectable non-small cell lung cancer. J Clin Oncol 17: 2692-2699, 1999.

185. Saunders MI, Dische S. Continuous hyperfractionated accelerated radiotherapy (CHART) in non-small cell carcinoma of the bronchus. Int J Radiat Oncol Biol Phys 19: 1211-1215, 1990.

186. Saunders M, Dische S, Barrett A, et al. Continuous hyperfractionated accelerated radiotherapy versus conventional radiotherapy in non-small cell lung cancer: a randomized multicentre trial. Lancet 350: 161-165, 1997.

187. Martini N, Kris M, Flehinger BJ, et al. Preoperative chemotherapy for stage IIIA (N2) lung cancer: The Sloan-Kettering experience with 136 patients. Ann Thorac Surg 55: 1365-1374, 1993.

188. Burkes RL, Shepherd FA, Ginsberg RJ, et al. Induction chemotherapy with MVP in patients with stage III (T1-3,N2,M0) unresectable non-small cell lung cancer. The Toronto experience. Proc Am Soc Clin Oncol 13: 327, 1994 (abstract).

189. Langer CJ, Curran WJ, Keller SM, et al. Report of phase II trial of concurrent chemoradiotherapy with radical thoracic irradiation (60 Gy), infusional fluorouracil, bolus cisplatin and etoposide for clinical stage IIIB and bulky IIIA NSCLC. Int J Rad Onc Biol Phys 26: 469-478, 1993.

190. Rusch VW, Albain KS, Crowley JJ, et al. Surgical resection of stage IIIA and IIIB non-small cell lung cancer after concurrent induction chemoradiotherapy. J Thorac Cardiovasc Surg 105: 97-106, 1993.

191. Albain K, Rusch V, Crowley J, Rice T, Turrisi A, Weick J, et al. Long term survival after concurrent cisplatin/etoposide plus chest radiotherapy followed by surgery in bulky stages IIIA (N2) and IIIB non-small cell lung cancer: 6-year outcomes from Southwest Oncology Group study 8805. Proc Am Soc Clin Oncol 18: A-1801, 1999.

192. Byhardt R, Scott C, Sause W, et al. Response, toxicity, failure patterns and survival in five Radiation Therapy Oncology Group (RTOG) trials of sequential and/or concurrent chemotherapy (CT) and radiation therapy (RT) for locally advanced non-small cell carcinoma of the lung (NSCLC). Proc 39th Ann Am Soc Ther Rad Oncol Mtg 195: 1997 (abstract 120).

193. Cartei G, Cartei F, Cantrone A, Cansarano D, Genco G, Tobaldin A, Interlandi G, Giraldi T. Cisplatin-cyclophosphamide-mitomycin combination chemotherapy with supportive care vs supportive care alone for treatment of metastatic non-small cell lung cancer. J Natl Cancer Inst 85: 794-800, 1993.

194. Non-Small Cell Lung Cancer Collaborative Group. Chemotherapy in non-small cell lung cancer: a meta-analysis using updated data on individual patients from 52 randomized clinical trials BMJ 311: 899-909, 1995.

195. Bonomi PD, Finkelstein DM, Ruckdeschel JC, et al. Combination chemotherapy versus single agents followed by combination chemotherapy in stage IV non-small cell lung cancer: a study of the Eastern Cooperative Oncology Group. J Clin Oncol 7: 1602-1613, 1989.

196. Klastersky J, Sculier JP, Lacroix H, et al. A randomized study comparing cisplatin or carboplatin with etoposide in patients with advanced non-small cell lung cancer: European Organization for Research and Treatment of Cancer Protocol 07861. J Clin Oncol 8: 1556-1562, 1990.

197. Gralla RJ, Casper ES, Kelsen DP, et al. Cisplatin and vindesine combination chemotherapy for advanced carcinoma of the lung: a randomized trial investigating two dosage schedules. Ann Intern Med 95: 414-420, 1981.

198. Klastersky J, Sculier JP, Ravez P, et al. A randomized study comparing a high and a standard dose of cisplatin in combination with etoposide in the treatment of advanced non-small cell lung carcinoma. J Clin Oncol 4: 1780-1786, 1986.

199. Shinkai T, Saijo N, Eguchi K, et al. Cisplatin and vindesine combination chemotherapy for non-small cell lung cancer: a randomized trial comparing two dosages of cisplatin. Jpn J Cancer Res 77: 782-789, 1986.

200. Wozniak AJ, Crowley JJ, Balcerzak SP, et al. Randomized trial comparing cisplatin with cisplatin plus vinorelbine in the treatment of advanced non-small cell lung cancer: a Southwest Oncology Group study. J Clin Oncol 16: 2459-2465, 1998.

201. Sandler A, Nemunaitis J, Dehnam C, et al. Phase III study of cisplatin (C) with or without gemcitabine (G) in patients with advanced non-small cell lung cancer (NSCLC). Proc Am Soc Clin Oncol 17: 454a, 1998 (abstract).

202. von Pawel J, von Roemeling R. Survival benefit from Triazone (tirapazamine) and cisplatin in advanced non-small cell lung cancer (NSCLC) patients final results

from the international phase III CATAPULT I trial. Proc Am Soc Clin Oncol 17: 454a, 1998 (abstract 1749).

203. Bonomi P, Kim K, Chang A, et al. Phase III trial comparing etoposide (E) cisplatin (C) versus taxol (T) with cisplatin-G-CSF (G) versus taxol-cisplatin in advanced non-small cell lung cancer. An Eastern Cooperative Oncology Group (ECOG) trial. Proc Am Soc Clin Oncol 15: 382, 1996 (abstract 1145).

204. Le Chevalier T, Brisgand D, Douillard JY, et al. Randomized study of vinorelbine and cisplatin versus vindesine and cisplatin versus vinorelbine alone in advanced non-small cell lung cancer: results of a European multicenter trial including 612 patients. J Clin Oncol 12: 360-367, 1994.

205. Peng R-P, Chen YM, Ming Liu J, Tsai C-M, Lin W-C, Yang K-Y, Whang Peng J. Gemcitabine versus the combination of cisplatin and etoposide in patients with inoperable non-small cell lung cancer in a phase II randomized study. J Clin Oncol 15(5): 2097-2102, 1997.

206. Manegold C, Bergman B, Chemaissani et al. Single agent gemcitabine versus cisplatin-etoposide: Early results of a randomized phase II study in locally advanced or metastatic non-small cell lung cancer. Ann Oncol 8(6): 525-529, 1997.

207. The Elderly Lung Cancer Vinorelbine Italian Study Group: Effects of vinorelbine on quality of life and survival of elderly patients with advanced non-small cell lung cancer. J Natl Cancer Inst 91: 66-72, 1999.

208. Murray N, Coy P, Pater J, Hodson I, Arnold A, et al. Importance of timing for thoracic irradiation in the combined modality treatment of limited-stage small-cell lung cancer. J Clin Oncol 11: 336-344, 1993.

209. Hansen HH. Management of small cell cancer of the lung. Lancet 339: 846-849, 1992.

210. Dearing MP, Steinberg SM, Phelps R, et al. Outcome of patients with small-cell lung cancer: effect of changes in staging procedures and imaging technology on prognostic factors over 14 years. J Clin Oncol 8: 1042-1049, 1990.

211. Albain KS, Crowley JJ, LeBlanc M, Livingston RB. Determinants of improved outcome in small cell lung cancer: an analysis of the 2850 patient Southwest Oncology Group data base. J Clin Oncol 8: 1563-1574, 1990.

212. Ihde DC, Glatstein EJ, Pass HI. Small-cell lung cancer, in DeVita VT Jr, Hellman S, Rosenberg SA (eds): Cancer: Principles and Practice of Oncology (ed 5). Philadelphia, PA, Lippincott-Raven, 1997, pp 911-950.

213. Livingston RB, McCracken JD, Trauft CJ, et al. Isolated pleural effusion in small cell lung carcinoma: favorable prognosis. Chest 81: 208-215, 1982.

214. Giannone L, Johnson DH, Hande KR, Greco FA. Favorable prognosis of brain metastases in small cell lung cancer. Ann Intern Med 106: 386-389, 1987.

215. Matthews MJ, Kanhouwa S, Pickren J, Robinette D. Frequency of residual and metastatic tumors in patients undergoing curative surgical resection for lung cancer. Cancer Chemother Rep 4: 63-67, 1973.

216. Williams CJ, McMillan I, Lea R, Mead G, Thompson J, Sweetenham J, Herbert A, Jeffreys M, Buchanan R, Whitehouse JM. Surgery after initial chemotherapy for localized small cell carcinoma of the lung. J Clin Oncol 5: 1579-1588, 1987.

217. Shields TW, Higgins GA, Matthews MJ, Heehn RJ. Surgical resection in the management of small cell carcinoma of the lung. J Thorac Cardiovasc Surg 84: 481-488, 1982.
218. Shepherd FA, Ginsberg RJ, Feld R, Evans WK, Johansen E. Surgical treatment for limited small cell lung cancer. The university of Toronto Lung Oncology Group experience. J Thorac Cardiovasc Surg 101: 385-393, 1991.
219. Shah SS, Thompson J, Goldstraw P. Results of operation without adjuvant therapy in the treatment of small-cell lung cancer. Ann Thorac Surg 54: 498-501, 1992.
220. Baldeyrou P, Marrash R, LeChevalier T, Arriagada R. L'endoscopie bronchique dans le bilan diagnostique et evolutif des cancers broncho-pulmonaires a petites cellules. Bull Cancer 74: 511-515, 1987.
221. Sagman U, Feld R, Evans WK, et al. The prognostic significance of pretreatment serum lactate dehydrogenase in patients with small-cell lung cancer. J Clin Oncol 9: 954-961, 1991.
222. Shepherd FA. Screening, diagnosis, and staging of lung cancer. Curr Opin Oncol 5: 310-322, 1993.
223. Hansen HH. Diagnosis in metastatic sites. In: Straus MJ, ed. Lung cancer clinical diagnosis and treatment. New York: Grune & Stratton, 185-200, 1983.
224. Newman SJ, Hansen HH. Frequency, diagnosis, and treatment of brain metastases in 247 consecutive patients with bronchogenic carcinoma. Cancer 33: 492-496, 1974.
225. Tritz DB, Doll DC, Ringenberg QS, et al. Bone marrow involvement in small cell lung cancer. Clinical significance and correlation with routine laboratory variables. Cancer 63: 763-766, 1989.
226. Levitan N, Byrne RE, Bromer RH, et al. The value of the bone scan and bone marrow biopsy in staging small cell lung cancer. Cancer 56(3): 652-654, 1985.
227. Ihde D, Simms E, Matthews M, Cohen MH, Bunn PA, Minna JD. Bone marrow metastases in small cell carcinoma of the lung. Blood 53: 677-686, 1978.
228. Zych J, Polowiec Z, Wiatr E, Broniek A, Rowinska-Zakrzewska E. The prognostic significance of bone marrow metastases in small cell lung cancer patients. Lung Cancer 10: 239-245, 1993.
229. Ihde DC, Hansen HH. Staging procedures and prognostic factors in small cell carcinoma of the lung. In: Greco FA, Oldham RK, Bunn PA, eds. Small cell lung cancer. New York: Grune & Stratton 261-283, 1981.
230. Mulshine JL, Makuch RW, Johnston-Early A, et al. Diagnosis and significance of liver metastases in small cell carcinoma of the lung. J Clin Oncol 2: 733-741, 1984.
231. Hirsch FR, Paulson OB, Hansen HH, Larsen SO. Intracranial metastases in small cell carcinoma of the lung, prognostic aspects. Cancer 51: 529-533, 1983.
232. Hirsch FR, Paulson OB, Hansen HH, Vraa-Jensen J. Intracranial metastases in small cell carcinoma of the lung, correlation of clinical and autopsy findings. Cancer 50: 2433-2437, 1982.
233. Nugent JL, Bunn PA, Matthews MJ, et al. CNS metastases in small cell bronchogenic carcinoma. Cancer 44: 1885-1893, 1979.

234. Crane JM, Nelson MJ, Ihde DC, et al. A comparison of computed tomography and radionuclide scanning for detection of brain metastases in small cell lung cancer. J Clin Oncol 2: 1017-1024, 1984.

235. Hardy J, Smith I, Cherryman G, et al. The value of computed tomographic scan surveillance in the detection and management of brain metastases in patients with small cell lung cancer. Br J Cancer 62: 684-686, 1990.

236. Akoun GM, Scarna HM, Milleron BJ, Bénichou MP, Herman DP. Serum neuron-specific enolase. A marker for disease extent and response to therapy for small-cell lung cancer. Chest 87: 39-43, 1985.

237. Jaques GJ, Bepler G, Holle R, Wolf M. Prognostic value of pretreatment carcinoembryonic antigen, neuron-specific enolase, and creatine kinase-BB levels in sera of patients with small cell lung cancer. Cancer 62: 125-134, 1988.

238. Joorgensen LGM, Osterlind K, Hansen HH, Cooper EH. The prognostic influence of serum neuron specific enolase in small cell l ung cancer. Br J Cancer 58: 805-807, 1988.

239. Gronowitz JS, Bergström R, Nou E, et al. Clinical and serologic markers of stage and prognosis in small cell lung cancer. A multivariate analysis. Cancer 66: 722-732, 1990.

240. Harding M, McAllister J, Hulks G, et al. Neurone specific enolase (NSE) in small cell l ung cancer: a tumour marker of prognostic significance? Br J Cancer 61: 605-607, 1990.

241. Heekstra R, Splintor TAW. Prognostic value of serum thymidine kinase, tissue polypeptide antigen and neuron specific enolase in patients with small cell lung cancer. Br J Cancer 64: 369-372, 1991.

242. Johnson PWM, Joel SP, Love S, et al. Tumour markers for prediction of survival and monitoring of remission in small cell lung cancer. Br J Cancer 67: 760-766, 1993.

243. Tokuraku M, Sato H, Murakami S, et al. Activation of precursor of gelatinase A/72 kDa type IV collagenase/MMP-2 in lung carcinomas correlates with the expression of membrane-type matrix metalloproteinase [MT-MMP] and with lymph node metastasis. Int J Cancer 64: 355-359, 1995.

244. Kawano N, Osawa H, Ito T, et al. Expression of gelatinase-A, tissue inhibitor of metalloproteinase-2, matrilysin, and trypsin(ogen) in lung neoplasms: An immunohistochemical study. Hum Pathol 28: 613-622, 1997.

245. Radic PA, Mathews MJ, Ihde DC, et al. The clinical behavior of "mixed" small cell/large cell bronchogenic carcinoma compared to "pure" small cell subtypes. Cancer 50: 2894-2902, 1982.

246. Aisner SC, Finkelstein DM, Ettinger DS, et al. The clinical significance of variant morphology small cell carcinoma of the lung. J Clin Oncol 8: 402-408, 1990.

247. Sehested M, Hirsch FR, Osterlind K, et al. Morphologic variations of small cell lung cancer: a histopathologic study of pretreatment and post treatment specimens in 104 patients. Cancer 57: 804-807, 1986.

248. Osterlind K, Andersen PK. Prognostic factors in small cell l ung cancer: Multivariate model based on 778 patients treated with chemotherapy with or without irradiation. Cancer Res 46: 4189-4194, 1986.

249. Ihde DC, Makuch RW, Carney DN, et al. Prognostic implications of stage of disease and sites of metastases in patients with small cell carcinoma of the lung treated with intensive combination chemotherapy. Am Rev Respir Dis 123: 500-507, 1981.

250. Wolf M, Holle R, Hans K, et al. Analysis of prognostic factors in 766 patients with small cell lung cancer: the role of sex as a predictor for survival. Br J Cancer 63: 986-992, 1991.

251. Spiegelman D, Maurer LH, Ware JH, et al. Prognostic factors in small-cell carcinoma of the lung: An analysis of 1,521 patients. J Clin Oncol 7: 344-354, 1989.

252. Chute JP, Venzon D, Hankins L, et al. Outcome of patients with small-cell lung cancer during 20 years of clinical research at the US National Cancer Institute. Mayo Clin Proc 72: 901-912, 1997.

253. Zelen M. Keynote address on biostatistics and data retrieval. Cancer Chemother Rep 4: 31-42,1973.

254. Aisner J. Extensive disease small-cell lung cancer: The thrill of victory; the agony of defeat. J Clin Oncol 14: 658-665, 1996.

255. Johnson DE, Turrisi AT, Chang AY, Blum R, Bonomi P, Ettinger D, Wagner H. Alternating chemotherapy and twice-daily thoracic radiotherapy in limited-stage small cell lung cancer: a pilot study of the Eastern Cooperative Group. J Clin Oncol 11: 879-884, 1993.

256. McCracken JD, Janaki LM, Crowley JJ, Taylor SA, Giri PG, Weiss GB, Gordon W Jr, Baker LH, Mansouri A, Kuebler JP. Concurrent chemotherapy/radiotherapy for limited small-cell lung carcinoma: a Southwest Oncology Group Study. J Clin Oncol 8: 892-898, 1990.

257. Bunn PA Jr, Lichter AS, Makuch RW, Cohen M, Veach SR, Matthews MJ, Johnston Anderson A, Edison M, Glatstein E, Minna JD, Ihde DC. Chemotherapy alone or chemotherapy with chest radiation therapy in limited stage small-cell lung cancer. A prospective, randomized trial. Ann Intern Med 106: 655-662, 1987.

258. Turrisi AT, Kim K, Blum R, Sause WT, Livingston RB, Komaki R, Wagner H, Aisner S, Johnson DH. Twice-daily compared with once-daily thoracic radiotherapy in limited small cell lung cancer treated concurrently with cisplatin and etoposide. N Engl J Med 340: 265-271, 1999.

259. Johnson BE, Salem C, Nesbitt J, et al. Limited stage small-cell 1 ung cancer (SCLC) treated with concurrent BID chest radiotherapy (RT) and etoposide/cisplatin (VP/Pt) followed by chemotherapy (CT) selected by in vitro drug sensitivity testing (DST). Proc Am Soc Clin Oncol 10: 240, 1991 (abstract).

260. Chute JP, Chen T, Feigal E, Simon R, Johnson BE. Twenty years of phase III trials for patients with extensive stage small cell lung cancer: perceptible progress. J Clin Oncol 17: 1794-1801, 1999.

261. Pignon J-P, Arriagada R, Ihde DC, et al. A meta-analysis of thoracic radiotherapy for small cell lung cancer. N Engl J Med 327: 1618-1624, 1992.

262. Takada M, Fukuoka M, Furuse K, et al. Phase III study of concurrent vs sequential thoracic radiotherapy (TRT) in combination with cisplatin (C) and etoposide (E) for limited stage (LS) small-cell lung cancer (SCLC): preliminary

results of the Japan Clinical Oncology Group (JCOG). Proc Am Soc Clin Oncol 15: 372, 1996 (abstract)

263. Murray N, Coy P, Pater JL, et al. The importance of timing for thoracic irradiation in the combined modality treatment of limited stage small cell lung cancer. J Clin Oncol 11: 336-344, 1993.

264. Auperin A, Arriagada R, Pignon J-P, LePechoux C, Gregor A, Stephens RJ, Kristjansen PEG, Johnson BE, Ueoka H, Wagner H, Aisner J. Prophylactic cranial irradiation for patients with small-cell lung cancer in complete remission. N Eng J Med 341: 476-484, 1999.

265. Fleck JF, Einhorn LH, Lauer RC, Schultz SM, Miller ME. Is prophylactic cranial irradiation indicated in small-cell lung cancer? J Clin Oncol 8: 209-214, 1990.

266. Gregor A, Cull A, Stephens RJ, et al. Prophylactic cranial irradiation is indicated following complete response to induction therapy in small-cell lung cancer: results of a multicentre randomized trial. Eur J Cancer 33: 1752-1758, 1998.

267. Komaki R, Byhardt RW, Anderson T, et al. What is the lowest effective biologic dose for prophylactic cranial irradiation? Am J Clin Oncol 8: 523-527, 1985.

268. Shepherd FA, Ginsberg RT, Feld R, Evans WK, Johansen E. Surgical treatment for limited small cell lung cancer. J Thorac Cardiovasc Surg 101: 385-393, 1991.

269. Jacoulet P, Depierre A, Moro D, Riviere A, Milleron B, Quoix E, et al. Long-term survivors of small cell lung cancer (SCLC): a French multicenter study. Ann Oncol 8(10): 1009-1014, 1997.

270. Heyne KH, Lippman SM, Lee JS, et al. The incidence of second primary tumors in long-term survivors of small cell lung cancer. J Clin Oncol 10: 1519-1524, 1992.

271. Lassen O, Osterlind K, Hansen M. Long-term survival in small cell lung cancer: post-treatment characteristics in patients surviving 5 to 18+ years - an analysis of 1,714 consecutive patients. J Clin Oncol 13: 1215-1220, 1995.

272. Sagman U, Lishner M, Maki E, et al. Second primary malignancies following diagnosis of small cell lung cancer. J Clin Oncol 10: 1525-1533, 1992.

273. Heyne KH, Lippman SM, Lee JJ, Lee JS, Hong WK. The incidence of second primary tumors in long term survivors of small cell lung cancer. J Clin Oncol 10: 1519-1524, 1992.

274. Richardson GE, Tucker MA, Venzon DJ, et al. Smoking cessation after successful treatment of small cell lung cancer is associated with fewer smoking-related second primary cancers. Ann Intern Med 119: 383-390, 1993.

275. Morstyn G, Ihde DC, Lichter AS, Bunn PA, Carney DN, Glatstein E, Minna JD. Small cell lung cancer 1973-1983: Early progress and recent obstacles. Int J Radiat Oncol Biol Phys 10: 515-539, 1984.

276. Murray N, Shah A, Osoba D, Page R, Karsai H, Grafton C, Goddard K, Fairey R, Voss N. Intensive weekly chemotherapy for the treatment of extensive-stage small cell lung cancer. J Clin Oncol 9: 1632-1638, 1994.

277. Grant SC, Kris MG. Phase II trials in small cell lung cancer: shouldn't we be doing better? J Natl Cancer Inst 84: 1058-1059, 1992.

278. Aisner J. Identification of new drugs in small cell lung cancer: phase II agents first? Cancer Treat Rep 71: 1131-1133, 1988.

279. Johnson DH. New drugs in the management of small cell lung cancer. 5: 221-231, 1989.

280. Ettinger DS, Finkelstein DM, Abeloff MD, Skeel RT, Stott PB, Frontiera MS, Bonomi P. Justification for evaluating new anticancer drugs in selected untreated patients with extensive stage small cell lung cancer: an Eastern Cooperative Oncology Group randomized study. J Natl Cancer Inst 84: 1077-1084, 1992.

281. Grant SC, Gralla RJ, Kris MG, Orazem F, Kitsis RA. Single agent chemotherapy trials in small cell lung cancer. 1970-1990: the case for studies in previously treated patients. J Clin Oncol 10: 484-498, 1992.

282. Ettinger DS, Finkelstein DM, Abeloff MD, Ruckdeschel JC, Aisner SC, Eggleston JC. A randomized comparison of standard chemotherapy versus alternating chemotherapy and maintenance versus no maintenance therapy for extensive stage small cell lung cancer: a phase III study of the Eastern Cooperative Oncology Group. J Clin Oncol 8: 230-240, 1990.

283. Fukuoka M, Furuse K, Saijo N, Nishiwaki Y, Ikegami H, Tamura T, Shimoyama M, Suemasu K. Randomized trial of cyclophosphamide, doxorubicin, and vincristine versus cisplatin and etoposide versus alternation of these regimens in small cell lung cancer. J Natl Cancer Inst 83: 855-861, 1991.

284. Roth BJ, Johnson DH, Einhorn LH, et al. Randomized study of cyclophosphamide, doxorubicin, and vincristine versus etoposide and cisplatin versus alternation of these two regimens in extensive small cell lung cancer: a phase III trial of the Southeastern Cancer Study Group. J Clin Oncol 10: 1-11, 1992.

285. Feld M, Evans WK, Coy P, Hodson I. Canadian multicenter randomized trial comparing sequential and alternating administration of two non-cross resistant chemotherapy combinations in patients with limited small cell carcinoma of the lung. J Clin Oncol 5: 1401-1409, 1987.

286. Maksymiuk AW, Jett JR, Earle JD, et al. Sequencing and schedule effects of cisplatin plus etoposide in small cell lung cancer: Results of a North Central Cancer Treatment Group randomized clinical trial. J Clin Oncol 12: 70-76, 1994.

287. Loehrer PJ, Sr, Ansari R, Gonin R, et al. Cisplatin plus etoposide with and without ifosfamide in extensive small cell lung cancer: A Hoosier Oncology Group study. J Clin Oncol 13: 2594-2599, 1995.

288. Rowland KM Jr, Loprinzi CL, Shaw EG, et al. Randomized double-blind placebo-controlled trial of cisplatin and etoposide plus megestrol acetate/placebo in extensive-stage small-cell lung cancer: A North Central Cancer Treatment Group study. J Clin Oncol 14: 135-141, 1996.

289. Miller AA, Herndon JE II, Hollis DR, et al. Schedule dependency of 21-day oral versus 3-day intravenous etoposide in combination with intravenous cisplatin in extensive stage small cell lung cancer: A randomized phase III study of the Cancer and Leukemia Group B. J Clin Oncol 13: 1871-1879, 1995.

290. Fukuoka M, Furuse K, Saijo N, et al. Randomized trial of cyclophosphamide, doxorubicin, and vincristine versus cisplatin and etoposide versus alternation of these regimens in small cell lung cancer. J Natl Cancer Inst 83: 855-861, 1991.

291. Johnson DH, Einhorn L, Birch R, et al. A randomized comparison of high dose versus conventional dose cyclophosphamide, doxorubicin and vincristine for

extensive stage small cell lung cancer: A phase III trial of the Southeastern Cancer Study Group. J Clin Oncol 5: 1731-1738, 1987.

SURGERY FOR NON-SMALL CELL LUNG CANCER

Jocelyne Martin, M.D.
Memorial Sloan-Kettering Cancer Center, New York, NY 10021 USA

Valerie Rusch, M.D.
Memorial Sloan-Kettering Cancer Center, New York, NY 10021 USA

INTRODUCTION

Surgery remains the primary curative treatment for patients with early stage non-small cell lung cancer (NSCLC). However, the proper use of surgical resection depends on a careful assessment of the extent of disease and of cardiopulmonary function. This chapter reviews the preoperative evaluation of patients with NSCLC and discusses the role of pulmonary resection in their management.

PREOPERATIVE EVALUATION

Assessment of risks

Patients with NSCLC who undergo evaluation for lung resection are usually smokers or former smokers whose habit increases the risk of vascular, cardiac and pulmonary diseases. Because lung resection remains the most effective treatment for patients with early stage NSCLC, the functional assessment of their cardiopulmonary reserve is very important.

Major complications occur in about 9% and minor complications in 19% of elective operations for lung cancer. The overall mortality is approximately 3% for lobectomies and 6% for pneumonectomies. The majority of complications are cardiopulmonary and are known to be related to several factors, including older age, diminished cardiopulmonary reserve, and the extent of resection, particularly a right pneumonectomy (1-3). Proper case selection and careful postoperative management help minimize the risk of complications.

Cardiac assessment

The preoperative cardiac assessment of patients scheduled for pulmonary resection may be complicated by the difficulty in distinguishing between respiratory symptoms caused by cardiac disease and those caused by primary pulmonary disease. Thoracic operations carry an intermediate to high risk of cardiac complications. As defined by The American College of Cardiology and The American Heart Association (ACC/AHA), this means a combined incidence of cardiac death, congestive heart failure and non-fatal myocardial infarction of approximately 5% (4).

The cardiac assessment begins with a complete history and physical examination, and EKG. It is important not only to identify the presence of heart disease but also to determine its severity, stability and prior treatment. The ACC/AHA have established clinical markers which predict perioperative cardiovascular risk. (Table 1).

*Table 1. **Clinical predictors of increased perioperative cardiovascular risks***

Major clinical predictors
    Recent myocardial infarction (less than 1 month)
    Unstable or severe angina (Class III or IV)
    Decompensated congestive heart failure
    Significant arrhythmias
        -AV block
        -Symptomatic ventricular arrhythmias
        -Supraventricular arrhythmias with uncontrolled ventricular rate
    Severe valvular disease

Intermediate clinical predictors
    Mild angina pectoris (Class I or II)
    Prior history of myocardial infarction by history or EKG
    Compensated or prior congestive heart failure
    Diabetes mellitus

Minor clinical predictors
    Advanced age (>70)
    Abnormal EKG
    Rhythm other than sinus
    History of stroke
    Uncontrolled systemic hypertension

**Modified from ACC/AHA Guidelines*

Patients who have had a complete coronary revascularization within the last five years and who do not have recurrent signs or symptoms can go directly to the surgery. This is also true for patients who have had a recent coronary evaluation (within two years), who have stable symptoms and no active ischemia. Coronary angiography should be considered in patients who have major clinical risk factors. Coronary interventions, including coronary artery bypass grafting, angioplasty and stenting, are almost never indicated solely to reduce the risk of cardiac complication associated with a surgery so the indications of such interventions are essentially the same as those for patients not undergoing surgery.

Patients who have minor or no risk factors and good functional capacity do not require further evaluation. A good functional capacity is characterized by the ability to perform normal daily activities meeting 4-METS demand such as climbing stairs, raking leaves or playing golf (4,5). Patients who have minor or intermediate risk factors but a poor functional capacity should undergo noninvasive testing. Many NSCLC patients fall into this category. Noninvasive techniques include exercise stress testing, dobutamine stress echocardiography and radionuclide myocardial perfusion imaging. The result of those tests determine further pre-operative management (6).

Pulmonary assessment

The initial pulmonary evaluation is based on a complete history and physical examination, review of radiographic imaging studies and pulmonary function testing. In addition to detecting symptoms of comorbid diseases, the history should elicit the patient's functional capacity for exercise. Cigarette smoking history, daily cough and sputum production and history of asthma also help determine pulmonary status.

All patients considered for thoracotomy should undergo pulmonary function testing as part of their pre-operative evaluation (7). Normal test results do not require further evaluation. Particular attention is paid to the FEV1 and DLCO which are considered normal when above 80% of the predicted value based on the age and height of the patient. Recently, emphasis has shifted toward the prediction of postoperative functions such as ppoFEV1 (predicted postoperative FEV1), ppoDLCO and ppoVO2max (8,9) (10,11). These predicted values are established by applying the results of split function studies from radionuclide perfusion lung scans using the following formula for a lobectomy or a pneumonectomy : ppoFEV1=pre-opFEV1 X (1-fractional contribution of the lung or the lobe to be removed) (12). The same technique is used to predict ppoDLCO and ppoVO2max. Bolliger (13) and Wyser (14) have developed an interesting algorithm for functional assessment of lung resection candidates, especially useful for patients considered to be intermediate or high-risk for postoperative complications. (Figure 1). The radionuclide study can also be conducted before the exercise testing with the same results, as demonstrated by Nakahara. (15).

See Figure 1 on page 120.

*Figure 1. Guidelines for pre-operative functional evaluation of lung resection candidates**

Recent experience with lung volume reduction surgery for patients with emphysema has led to re-evaluation of traditional approaches to preoperative evaluation. A few patients whose poor pulmonary function would ordinarily preclude pulmonary resection can now undergo surgery if their tumor is located in an area of poorly perfused, relatively non-functional lung tissue. The pulmonary resection then also acts as a lung volume reduction operation (16,17)

Predicting complications after pulmonary resection

Various formulas have been developed to predict mortality and complications after thoracic surgery. The CPRI (cardiopulmonary risk index), developed by Epstein and colleagues from retrospective data, combines a cardiac risk index (adapted from Goldman's criteria) and a pulmonary risk index. Initially it seemed to correlate with complication and death rates (18,19). However, when prospectively applied to a large population this index failed to predict outcome reliably (20). Pierce and al proposed the use of the predicted postoperative product (PPP) as the best predictor of surgical mortality (21). The PPP is the algebraic product of the ppoFEV1% and the ppoDLCO%. This concept is attractive because it incorporates elements of ventilatory function, gas exchange, lung perfusion and proportion of lung to be resected. Their results were poor when trying to predict complication rates. Based on Pierce's methodology, Melendez et al constructed the predictive respiratory quotient (PRQ), $PRQ=(ppoFEV1\%)X(ppoDLCO\%)^2/ \text{A-a } PO2$ (22). By adding the alveolar-arterial oxygen gradient in the equation, PRQ seems to predict the outcome better than other previously devised indexes. However, this proposed index also needs to be validated prospectively.

Preparation of high-risk patients for thoracic surgery

Adequate preparation for thoracic surgery requires that the pulmonary function of each patient be maximized in order to reduce the risk of operative complications (23,24). All patients should be encouraged to quit smoking at least two to four weeks prior to surgery to decrease airway inflammation and pulmonary secretion production. In patients with reactive airways, bronchodilator treatment should be optimized and corticosteroid therapy (inhaled or occasionally short course systemic therapy) is often helpful. Antibiotic therapy is sometimes needed to treat chronic bronchitis, or postobstructive pneumonitis caused by the primary tumor.

The type of pulmonary rehabilitation usually offered to COPD patients and to patients being considered for lung transplantation or lung volume reduction surgery can also benefit lung cancer patients (25,26). Programs of supervised exercise for muscle training and pulmonary toilet, techniques for medication compliance, and nutritional support may improve surgical outcome. However, the potential benefit of preoperative rehabilitation, though a logical extension of the experience in patients with benign disease, is not as well proven in lung cancer patients.

CLINICAL STAGING

All patients with NSCLC should be thoroughly evaluated to determine whether extrathoracic metastases are present using a standardized approach to preoperative assessment. Guidelines for this have been developed by several institutions that care for large numbers of lung cancer patients (27,28).

Noninvasive clinical staging

The first step is a clinical evaluation to detect locoregional invasion and extrathoracic metastases. The most common sites of metastatic disease at diagnosis are the brain, bones, liver and adrenals, in that order. The clinical evaluation should be oriented accordingly(29). The history should then particularly elicit constitutional symptoms such as weight loss, musculoskeletal pain or neurological symptoms (30). Signs that can be found on physical examination include cervical or supraclavicular lymphadenopathy, hoarseness, superior vena cava syndrome, bone tenderness, hepatomegaly, focal neurologic signs or soft tissue mass among others. Routine blood tests are drawn to rule out elevated calcium level or increased hepatic enzymes. A normal clinical evaluation indicates that the likelihood of finding metastases on further investigation is low. Abnormal findings on clinical evaluation warrant further investigation by appropriate imaging studies because metastatic disease will be documented in approximately half of these patients (31).

Chest X-Ray and CT scan of the chest and upper abdomen, including the adrenals, are the most common imaging studies done prior to diagnosis. Although CT scan defines the extent of the primary tumor and may diagnose metastatic disease to the liver and adrenals, it has only a 65% accuracy in detecting mediastinal nodal metastases. MRI has no advantage over CT in this regard (32-35).

After preliminary screening, staging recommendations are subsequently more individualized and are based on the patient's signs and symptoms and laboratory and imaging results. When clinically indicated, an ultrasound or CT of the liver with contrast, CT scan with contrast or MRI of the brain, or a radionuclide bone scan may be performed, all with or without biopsy.

Invasive clinical staging

The most important reason to use invasive techniques for clinical staging is to determine the likelihood of a complete resection (R0), and avoid primary surgical treatment in patients who have mediastinal node metastases. This is especially important since the widespread acceptance of induction therapy in such patients. Preoperative identification of T4 disease is more difficult and sometimes may not be identified until the time of the surgery.

Bronchoscopy

Flexible bronchoscopy is a good technique for the evaluation and staging of lung cancers. It allows visual assessment of an endobronchial tumor, and biopsy for tissue diagnosis. It helps plan the pulmonary resection, may identify an unexpected second primary tumor and permits evaluation of vocal cord function. However, bronchoscopy has a limited role in the assessment of mediastinal lymph nodes. Trans-bronchial biopsy of enlarged lymph nodes causing extrinsic airway compression has an overall sensitivity of 50%, even when guided by a prior chest CT scan (36,37), and is much less reliable than mediastinoscopy.

Mediastinoscopy

Cervical mediastinoscopy is the most commonly employed invasive staging procedure. The sensitivity (87%), specificity (100%) and accuracy (95%) of mediastinoscopy make it the best staging modality available today(34). Patients should undergo mediastinoscopy if they have enlarged mediastinal nodes (1 cm or greater in diameter by CT scan). However, cervical mediastinoscopy does not provide good access to lymph nodes in the aorto-pulmonary window. These nodes are particularly important in patients with left upper lobe tumors because they are usually the first site of regional metastases.

The extended mediastinoscopy, described by Ginsberg in 1987, provides access to these nodes (38). Through the standard cervical mediastinoscopy incision, the mediastinoscope is passed over the aortic arch between the innominate and left carotid arteries. Atherosclerosis of the aorta contraindicates this difficult technique and experience is required for this procedure to be successful. For these reasons, anterior or parasternal mediastinotomy (Chamberlain procedure) through the bed of the left second costal cartilage or second rib interspace is the more popular approach to biopsying the aortopulmonary window (levels 5 and 6) lymph nodes.

Scalene lymph node biopsy

Scalene lymph node biopsy was widely used before the development of cervical mediastinoscopy. It has largely been abandoned in favor of needle aspiration of palpable nodes. In 1996, Lee and Ginsberg reassessed the potential utility of this technique in detecting scalene node metastases, which are generally considered a contraindication to surgical resection (39). When N2 or N3 disease was suspected clinically, they performed an ipsilateral scalene lymph node biopsy through the cervical mediastinoscopy incision using the mediastinoscope to reach the scalene fat pad. Microscopic scalene lymph node metastases were identified in 15% of patients staged as having N2 disease and in 68% of patients found to have N3 disease by mediastinoscopy. Therefore a small but definite percentage of patients thought to have only N2 disease by mediastinoscopy will benefit from this additional staging procedure, and will avoid a subsequent inappropriate pulmonary resection.

Thoracoscopy

Thoracoscopy or VATS (video assisted thoracic surgery) is another technique used to stage the ipsilateral hemithorax. Paratracheal and hilar lymph nodes can be biopsied. In the left hemithorax, thoracoscopy is particularly useful for accessing the preaortic and aortopulmonary nodes. Thoracoscopy also allows evaluation of lymph nodes that can not be assessed with any other surgical staging method: posterior mediastinal, inferior pulmonary ligament and paraesophageal nodes (40). The anterior mediastinum is still best assessed by cervical mediastinoscopy, and thoracoscopy may be utilized when other surgical staging procedures have failed to define the status of locoregional involvement. In addition, VATS may be helpful in evaluating whether the primary tumor directly invades mediastinal structures (T4 disease) and whether pleural metastases are present.

Transesophageal ultrasound

Transesophageal ultrasound with needle aspiration biopsies of deep subcarinal and posterior paraesophageal mediastinal lymph nodes may improve the preoperative evaluation of patients with suspicious contralateral posterior mediastinal or bulky subcarinal nodes but its current role is still not fully defined (41,42).

Future directions

A relatively new imaging modality, the FDG-PET (positron emission tomography with 2-fluorine-18-fluorodeoxyglucose) is under investigation to assess its ability in improving non-invasive staging. Small single institution studies suggest that PET-FDG is more accurate than CT in detecting mediastinal nodal metastases. However, like all radionuclide imaging studies, PET lacks spatial resolution. Whether the combined analysis of the mediastinum by CT with PET can potentially replace mediastinoscopy remains to be seen and the subject of ongoing multi-institutional trials. PET may be more accurate than CT in detecting metastatic disease in some sites such as bone marrow, the adrenals or the liver, but this also requires further investigation (43-45). Conversely it may be less accurate than CT or MRI in detecting brain metastases.

The use of molecular markers performed on biopsies of the primary tumor or mediastinal nodes is not yet part of the clinical staging of lung cancer patients (46). However, in the future, such markers may contribute to the selection of treatment.

A table summarizing preoperative staging modalities is shown in Table 2. The selection of these modalities must be individualized for each patient, and will evolve in the future as new technologies emerge and a better understanding of tumor biology is achieved. In general, patients considered to have a clinical Stage I tumor do not require an extensive evaluation for metastatic disease because the yield in such cases is low. However, clinical Stage II and especially Stage III patients should undergo a meticulous evaluation for mediastinal and distant metastases.

Table 2. **Preoperative evaluation for clinical staging**

Recommended for all patients	
	History and physical examination
	Complete blood count
	Serum electrolytes, calcium, liver enzymes, creatinine
	Chest radiograph
	CT scan of the chest including adrenals
	*Pathologic confirmation of malignancy
Recommended for selected patients	
Non invasive	CT scan of liver/ultrasound
	CT scan of brain/MRI
Invasive :	Bronchoscopy +/- Transbronchial needle biopsy
	Mediastinoscopy +/- Parasternal mediastinotomy
	Thoracoscopy
	Adrenal, liver or other biopsy to rule out metastasis
	? Scalene lymph node biopsy
	? Transesophageal lymph node biopsy
Future :	
	PET-FDG scan
	Molecular markers

**May not be necessary in cases where the patient will undergo surgical resection regardless of the outcome of the biopsy.*

SURGICAL MANAGEMENT

Stage I and II NSCLC are best treated by surgical resection. Specific groups of patients with stage III disease also benefit from pulmonary resection, usually in combination with other treatment modalities. The goals of surgery are to remove the primary tumor completely and to stage it definitively. The guiding principles of an adequate oncologic operation are a microscopically complete (RO) resection; an en bloc removal of tumor with resection, when necessary, of involved adjacent structures (e.g. chest wall); and complete peribronchial, hilar and mediastinal nodal sampling or dissection.

The operation should provide microscopically negative vascular and bronchial margins. Margins should be assessed by frozen-section analysis and re-excision performed if positive margins are encountered. All lymph nodes removed should be appropriately identified and labeled by the surgeon for the pathologist.

Stage I and II disease

The extent of pulmonary resection is dictated by the location and the size of the primary tumor and by whether there is involvement of the adjacent bronchopulmonary nodes. Depending on these factors, a lobectomy, a bilobectomy, or a pneumonectomy is the appropriate operation and should provide microscopically negative margins.

Lesser resections by wedge excision or segmentectomy have been advocated by some for early stage tumors in retrospective studies. The North American Lung Cancer Study Group performed a randomized clinical trial comparing lobectomy to lesser resection by wedge or segmentectomy in peripheral stage IA carcinoma (47). Patients undergoing limited resection experienced a higher rate of locoregional recurrence. The risk of distant metastases was unaffected by the type of pulmonary resection. The death rate from cancer was lower in the lobectomy group but the observed difference did not reach statistical significance. Although lobectomy patients had a greater decrease in pulmonary function during the initial postoperative period, there was no significant difference in pulmonary function between the two patient groups long term. Limited pulmonary resections should then be confined to patients with very limited pulmonary reserve who might not otherwise tolerate the early decrease in lung function accompanying a lobectomy. Such patients should be carefully evaluated to determine whether lobectomy might actually benefit them by also allowing lung volume reduction (16). They should be monitored closely after surgery for possible local recurrence, usually by serial CT scans.

Tumors confined to the lung or bronchus with involvement of hilar or broncho-pulmonary lymph nodes (T1-2,N1) make up approximately 10% of all resected lung cancers (48). The Memorial Sloan-Kettering Cancer Center reviewed its experience with stage II NSCLC and noted that 83% of patients with T1N1 lesions had adenocarcinomas whereas in T2N1 lesions squamous cell and adenocarcinoma histologies were of equal frequency. The procedure of choice to encompass all disease in most cases is a lobectomy, but in some cases a bilobectomy or a pneumonectomy will be required.

Clinical staging of mediastinal nodes is inaccurate and should not be substituted for careful intraoperative staging. Complete en bloc mediastinal lymph node dissection is advocated by some groups as the most accurate means of staging (49,50). For right-sided tumors, this involves en bloc removal of the entire subcarinal packet of nodes (level 7 nodes) and en bloc removal of all paratracheal lymph nodes located between the trachea posteriorly, the superior vena cava anteriorly, the innominate artery superiorly, and the tracheo-bronchial angle inferiorly (level 4R nodes). For left-sided tumors, the dissection includes en bloc removal of the subcarinal nodes and of the subaortic and periaortic nodes (levels 5 and 6 nodes). If technically accessible, the left tracheobronchial angle nodes (level 4L nodes) are also removed. Whether this extensive dissection results in more accurate staging than simply sampling lymph nodes from each one of the levels remains controversial and is under investigation in a nationwide randomized trial. No survival or local recurrence advantage have been shown until now but there is no doubt that a meticulous pathologic staging provides accurate prognostic information and allows appropriate decisions to be made regarding the use of postoperative adjuvant therapy (48). No matter which method is chosen, each lymph node group should be identified by the surgeon and submitted appropriately labeled to the pathologist using standard nomenclature and numbering system.

Tumors with direct extension into the chest wall, diaphragm, or pericardium (T3 tumors) should undergo resection of the adjacent involved structure en bloc with the pulmonary resection (51). Reconstruction is performed as necessary. Tumors that have extensive endobronchial component can sometimes be completely removed by a lobectomy with segmental resection of the bronchus (sleeve resection), thereby preserving lung function. These options are discussed below.

Stage III disease

Many of these locally advanced tumors, particularly T3 and/or N2 diseases (stage IIIA), are amenable to combined modality therapy that includes surgery. However, very few stage IIIB cases will be considered for operation by most thoracic surgeons. The most controversial and complex part of treatment of lung cancer is probably the management of patients with IIIA-N2 disease and the first step in almost all cases of stage III disease will be to perform a mediastinoscopy to determine whether mediastinal lymph node metastases are present.

Tumors invading the chest wall

Although the majority of resectable lung cancers are confined to the pulmonary parenchyma, approximately 5% will invade the parietal pleura or the chest wall. Even with chest wall invasion, a significant number of these patients are amenable to treatment by resection. Factors consistently found to influence prognosis are the extent of nodal involvement and the completeness of the resection. The depth of chest wall invasion is probably not a significant independent prognostic factor if the resection is complete (52).

Now that reconstruction of the chest wall with appropriate prosthetic material is standard practice, en bloc and extrapleural resections are associated with similar surgical mortality rates that are related to the extent of the underlying pulmonary resection, and not to the extent of the chest wall resection itself.

The importance of complete resection in these patients is illustrated by the experience at Memorial Sloan-Kettering Cancer Center, where 334 patients with carcinoma of the lung invading the chest wall were treated surgically from 1974 to 1993 (52). The 175 patients who had a complete resection (R0) experienced an overall 5-year survival of 32%, whereas those who had incomplete resection with microscopic (R1) or macroscopic residual disease (R2) had an overall 5-year survival of 4%. None of the patients who had exploration only survived 5 years. Postoperative adjuvant radiation did not improve survival, a finding which has been confirmed in other series (53).

These tumors can be resected en bloc or via an extrapleural approach. The Memorial series suggests that some patients whose tumors clinically involve the parietal pleura can be adequately treated by an extrapleural mobilization of the tumor without an en bloc resection of the chest wall, providing the pleural margins are histologically negative. However, the decision to omit chest wall resection requires considerable experience and careful intraoperative evaluation of tumor extent. If the tumor is fixed or if there is any doubt as to the possibility of malignancy extending into the deep tissues, an en bloc resection must be performed. It should be noted that many authors such as DeMeester and Pairolero advocate en bloc resection of the chest wall in all cases (54,55). Using either approach, histologically negative margins must be obtained in order to achieve long-term survival.

The presence of hilar or mediastinal nodes adversely affects survival despite a complete resection. The 5-year survival of patients with T3N0 disease who have a R0 resection is 49%, whereas it is 27% for T3N1 tumors and only 15% for completely resected T3N2 tumors (52). Because effective induction therapy is now available for locally advanced NCSLC, a mediastinoscopy should be considered in the preoperative assessment of patients with suspected chest wall involvement.

Small chest wall defects of two ribs or less may not require reconstruction, especially if situated posteriorly, beneath the scapula. However, most anterior and lateral defects require reconstruction as do posterior defects located at or before the tip of the scapula. Some surgeons, particularly the Mayo Clinic group, routinely use a 2 mm. thickness Gore-Tex patch (56). However, other groups, including Memorial Sloan-Kettering Cancer Center, advocate the use of Marlex mesh methyl methacrylate sandwich prosthesis because it provides absolute stability and can be molded to the contour of the chest wall even for very large anterolateral defects (57).

Superior sulcus tumors

Superior sulcus tumors (Pancoast tumors) represent a subset of carcinoma of the lung invading the chest wall. Because of their unique location in the pleural apex, they invade surrounding tissues early. Superior sulcus tumors are generally defined as T3 tumors but invasion of brachial plexus, mediastinal structures, or vertebral bodies is classified as T4. The staging of lymph node involvement and distant metastases is the same as for other NSCLC tumor subsets but some surgeons including Spaggiari think that supraclavicular (scalene) metastases are the most direct and first site of nodal metastases and should be considered as N1 nodes (58). In the absence of distant metastases, these tumors are by definition either stage IIB, IIIA or IIIB because of the status of the primary tumor.

Patients with tumors of the superior sulcus are often symptomatic from the onset. Characteristic symptoms and signs include: shoulder and arm pain radiating to the inner aspect of the upper arm and fourth and fifth fingers caused by involvement of the lower brachial plexus (mainly T1 and C8 nerve roots); atrophy and weakness of the muscles of the hand; Horner's syndrome caused by involvement of the sympathetic chain, including the stellate ganglion; and local rib erosion or vertebral body infiltration. These signs and symptoms define the typical Pancoast syndrome, described in 1924 (59). T3 Pancoast tumors will manifest only some of these symptoms, typically pain and numbness radiating down the arm and hand, whereas T4 tumor usually manifest all of these characteristics.

Most NSCLC of the superior sulcus are initially diagnosed by percutaneous transthoracic needle biopsy and are either squamous cell or adenocarcinomas. Magnetic resonance imaging is helpful in defining involvement of the brachial plexus, subclavian vessels, vertebral bodies and spinal canal.

Tumors of the superior sulcus were for a long time considered unresectable and incurable. However, in 1961 Shaw and Paulson first described the use of preoperative radiation therapy (3000 cGy in 10 fractions) followed by surgical resection. They documented long-term survival in approximately 30% of patients and as a result this approach became a standard of care for many years (60). However, the recent widespread use of induction chemotherapy and chemoradiation for Stage IIIA (N2) NSCLC has prompted investigations of this approach for tumors of the superior sulcus. An intergroup North American trial testing induction chemoradiation has recently been completed and is being analyzed.

The overall 5-year survival rate for resected patients remains approximately 30%, emphasizing the need to test novel therapies in this group of NSCLC patients. Survival is worse for patients with T4 tumors, N2 and N3 disease, Horner's syndrome and incomplete resection (61,62). It must be emphasized again that mediastinoscopy should be performed before surgical resection in any patient suspected to have N2 disease preoperatively. Contraindication to surgery vary from group to group but T4N2 is considered an absolute contraindication to operation (58). Other contraindications may include extensive involvement of the brachial plexus and paraspinal region, invasion of soft tissue of the neck and N2 disease (63).

Several technical approaches for the resection of superior sulcus tumors have been introduced since Paulson's original description of an extended posterolateral thoracotomy (64). (Figure 2) This classic incision is preferred for tumors arising posteriorly in the lung apex. For anteriorly located tumors, where adherence to the subclavian vessels is suspected, an anterior approach is often appropriate. Dartevelle described an anterior transcervical-thoracic approach also called transclavicular (65). (Figure 3) When using an anterior access, a combined posterolateral thoracotomy may be necessary to complete the resection when the tumor also invades the posterior chest wall. Spaggiari et al recently proposed the use of a transmanubrial osteomuscular sparing approach combined with an antero-lateral muscle-sparing thoracotomy (66). (Figure 4) This incision has some advantages over Dartevelle's approach including better exposure to facilitate pulmonary resection and lymph node dissection. The clavicle and its muscular insertions are also preserved. Another variant is the combination of a partial sternotomy, an anterior thoracotomy or so-called hemiclamshell incision along with a neck incision along the anterior border of the sternocleidomastoid muscle (67). (Figure 5)

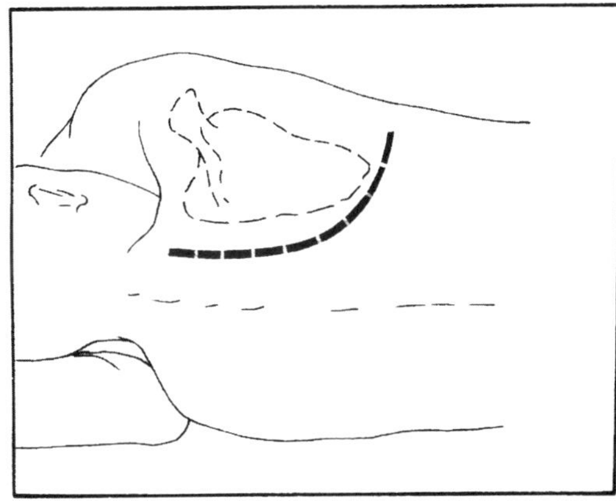

Figure 2. Extended posterolateral incision. From Cooper JD, Urschel JC Jr. Superior pulmonary sulcus carcinoma resection: Posterior approach. In Atlas of Thoracic Surgery. New York: Churchill Livingstone, 1995, p. 181.

All these procedures are potentially appropriate as long as several principles are followed : 1) removal of the pulmonary component by at least a lobectomy (versus a wedge resection) (61; 63), 2) en bloc resection including chest wall and adjacent structures (nerve roots, subclavian artery or vein, vertebral body) to achieve complete resection, 3) the addition of external radiation either preoperatively or postoperatively. The addition of preoperative chemotherapy or chemoradiation may improve the rates of resectability and overall survival but the routine use of this approach awaits the results of ongoing clinical trials.

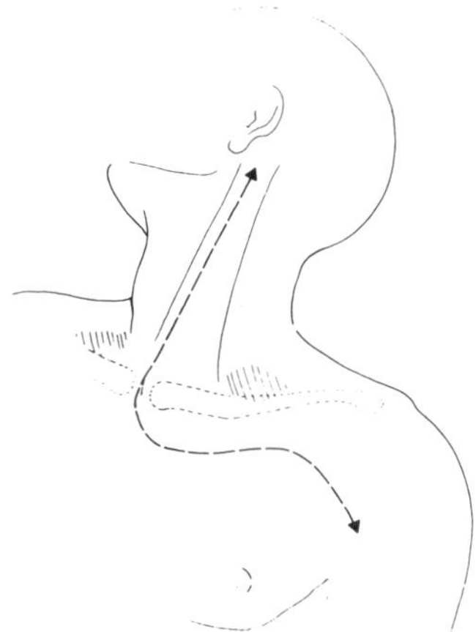

Figure 3. Transclavicular approach. From: Macchiarini P, Dartevelle P, Chapelier A et al. Technique for resecting primary and metastatic nonbronchogenic tumors of the thoracic outlet. Ann Thorac Surg 1993;55:p.613.

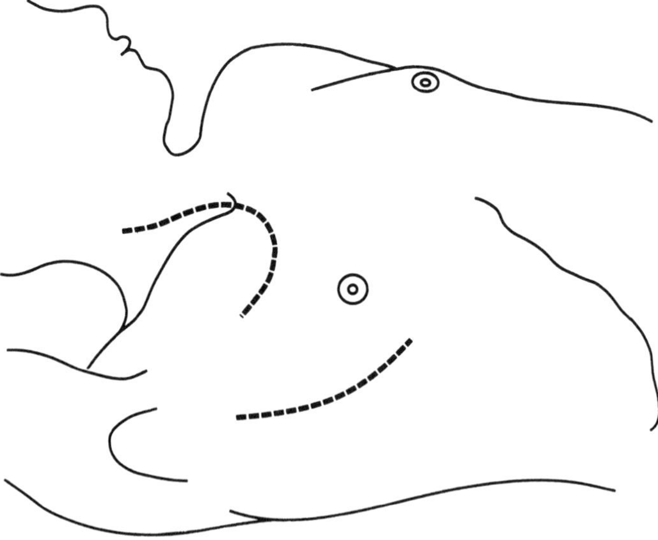

Figure 4. Transmanubrial approach. From: Spaggiari L, Pastorino U. Transmanubrial approach with antero-lateral thoracotomy for apical chest tumor. Ann Thorac Surg 1999;68:p.591.

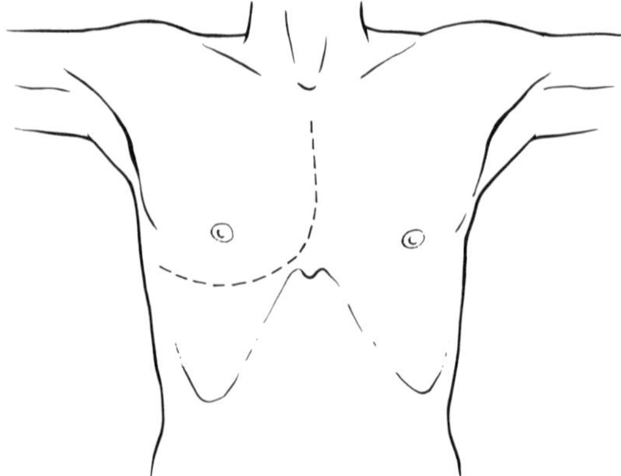

Figure 5. Hemiclamshell. From: Bains MS, Ginsberg RJ, Jones WG, et al. The clamshell incision: An improved approach to bilateral pulmonary and mediastinal tumor. Ann Thorac Surg 1994;58: p.31.

Tumor invading the mediastinal pleura, the pericardium or diaphragm

There are few reports describing the results of surgical resection of tumors invading only the mediastinal pleura, pericardium or diaphragm (T3 disease). Studies often pool data from T3 and T4 tumors making stage-specific interpretation difficult. However, the extent of mediastinal involvement (T3 versus T4) does appear to influence resectability and survival independent of N status (68). Overall, complete resection of T3 tumors invading the pericardium or mediastinal pleura is associated with a 5-year survival of 30% (69,70). When the N status is taken into consideration the 5-year survival for T3N0 tumors is approximately 45%, as compared to 37% for T3N1 and 0% for T3N2 tumors (70). These results underscore the importance of performing a mediastinoscopy to exclude the presence of N2 disease prior to resection of T3 mediastinal tumors.

To our knowledge, only one small report is available on the management of lung cancer directly invading the diaphragm (71). This appears to be a particularly unusual presentation of NSCLC. A review of the Memorial Sloan-Kettering Cancer Center database from 1974 to 1995 identified only 8 patients who had exploratory thoracotomy for resection of NSCLC invading the diaphragm, representing 0.17% of all patients undergoing thoracotomy at that institution. Four of these patients were also found to have N2 disease and their survival was extremely poor, with a median of only 92 weeks. The cancer-specific survival of the 4 patients who had N0 disease could not be defined because 3 of them died of unrelated causes and the fourth patient was still alive with no evidence of disease at 69 weeks postoperatively. Again, mediastinoscopy to detect N2 disease is clearly very important to avoid resection in patients who will not benefit from it.

Tumors in proximity to carina

Patients who have tumors located within 2 cm of the carina also benefit from surgical resection. In those cases where the tumor is in proximity to the carina without invading it, a sleeve lobectomy is often an appropriate alternative to pneumonectomy. Sleeve resections allow conservation of lung tissue and can be performed when the primary tumor involves a major lobar orifice (usually the right upper lobe) and does not have a significant peribronchial component. A sleeve resection entails the resection of a portion of the mainstem bronchus and the lobar orifice with anastomosis of the residual distal bronchus to the proximal mainstem bronchus. Although originally performed only for low-grade tumors, sleeve resections are now recognized to yield long-term survival equivalent to that of standard lobectomy or pneumonectomy. The operative mortality is 2 to 5% (less than a pneumonectomy) and the complication rate is approximately the same as after a pneumonectomy (72-74).

In a review of 142 cases, Mehran and Deslauriers suggest that sleeve resection is adequate for patients with resectable lung cancer and N0 or N1 status (73). For patients with N0 status, the 5- and 10-year survivals were 57% and 46%, and were 46% and 27% for patients with N1 disease. N2 disease significantly worsened the prognosis, with no patient surviving 5 years. Faber has suggested that sleeve lobectomy should be the operation of choice when the extent of the tumor permits, even if the patient can tolerate a pneumonectomy and this is now a generally accepted recommendation (72).

N2 disease

Considerable controversy exists regarding the ideal treatment of stage IIIA-N2 disease. Reported 5-year survival rates after resection for N2 disease are usually 20-30% but range from 0 to 40%. Many series report an inappropriately optimistic view of the benefit of surgical resection for N2 disease because they focus on highly selected groups of patients.

The experience reported by Martini and Flehinger in 1983 places surgical resection for N2 disease in perspective because it examines the outcome of treatment of all patients with N2 disease, not just a small subset (75). From 1974 to 1981, 1598 patients were seen with non-small cell lung cancer, of whom 706 had mediastinal nodal metastases. Only 151 patients, or 21% of all patients with N2 disease, had technically complete resections of the primary tumor and all accessible mediastinal lymph nodes. The survival rate of these 151 patients was 29% at 5 years. Moreover, the subset of 33 patients who had clinical N2 disease (mediastinal nodal involvement extensive enough to be visible on chest radiograph or at bronchoscopy) had only an 8% survival rate at 3 years. Thus, only 16.7% of all patients really benefited in the long term from surgical resection.

With respect to mediastinal lymph node involvement, several prognostic factors have been identified. The outcome is especially poor for patients who have clinical N2 disease (mediastinal adenopathy visible on chest X-ray), for patients with multiple levels of mediastinal nodal metastases, extracapsular nodal disease, and for large primary tumors (76,77). The survival also seems to be worse for patients whose N2 disease is established at mediastinoscopy than in patients with a negative mediastinoscopy found to have N2 disease at subsequent thoracotomy (78,79). Patients who have left upper lobe tumors with nodal metastases confined to the aortopulmonary window nodes also appear to have a more favorable prognosis with a 5-year survival of approximately 40% (79,80). Today, most surgeons will only consider resection for patients who have a T1 or T2 primary tumor and single-level, intra-nodal N2 disease, in the setting of a negative mediastinoscopy.

Although a few patients with minimal N2 disease benefit from surgical resection as their primary form of treatment, most patients have more extensive nodal involvement and are not surgical candidates. Until the 1980s, the standard treatment for such patients was radiation. The survival after radiation is harder to interpret than after surgical resection because most series include a mixture of stage IIIA and IIIB patients and do not define the precise extent of nodal involvement. Sequential trials by the Radiation Therapy Oncology Group showed that high-dose, continuous irradiation yields the best chance of local control (81). Distant metastatic disease, however, is the dominant form of relapse after radiation, just as it is after surgical resection. For this reason, chemotherapy has been investigated as adjuvant postoperative therapy in patients with N2 disease. Unfortunately, multiple prospective clinical trials have failed to show a survival benefit for adjuvant chemotherapy (82). The poor long-term survival, the risk of distant metastatic disease, and the development of well tolerated chemotherapy regimens prompted investigation of preoperative or so-called neoadjuvant therapy for stage III non-small cell lung cancer.

Many trials have now explored various neoadjuvant regimens. Chemotherapy is now the primary treatment for most patients with stage IIIA-N2 disease, with surgical resection, radiation, or both added to optimize control of locoregional disease. This is discussed in detail in another chapter.

Locally advanced tumors-T4 or N3

Patients presenting with supraclavicular or contralateral mediastinal lymph node metastases (N3), invasion of the spine, trachea, carina, esophagus, aorta or heart, or malignant pleural effusion (T4) are generally considered inoperable. Most of these patients are candidates for radiation, chemotherapy, or both. Only a few may be considered for surgical resection.

Tumor invading the carina

Reports of resection of lesions extending to or invading the carina have shown a 5-year survival of approaching 20% in carefully selected patients (65). However, pneumonectomy with tracheal sleeve resection and direct anastomosis of the contralateral mainstem bronchus to the trachea (sleeve resection) is associated with 10 to 30% operative mortality and complication rates of 40% (83,84). Sleeve pneumonectomy should therefore be reserved for young healthy patients with completely resectable tumors and should be performed by thoracic surgeons and anesthesiologists experienced in airway surgery. Mediastinal nodal metastases diagnosed by mediastinoscopy, are considered a contraindication to carinal resection because they are associated with an extremely poor survival (83).

Tumor invading the mediastinum

T4 tumors invading the mediastinal structures, especially the aorta, esophagus, or vertebral body can be completely resected in highly selected cases (85). Incomplete resection does not improve survival. Of 44 patients at Memorial Sloan-Kettering Cancer Center who had tumors invading the mediastinum, only 8 underwent a complete resection, and only 1 patient was alive 5 years postoperatively (68). Based on these findings, most T4 tumors invading the mediastinum should be considered for combined modality therapy (86).

N3 disease

Contralateral mediastinal and supraclavicular lymph node disease have traditionally been considered to be absolute contraindications to surgical resection because of poor long-term survival. The initial experience with induction therapy followed by surgical resection suggested that complete resection rates and short-term survival might be similar to those seen for N2 disease. In a prospective Phase II trial of induction chemoradiation and surgical resection performed by the Southwest Oncology Group, 7 of 9 patients with contralateral mediastinal nodes, and 7 of 18 patients with supraclavicular nodes were completely resected (87). However, the long-term survival of these patients was very poor, suggesting that such patients are best treated non-surgically (88). In a German phase II trial with preoperative chemoradiation therapy followed by surgical resection, 13 of 18 patients with involved mediastinal N3 nodes on initial assessment were free of mediastinal disease on repeat mediastinoscopy and thoracotomy (89). However, the long-term results in this trial were not provided and the benefit of adding surgical resection to chemoradiation is at present highly questionable.

Stage IV

In general, stage IV NSCLC is not managed surgically. However, when locoregional control of the lung tumor is achieved, solitary site metastatic disease may be amenable to surgical resection. It is especially indicated for solitary brain and adrenal metastases. Patients with solitary brain metastases who undergo surgical resection and radiation live longer, have fewer recurrences in the brain and have better quality of life than similar patients treated with radiation alone (90). The 1-year and median survival after resection of a solitary brain metastasis are reported to be 55% and 14 months respectively (91). In our institution, the management of solitary brain metastasis is as follows: if a brain lesion is detected and the search for the primary is negative, the cranial metastasis is resected. Resection of a metachronous metastasis is also the treatment of choice if no other site of recurrence is present. When synchronous brain and lung lesions are detected, if both are resectable, craniotomy is done first followed by thoracotomy. If either brain or lung tumor is suspected to be unresectable, surgical treatment is first directed to the site where resectability is questioned most. If one or the other is unresectable, non-surgical therapy is recommended. Postoperative brain irradiation usually follows resection of brain metastases (92). The survival of patients with a metachronous metastasis is more favorable than that of patients with synchronous metastases, and is approximately 15 to 20% at 5 years

POST-RESECTION FOLLOW-UP

Complete resection is the therapy of choice for localized NSCLC. Determinants of survival are the stage of the cancer and its complete resectability. The 5-year survivals following complete resection are approximately 80% in stage IA, 70% in stage IB, 50% in stage II and 25-30% in stage IIIA (92,93). Recurrences after apparently complete resection develop in approximately 25-30% of patients with stage I disease, in 50% of those with stage II and in 70-80% in stage III over the following 5 years (48,93). Locoregional recurrences and distal metastases are detected most frequently in the first 24 months after operation. Recurrences of the original primary tumor are infrequent after 5 years. Systemic relapse is more common than locoregional disease and is seen in 70% of patients (48,93,94).

The risk of developing a second lung cancer or other aerodigestive tumor in patients who have been treated for NSCLC is approximately 10-fold higher than for other adult smokers. The risk of developing a second lung cancer is approximately 2.5% per patient per year, and approximately one half of the patients who develop a second NCSLC can have their tumor resected. The survival of patients treated by resection for their second primary lung cancer is similar to patients who have been treated for a first NSCLC, stage for stage (95,96). It has also been shown that the chance of developing a second cancer is greater than the chance of a recurrence after 5 years from the initial resection.

In 1975, Martini and Melamed developed clinical criteria to differentiate a second lung primary from a recurrence (97). (Table 3)

Table 3. **Criteria for the diagnosis of multiple metachronous lung cancers**

I. Different histologic types	

II. Same histologic type if:	a) Disease-free interval between cancers is at least 2 years or
	b) Originate from carcinoma in situ or
	c) Second cancer in different lobe or lung but:
	    1. No carcinoma in lymphatics common to both
	    2. No extrapulmonary metastases at time of diagnosis

The effectiveness of routine follow-up has never been studied in a prospective manner and it has never been demonstrated that follow-up improves the survival of patients with recurrent disease, despite the fact that earlier detection may occur in some cases (98). Data are thus insufficient to support firm recommendations for postoperative monitoring. However, the practice in our center is quite similar to the guidelines suggested by the National Comprehensive Cancer Network and the American Society of Clinical Oncology (28,99). After the immediate postoperative period, a visit is scheduled every 3 months for the first year, every 4 months for the second, every 6 months for the third and forth years, and once a year thereafter. In addition to symptoms of complications related to the surgery, specific symptoms of locoregional recurrence are sought: recurrent or new chest pain, persistent cough, hemoptysis, hoarseness or symptoms of superior vena cava obstruction. Non specific signs such as weight loss and anorexia may herald recurrent disease. Visual disturbances, mental changes, seizures, speech or gait disturbances or new skeletal pain suggest distant metastases. Physical examination may reveal supraclavicular adenopathies, abnormal lung sounds, enlarged liver or chest wall recurrence. Each visit includes a chest radiograph that has to be compared with previous ones. Additional imaging studies are ordered only if suspicious signs, symptoms or radiographic changes are found.

Although blood tests are not routinely performed, serial CEA (carcinoembryonic antigen) assessment may be valuable in patients with adenocarcinoma in whom the antigen was elevated prior to surgery and normalized shortly after. Surveillance bronchoscopy is reserved for patients with known severe dysplasia or carcinoma in situ at the resection margin or patients with signs suggesting recurrent disease. Low-dose helical chest CT scan, presently under investigation for screening of lung cancer, has the potential to detect second primary lung cancers early and at a lower cost than standard CT (100). The role of sputum cytology coupled with monoclonal antibody staining for the early detection of second primary lung cancers is also currently under investigation. However, the optimal methods for follow-up of NSCLC patients after resection both for the detection of recurrent disease and second primary lung cancers require further investigation.

CONCLUSION

Surgical resection remains the mainstay of treatment for patients with early stage NSCLC. However, it is essential that patients be properly staged and their cardiopulmonary function carefully evaluated preoperatively. Surgical resection alone is no longer the accepted treatment for most patients with locally advanced (Stage III) NSCLC with nodal metastases (N2 or N3 disease) because combined modality regimens incorporating surgery have led to improved survival in this group of patients. However, some patients with tumors that are locally advanced by T status (T3 or T4) benefit from surgical resection if nodal metastases are not present. Surgical resection is occasionally useful in the treatment of Stage IV NSCLC, primarily for the resection of isolated metastases. The role of surgical resection in NSCLC continues to evolve as a better understanding of the disease, and of tumor biology emerge, and better systemic therapy becomes available.

REFERENCES

1. Nagasaki F, Flehinger BJ, Martini N. Complications of surgery in the treatment of carcinoma of the lung. Chest 82:25-9, 1982.
2. Deslauriers J, Ginsberg RJ, Dubois P, Beaulieu M, Goldberg M, Piraux M. Current operative morbidity associated with elective surgical resection for lung cancer. Can.J.Surg. 32:335-9, 1989.
3. Ginsberg RJ, Hill LD, Eagan RT, et al. Modern thirty-day operative mortality for surgical resections in lung cancer. J.Thorac.Cardiovasc.Surg. 86:654-8, 1983.
4. Ritchie JL, ACC/AHA Task Force on Practice Guidelines. ACC/AHA Guidelines for perioperative cardiovascular evaluation for noncardiac surgery. Circulation. 1996;93:1280-317, 1996.
5. Teplick R. Preoperative cardiac assessment of the thoracic surgical patient. Chest Surg Clin N Amer 7:655-94, 1997.
6. Eagle KA, Coley CM, Newell JB, et al. Combining clinical and thallium data optimizes preoperative assessment of cardiac risk before major vascular surgery. Ann Int Med 110:859-66, 1989.
7. Zibrak JD, O'Donnell CR, Marton K. Indications for pulmonary function testing. Ann Int Med 112:763-71, 1990.
8. Nakahara K, Ohno K, Hashimoto J, et al. Prediction of postoperative respiratory failure in patients undergoing lung resection for lung cancer. Ann Thorac Surg 46:549-52, 1988.
9. Ferguson MK, Reeder LB, Mick R. Optimizing selection of patients for major lung resection. J Thorac Cardiovasc Surg 109:275-83, 1995.
10. Wang J, Olak J, Ferguson MK. Diffusing capacity predicts operative mortality but not long-term survival after resection for lung cancer. J Thorac Cardiovasc Surg 117:581-7, 1999.
11. Bolliger CT, Wyser C, Roser H, Solèr M, Perruchoud AP. Lung scanning and exercise testing for the prediction of postoperative performance in lung resection candidates at increased risk for complications. Chest 108:341-8, 1995.

12. Wernly JA, DeMeester TR, Kirchner PT, Myerowitz PD, Oxford DE, Golomb HM. Clinical value of quantitative ventilation-perfusion lung scans in the surgical management of bronchogenic carcinoma. J Thorac Cardiovasc Surg 80:535-43, 1980.

13. Bolliger CT, Perruchoud AP. Functional evaluation of the lung resection candidate. Eur Respir J 11:198-212, 1998.

14. Wyser C, Stulz P, Solèr M, et al. Prospective evaluation of an algorithm for the functional assessment of lung resection candidates. Am J Respir Crit Care Med 159:1450-6, 1999.

15. Nakahara K, Miyoshi S, Nakagawa K. A method for predicting postoperative lung function and its relation to postoperative complications in patients with lung cancer. 1992 update. Ann Thorac Surg 54:1016-7, 1992.

16. McKenna Jr. RJ, Fischel RJ, Brenner M, Gelb AF. Combined operations for lung volume reduction surgery and lung cancer. Chest 110:885-8, 1996.

17. Cooper JD, Patterson GA, DeMeester SR, Yusen RD, Lefrak SS. Lobectomy combined with lung volume reduction for high risk lung cancer patients with severe emphysema. Chest 110:49S, 1996[Abstract].

18. Epstein SK, Faling LJ, Daly BDT, Celli BR. Predicting complications after pulmonary resection. Preoperative exercise testing vs. a multifactorial cardiopulmonary risk index. Chest 104:694-700, 1993.

19. Epstein SK, Faling LJ, Daly BDT, Celli BR. Inability to perform bicycle ergometry predicts increased morbidity and mortality after lung resection. Chest. 107:311-6, 1995.

20. Melendez JA, Carlon VA. Cardiopulmonary risk index does not predict complications after thoracic surgery. Chest 114:69-75, 1998.

21. Pierce RJ, Copland JM, Sharpe K, Barter CE. Preoperative risk evaluation for lung cancer resection: Predicted postoperative product as a predictor of surgical mortality. Am J Respir Crit Care Med 150:947-55, 1994.

22. Melendez JA, Barrera R. Predictive respiratory complication quotient predicts pulmonary complications in thoracic surgical patients. Ann Thorac Surg 66:220-4, 1998.

23. Bisson A, Stern M, Caubarrerre I. Preparation of high-risk patients for major thoracic surgery. Chest Surg Clin N Amer 8:541-55, 1998.

24. Reilly JJ. Preoperative evaluation of patients. Chest 112:206S-8S, 1997.

25. Lacasse Y, Wong E, Guyatt GH, King D, Cook DJ, Goldstein RS. Meta-analysis of respiratory rehabilitation in chronic obstructive pulmonary disease. Lancet. 348:1115-9, 1996.

26. Nomori H, Kobayashi R, Fuyuno G, Morinaga S, Yashima H. Preoperative respiratory muscle training. Assessment in thoracic surgery patients with special reference to postoperative pulmonary complications. Chest. 104:1782-8, 1994.

27. Jett J, Feins R, Kvale P, et al. Pretreatment evaluation of non-small cell lung cancer. Am J Respir Crit Care Med 156:320-32, 1997.

28. Winn RJ, Brown NH, Botnick WZ. A comparison of the NCCN and ASCO lung cancer guidelines. Oncology 13:35-9, 1999.

29.   Quint LE, Tummala S, Brisson LJ, et al. Distribution of distant metastases from newly diagnosed non-small cell lung cancer. Ann Thorac Surg 62:246-50, 1996.

30.   Guyatt GH, Cook DJ, Griffiths LE, et al. Surgeons' assessment of symptoms suggesting extrathoracic metastases in patients with lung cancer. Ann Thorac Surg 68:309-15, 1999.

31.   Silvestri GA, Littenberg B, Colice GL. The clinical evaluation for detecting metastatic lung cancer. A meta-analysis. Am J Respir Crit Care Med 152:225-30, 1995.

32.   Webb WR, Gatsonis C, Zerhouni EA, et al. CT and MR imaging in staging non-small cell bronchogenic carcinoma: Report of the Radiologic Diagnostic Oncology Group. Radiology 178:705-13, 1991.

33.   Martini N, Heelan R, Westcott J, et al. Comparative merits of conventional, computed tomographic, and magentic resonance imaging in assessing mediastinal involvement in surgically confirmed carcinoma. J Thorac Cardiovasc Surg 90:639-48, 1985.

34.   Patterson GA, Ginsberg RJ, Poon PY, et al. A prospective evaluation of magnetic resonance imaging, computed tomography, and mediastinoscopy in the preoperative assessment of mediastinal node status in bronchogenic carcinoma. J Thorac Cardiovasc Surg 94:679-84, 1987.

35.   McLoud TC, Bourgouin PM, Greenberg RW, et al. Bronchogenic carcinoma: Analysis of staging in the mediastinum with CT by correlative lymph node mapping and sampling. Radiology 182:319-23, 1992.

36.   Arroliga AC, Matthay RA. The role of bronchoscopy in lung cancer. Clin Chest Med 14:87-98, 1993.

37.   Wang K-P. Transbronchial needle aspiration and percutaneous needle aspiration for staging and diagnosis of lung cancer. Clin Chest Med 16:535-52, 1995.

38.   Ginsberg RJ, Rice TW, Goldberg M, Waters PF, Schmocker BJ. Extended cervical mediastinoscopy. A single staging procedure for bronchogenic carcinoma of the left upper lobe. J Thorac Cardiovasc Surg 94:673-8, 1987.

39.   Lee JD, Ginsberg RJ. Lung cancer staging: The value of ipsilateral scalene lymph node biopsy performed at mediastinoscopy. Ann Thorac Surg 62:338-41, 1996.

40.   Mentzer SJ, Swanson SJ, DeCamp MM, Bueno R, Sugarbaker DJ. Mediastinoscopy, thoracoscopy and video-assisted thoracic surgery in the diagnosis and staging of lung cancer. Chest 112:239S-41S, 1997.

41.   Gress FG, Savides TJ, Sandler A, et al. Endoscopic ultrasonography, fine-needle aspiration biopsy guided by endoscopic ultrasonography, and computed tomography in the preoperative staging of non-small cell lung cancer: A comparative study. Ann Int Med 127:604-12, 1997.

42.   White P, Jr., Ettinger DS. Tissue is the issue: Is endoscopic ultrasonography with or without fine-needle aspiration biopsy in the staging of non-small cell lung cancer an advance? Ann Int Med 127:643-5, 1997.

43.   Steinert HC, Hauser M, Allemann F, et al. Non-small cell lung cancer: Nodal staging with FDG PET versus CT with correlative lymph node mapping and sampling. Radiology 202:441-6, 1997.

44. Vansteenkiste JF, Stroobants SG, De Leyn PR, et al. Mediastinal lymph node staging with FDG-PET scan in patients with potentially operable non-small cell lung cancer. A prospective analysis of 50 cases. Chest 112:1480-6, 1997.

45. Weder W, Schmid RA, Bruchhaus H, Hillinger S, von Schulthess GK, Steinert HC. Detection of extrathoracic metastases by positron emission tomography in lung cancer. Ann Thorac Surg 66:886-93, 1998.

46. Miyake M, Adachi M, Huang C-L, Higashiyama M, Kodama K, Taki T. A novel molecular staging protocol for non-small cell lung cancer. Oncogene 18:2397-404, 1999.

47. The Lung Cancer Study Group., Ginsberg RJ, Rubinstein LV. Randomized trial of lobectomy versus limited resection for T1 N0 non-small cell lung cancer. Ann Thorac Surg 60:615-23, 1995.

48. Martini N, Burt ME, Bains MS, McCormack PM, Rusch VW, Ginsberg RJ. Survival after resection of stage II non-small cell lung cancer. Ann Thorac Surg 54:460-6, 1992.

49. Izbicki JR, Thetter O, Habekost M, et al. Radical systematic mediastinal lymphadenectomy in non-small cell lung cancer: A randomized controlled trial. Br J Surg 81:229-35, 1994.

50. Graham ANJ, Chan KJM, Pastorino U, Goldstraw P. Systematic nodal dissection in the intrathoracic staging of patients with non-small cell lung cancer. J Thorac Cardiovasc Surg 117:246-51, 1999.

51. McCaughan BC, Martini N, Bains MS, McCormack PM. Chest wall invasion in carcinoma of the lung. Therapeutic and prognostic implications. J Thorac Cardiovasc Surg 89:836-41, 1985.

52. Downey RJ, Martini N, Rusch VW, Bains MS, Korst RJ, Ginsberg RJ. Extent of chest wall invasion and survival in patients with lung cancer. Ann Thorac Surg 68:188-93, 1999.

53. Pitz CCM, de la Rivière AB, Elbers HRJ, Westermann CJJ, van den Bosch JMM. Surgical treatment of 125 patients with non-small cell lung cancer and chest wall involvement. Thorax 51:846-50, 1996.

54. Albertucci M, DeMeester TR, Rothberg M, Hagen JA, Santoscoy R, Smyrk TC. Surgery and the management of peripheral lung tumors adherent to the parietal pleura. J Thorac Cardiovasc Surg 103:8-13, 1992.

55. Pairolero PC, Arnold PG. Chest wall tumors. Experience with 100 consecutive patients. J Thorac Cardiovasc Surg 90:367-72, 1985.

56. Deschamps C, Tirnaksiz BM, Darbandi R, et al. Early and long-term results of prosthetic chest wall reconstruction. J Thorac Cardiovasc Surg 177:588-92, 1999.

57. McCormack P, Bains MS, Beattie EJ, Jr., Martini N. New trends in skeletal reconstruction after resection of chest wall tumors. Ann Thorac Surg 31:45-52, 1981.

58. Spaggiari L, Rusca M, Carbognani P, Solli P. Hemivertebrectomy for apical chest tumors: Is risk justified by the outcome? Ann Thorac Surg 65:1515-7, 1998.

59. Pancoast HK. Henry K. Pancoast describes suprior pulmonary sulcus tumor. Surgical Rounds. January:29-32, 1980.

60. Shaw RR, Paulson DL, Kee JL, Jr. Treatment of the superior sulcus tumor by irradiation followed by resection. Ann Surg 7:29-40, 1961.

61. Ginsberg RJ, Martini N, Zaman M, et al. Influence of surgical resection and brachytherapy in the management of superior sulcus tumor. Ann Thorac Surg 57:1440-5, 1994.

62. Hagan MP, Choi NC, Mathisen DJ, Wain JC, Wright CD, Grillo HC. Superior sulcus lung tumors: Impact of local control on survival. J Thorac Cardiovasc Surg 117:1086-94, 1999.

63. Rusch VW, Parekh KR, Leon L, et al. Factors determining outcome after surgical resection of T3 and T4 lung cancers of the superior sulcus. J Thorac Cardiovasc Surg "in press", 2000.

64. Paulson DL. Extended resection of bronchogenic carcinoma in the superior pulmonary sulcus. Surgical Rounds January:10-21, 1980.

65. Mathisen DJ, Grillo HC. Carinal resection for bronchogenic carcinoma. J Thorac Cardiovasc Surg 102:16-23, 1991.

66. Spaggiari L, Pastorino U. Transmanubrial approach with antero-lateral thoracotomy for apical chest tumor. Ann Thorac Surg 68:590-3, 1999.

67. Bains MS, Ginsberg RJ, Jones WG, et al. The clamshell incision. An improved approach to bilateral pulmonary and mediastinal tumor. Ann Thorac Surg 58:30-3, 1994.

68. Martini N, Yellin A, Ginsberg RJ, et al. Management of non-small cell lung cancer with direct mediastinal involvement. Ann Thorac Surg 58:1447-51, 1994.

69. Nakahashi H, Yasumoto K, Ishida T, et al. Results of surgical treatment of patients with T3 non-small cell lung cancer. Ann Thorac Surg 46:178-81, 1988.

70. Pitz CCM, de la Rivière AB, Elbers HRJ, Westermann CJJ, van den Bosch JM. Results of resection of T3 non-small cell lung cancer invading the mediastinum or main bronchus. Ann Thorac Surg 62:1016-20, 1996.

71. Weksler B, Bains M, Burt M, et al. Resection of lung cancer invading the diaphragm. J Thorac Cardiovasc Surg 114:500-1, 1997.

72. Faber LP, Jensik RJ, Kittle CF. Results of sleeve lobectomy for bronchogenic carcinoma in 101 patients. Ann Thorac Surg 37:279-85, 1984.

73. Mehran RJ, Deslauriers J, Piraus M, Beaulieu M, Guimont C, Brisson J. Survival related to nodal status after sleeve resection for lung cancer. J Thorac Cardiovasc Surg 107:576-82, 1994.

74. Suen H-C, Meyers BF, Guthrie T, et al. Favorable results after sleeve lobectomy or bronchoplasty for bronchial malignancies. Ann Thorac Surg 67:1557-62, 1999.

75. Martini N, Flehinger BJ, Zaman MB, Beattie EJ, Jr. Results of resection in non-oat cell carcinoma of the lung with mediastinal lymph node metastases. Ann Surg 198:386-97, 1983.

76. Martini N, Flehinger BJ. The role of surgery in N2 lung cancer. Surg Clinics N Amer 67:1037-49, 1987.

77. Suzuki K, Nagai K, Yoshida J, Nishimura M, Takahashi K, Nishiwaki Y. The prognosis of surgically resected N2 non-small cell lung cancer: The importance of clinical N status. J Thorac Cardiovasc Surg 118:145-53, 1999.

78. Pearson FG, Delarue NC, Ilves R, Todd TRJ, Cooper JD. Significance of positive superior mediastinal nodes identified at mediastinoscopy in patients with resectable cancer of the lung. J Thorac Cardiovasc Surg 83:1-11, 1982.

79. Okada M, Tsubota N, Yoshimura M, Miyamoto Y, Matsuoka H. Prognosis of completely resected pN2 non-small cell lung carcinomas: What is the significant node that affects survival? J Thorac Cardiovasc Surg 118:270-5, 1999.

80. Patterson GA, Piazza D, Pearson FG, et al. Significance of metastatic disease in subaortic lymph nodes. Ann Thorac Surg 43:155-9, 1987.

81. Perez CA, Pajak TF, Rubin P, et al. Long-term observations of the patterns of failure in patients with unresectable non-oat cell carcinoma of the lung treated with definitive radiotherapy. Report by the Radiation Therapy Oncology Group. Cancer. 59:1874-81, 1987.

82. Keller SM, Adak S, Wagner H, et al. Prospective randomized trial of postoperative adjuvant therapy in patients with completely resected stages II and IIIA non-small cell lung cancer: An intergroup trial (E3590). Proc ASCO. 18:465a, 1999[Abstract].

83. Deslauriers J, Jacques LF. Sleeve pneumonectomy. Chest Surg Clin N Amer 5:297-313, 1995.

84. Mitchell JD, Mathisen DJ, Wright CD, et al. Clinical experience with carinal resection. J Thorac Cardiovasc Surg 117:39-53, 1999.

85. Klepetko W, Wisser W, Birsan T, et al. T4 lung tumors with infiltration of the thoracic aorta: Is an operation reasonable? Ann Thorac Surg 67:340-4, 1999.

86. Rendina EA, Venuta F, De Giacomo T, et al. Induction chemotherapy for T4 centrally located non-small cell lung cancer. J Thorac Cardiovasc Surg 117:225-33, 1999.

87. Albain KS, Rusch VW, Crowley JJ, et al. Concurrent cisplatin/etoposide plus chest radiotherapy followed by surgery for stages IIIA (N2) and IIIB non-small cell lung cancer: Mature results of Southwest Oncology Group Phase II study 8805. J Clin Oncol 13:1880-92, 1995.

88. Albain K, Rusch V, Crowley J, et al. Long-term survival after concurrent cisplatin/etoposide (PE) plus chest radiotherapy (RT) followed by surgery in bulky, stages IIIA (N2) and IIIB non-small cell lung cancer (NSCLC): 6-year outcomes from Southwest Oncology Group study 8805. Proc ASCO 18:467a, 1999 [Abstract].

89. Eberhardt W, Wilke H, Stamatis G, et al. Preoperative chemotherapy followed by concurrent chemoradiation therapy based on hyperfractionated accelerated radiotherapy and definitive surgery in locally advanced non-small cell lung cancer: Mature results of a Phase II trial. J Clin Oncol 16:622-34, 1998.

90. Patchell RA, Tibbs PA, Walsh JW, et al. A randomized trial of surgery in the treatment of single metastases to the brain. N Engl J Med 322:494-500, 1990.

91. Burt M, Wronski M, Arbit E, et al. Resection of brain metastases from non-small-cell lung carcinoma. Results of therapy. J Thorac Cardiovasc Surg 103:399-411, 1992.

92. Martini N. Surgical treatment of non-small cell lung cancer by stage. Sem Surg Onc 6:248-54, 1990.

93. Martini N, Bains MS, Burt ME, et al. Incidence of local recurrence and second primary tumors in resected stage I lung cancer. J Thorac Cardiovasc Surg 109:120-9, 1995.

94. Thomas P, Rubinstein L, The Lung Cancer Study Group. Cancer recurrence after resection: T1 N0 non-small cell lung cancer. Ann Thorac Surg 49:242-7, 1990.

95. Johnson BE. Second lung cancers in patients after treatment for an initial lung cancer. J Natl Cancer Inst 90:1335-45, 1998.

96. Johnson BE, Cortazar P, Chute JP. Second lung cancers in patients successfully treated for lung cancer. Semin Oncol 24:492-9, 1997.

97. Martini N, Melamed MR. Multiple primary lung cancers. J Thorac Cardiovasc Surg 70:606-12, 1975.

98. Walsh GL, O'Connor M, Willis KM, et al. Is follow-up of lung cancer patients after resection medically indicated and cost-effective? Ann Thorac Surg 60:1563-72, 1995.

99. Downey RJ. Follow-up of patients with completely resected lung cancer. Chest 115:1487-8, 1999.

100. Henschke CI, McCauley DI, Yankelevitz DF, et al. Early lung cancer action project: Overall design and findings from baseline screening. Lancet 354:99-105, 1999.

Figure 1-   Guidelines for pre-operative functional evaluation of lung resection candidates*

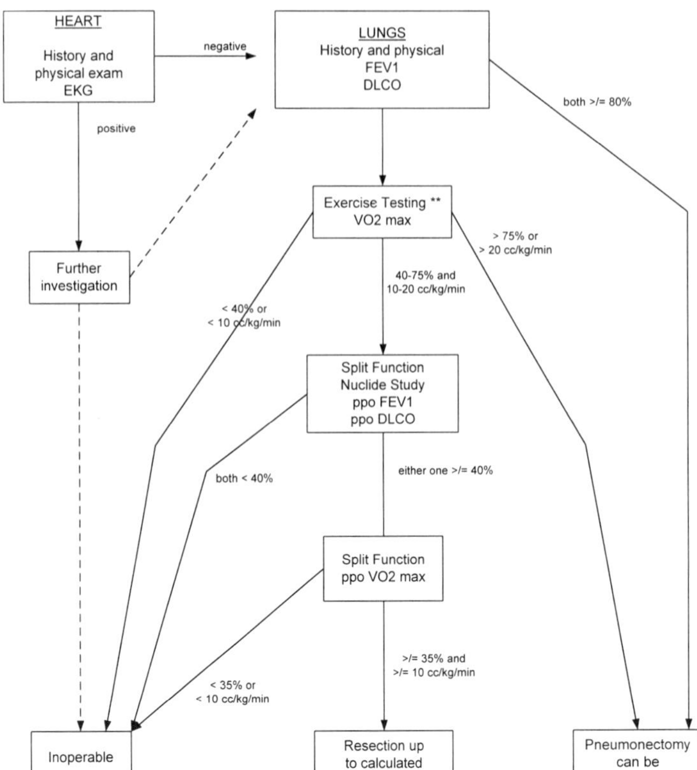

* Modified from Bolliger and Nakahara
** Exercise testing can be interchanged with split funciton testing

RADIATION THERAPY FOR NON-SMALL CELL LUNG CANCER (NSCLC)

Hak Choy, M.D.
Vanderbilt University Medical Center, Nashville, TN 37232 USA

Anuradha Chakravarthy, M.D.
Vanderbilt University Medical Center, Nashville, TN 37232 USA

Jae-Sung Kim, M.D.
Vanderbilt University Medical Center, Nashville, TN 37232 USA

INTRODUCTION

The year 1995 marked the centennial of Roentgen's landmark discovery of x-rays in 1895 (1). "A new kind of ray", which was emitted by a gas discharge tube, could blacken photographic film. Almost immediately, its applications to medicine were recognized. It was used to locate a piece of knife in the backbone of a sailor who had been paralyzed until the fragment could be located and removed. X-rays were first used therapeutically in 1897 when Leopold Freund, a German surgeon, successfully irradicated a hairy mole using the new technique (2). By 1934 Coutard developed a protracted, fractionated scheme for the successful treatment of laryngeal cancer (3).

The absorption of energy from radiation in biological materials can lead to the raising of an electron in an atom to a higher energy level. If the radiation has sufficient energy, it can cause the electron to be ejected from the atom; this is called ionization (therefore, the term ionizing radiation). Over the next 100 years, technical advances in the use of ionizing radiation would allow the development of high-energy photons to prevent skin reactions from being the dose-limiting toxicity. Electrons would also be developed which could target superficial structures while sparing deeper organs. The Curies discovered radium in 1898, initiating the development of brachytherapy (4). The use of brachytherapy began with the use of ^{226}Radium needles and tubes, however, over time newer, safer isotopes were discovered and continue to be in use today. Most current applications of radiation utilize one of two forms of electromagnetic radiation, x-rays and gamma rays. X-rays are produced outside the nucleus by an electrical device that accelerates electrons to high energy and then stops them abruptly on a target such as tungsten. Part of the kinetic energy of the electrons is then converted into x-rays. Gamma rays, on the other hand, are produced intranuclearly by radioactive isotopes, such as

Cobalt. The excess energy is given off as the nucleus breaks up and tries to reach a stable form and is released as gamma rays.

The biological effects of radiation result primarily in damage to DNA, the basic building block of all living creatures. When any form of radiation, x-ray or gamma-rays, interacts with cells, it can cause the atoms of the DNA itself to become excited, leading ultimately to strand breaks that cannot be repaired, resulting in cell death. These are the direct effects of radiation. There can also be indirect effects when radiation interacts with other atoms or molecules in the cell (particularly water) to produce free radicals that can diffuse and subsequently damage critical targets such as DNA. Almost two-thirds of the biological damage produced by radiation is due to these indirect effects. It is these indirect effects that can be modified by radiation sensitizers and protectors.

The aim of therapy should be decided from the onset of treatment. The goal can be curative when there is the possibility of long-term survival after adequate therapy, even if that possibility is extremely small (i.e. medically inoperable early stage lung cancer, locally advanced lung cancer). It can also be palliative, where there is no chance of survival regardless of dose, yet symptoms can be relieved (i.e. metastatic lung cancer). In the curative setting, both the patient and the physician are willing to take a risk of significant side effects, whereas, iatrogenically induced side effects are less acceptable in the palliative setting. In this chapter, we will provide an overview for the role of radiation therapy in the management of non-small cell lung cancer.

MEDICALLY INOPERABLE STAGE I/II NSCLC

For technically and medically operable patients with clinical stage I and II non-small cell lung cancer (NSCLC), surgery remains the treatment of choice with 5-year survival rates of 24 – 61% for clinically staged patients (5). However, not all patients with operable tumors are candidates for surgery, for example: chronic tobacco abuse often causes cardiopulmonary dysfunction making patients who would anatomically and biologically be suitable candidates for surgery, medically inoperable, and occasionally, patients refuse surgery. During the past decade, several institutions have reported their results using radical radiotherapy for patients with clinically staged, medically inoperable, stage I and II, non-small cell lung cancer. They have generally concluded that this represents a reasonable treatment option for patients whose cancer is medically inoperable or who refuse surgery. In comparing the results of surgical and non-surgical therapy in these patients, it is essential to be aware of the potential biases in comparing clinically versus surgically staged patients. Surgical series have reported outcomes based on both preoperative clinical staging and operative pathological staging. Mountain (5) in an article describing a database of 5319 patients reported 5-year survivals based on clinical and surgical staging, with marked improvement for the surgically staged patients in most TNM subgroups. Although radiographic overstaging does occur, the more common problem is the presence of microscopic N1 or N2 disease, resulting in the surgical upstaging of patients who were clinically N0.

Overview of Results

Table 1 summarizes the results of radical radiotherapy for patients with early-stage NSCLC. There is considerable variation in patient characteristics (median age, performance status, weight loss), tumor characteristics (pathologic and clinical staging) and treatment characteristics (fractional dose, fractionation schedule, and volume treated, etc. Despite these limitations, a few general conclusions can be deduced from reviewing this data.

Table 1. Outcome of radiotherapy for patients with clinically early-stage non-small cell lung cancer

Investigators	No. of Patients	Stage (Clinical)	Dose (Gy)	Median	2-year Surv. (%)	5-year Surv. (%)	Local Failure (%)
Haffty et al, 1988[2]	43	T1-2, N0-1	54 – 59	28 mo	60	21	39
Noordikj et al, 1988[3]	50	T1-2, N0	60	25 mo	56	16	70
Zhang et al, 1989[4]	44	T1-2, N0-2	55 – 70	>36 mo	55	32	n/a
Talton et al, 1990[5]	77	T1-3, N0	60	17 mo	36	17	n/a
Sandler et al, 1991[6]	77	T1-2, N0	60	20 mo	30	10	56
Ono et al, 1991[7]	38	T1, N0	60 – 70	40 mo	68	42	n/a
Dosoretz et al, 1992[8]	152	T1-3, N0-1	50 – 70	17 mo	40	10	70
Krol et al, 1996[9]	108	T1-2, N0	60 – 65	24 mo	50	15	66
Kupelian et al, 1996[10]	71	T1-4, N0	median 63	16 mo	30	12	44
Sibley et al, 1998[11]	141	T1-2, N0	50 – 80	18 mo	39	13	42

Radiotherapy can produce long-term survival in a proportion of these patients, ranging from 10% for patients with later stage disease to 42% for patients with T1 N0 M0 disease. Several studies have shown a correlation between survival and decreasing tumor size. In a retrospective review of 77 patients, the actuarial 3-year disease-specific survival was 30% for patients with Stage I tumors treated with definitive radiation and dropped to 17% for tumors 3-6 cm in size (6). In another retrospective review of 50 patients with T1-2, N0 NSCLC, treated with curative intent, the crude 5-year survival results were 38% in patients with tumors less than 2 cm in size vs. 0% for patients with tumors larger than 4 cm (7). In a retrospective review of 152 patients with medically inoperable NSCLC, the overall 5-year survival was 10%. The 2-year disease-free survival, however, was 55% for T1 tumors compared to 20-25% for T2, T3 tumors (p=. 006). There was also a decreased local and distant failure rate seen in patients with T1 disease treated with doses greater than 65 Gy. Although surgery remains the treatment of choice for early stage NSCLC, in patients who are medically inoperable or refuse surgery, definitive radiation should be considered, especially in patients with smaller tumors. Local failure within the irradiated volume is frequent, with the best series reporting 30% local failure for T1 lesions, rising to 70% for T2 lesions. Local failure rates after surgery, even with limited resections are less than 20%. These high local failure rates suggest that the difference in survival between the surgical and radiotherapeutic series is not solely due to stage imbalance but in part reflects the inferior local control achieved with radiotherapy only. These failure rates also suggest that improved radiotherapy techniques for target volume delineation, dose delivery, and fractionation may result in improved local control and survival.

Failure Patterns Related to the Radiation Dose and Treatment Volume

Zhang et al. (8) reported improved local control and survival with higher doses of radiation. Patients receiving 55 to 61 Gy had a 5-year survival of 27%(6/22), compared with 36% (8/22) for those receiving 69 to 70 Gy. Local recurrence was seen in 8 of 22 patients (36%) in the low-dose group, compared with 4 of 22 patients (18%) in the high-dose group. Dosoretz et al also observed a decrease in local failure with increasing dose, especially at the highest dose level. This was especially true for the smaller tumors (9). Actuarial local failure rates, however, are greatly affected by competing events such as intercurrent death and distant metastases. Gelman et al (10) recommended that a multinomial regression analysis be used to analyze local failure in an effort to minimize the effect of these confounding variables. This type of analysis was performed by Sibley et al (11) who found that higher doses were associated with improved local control on multivariate analysis (p=0.07). Studies that have examined a range of doses have consistently found advantages in either local control or disease free survival when higher doses are used. This has not been associated with an increased rate of morbidity in any reported series to date. In a review of 10 studies, Sibley et al (11) reported complication rates of less than 2% with no serious acute or late morbidity. Most of these studies utilized prophylactic irradiation. It is therefore expected that if prophylactic nodal irradiation were eliminated, there would be a further reduction in the incidence of complications. The optimal treatment volume in medically inoperable lung carcinoma remains controversial. Krol et al (12) have advocated the use of radiotherapy fields that omit prophylactic nodal coverage because regional failure is uncommon. From estimates of surgical upstaging, "postage stamp" fields would be expected to miss locoregional disease in approximately 25% of cases (13). However, given the magnitude of compromising events (i.e., intercurrent death, distant metastases, and local failure), isolated regional failure is expected to be an unlikely event. This is supported by the regional only failure rates of 3% reported by Krol et al (12) and 7% reported by Sibley et al (11). The majority of patients are medically inoperable due to pulmonary compromise, and comprehensive nodal treatment may carry a significant risk. In addition, large fields may limit patient tolerance to radiotherapy and may ultimately limit the dose that could be given to the primary lesion. Because local failure rates of up to 50% have been reported, comprehensive nodal irradiation becomes difficult to justify.

Rationale for Dose Escalation

Radiotherapy for stage I, II NSCLC lung cancer appears to provide a poorer outcome than surgery. There are several reasons for this, including clinical versus pathologic staging, and more importantly, age and performance status differences. However, the local only failure rates of 50% in many radiotherapy series stands in stark contrast to the 5–20% local failure rates in surgical series. These differences cannot easily be explained by difference in performance status, age, or extent of mediastinal staging and highlight the need for more effective local therapy. Reluctance to escalate the dose in stages I & II lung cancer cannot be attributed to a high rate of complications in this infirmed population, because the complication rate is less than 2%. Although it is certainly true that there is a high rate of intercurrent death among these medically inoperable lung cancer patients, a consistent finding in most studies of medically inoperable lung cancer is that the majority of patients die of uncontrolled lung cancer. The importance of local control on survival has been described in patients with T1 medically inoperable lung cancer (14,15). Survival is significantly improved in both T1 N0 and T2 N0 patients who are locally controlled with a 5- year cause-specific survival rate of 46% versus 12% for uncontrolled tumors (p=0.03)(11). In conclusion, the published retrospective data suggest that local control and outcome may be improved with high dose radiotherapy without significant risk of complications.

The Role of Post-Operative Radiation in Resectable NSCLC

The role of adjuvant radiation was examined in a randomized study of 210 RTOG patients with Stage II/III squamous cell carcinoma of the lung. Following surgery, patients received 50Gy in 25 fractions or no further therapy. This study showed a significant decrease in local recurrence (3% vs 41%, p< .05) in node-positive patients, however, with no difference in overall survival (15). The lack of a survival benefit may have been due in part to the fact that over two-thirds of first failures were systemic, not local, and therefore would not be expected to change with the addition of radiation alone. A meta-analysis of 9 randomized studies of postoperative radiation versus surgery alone has shown a trend towards a benefit in overall survival with the addition of radiation in N2 patients (16). Although the difference in overall survival with the addition of radiation was not statistically significant in N2 patients (16), post-operative radiation in patients with pathologically documented N2 disease remains the standard of care. There was, however, a significant adverse effect to the addition of postoperative radiation on survival, reducing it from 55 to 48%. Subgroup analyses showed this adverse effect was the greatest for Stage I/II, N0-1 disease. Outside of a study setting, there is no role for post-operative radiation in Stage I/II, N0-1 disease.

Given the high rates of distant failure, it would be logical to consider the addition of chemotherapy to radiation to help improve the results of adjuvant therapy. Unfortunately, preliminary results of a recently closed intergroup trial (ECOG 3590) adjuvant radiotherapy versus adjuvant radiation therapy plus cisplatin plus etoposide did not show a statistically significant benefit of chemoradiotherapy to radiation alone. Median survival in the chemoradiotherapy arm was 38.6 months compared to 41.1 months in the RT only arm (p=.99). Analysis of the stratified subgroups showed no subgroup to benefit from adjuvant chemoradiotherapy (17). The role of post-operative adjuvant therapy, consisting of radiation with or without chemotherapy, or chemotherapy alone remains to be defined.

Role of Neoadjuvant Radiation, With/Without Chemotherapy in Marginally Resectable NSCLC

N2 disease can be divided into those that are (1) not visible by preoperative CT scans and found only at the time of mediastinoscopy or pathologic evaluation of the resected specimen (2) multiple levels of nodal involvement seen on preoperative staging (3) bulky mediastinal disease. Patients with N2 disease that is visible by CT or found at mediastinoscopy are ideal candidates for consideration of neoadjuvant chemoradiation with the hopes of potential downstaging and surgical resection. Bulky mediastinal nodes, on the other hand, are perhaps better treated with primary chemoradiation.

Martini and colleagues had observed (18) that patients with clinically evident (by chest x-ray) mediastinal nodal involvement had a 3 year survival rate of only 9%. Whereas for those patients whose metastatic lymph nodes were found at the time of surgery, the survival rate was 50%. Due to the poor outcome of patients with clinically evident N2 disease, pre-operative (induction therapy or neoadjuvant therapy) has been tried using radiation with or without chemotherapy.

Several recent studies suggest that neoadjuvant therapy consisting of chemotherapy with or without radiation can convert patients who are marginally resectable to curatively resectable patients. A prospective, multi-institutional, phase II study of Stage III A/B patients has shown neoadjuvant chemoradiation to be well tolerated, and associated with a high response and resectablility rates. Induction therapy utilized two cycles of Cisplatin and etoposide with concurrent radiation to a total dose of 45 Gy. Resection was attempted 3-5 weeks following induction therapy. Fifty-five of the 75 patients (73%) were able to undergo complete resection. Eleven of 55 (20%) underwent complete pathologic response and 20/55 (36%) had only rare microscopic residual on pathologic specimens. The 2-year survival of 40% is significantly better than historical controls (19).

In a randomized study of preoperative chemotherapy (cyclophosphamide, etoposide, and Cisplatin) followed by surgery to surgery alone, the median survival of patients in the combined modality arm was 64 months vs. 11 months for patients who had surgery alone (p< .008). The 5-year survival was 36% for the combined modality therapy compared to 15% for surgery alone (20).

In a second randomized study of preoperative chemotherapy (ifosphamide, mitomycin, Cisplatin for 3 cycles) followed by surgery to surgery alone, the median survival was improved (26 vs. 8 months, p .001) with preoperative chemotherapy (21).

Although there are no randomized studies comparing neoadjuvant chemotherapy to neoadjuvant chemoradiation, the higher complete pathologic responders (11%) with neoadjuvant chemoradiation over chemotherapy (5%) suggests a potential advantage to the combination even in the neoadjuvant setting. A large intergroup trial (RTOG 9309) is currently ongoing to determine if surgery provides an additive effect to primary chemoradiation in this group of patients.

Role of Radiation in Locally Unresectable Lung Cancer

Patients with clinical T4, and/or bulky N2 disease who do not have evidence for metastatic disease are considered to have locally unresectable disease. A recent analysis of 1592 patients on four RTOG studies showed that performance status, weight loss > 5%, age > 60 years, pleural effusion, and higher T and N stages all predicted for poorer outcome (22). Until recently, most patients with locally advanced NSCLC were treated with radiotherapy alone, which provides good palliative effects, however has marginal survival benefits. Chemotherapy alone also appears to be ineffective for the management of locally advanced NSCLC. Kubota and his colleagues from Japan conducted a phase III randomized trial comparing sequential chemotherapy and radiation to chemotherapy alone and found substantially lower survival rates with chemotherapy alone in comparison to chemotherapy plus radiation (23).

Table 2. Chemotherapy alone vs. chemoradiation for locally advanced lung cancer

	Median S **(Days)**	**2-YS** **(%)**	**3-YS** **(%)**	**5-YS** **(%)**
Chemo + RT	461	36	29	9.7
Chemo	447	9	3.1	3.1

Given this study we recommend that patients with locally advanced non-small cell lung cancer always be evaluated by a medical, as well as a radiation oncologist. Only patients, who are judged by the radiation oncologist to be ineligible for radiation on the basis of tumor size, lung volume to be treated, or pulmonary function tests should be offered palliative chemotherapy alone. The only exception would be patients with malignant pleural effusions whose prognosis is similar to patients with distant metastatic disease. Patients, who in the judgment of the treating medical oncologist are ineligible for chemotherapy on the basis of performance status, underlying medical condition, and degree of weight loss should be considered for palliative radiation alone in the setting of locally advanced lung cancer.

Induction CT Followed by RT

Induction chemotherapy followed by radiation has the theoretical advantage of downsizing the primary tumor to allow a smaller volume of radiation. It also allows full doses of both modalities to be delivered. Given that the likely cause of death is distant metastases, induction chemotherapy allows the systemic portion of therapy to begin immediately. One of the first studies to establish the value of adding chemotherapy to radiation in the management of locally advanced lung cancer was CALGB 8433. This study of good performance status patients with <5% weight loss found that with the addition of two cycles of induction chemotherapy consisting of cisplatin $100mg/m^2$ on D1, 29 and vinblastine 5 mg/m^2 on D1, 8,15,22 and 29 survival was doubled.

Conventional radiation (60 Gy in 30 fractions over 6 weeks) was started on day 50 for patients on the induction chemotherapy arm and immediately for patients on the radiation alone arm. The significant survival advantage led to early closure of the study (24).

Although the remaining trials of combined modality therapy to radiation alone did not show as much benefit, they did confirm the value of platinum-based chemotherapy with thoracic radiation over radiation alone (Table 3). RTOG 8808 was a study to confirm the findings of the CALGB8433 trial. Two of the treatment arms were the same as that of the CALGB8433. A third arm asked whether hyperfractionated radiation alone (1.2 Gy twice daily, five days/week for a total of 69.6 Gy) would be equivalent to induction chemotherapy followed by radiation using standard fractionation. The overall survival showed a statistically significant benefit to induction chemotherapy over radiation alone and that hyperfractionated radiation was equivalent to the radiation alone arm (25).

The third large randomized study of induction chemotherapy utilized definitive radiation consisting of 65Gy in 26 fractions given over 45 days with induction chemotherapy consisting of the combination of Vindesine, cisplatin, lomustine and cyclophosphamide for three cycles before and after radiation. Although the 2-year survival was

Table 3. Randomized Trials of Induction Chemotherapy followed by Radiation.

Author	Treatment	Medn S	2YS	5YS	p-value
Dillman[24]	CDDP/Vbl→RT	13.7	26	17	.012
CALGB8433	RT only	9.6	13	6	
Sause[22,25]	CDDP/Vbl→RT	13.7	31	8	.04*
ECOG4588	RT only	11.4	20	5	
	HRT	12.2	24	6	
Le Chevalier[26]	VCPC→RT→VCPC	12	21	6	.02
	RT	10	14	3	

**CDDP/Vbl→RT vs RT only, 2 YS - 2-year survival, 5 YS - 5-year survival*

significantly improved, the percentage of patients surviving at 5 years was only 6% for the combined modality arm vs 3% for the radiation alone arm. An analysis of the patterns of failure shows that although distant metastatic progression was significantly decreased, (70% vs 49%, p<0.001), local failure occurred in 92% of patients at 5 years (27).

Concurrent Chemotherapy and Radiation

There are a number of theoretical advantages to the concurrent use of chemotherapy and radiation. These include the use of cytotoxic agents as soon as possible to eradicate potential micrometastases. Depending on the agents used, concurrent chemotherapy may also act as a radiosensitizer and, thereby, maximize effects on local control. Unfortunately, the disadvantage includes the possibility of increased side effects leading to decreased doses of chemotherapy as well as radiation.

The EORTC randomized patients receiving split course radiation (30 Gy in 10 fractions followed by a 3-4 week break and an additional 25 Gy in 10 fractions) to either chemotherapy and concurrent radiation using either weekly cisplatin 30 mg/m2/week or daily cisplatin 6 mg/m^2/day during the course of radiation, or to radiation alone. The same total dose of platinum was used in both chemotherapy arms. There was a significant improvement in 2-year survival between the daily cisplatin arm over radiation alone (26% vs 13%, p = .009). Although the doses of cisplatin used in this study were adequate for radiosensitization, they were much lower than those required for systemic control. An analysis of failure patterns revealed that the survival benefit noted in the weekly cisplatin arm was due to improved local control (28). In a phase II study by SWOG (29), two cycles of cisplatin (50 mg/m^2 D1, 8 q 28days) and etoposide (50mg/m^2 D1, 5 q28days) were given with radiation (61.2 Gy in 34 fractions). The encouraging median survival of 13 months and 3 year survival of 26% suggest that concurrent chemoradiotherapy may lead to better results over sequential treatment. SWOG (S9909) is planning a randomized study to further evaluate this question.

Chemotherapy and Radiation is Superior to RT Only
Negative Studies of combined modality therapy
Although there have been randomized studies that have not shown a survival advantage to the addition of chemotherapy to radiation, many have been small and lacked the statistical power to measure a difference. Moreover, many used sub-optimal chemotherapy (30,31,32,33,34). Despite these negative trials, 3 separate meta-analyses have found a small but statistically significant survival advantage to the addition of chemotherapy to thoracic radiation in the management of locally advanced NSCLC (35,36,37). Non-small Cell Lung Cancer Collaborative Group found that trials using cisplatin-based therapy provided the greatest benefit with a 13% reduction in the risk of death and an absolute benefit of 4% (confidence interval, 1-7%) at two years and 2% (CI 1-4%, at 5 years) (35). Pritchard concluded that the median survival improved from 10.3 to 12 months (37). These studies have helped to establish that for patients with good performance status and little cancer-related weight loss, there is a survival advantage to combined modality therapy over thoracic RT alone. Questions that remain include the sequencing of chemotherapy with radiation, the specific drugs to be used, the dose and intensity of the drugs and the radiation, the best way to maximize tumor control while at the same time decreasing normal tissue toxicity of aggressive combined modality approaches.

CHEMORADIATION: SEQUENTIAL VS CONCURRENT: WHICH IS BETTER?

Non-randomized studies:
A retrospective analysis using data from 461 patients in five completed RTOG studies has found that the overall response rate is improved in patients receiving concurrent over sequential therapy. The 3-year survival was 17% (standard fractionation radiation) and

25% (hyperfractionated radiation) compared to 15% in patients treated with sequential chemotherapy and radiation. (Table 4) (38).

Table 4. Combined Response and Toxicity Analysis from five RTOG Lung Studies: Sequential vs Concurrent Chemoradiotherapy

	CT→RT	CT→CT + RT	CT + HFX RT
Overall response rate	63%	77%	79%
3YS	15%	17%	25%
Severe non-hematological toxicities	27%	34%	55%
Severe esophagitis	1.3%	6%	34%

Randomized Studies of Sequencing

There are three randomized studies that have recently completed accrual, which compare sequential to concurrent chemoradiotherapy. These are summarized in Table 5. The West Japan Lung Cancer Group trial randomized 344 patients to two treatment arms. One involved concurrent 2 cycles of chemotherapy (mitomycin $8mg/m^2$ D1, vindesine $3mg/m^2$ D1, 8 and cisplatin 80 mg/m^2 D1) given every 28 days along with split course radiation (30 Gy/10 fractions followed by a 3-4 week break and 25 gy/10 fraction, total = 55 Gy). The second arm involved the same chemotherapy followed by continuous course radiation. The overall response rates were superior in the current arm over the sequential arm, 84% vs 66.4 %. Median survival also showed a statistically significant improvement with concurrent chemotherapy and split-course RT over the same chemotherapy given before continuous course RT (16.5 vs. 13.3 months, p=. 0473) (39).

Table 5. Randomized studies of sequential vs Concurrent Chemoradiation

	Regimen	Median Survival (months)	p-value
West Japan [39]	MMC, vindesine, P + RT(split)	16.5	.0473
	MMC,vindesine,P→RT (continuous)	13.3	
CALGB 9130 [40]	Vinblastine/P→RT	10 (4YS)	NS
	Vinblastine/P→RT with weekly carboplatin	13 (4YS)	
RTOG 9410 [41]	Vinblastine/P→RT	14.6	
	Vinblastine/P + RT(std)	17.0	0.08
	Etoposide/P + RT (hfxn)	15.6	0.31

4 YS - 4-year survival

The CALGB trial showed improved complete response rate with decreased local failure rate within the boost volume with concurrent weekly carboplatin and thoracic RT compared sequential chemo-RT. However there was no statistical difference in overall survival between two group (40).

The RTOG trial has randomized 611 patients to one sequential combined modality treatment arm or to two concurrent combined modality treatment arms. These preliminary survival results for the concurrent chemoradiation arm are promising and strongly support the continued investigation of concurrent strategies for patients with locally advanced NSCLC (41).

Sequential vs Concurrent: Patterns of Failure

Although the best sequencing is still under investigation, an analysis of the failure patterns between sequential vs concurrent therapy suggests a difference between these two strategies. Sequential trials delay or decrease the development of systemic disease, whereas concurrent regimens enhance local control. An indirect comparison of RTOG studies comparing sequential to concurrent chemoradiation trials reveals an improvement in overall response, in-field progression-free survival, as well as, 3-year overall survival for patients on concurrent chemoradiation trials. Although not randomized, these studies (8808, 8804, 9204, 9015, 9106) employed similar eligibility criteria. All patients had pathologically confirmed inoperable or unresectable NSCLC, Karnofsky Performance Status 50% or higher an no prior therapy for NSCLC. The sequential studies include RTOG 88-08 (25). It required induction chemotherapy consisting of cisplatin ($100mg/m^2$) D1, 29 and $5mg/m^2$ vinblastine for 5 weeks beginning on D1. This was followed by radiation Day 50. Protocol 8804 used the same induction regimen, but added cisplatin ($75 mg/m^2$) concurrently with standard radiation on day 50, 71 and 92 (42). Protocol 90-15 combined cisplatin ($75mg/m^2$) days 1, 29 and 50, and $5mg/m^2$ Vinblastine weekly for 5 weeks concurrently with Hyperfractionated radiation therapy (69.6 Gy, 1.2 Gy twice daily, 5 days per week for 6 weeks) (43).

Protocol 9106 combined cisplatin ($50mg/m^2$ days 1 and 8) and oral etoposide (100 mg/day in 2 divided doses, days 1-14) concurrent with the same hyperfractionated radiation regimen as in RTOG 9015. Cisplatin and etoposide were repeated beginning day 29.[77] Protocol 92-04 was a randomized Phase II comparison of the regimens piloted in RTOG 8804 and 9106 (44). Table 6 summarizes the overall response, 3-year progression-free survival, 3-year in-field progression-free survival and 3- year overall survival for these trials, The improvement in overall survival and especially 3-year in-files progression free survival suggests that concurrent chemoradiation may be superior to sequential therapy in enhancing local tumor control.

Table 6. Indirect Comparison of RTOG Trials of Chemoradiation Sequencing.

	Sequential CT/RT	Induction CT Concurrent CT/RT	Concurrent CT/RT
	(8808)	(8804,9204)	(9015,9106,9204)
OR	63%	77%	79%
3-yr PFS	7%	15%	15%
3-yr in field PFS	9%	17%	20%
3-yr OS	15%	17%	25%

*OR - Overall response	PFS - Progression-free survival*
OS - Overall survival

RECURRENT NSCLC FOLLOWING SURGERY

A solitary pulmonary metastasis is extremely uncommon from lung cancer. Therefore, patients who develop solitary lung metastasis following previous resection or treatment with primary chemoradiation should be treated as second primary lung cancers unless proven otherwise. Thus if the first primary tumor is well-controlled and restaging evaluation does not reveal metastatic disease, the second primary lung tumor should be resected, if possible. Adjuvant radiation therapy will depend on pathologic findings, as well as, the prior treatment (45,46).

Mediastinal or endobronchial recurrence following curative resection of NSCLC can be treated with radiation for palliation of obstructive symptoms.

RT FOR SUPERIOR VENA CAVA SYNDROME (SVCS)

Obstruction of the blood flow through the superior vena cava is due to intrathoracic malignancy in almost 90% of cases. Lung cancer is the most common malignant cause accounting for 90% of cases. Although it occurs in less than 5% of all patients with lung cancer (47), it is an important syndrome that requires recognition and management. The rapidity of symptoms is an important determinant of the type of clinical syndrome produced. Rapid occlusion produces acute and at times dramatic clinical signs. Gradual occlusion allows time for the development of extensive collateral vessels mitigating the clinical signs and symptoms. The most common presenting symptoms and signs are dyspnea, facial swelling, cough, orthopnea, and distension of the veins of the neck and chest wall. Although SVCS has long been considered a medical emergency, in general the only threat to the patient's life is when the airway is impeded either from the mass itself or from laryngeal edema, secondary to venous hypertension or from raised intracranial pressure. Irradiating patients without obtaining a tissue diagnosis is usually unneccessary (48,49). The prognosis of this syndrome is strongly correlated with that of its underlying cause. The chest radiograph is usually, although not invariably, abnormal. CT and MRI scanning provide valuable anatomic detail and staging information as well as vital detail for treatment planning. As many patients present prior to an established tissue diagnosis (18), the acquisition of tissue is a key issue. A substantial proportion of tissue diagnoses may be obtained by judicious use of tests such as a sputum cytology, thoracentesis, bone marrow and lymph node biopsy. However, bronchoscopy, mediastinoscopy, and even thoracotomy may be required and are usually successful. Before instituting radiotherapy general medical maneuvers such as oxygen support, bed rest with elevation of the head of the bed, and corticosteroids, may be used as temporizing measures. The optimal initial management for the patient with SCLC or lymphoma presenting with SVCS is generally combination chemotherapy, although radiotherapy has been used in selected series. There is no difference in outcome or in time to resolution between the two but chemotherapy offers the advantage of simultaneously treating the systemic disease and the avoidance of large field irradiation to the heart and the lung. Resolution of the syndrome is prompt (7 to 10 days) and is achieved in 43 to 100% of cases (50). Radiation is generally central to the management of the patient with NSCLC presenting with SVCS. Initial treatment with two to four fractions of 300 to 400 cGy has been advocated, based on limited evidence suggesting a more prompt response with this schedule (47). However the optimal fractionation schedule in SVCS has not been established and there are no clinical data to suggest a dose response in terms of the final dose required. We generally treat patients with NSCLC presenting with SVCS with 3900 cGy in 13 fractions. The treatment volume includes the tumor, ipsilateral supraclavicular node, adjacent mediastinum and hilar nodes.

PALLIATIVE TREATMENT OF STAGE IV NSCLC

Patients with Stage IV disease are generally treated with chemotherapy. Numerous studies have examined the role of palliative chemotherapy to best supportive care in NSCLC. They have come up with the same conclusions. There is a small but real benefit to the addition of chemotherapy over best supportive care. A recent meta-analysis suggests a possible 10% benefit at one year to Cisplatin containing regimens (35). Patient selection is of major importance and the patients most likely to benefit from such aggressive treatment measures, include those with ECOG performance status level 1-2. The ASCO guidelines provide an overview for patient selection (51).

The majority of patients who are of poor performance status can benefit from the use of radiation alone to relieve the local symptoms of lung cancer. These include obstructive symptoms from tracheal or esophageal compression including cough, and shortness of breath. The appropriate dose and fractionation scheme remains unclear. In a study of 369 patients, The Medical Research Council randomized patients to 17 Gy in two fractions given 1 week apart, 30 Gy in 10 fractions, or 27 Gy in 6 fractions. As assessed by patient and treating physician, the quality of life deteriorated slightly during treatment primarily due to treatment related dysphagia, but then improved. Hemoptysis, chest pain, and anorexia disappeared for a time in over 50% of patients and cough in 37% of patients. There was no difference in survival between the groups and, therefore, the authors recommended 8.5Gy X 2 fractions, given one week apart (52). However, a second randomized study of 291 patients performed in Japan, , found that although response rates were approximately the same, the slower fractionation schema provided superior symptom palliation. Patients were randomized to 45 Gy/18 fractions/ 4 ½ weeks or 31.2 Gy/4 fractions/4 weeks. Although the tumor response was similar (53% vs. 50%), the extended course was superior in terms of symptom palliation (71% vs. 54%, p< 0.02). Both arms were equally well tolerated (53). In patients with poor performance status who do not qualify for clinical trials, we generally recommend 3900 cGy/ 13 fractions.

Pain from direct invasion or from metastatic disease to bone can be palliated in over 60% of patients. In patients with symptomatic bony metastases, we generally recommend 3000 cGy/10 fractions.

In the patients with multiple brain metastases from non-small cell lung cancer, we also recommend 3000 cGy/10 fractions. For those patients, however, with a single brain lesion and resectable lung cancer, we would treat both lesions surgically and add postoperative radiation to the lung if warranted by pathologic findings. We would treat the whole brain with 250cGy/fraction for 15 fractions, followed by a boost of 3 fractions to the tumor a total dose of 4500cGy to help prevent the long term sequelae of brain irradiation (54,55). Patients who develop a single brain metastasis after surgical resection or primary chemoradiation for localized lung cancer, surgical resection of the brain metastasis and postoperative whole brain irradiation should be considered (56). Selected patients with either single or a few small metastases can be considered for whole brain radiation with radiosurgical boost. Unresectable lesions may be treated with radiosurgery (57).

Approximately half of the patients treated with resection and postoperative radiation to the whole brain for a single metastatic lesion will recur. If the patient still has a good performance status and no evidence of widespread progressive metastatic disease, reoperation or radiosurgery can be considered for palliation.

DOSE AND FRACTIONATION

Curative Dose

RTOG studies of lung cancer have demonstrated that intrathoracic failure rate is dose-dependent. A local failure rate of 52% was seen with 40Gy continuous radiation, 44% with 40 Gy split-course radiation, and 33% with 60 Gy continuous course (58). Given the high intrathoracic failure rates with conventional radiotherapy, altered fractionation schedules have been developed to improve local control. A phase II study using hyperfractionation (1.2 Gy bid) randomized patients to 60, 64.8, 69.6, 74.4, and 79.2 Gy. Among the patients with good performance status, and less than 5% weight loss, the survival was significantly improved with higher doses (69.6 Gy, 1.2 bid) over 60 Gy given in standard fractionation. There was, however, no difference in survival among the three highest total dose arms (59). Outside of a protocol setting, the current recommendations would be 60Gy at 2Gy/fraction given over 6 weeks.

Altered Fractionation

While some investigators have tried to improve local control by adding radiosensitizing chemotherapy to radiation, others have tried to improve radiation's effect by altering fractionation. Dividing a dose into a number of fractions spares normal tissues due to the repair of sublethal damage between dose fractions and cellular repopulation. At the same time, fractionation increases tumor damage by allowing reoxygenation and reassortment of cells into more sensitive portions of the cell cycle. Fraction size is the dominant factor in determining late effects, while overall treatment time has little effect. Fraction size and overall treatment time are important in determing the response of acutely responding tissues such as tumors. Hyperfractionation, or the delivery of multiple doses using smaller dose per fraction tries to separate early from late effects. The overall treatment time remains the same, approximately 6-8 weeks, but since two or three fractions per day are used, the total number of fractions can be 60-80. The dose must increase, since the dose per fraction is decreased, and tumor effects are improved while late effects are spared.

An alternative strategy uses accelerated treatment, which involves approximately conventional doses using approximately conventional dose/fraction but decreases the overall treatment time by almost half. This reduces repopulation of rapidly proliferating tumor cells and, thereby, improves tumor effects but at the cost of significant acute effects on normal tissues. There is little or no change on late tissue effects. Table 7 summarizes some of the studies of altered fractionation alone.

Table 7. Hyperfractionation Alone in the management of locally advanced lung cancer

Regimen	Dose/fxn	Fxn #	Duration	Total dose	1YS	2YS	MS
CHART[60]	1.5Gy tid RT std fxn	36	12days	54Gy	63% 55%	29% 20%	NA
HART E4593 [62]	1.5-1.8Gy tid	36	16days	57.6Gy	57%	NA	13months

Fxn- fraction, MS - median survival, std - standard, 1 YS - 1-year survival, 2 YS - 2-year survival

CHART (continuous hyperfractionated accelerated radiation therapy) takes advantage of smaller fraction size to spare normal tissue toxicity while shortening the duration of treatment and thereby not allowing tumor cell repopulation during the normal breaks of standard fractionation. 563 patients were randomized to CHART (1.5 Gy/fraction, 3 fractions/day, 36 fractions for a total dose of 54Gy over 12 days) or standard fraction radiation (2Gy/fraction, 1 fraction/day, 30 fractions, for a total dose of 60 Gy over 6 weeks). There was an improvement in 1-year survival (63% vs 55%) and 2-year survival (29% vs 20%) to the hyperfractionated arm (60). Remarkably despite this aggressive radiation the short and long-term toxicities were equivalent (61). An analysis of the patterns of failure showed that the improved survival was due to a decrease in local progression. Unfortunately, this study has been criticized as it had included medically inoperable Stages I/II disease and a large percentage of patients with squamous cell cancer, a histology known for its higher propensity for local progression over systemic disease.

HART (Hyperfractionated accelerated radiation therapy) uses the same principals as CHART except that it does not involve treatment over the weekends. In ECOG 4593, a phase II study of hyperfractionated radiation, 30 patients were treated with 1.5-1.8 Gy/fraction, 3 fractions/day, 36 fractions for a total dose of 57.6 Gy over 16 days. With a median follow up of 19 months, median survival was 13 months and 1-year survival 57%. These survivals are similar to those achieved in the combined modality arms of CALGB8433 (62).

Since hyperfractionated radiation has shown results comparable to the combined modality arms utilizing chemotherapy and radiation, the next question in the management of locally advanced lung cancer is whether results could be improved with the combination of hyperfractionated radiation and chemotherapy. Table 8 summarizes some of the trials of combined modality therapy utilizing hyperfractionation.

VOLUME, PORTALS, BEAM ARRANGEMENTS

The volume to be treated and the radiation portal are determined by the size, stage, and location of the primary as well as the involved or at risk lymph nodes.

Table 8. Hyperfractionated radiation with chemotherapy

Author	Type	Regimen	CT	MS (mo)	1YS	2YS
Byhardt[38]	Phase II	RT bid with CT	Vinblastine Cisplatin	12.2	54%	28%
Choy[63]	Phase II	RT bid with CT	Paclitaxel Carboplatin			
R T O G 9106 Lee JS[64]	Phase II	RT bid with CT	Cisplatin Etoposide po	18.9	67%	35%
R T O G 9410[41]	Phase III	CMT, std CMT,hyperfxn				
R T O G 9204 Komaki[44]	Phase III	I: CT→std RT/P II: CT + hfxn RT	I:P,vinblastine II: P, VP16	15.5 14.4	65% 58%	

MS - median survival, 1 YS - 1-year survival, 2 YS - 2-year survival, hfxn -   hyperfractionated radiation therapy

Primary Radiation for Early Stage, Medically Inoperable NSCLC

The volume to be treated includes the tumor mass. In patients with poor pulmonary function tests and peripherally located lesions, we limit the treatment to the mass alone. In patients who have centrally located lesions, whose mediastinum can be easily incorporated without a significant increase in the amount of lung volume treated, we include both the mass and mediastinum in the original volume to 4000 cGy. This is followed by a cone down to mass alone, off cord, for the remaining 2000 cGy.

Primary Radiation (With/Without Chemotherapy) for Unresectable NSCLC

For patients with good performance status, we advocate the use of combined modality therapy. For patients who have poor performance status, radiation alone is sometimes utilized. For patients who will be receiving concurrent chemotherapy, the radiation and chemotherapy begins on day 1. The initial volume consists of the mediastinum and primary tumor followed by a boost to the tumor alone. The initial volume receives 2 Gy, 5 days a week, for 20 fractions for a total dose of 40Gy. The boost volume receives 2Gy, 5 days a week for 10 fractions for an additional 20 Gy for a total tumor dose of 60Gy.

The treatment portals are designed with 2-cm margins around the gross tumor and approximately 2-cm margin around electively treated regional lymph nodes. Irregularly shaped fields are preferred and as much normal heart and lung is blocked with secondary blocking. On occasion, the entire lung must be treated when atelectesis or pneumonitis complicates the lesion when it is not possible to determine the boundaries of the primary tumor. Such patients are rescanned following the initial 2 weeks (20Gy) of therapy. Often, following a few weeks of therapy, the lung expands and the tumor volume can now be determined.

The initial volume includes the tumor and regional lymph nodes. The regional lymph nodes vary with the location of the tumor. Only patients who have upper lobe or main stem bronchus tumor require inclusion of the ipsilateral supraclavicular nodes. Ipsilateral hilar nodes are always treated with a 2-cm margin. The superior mediastinal nodes are always treated with a 2-cm margin. The inferior mediastinal nodes to the diaphragm (to bottom of T10) are included only in patients with lower lobe lesions. Otherwise, the inferior border of the field is usually 5 cm below the bifurcation of the carina or 2 vertebral bodies below the carina. Contralateral hilar lymph nodes are included, with a 1-cm margin, only in patients with contralateral mediastinal, subcarinal, or contralateral hilar involvement.

All patients then go to the boost volume, which includes the tumor and mediastinum. This includes the tumor and ipsilateral mediastinum with a 2-cm margin. The boost volume should include less than 50% of the ipsilateral total lung volume. Multiple beams and oblique portals can be used to deliver adequate tumor dose while maintaining the spinal cord dose below 4500 cGy. We do not recommend the use of posterior spinal blocks as this causes substantial underdosage of the mediastinum. Compensating filters or wedges can be used to correct for the sloping contour of the chest and avoid higher doses of radiation to the cervical and upper thoracic spinal cord.

It is important not to exceed normal tissue tolerances for any of the sensitive structures in the thorax. These include the heart, lung, and spinal cord. It is important to limit the radiation dose to the entire lung volume to less than 20 Gy. The spinal cord to 45 Gy. No more than 50% of the cardiac volume should get more than 35 Gy. Megavoltage equipment is required so that doses to normal structures can be reduced while still treating deep-seated tumors. We generally use 18MV photons for both the initial AP-PA fields, as well as the oblique fields.

Neoadjuvant Chemoradiation for Locally Advanced Lung Cancer

The portals, target volumes are the same as that described for locally unresectable patients. The total dose, however, is usually 4500-5040 cGy.

Post-Operative Chemoradiation for Resectable NSCLC

The target volume for resected NSCLC includes the mediastinal and ipsilateral hilar nodes. The tumor bed is included only if invasion of the parietal pleura or positive

margins is documented. Anatomic landmarks rather than the preoperative appearance of the tumor, therefore, determine the target volume. The target volume consists of the ipsilateral hilum, mediastinal and bilateral paratracheal nodes. Neither the contralateral hilum nor the supraclavicular fossa is routinely included. If, however, it is necessary to treat the tumor bed for a T3 lesion of the upper lobe, the supraclavicular fossa may be included. Although the exact field borders will vary depending on the anatomy and postoperative shift of mediastinal structures, these are the general guidelines:
Superior border: lung apex, approximately C5 for patients with N1 disease. Ipsilateral supraclavicular fossae for N2 disease.

Inferior border: 5 cm below carina for upper lobe lesions and 8 cm below carina for lower or middle lobe lesions. Any patient with histologically positive subcarinal nodes should have the inferior border 8-cm below the carina.

Ipsilateral border: 2cm beyond the lateral edge of the vertebral body to include the ipsilateral hilum with a 2-cm margin. In patients who have undergone pneumonectomy, the bronchial stump and associated peribronchial nodes should be included with margins based on the preoperative CT scan.

Contralateral border: 2-cm lateral to the lateral edge of the vertebral body.

The initial field is given with parallel-opposed AP-PA fields, to a dose of 36-42 Gy of the planned total dose of 5400 cGy. The remainder of the treatment is to the same target volume but with field arrangements to exclude the spinal cord and keep the total cord dose to less than 45 Gy. Oblique fields with angles usually between 20-40 degrees are used, with medial borders defined by the ipsilateral pedicle of the spine and including the subcarinal space and contralateral main stem bronchus. Lateral fields should be avoided as they increase the dose to the normal lung tissue. The entire volume will receive 50.4 Gy/28 fraction/6 weeks. For patients with gross nodal disease, the nodes will be boosted to 5400 cGy.

RT TECHNIQUE: 3D CONFORMAL

The use of multiple non-coplanar beams allows improved tumor volume definition (65). A pilot trial conducted by Washington University investigators shows grade 3 or higher radiation pneumonitis increases with increasing percentage of normal lung to doses over 20.0Gy. There is also an ongoing prospective trial at the University of Michigan in which total RT doses are partitioned according to the percentage of the entire lung volume receiving more than 20.0 Gy. The current prescribed dose in this study is 100.0 Gy. The RTOG is currently evaluating the potential of a phase III trial comparing maximum-tolerated doses of three-dimensional conformal RT to standard dose RT.

Side Effects of Therapy
Acute side effects usually begin in the second or third week of treatment. Dermatitis is rarely severe. It is treated with aloe vera gel or wool wax alcohol (Aquaphor).

Esophagitis, following radiation alone, is usually mild to moderate pain with swallowing, which may require changing to a semi-solid diet, liquid analgesics, and antacids. In trials of radiation combined with chemotherapy, esophagitis is often the dose-limiting toxicity. The acute symptoms of esophagitis usually resolve 2-3 weeks following therapy completion. Chronic esophagitis is rare, but can be seen 1-5 years after completion of therapy and includes stenosis, stricture, or tracheoesophageal fistula. The extent of esophagitis is a function of dose, technique, use of chemotherapy, and length of esophagus treated (60).

Radiation pneumonitis is the most significant side effect from radiation to the lung. It can be fatal in a small percentage of patients. It is a function of the amount of lung irradiated, concurrent use of chemotherapy, total dose, and fractionation. It is often difficult to diagnose, as it is a diagnosis of exclusion. Patients often present with low grade fever, tachycardia, dyspnea, and hypoxia. Radiographs initially show an infiltrate that corresponds to the treated port. Often a CT scan in the correct clinical setting can be diagnostic as it reveals a geometrically shaped infiltrate corresponding to the treated port. It can develop 3-6 months following treatment completion. After other etiologies such as recurrent disease and infection have been ruled out, patients are treated with prednisone (1mg/kg/day) and tapering gradually while monitoring symptoms. This taper can often take 2-3 months. Patients, who have received radiation to the lung and receive steroids for other reasons, can develop radiation pneumonitis when the steroids are tapered. Often patients are prophylaxed with trimethoprim-sulfamethoxazole during prednisone to prevent superinfection with Pneumocystis carinii.

INTENSITY MODULATED RADIATION THERAPY (IMRT)

Conventional radiation therapy is delivered with beams of uniform intensity across the treatment field. Simple beam modifiers such as wedges and compensators are often used to account for missing tissue, and in some instances, to shape dose distribution. While this approach works well for simple, regularly shaped target volumes, it is limited for complex target shapes or for geometries in which the planning target volume (PTV) is in close proximity to critical organs. In the 3-dimensional paradigm, these limitations are overcome by employing non-uniform beam fluence distributions for a selected number of beams, or via arc therapy. The dose distribution is produced by dividing each beam into tiny subdivisions called "beamleats" with each beamlet's intensity being determined by a computer optimization algorithm. The development of the multileaf collimator (MLC) and sophisticated computer control systems, have made it possible to use the MLC in a dynamic mode, and has spurred the development of Intensity Modulated Radiation Therapy (IMRT).

There are 3 kinds of IMRT types generally classified to date. The first is tomotherapy IMRT proposed by Mackie et al (67). Tomotherapy" which literally means "slice therapy" is IMRT delivered using a narrow slit beam. A slit mini-MLC system (called MIMiC) of the type proposed by Mackie et al is now commercially available (Peacock, Nomos Corporation, Sewickley, PA). The Peacock system's MIMiC is mounted on to a conventional low energy megavoltage medical linear accelerator, and treatment is delivered slice by slice using arc rotations (68). The beam is collimated to a narrow slit, and beamlets of varying intensity are created by driving the MIMiC's leaves in and out of the radiation beam's path as the gantry rotates around the patient. A complete treatment is accomplished by sequential delivery to adjoining axial slices.

The second approach is to use a conventional MLC, used in a dynamic mode. It provides a full field approach to IMRT, compared to the slit-field approach of tomotherapy. For a fixed gantry position, the gap formed by each pair of opposing MLC leaves is swept across the target volume under computer control with the radiation beam on to produce the desired fluence profiles. The setting of the gap opening and its speed for each MLC leaf pair are determined by a technique first introduced by Convery et al (69) and extended by Bortfeld et al (70) and Spirou et al (71). Another approach uses a sequence of static MLC fields (typically called "segments" or "subfields") that are set up and delivered at each orientation of the gantry under complete control. This method is sometimes referred to as "step and shoot" or "stop and shoot" and the leaf sequences can be determined by the method suggested by Bortfeld et al (72). In this approach, the linear accelerator is switched on and off for a predefined number of monitor units for each subfield automatically, under computer control. This allows a completely automated treatment delivery of all subfields of all beams of a treatment plan, including gantry rotation. Most medical linear accelerator manufacturers now offer this type of computer control feature. Thus, widespread implementation of this form of IMRT is anticipated over the next several years.

The third MLC approach, called intensity modulated arc therapy (IMAT), has been suggested by Yu et al (73,74). In this case, multiple superimposing arcs are used with the beam aperture changing shape during gantry rotation under computer control, with the radiation beam on to produce the desired fluence profiles. The cumulative fluence distribution of all the arcs generates the desired dose distribution.

Finally, a physical compensation filter approach can also be used to deliver IMRT. Filters designed using 3-dimensional radiotherapy planning are capable of compensating not only for the missing tissue, but also for internal tissue heterogeneities. Filters can be designed by calculating the thickness along a ray line, using an effective attenuation coefficient for the filter material and dose-ratio parameters for effective depths that generate the desired IMRT fluence profile when the filter is placed in the radiation beam. Stein et al are investigating the use of physical modulators fabricated using a low-melting point alloy poured into foam molds, which are cut using a computer controlled cutter (75). In addition, Dubal et al recently described a compensating filter approach for IMRT for the treatment of breast cancer (76).

ENDOBRONCHIAL BRACHYTHERAPY

Recurrent endobronchial tumors present a difficult therapeutic problem. Most often these patients present with endobronchial disease following a definitive course of external beam irradiation. The most common method of treatment include endobronchial excision of the tumor or laser coagulation The improvement obtained from these procedures is usually limited to 3 or 4 months, and repeated treatments become more difficult and less effective. In recent years, there has been a rapid increase in the use of endobronchial brachytherapy to treat endobronchial recurrence or as a way to boost the initial treatment for primary NSCLC. Two technological developments including the introduction of the high-dose-rate (HDR) remote afterloading device and the advent of fiberoptic bronchoscopy with its widespread utilization have led to the increased utilization of endobronchial brachytherapy. Endobronchial brachytherapy is often used for palliative purposes in patients with recurrent endobronchial disease after prior external beam irradiation, to relieve life-threatening complications, such as hemoptysis and airway obstruction with associated atelectasis and pneumonia. Endobronchial brachytherapy is less frequently used in combination with external beam irradiation to deliver an additional boost with curative intent to the primary endobronchial lesion in patients with poor lung function precluding surgical resection. There are now numerous studies in the literature that support the use of endobronchial HDR brachytherapy to palliate local symptoms such as cough, dyspnea, and hemoptysis. Overall response rates (clinical, radiological and bronchoscopic), reported in over 1,000 patients treated with HDR endobronchial brachytherapy, are in the range of 80-90%, with most cases considered a complete response (77,78). Hemoptysis appears to be particularly responsive. Cough and dyspnea can also be palliated in more than 50% of cases. The effectiveness of treatment depends on a number of factors, with radiation dose being the most important. Doses higher than 1,000 cGy at 1 cm from the source may give slightly better response rates but at the cost of increased morbidity, especially fatal hemoptysis (79,80). An analysis of reports from the literature suggests that HDR endobronchial irradiation can provide significant palliation of severe symptoms caused by primary or recurrent endobronchial disease (81,82,83). Patient condition, tumor extent, and dose of HDR therapy affect the incidence of morbidity. The optimal approach, however, remains unclear, especially in terms of dose per fraction and number of fractions. We believe that no more than 10 Gy, prescribed to a depth of 1 cm from the central axis of the source, should be given in a single application. In debilitated patients or patients who have previously received large doses of external beam irradiation, a dose of 5 Gy per application, delivered every week for three weeks is recommended. We feel that when HDR is available, it is the preferred method of treatment because it provides advantages in patient comfort, convenience, and safety. Until more is known about mucosal tolerance, we choose to be conservative with fraction size and prescription point.

REFERENCES

1. W. C. Roentzen. "On a New Kind of Rays (Preliminary Communication)"- Translation of a paper read before the Physikalische-Medicinischen Gesellschaft of Wurzburg on December 28, 1895. *British Journal of Radiology* 4 (32), 1931.
2. H.D. Kogelnik. Inauguration of radiotherapy as a new scientific speciality by Leopold Freund 100 years ago [see comments]. *Radiother.Oncol.* 42 (3):203-211, 1997.
3. H. Coutard. Pinciples of x-ray therapy of malignant diseases. *Lancet* 2:1-8, 1934.

4.   P Curie, M. P. Curie, and G. Bemont. Sur Une Nouvell Substance Fortement Radioactive Contenue dans la Peckblende (Note presented by M. Becquerel). *Complete Rendition of Academy of Sciences (Paris)* 127:1215-1217, 1898.

5.   C. F. Mountain. Revisions in the International System for Staging Lung Cancer [see comments]. *Chest* 111 (6):1710-1717, 1997.

6.   H. M. Sandler, W. J. Curran, Jr., and A. T. Turrisi, III. The influence of tumor size and pre-treatment staging on outcome following radiation therapy alone for stage I non-small cell lung cancer. *Int.J.Radiat.Oncol.Biol.Phys.* 19 (1):9-13, 1990.

7.   E. M. Noordijk, Clement E. Poest, J. Hermans, A. M. Wever, and J. W. Leer. Radiotherapy as an alternative to surgery in elderly patients with resectable lung cancer. *Radiother.Oncol.* 13 (2):83-89, 1988.

8.   H. X. Zhang, W. B. Yin, L. J. Zhang, Z. Y. Yang, Z. X. Zhang, M. Wang, D. F. Chen, and X. Z. Gu. Curative radiotherapy of early operable non-small cell lung cancer. *Radiother.Oncol.* 14 (2):89-94, 1989.

9.   D. E. Dosoretz, M. J. Katin, P. H. Blitzer, J. H. Rubenstein, S. Salenius, M. Rashid, R. A. Dosani, G. Mestas, A. D. Siegel, and T. T. Chadha. Radiation therapy in the management of medically inoperable carcinoma of the lung: results and implications for future treatment strategies [see comments]. *Int.J.Radiat.Oncol.Biol.Phys.* 24 (1):3-9, 1992.

10. R. Gelman, R. Gelber, I. C. Henderson, C. N. Coleman, and J. R. Harris. Improved methodology for analyzing local and distant recurrence [see comments]. *J.Clin.Oncol.* 8 (3):548-555, 1990.

11. G. S. Sibley, T. A. Jamieson, L. B. Marks, M. S. Anscher, and L. R. Prosnitz. Radiotherapy alone for medically inoperable stage I non-small-cell lung cancer: the Duke experience. *Int.J.Radiat.Oncol.Biol.Phys.* 40 (1):149-154, 1998.

12. A. D. Krol, P. Aussems, E. M. Noordijk, J. Hermans, and J. W. Leer. Local irradiation alone for peripheral stage I lung cancer: could we omit the elective regional nodal irradiation? *Int.J.Radiat.Oncol.Biol.Phys.* 34 (2):297-302, 1996.

13. T. Naruke, T. Goya, R. Tsuchiya, and K. Suemasu. Prognosis and survival in resected lung carcinoma based on the new international staging system [published erratum appears in J Thorac Cardiovasc Surg 1989 Mar;97(3):350]. *J.Thorac.Cardiovasc.Surg.* 96 (3):440-447, 1988.

14. D. E. Dosoretz, D. Galmarini, J. H. Rubenstein, M. J. Katin, P. H. Blitzer, S. A. Salenius, R. A. Dosani, M. Rashid, G. Mestas, and S. E. Hannan. Local control in medically inoperable lung cancer: an analysis of its importance in outcome and factors determining the probability of tumor eradication. *Int.J.Radiat.Oncol.Biol.Phys.* 27 (3):507-516, 1993.

15. Effects of postoperative mediastinal radiation on completely resected stage II and stage III epidermoid cancer of the lung. The Lung Cancer Study Group. *N.Engl.J.Med.* 315 (22):1377-1381, 1986.

16. Postoperative radiotherapy in non-small-cell lung cancer: systematic review and meta-analysis of individual patient data from nine randomised controlled trials. PORT Meta-analysis Trialists Group [see comments]. *Lancet* 352 (9124):257-263, 1998.

17. S. M. Keller. ECOG: Phase III comparison of thoracic radiotherapy alone Vs combined with CDDP/VP-16 chemotherapy as postoperative adjuvant therapy for Stage II/IIIA non-scall cell lung cancer, Closed 02/04/97. PASCO, 1999.

18. N. Martini, M. G. Kris, R. J. Gralla, M. S. Bains, P. M. McCormack, L. R. Kaiser, M. E. Burt, and M. B. Zaman. The effects of preoperative chemotherapy on the resectability of non- small cell lung carcinoma with mediastinal lymph node metastases (N2 M0). *Ann.Thorac.Surg.* 45 (4):370-379, 1988.

19. V. W. Rusch, K. S. Albain, J. J. Crowley, T. W. Rice, V. Lonchyna, R. McKenna, Jr., R. B. Livingston, B. R. Griffin, and J. R. Benfield. Surgical resection of stage IIIA and stage IIIB non-small-cell lung cancer after concurrent induction chemoradiotherapy. A Southwest Oncology Group trial. *J.Thorac.Cardiovasc.Surg.* 105 (1):97-104, 1993.

20. J. A. Roth, F. Fossella, R. Komaki, M. B. Ryan, J. B. Putnam, Jr., J. S. Lee, H. Dhingra, L. De Caro, M. Chasen, and M. McGavran. A randomized trial comparing perioperative chemotherapy and surgery with surgery alone in resectable stage IIIA non-small-cell lung cancer [see comments]. *J.Natl.Cancer Inst.* 86 (9):673-680, 1994.

21. Rosell R, Gomez-Codina J, Camps C, Maestre J, Padille J, Canto A, Mate JL, Li S, Roig J, Olazabal A, et al. A randomized trial comparing preoperative chemotherapy plus surgery with surgery alone in patients with non-small cell lung cancer. N Engl J Med 330:153-158, 1994.

22. T. Sause, P. Koselar, S. Taylor, D. Johnson, R. Livingston, R. Komaki, B. Emami, W. Curran, R. Byhardt, B. Fisher, and A. T. Turrisi. Five-year Results; Phase III trial of regionally advanced unresectable non-small cell lung cancer, RTOG 8808, ECOG 4588, SWOG 8992. *Proceeding of the American Society of Clinical Oncology* 1998:1743, 1998. (Abstract)

23. K. Kubota, K. Furuse, M. Kawahara, N. Kodama, M. Yamamoto, M. Ogawara, S. Negoro, N. Masuda, M. Takada, and K. Matsui. Role of radiotherapy in combined modality treatment of locally advanced non-small-cell lung cancer. *J.Clin.Oncol.* 12 (8):1547-1552, 1994.

24. R. O. Dillman, S. L. Seagren, K. J. Propert, J. Guerra, W. L. Eaton, M. C. Perry, R. W. Carey, E. F. Frei, III, and M. R. Green. A randomized trial of induction chemotherapy plus high-dose radiation versus radiation alone in stage III non-small-cell lung cancer [see comments]. *N.Engl.J.Med.* 323 (14):940-945, 1990.

25. W. T. Sause, C. Scott, S. Taylor, D. Johnson, R. Livingston, R. Komaki, B. Emami, W. J. Curran, R. W. Byhardt, and A. T. Turrisi. Radiation Therapy Oncology Group (RTOG) 88-08 and Eastern Cooperative Oncology Group (ECOG) 4588: preliminary results of a phase III trial in regionally advanced, unresectable non-small-cell lung cancer. *J.Natl.Cancer Inst.* 87 (3):198-205, 1995.

26. T. Le Chevalier, R. Arriagada, E. Quoix, P. Ruffie, M. Martin, M. Tarayre, M. J. Lacombe-Terrier, J. Y. Douillard, and A. Laplanche. Radiotherapy alone versus combined chemotherapy and radiotherapy in nonresectable non-small-cell lung cancer: first analysis of a randomized trial in 353 patients [see comments]. *J.Natl.Cancer Inst.* 83 (6):417-423, 1991.

27. R. Arriagada, T. Le Chevalier, and E Rekacewicz. Cisplatin-Based Chemoradiotherapy in Patients with Locally Advanced Non-Small Cell Lung Cancer(NSCLC: Late Analysis of a French Randomized Trial (abstract). *Proceeding of the American Society of Clinical Oncology* 16:446a, 1997. (Abstract)

28. C. Schaake-Koning, Bogaert W. van den, O. Dalesio, J. Festen, J. Hoogenhout, P. van Houtte, A. Kirkpatrick, M. Koolen, B. Maat, and A. Nijs. Effects of concomitant cisplatin and radiotherapy on inoperable non- small-cell lung cancer [see comments]. *N.Engl.J.Med.* 326 (8):524-530, 1992.

29. K. S. Albain, V. W. Rusch, J. J. Crowley, T. W. Rice, A. T. Turrisi, III, J. K. Weick, V. A. Lonchyna, C. A. Presant, R. J. McKenna, and D. R. Gandara. Concurrent cisplatin/etoposide plus chest radiotherapy followed by surgery for stages IIIA (N2) and IIIB non-small-cell lung cancer: mature results of Southwest Oncology Group phase II study 8805. *J.Clin.Oncol.* 13 (8):1880-1892, 1995.

30. K. Mattson, L. R. Holsti, P. Holsti, M. Jakobsson, M. Kajanti, K. Liippo, M. Mantyla, S. Niitamo-Korhonen, V. Nikkanen, and E. Nordman. Inoperable non-small cell lung cancer: radiation with or without chemotherapy. *Eur.J.Cancer Clin.Oncol.* 24 (3):477-482, 1988.

31. P. van Houtte, J. Klastersky, A. Renaud, J. Michel, G. Vandermoten, H. Nguyen, J. P. Sculier, J. Devriendt, and P. Mommen. Induction chemotherapy with cisplatin, etoposide and vindesine before radiation therapy for nonsmall-cell lung cancer. A randomized study. *Antibiot.Chemother.* 41:131-137, 1988.

32. L. Crino, P. Latini, M. Meacci, E. Corgna, E. Maranzano, S. Darwish, V. Minotti, A. Santucci, and M. Tonato. Induction chemotherapy plus high-dose radiotherapy versus radiotherapy alone in locally advanced unresectable non-small-cell lung cancer. *Ann.Oncol.* 4 (10):847-851, 1993.

33. A. Planting, P. Helle, P. Drings, O. Dalesio, A. Kirkpatrick, G. McVie, and G. Giaccone. A randomized study of high-dose split course radiotherapy preceded by high-dose chemotherapy versus high-dose radiotherapy only in locally advanced non-small-cell lung cancer. An EORTC Lung Cancer Cooperative Group trial [see comments]. *Ann.Oncol.* 7 (2):139-144, 1996.

34. R. F. Morton, J. R. Jett, W. L. McGinnis, J. D. Earle, T. M. Therneau, J. E. Krook, T. E. Elliott, J. A. Mailliard, R. A. Nelimark, and A. W. Maksymiuk. Thoracic radiation therapy alone compared with combined chemoradiotherapy for locally unresectable non-small cell lung cancer. A randomized, phase III trial [see comments]. *Ann.Intern.Med.* 115 (9):681-686, 1991.

35. Chemotherapy in non-small cell lung cancer: a meta-analysis using updated data on individual patients from 52 randomised clinical trials. Non-small Cell Lung Cancer Collaborative Group [see comments]. *BMJ* 311 (7010):899-909, 1995.

36. P. Marino, A. Preatoni, and A. Cantoni. Randomized trials of radiotherapy alone versus combined chemotherapy and radiotherapy in stages IIIa and IIIb nonsmall cell lung cancer. A meta-analysis [see comments]. *Cancer* 76 (4):593-601, 1995.

37. R. S. Pritchard and S. P. Anthony. Chemotherapy plus radiotherapy compared with radiotherapy alone in the treatment of locally advanced, unresectable, non-small-cell lung cancer. A meta-analysis [published erratum appears in Ann Intern Med 1997 Apr 15;126(8):670]. *Ann.Intern.Med.* 125 (9):723-729, 1996.

38. R. W. Byhardt, C. Scott, W. T. Sause, B. Emami, R. Komaki, B. Fisher, J. S. Lee, and C. Lawton. Response, toxicity, failure patterns, and survival in five Radiation Therapy Oncology Group (RTOG) trials of sequential and/or concurrent chemotherapy and radiotherapy for locally advanced non-small-cell carcinoma of the lung. *Int.J.Radiat.Oncol.Biol.Phys.* 42 (3):469-478, 1998.

39. K. Furose, M. Fukuoka, and M. Takada. A Randomized Phase II Study of Concurrent vs. Sequential Thoracic Radiotherapy in Combination with Mitomycin, Vindesine adn Cisplatin in Unresectable Stage III NSCLC: Preliminary Analysis. *Proceeding of the American Society of Clinical Oncology* 16: 1999. (Abstract)

40. G. Clamon, J. Herndon, R. Cooper, A. Y. Chang, J. Rosenman, and M. R. Green. Radiosensitization with carboplatin for patients with unresectable stage III non-small-cell lung cancer: a phase III trial of the Cancer and Leukemia Group B and the Eastern Cooperative Oncology Group [see comments]. *J.Clin.Oncol.* 17 (1):4-11, 1999.

41. Curran WJ, Scott C, Langer C, Komaki R, Lee JS, Hauser S, Movsas B, Wasserman T, Rosenthal S, Byhardt R, Sause W, Cox J. Phase III comparison of sequential vs. concurrent chemoradiation for patients (pts) with unresected stage III non-small cell lung cancer (NSCLC): Initial report of Radiation Therapy Oncology Group (RTOG) 9410. PASCO 2000 Abstract No. 1891.

42. W. T. Sause, C. Scott, S. Taylor, D. Johnson, R. Livingston, R. Komaki, B. Emami, W. J. Curran, R. W. Byhardt, and A. T. Turrisi. Radiation Therapy Oncology Group (RTOG) 88-08 and Eastern Cooperative Oncology Group (ECOG) 4588: preliminary results of a phase III trial in regionally advanced, unresectable non-small-cell lung cancer. *J.Natl.Cancer Inst.* 87 (3):198-205, 1995.

43. Byhardt, C. B. Scott, D. S. Ettinger, W. J. Curran, R. L. Doggett, C. Coughlin, C. Scarantino, M. Rotman, and B. Emami. Concurrent hyperfractionated irradiation and chemotherapy for unresectable nonsmall cell lung cancer. Results of Radiation Therapy Oncology Group 90-15. *Cancer* 75 (9):2337-2344, 1995.

44. R. Komaki, C. Scott, D. Ettinger, J. S. Lee, F. V. Fossella, W. Curran, R. F. Evans, P. Rubin, and R. W. Byhardt. Randomized study of chemotherapy/radiation therapy combinations for favorable patients with locally advanced inoperable nonsmall cell lung cancer: Radiation Therapy Oncology Group (RTOG) 92-04. *Int.J.Radiat.Oncol.Biol.Phys.* 38 (1):149-155, 1997.

45. T. A. Salerno, D. D. Munro, P. E. Blundell, and R. C. Chiu. Second primary bronchogenic carcinoma: life-table analysis of surgical treatment. *Ann.Thorac.Surg.* 27 (1):3-6, 1979.

46. A. Yellin, L. R. Hill, and J. R. Benfield. Bronchogenic carcinoma associated with upper aerodigestive cancers. *J.Thorac.Cardiovasc.Surg.* 91 (5):674-683, 1986.

47. B. A. Armstrong, C. A. Perez, J. R. Simpson, and M. A. Hederman. Role of irradiation in the management of superior vena cava syndrome. *Int.J.Radiat.Oncol.Biol.Phys.* 13 (4):531-539, 1987.

48. C. P. Escalante. Causes and management of superior vena cava syndrome. *Oncology (Huntingt)* 7 (6):61-68, 1993.

49. D. E. Schraufnagel, R. Hill, J. A. Leech, and J. A. Pare. Superior vena caval obstruction. Is it a medical emergency? *Am.J.Med.* 70 (6):1169-1174, 1981.

50. A. M. Maddox, M. Valdivieso, J. Lukeman, T. L. Smith, H. E. Barkley, M. L. Samuels, and G. P. Bodey. Superior vena cava obstruction in small cell bronchogenic carcinoma. Clinical parameters and survival. *Cancer* 52 (11):2165-2172, 1983.

51. Clinical practice guidelines for the treatment of unresectable non- small-cell lung cancer. Adopted on May 16, 1997 by the American Society of Clinical Oncology. *J.Clin.Oncol.* 15 (8):2996-3018, 1997.

52. Inoperable non-small-cell lung cancer (NSCLC): a Medical Research Council randomised trial of palliative radiotherapy with two fractions or ten fractions. Report to the Medical Research Council by its Lung Cancer Working Party. *Br.J.Cancer* 63 (2):265-270, 1991.

53. P. Teo, T. H. Tai, D. Choy, and K. H. Tsui. A randomized study on palliative radiation therapy for inoperable non small cell carcinoma of the lung. *Int.J.Radiat.Oncol.Biol.Phys.* 14 (5):867-871, 1988.

54. L. Mandell, B. Hilaris, M. Sullivan, N. Sundaresan, D. Nori, J. H. Kim, N. Martini, and Z. Fuks. The treatment of single brain metastasis from non-oat cell lung carcinoma. Surgery and radiation versus radiation therapy alone. *Cancer* 58 (3):641-649, 1986.

55. L. M. DeAngelis, L. R. Mandell, H. T. Thaler, D. W. Kimmel, J. H. Galicich, Z. Fuks, and J. B. Posner. The role of postoperative radiotherapy after resection of single brain metastases. *Neurosurgery* 24 (6):798-805, 1989.

56. Patchell RA, Tibbs PA, Walsh JW, Dempsey RJ, Maruyama Y, Kryscio RJ, Markesbery WR, Macdonald JS, Young B. A randomized trial of surgery in the treatment of single metastases to the brain. N Engl J Med 22:322:494-500, 1990.

57. Alexander E 3rd, Moriarty TM, Davis RB, Wen PY, Fine HA, Black PM, Kooy HM, Loeffler JS. Stereotactic radiosurgery for the definitive, noninvasive treatment of brain metastases. J Natl Cancer Inst 87:34-40, 1995.

58. C. A. Perez, M. Bauer, S. Edelstein, B. W. Gillespie, and R. Birch. Impact of tumor control on survival in carcinoma of the lung treated with irradiation [published erratum appears in Int J Radiat Oncol Biol Phys 1986 Nov;12(11):2057]. *Int.J.Radiat.Oncol.Biol.Phys.* 12 (4):539-547, 1986.

59. J. D. Cox, N. Azarnia, R. W. Byhardt, K. H. Shin, B. Emami, and T. F. Pajak. A randomized phase I/II trial of hyperfractionated radiation therapy with total doses of 60.0 Gy to 79.2 Gy: possible survival benefit with greater than or equal to 69.6 Gy in favorable patients with Radiation Therapy Oncology Group stage III non-small-cell lung carcinoma: report of Radiation Therapy Oncology Group 83-11. *J.Clin.Oncol.* 8 (9):1543-1555, 1990.

60. M. Saunders, S. Dische, A. Barrett, A. Harvey, D. Gibson, and M. Parmar. Continuous hyperfractionated accelerated radiotherapy (CHART) versus conventional radiotherapy in non-small-cell lung cancer: a randomised multicentre trial. CHART Steering Committee [see comments]. *Lancet* 350 (9072):161-165, 1997.

61. A. J. Bailey, M. K. Parmar, and R. J. Stephens. Patient-reported short-term and long-term physical and psychologic symptoms: results of the continuous hyperfractionated accelerated [correction of acclerated] radiotherapy (CHART)

randomized trial in non- small-cell lung cancer. CHART Steering Committee. *J.Clin.Oncol.* 16 (9):3082-3093, 1998.

62. M. P. Mehta, S. P. Tannehill, S. Adak, L. Martin, D. G. Petereit, H. Wagner, J. F. Fowler, and D. Johnson. Phase II trial of hyperfractionated accelerated radiation therapy for nonresectable non-small-cell lung cancer: results of Eastern Cooperative Oncology Group 4593. *J.Clin.Oncol.* 16 (11):3518-3523, 1998.

63. Choy H, Devore RF 3rd, Hande KR, Porter LL, Rosenblatt P, Yunus F, Schlabach L, Smith C, Shyr Y, Johnson DH. A phase II study of paclitaxel, carboplatin, and hyperfractionated radiation therapy for locally advanced inoperable non-small cell lung cancer (a Vanderbilt Cancer Center Affiliate Network Study). Int J Radiat Oncol Biol Phys 47:931-937, 2000.

64. J. S. Lee, C. Scott, R. Komaki, F. V. Fossella, G. S. Dundas, S. McDonald, R. W. Byhardt, and W. J. Curran, Jr. Concurrent chemoradiation therapy with oral etoposide and cisplatin for locally advanced inoperable non-small-cell lung cancer: radiation therapy oncology group protocol 91-06. *J.Clin.Oncol.* 14 (4):1055-1064, 1996.

65. M. V. Graham, M. Jahanzeb, C. M. Dresler, J. D. Cooper, B. Emami, and J. E. Mortimer. Results of a trial with topotecan dose escalation and concurrent thoracic radiation therapy for locally advanced, inoperable nonsmall cell lung cancer. *Int.J.Radiat.Oncol.Biol.Phys.* 36 (5):1215-1220, 1996.

66. A. Vanagunas, P. Jacob, and E. Olinger. Radiation-induced esophageal injury: a spectrum from esophagitis to cancer. *Am.J.Gastroenterol.* 85 (7):808-812, 1990.

67. T. R. Mackie, T. Holmes, S. Swerdloff, P. Reckwerdt, J. O. Deasy, J. Yang, B. Paliwal, and T. Kinsella. Tomotherapy: a new concept for the delivery of dynamic conformal radiotherapy. *Med.Phys.* 20 (6):1709-1719, 1993.

68. M. P. Carol. Integrated 3D conformal plannin/multivane intesity modulatin delivery system for radiotherapy. In: *3D Radiaiton Treatemtn Planning and Conformal Therapy*, edited by J. A. Purdy and B. Emami, Madison, WI:Medical Physics Publishing, 1995, p. 435-445.

69. D. J. Convery and M. E. Rosenbloom. The generation of intesity-modulated fields for the conformal radiotherapy by dynamic collimation *Physics in medicine & biology* 37:1359, 1992.

70. T. Bortfeld, A. L. Boyer, W. Schlegel, D. L. Kahler, and T. J. Waldron. Realization and verification of three-dimensional conformal radiotherapy with modulated fields [see comments]. *Int.J.Radiat.Oncol.Biol.Phys.* 30 (4):899-908, 1994.

71. S. V. Spirou and C. S. Chui. Generation of arbitrary intensity profiles by dynamic jaws or multileaf collimators. *Med.Phys.* 21 (7):1031-1041, 1994.

72. T. Bortfeld, D. L. Kahler, and T. J. Waldron. X-ray field compensation with multi-leaf collimaters *Int.J.Radiat.Oncol.Biol.Phys.* 28:723, 1994.

73. C. X. Yu, M. J. Symons, M. N. Du, A. A. Martinez, and J. W. Wong. A method for implementing dynamic photon beam intensity modulation using independent jaws and a multileaf collimator. *Phys.Med.Biol.* 40 (5):769-787, 1995.

74. C. X. Yu. Intensity-modulated arc therapy with dynamic multileaf collimation: an alternative to tomotherapy. *Phys.Med.Biol.* 40 (9):1435-1449, 1995.

75. J. Stein, K Hartwig, S Levegrun, and et al. Intesity-modulated treatments: Compensators vs. multi-leaf modulation. In: *XII International conference on the*, edited by D. D. Leavitt and G. Starkschall, 1999.
76. Dubal N, Chans, Cullip T, et al. Intensity modulation for tangential breast treatment. Int J Radiat Oncol Biol Phys 42:127, 1998.
77. Mehta M, Petereit D, Chosey L, et al. Sequential comparison of low dose rate and hyperfractionated high dose rate endobronchial radiation for malignant airway occlusion. Int J Radiat Oncol Biol Phys 23:133, 1992.
78. Speiser B. Remote afterloading brachytherapy for the local control of endobronchial carcinoma. Int J Radiat Oncol Biol Phys 25:579, 1993.
79. Taulelle M, Chauvet B, Vincent P, et al. High dose rate endobronchial brachytherapy; results and complications in 189 patients. 11:162, 1998.
80. Hennequin C, Tredanial J, Durdux C, et al. Endobronchial brachytherapy: the Saint Louis Hospital experience. Cancer Radiother 1:159, 1997.
81. Gollins SW, Ryder WDJ, Burt PV, et al. Massive haemoptysis death and other morbidity associated with high dose rate inraluiminal radiotherapy for carcinoma of the bronchus. Radiother Oncol 39:105, 1996.
82. Huber RM, Fischer R, Hautmann H, et al. Does additional brachytherapy improve the effect of external irradiation? A prospective, randomized study in central lung tumors. Int J Radiat Oncol Biol Phys 43:533, 1997.
83. Ornadel D, Duchesene G, Wall P, et al. Defining the roles of high dose rate endobronchial brachytherapy and laser resection for recurrent bronchial malignancy. In Hansen HH (ed): Lung Cancer 16, pp 203-213, New York, NY, Elsevier, 1997.

COMBINED MODALITY THERAPY FOR EARLY STAGE OPERABLE AND LOCALLY ADVANCED POTENTIALLY RESECTABLE NON-SMALL CELL LUNG CARCINOMA

Joseph I. Clark, M.D.
Loyola University Medical Center, Maywood, IL 60153 USA

Kathy S. Albain, M.D.
Loyola University Medical Center, Maywood, IL 60153 USA

INTRODUCTION

Surgical resection of non-small cell lung carcinoma (NSCLC) remains the primary treatment for early stage disease, that is, stage I and II disease. Yet, the vast majority of patients with lung cancer present with either distant metastatic disease (stage IV) or locally advanced NSCLC (stage IIIA and IIIB). Today, despite modest gains in outcome in patients with early stage disease, using improved surgical techniques, better preoperative risk assessment, and advances in thoracic anesthesia, a significant proportion of these patients will eventually succumb to their disease due to local and/or distant recurrence. For those patients with locally advanced NSCLC, defined either by the presence of mediastinal nodal involvement or a primary tumor that invades key thoracic elements (chest wall, vertebral body, great vessels) surgical resection of this tumor is either difficult (T3) or impossible (T4). Therefore, a combined modality approach to the treatment of most operable or potentially resectable non-small cell lung cancers has been actively pursued by clinical investigators.

The proper role for chemotherapy with or without radiotherapy (RT) applied as induction therapy before attempted resection or as adjuvant "consolidation" treatment after definitive surgical resection in NSCLC remains undefined (1-7). It is, however, generally recognized that eradication of systemic micrometastases is crucial to the success of any local approach. Therefore, the goal of combined modality investigational trials is to simultaneously optimize control of local bulk disease and distant micrometastases through the use of systemic chemotherapy with or without RT. Definitive local control is therefore pursued via surgical resection, followed then by variable postoperative therapy directed at residual local and/or distant disease. Standard postoperative therapeutic methods utilizing adjuvant chemotherapy with or without RT have not yet been established but are still under investigational study (8). Induction therapy on the other hand has the advantage of inducing cytoreduction of distant and local disease, improving resection rates for technically difficult cases, potentially sparing normal lung tissue, providing a sense of "chemosensitivity" for a particular individual's disease, and ultimately improving survival. Also, compliance with the delivery of systemic chemotherapy may be better in the induction period than as postoperative treatment.

Despite the theoretical advantage of a combined modality approach to the treatment of potentially resectable NSCLC, as well as its possible role in de novo resectable disease, such benefits must be weighed against potential risks of increased morbidity and mortality. Postoperative challenges include standard risks of thoracotomy, with the possibility of delayed wound healing, development of broncho-pleural fistula, infection, etc., therefore delaying initiation and potential tolerance of the planned postoperative adjuvant therapy. Whereas, induction programs may result in postoperative pulmonary complications and treatment-related deaths, technical challenges during thoracotomy due to radiation fibrosis, prolonged recovery from surgery, and suppressed immune function from the induction therapy.

Objectives

The objectives of this review are to provide a perspective on two pertinent questions. That is: 1) does surgical resection after induction chemotherapy plus RT (chemoRT) improve outcome over chemoRT alone in patients who present with advanced stage or bulky disease [T3 and/or bulky N2 disease on computerized tomography (CT) scan or chest radiograph]? And 2) does induction or postoperative adjuvant chemotherapy with or without RT improve survival over the standard approach of surgery alone in patients with early stage or nonbulky disease [T2 or T3N0; T1, T2, T3N1; and T1, T2 or T3N2 ("minimal" – defined as either non-enlarged N2 nodes on CT scan, or unexpected microscopic N2 nodal involvement after a normal preoperative CT scan of the mediastinum)]? Initial surgical resection has been the standard of care for the patients with earlier stage, nonbulky disease, where the amount of mediastinal disease is critical in determining potential for cure after surgical resection (9-11). The standard of care for patients with advanced/bulky stage IIIA or IIIB NSCLC is one of several published programs of chemoRT, administered either concurrently or sequentially, that have demonstrated a significant benefit over RT alone (1,5,12,13).

SURGERY AFTER INDUCTION THERAPY FOR LOCALLY ADVANCED BUT POTENTIALLY RESECTABLE NSCLC

Radiation Therapy

Initial studies using induction therapy for locally advanced NSCLC tested the value of preoperative RT alone. That is, an attempt was made to convert unresectable NSCLC to resectable disease. These early studies, conducted in the 1950's through the early 1970's, established that, although feasible, radiation therapy alone as induction therapy was inadequate (14-18). These trials were performed without the benefit of modern staging technologies. Initial results, however, were intriguing in that up to 15% of patients were reported to have pathologic complete responses. Unfortunately, operative morbidity rates rose when RT doses of greater than 40 Gy were administered. Subsequent randomized trials were disappointing since no survival benefit was demonstrated (19,20). Thus, based on these more recent studies, RT alone is no longer recommended as the sole induction modality prior to surgery.

Early Induction Trials

Initial studies using neoadjuvant or induction systemic chemotherapy with or without sequential RT prior to surgery in potentially resectable NSCLC were first conducted in the 1980's (21-25). Various cisplatin-based chemotherapy regimens were employed in these small trials that accrued a heterogeneous range of stage subsets and did not necessarily require histologic staging of mediastinal nodal status (Table 1). Induction therapy produced response rates of approximately 40% to 80% and resection rates were highly variable ranging from 14% to 88%. Median and 3-year survival rates varied widely from 8 to 32 months and 8% to 34% respectively. Definitive conclusions regarding efficacy of this approach or comparison across trials are difficult to make given the heterogeneous nature of the patients accrued to these studies. These pivotal studies did however demonstrate the general safety of surgery following induction therapy and with some promising survival data led to the design of second generation trials.

Chemotherapy

The next generations of studies testing the role of preoperative chemotherapy in locally advanced disease, were in general, larger, enrolled more restricted stage subsets and in most instances required pathologic documentation of nodal disease. Table 2 represents a summary of selected phase II trials of induction chemotherapy (26-31). The response rates to induction therapy in these trials ranged from 60% to 78%, with complete resection rates between 31% and 68% and an overall long-term survival of 17% to 34%. Once again, the variable outcomes in these trials represent some of the difficulty in interpreting different phase II trials. Although cisplatin-based induction regimens were used in all trials, the different combinations used and the inconsistent use of postoperative adjuvant chemotherapy with or without radiation contribute somewhat to this difficulty of interpretation. In addition, the Toronto (28), Dana Farber (29) and Cancer and Leukemia Group B (CALGB) (30) series included only patients with surgically staged IIIA N2 disease that was confirmed by mediastinoscopy. On the other hand, both the Memorial Sloan-Kettering (IIIA N2) (26) and Roswell Park (IIIA N0-2, IIIB) (27) series included patients who were not consistently surgically staged prior to initiating induction chemotherapy. Therefore, the heterogeneity in patient populations included in these trials with potentially different long-term prognosis limits the ability to generalize these results to a specific patient population.

Table 1. Initial Phase II Induction Trials for Stage III NSCLC

Reference	Number of patients	Chemotherapy	Response rate (%)	Complete resection rate (% initial n)	Median survival (months)	Long-term survival
Skarin et al, 1989[21]	41	CAP	43	88	32	31%, 3-year
Eagan et al, 1987[22]	39	CAP	51	33	11	8%, 2-year
Bitran et al, 1986[23]	21	VdEP	70	14	8	34%, 1-year
Elias et al, 1994[24]	54	CAP	39	56	18	22%, 5-year
Darwish et al, 1994[25]	42	EP	82	72	24	24%, 3-year

C, cyclophosphamide; A, doxorubicin; P, cisplatin; Vd, vindesine; E, etoposide 5-FU, 5-fluorouracil; NR, not reported

In two randomized phase II trials, improvements in either tumor downstaging or survival were not seen in the preoperative chemotherapy arms (31,32). In a Lung Cancer Study Group trial, induction chemotherapy using mitomycin, vinblastine and cisplatin was compared to preoperative RT in 67 patients with surgically staged unresectable N2 or T4 disease (31). Toxicity was quite high in both arms, with an overall perioperative death rate of 18%. No obvious difference was observed in radiologic or pathologic response. The second trial reported in 1990 by Dautzenberg et al, was a randomized phase II trial evaluating the preoperative regimen of cisplatin, cyclophosphamide and vinblastine (32). Unfortunately, enrollment onto this trial stopped after only 26 patients were enrolled due to a high rate, i.e. 36%, of disease progression during induction chemotherapy. Small numbers of patients enrolled onto this trial make it difficult to formulate definitive conclusions.

Induction Chemoradiotherapy in Locally Advanced, Potentially Operable Stage III NSCLC

The standard of care for patients with advanced/bulky stage IIIA or IIIB NSCLC is one of several published programs of chemoRT, administered either concurrently or

Table 2. Second-Generation Induction Chemotherapy Trials in Stage III NSCLC

Reference	Number of patients	Chemotherapy	Response rate (%)	Complete Resection* (%)	Treatment Mortality (%)	Median survival (months)	Long-term survival
Martini et al, 1993[26]	136	MVP	78	65	5	19	17%, 5-year
Takita et al, 1995[27]	41	PACCO	60	42	2	18	NR
Burkes et al, 1994[28]	55	MVP	71	51	15	21	34%, 5-year
Elias et al, 1997[29]	34	PFL	65	62	0	18	18%, 4-year
Sugarbaker et al, 1995[30]	74	VP	64[#]	31	5.4	15	23%, 3-year
Wagner et al, 1994[31]	28	MVP	46	68	17	12	27%, 4-year

** Percent of all evaluable patients; [#] Includes stable disease; MVP = mitomycin, vinblastine, cisplatin; PACCO = cisplatin, doxorubicin, cyclophosphamide, CCNU, vincristine; PFL = cisplatin, 5-fluorouracil, leucovorin (continuous infusion); VP = vinblastine, cisplatin; NR = not reported*

sequentially, that have demonstrated a significant benefit over RT alone (1,5,12,13). Whether preoperative therapy in these stage III patients should involve chemotherapy and RT or chemotherapy alone has not been well studied. In a phase II induction trial performed by the CALGB, using chemotherapy alone, the major site of disease progression during induction therapy was within the thorax (33). These observations support the potential role of RT, in combination with systemic chemotherapy, to maximize local control and tumor downstaging prior to surgery. However, as reported by Shepherd in an overview of the phase II experience with induction therapy, no clear benefit was observed when combining both chemotherapy and RT preoperatively (34).

The rationale for induction chemoRT in potentially operable stage III disease is best understood in the context of data from combined modality approaches for unresectable disease. The majority of early studies that suggested a benefit on survival for combined chemoRT in inoperable NSCLC used a sequential schedule (13,35,36). Theoretical concerns however, suggest that this may not represent the optimal scheduling of these modalities. That is, it is conceivable that the potential for increased tumor cell repopulation during radiation exists; selection of drug-resistant cells and the stimulation of metastases may occur with the sequential approach (37). It is felt therefore, that these potential adverse outcomes are less likely with a concurrent chemoRT approach. The potential for overlapping toxicities however is a potential drawback. Data exists, as well, suggesting that while distant metastases are decreased with a sequential combined chemoRT approach, local control remains suboptimal (38). Randomized phase III trials using concurrent chemoRT or chemotherapy plus hyperfractionated RT schedules have been associated with improved local control and survival in patients with advanced inoperable stage III NSCLC (39-41). A recently updated trial confirmed this theoretical advantage in which patients with unresectable stage III NSCLC were randomized between sequential chemoRT vs. concurrent therapy (42). A survival benefit was observed for those patients receiving the concurrent treatment.

Based on this data, it was logical to test concurrent combined modality therapy as induction therapy. Selected phase II trials incorporating concurrent chemoRT strategies are summarized in Table 3 (43-48). These trials are relatively homogeneous in that four of the five trials required surgical staging prior to the initiation of treatment (44-48). Three of the trials however include patients with more advanced disease than the previously described phase II studies, i.e. those with stage IIIB (T4 or N3) disease (44-46). Roughly 67% of all patients included in these trials had clinically apparent mediastinal nodal disease as defined by lymph nodes greater than 1 cm on radiographic computed tomography imaging. Across all five of these studies, complete resection rates and overall survival was comparable to the phase II trials of induction chemotherapy alone, as described above, despite the advanced nature of these patients' disease. Local control was good, whereas the majority of relapses were distant. In the Southwest Oncology Group (SWOG) 8805 trial, the initial relapse sites were locoregional in 11%, distant in 61% and combined in 28% (44,48). Forty percent ultimately relapsed in the central nervous system. Hyperfractionated RT did not appear to add to treatment related mortality, while response and overall survival rates were comparable to those observed with conventional RT schedules.

Induction chemoRT administered concurrently compared to chemotherapy alone has only been tested in one randomized trial to date (49). In this trial, Fleck et al, randomized 69 patients with stage IIIA (N2) or IIIB (T4) to either preoperative concurrent cisplatin and 5-fluorouracil with RT (30Gy) or to induction cisplatin, mitomycin and vinblastine alone. Results of this trial revealed a statistically significant advantage in favor of the concurrent arm with regard to response rate (67% vs. 44%, p=0.02), resectability rate (52% vs. 31%, p=0.03), and freedom from progression (40% vs. 21%, p=0.04). Overall survival was not reported in this early report however and this study has only been published in abstract form. A second randomized trial is being conducted by German investigators comparing induction chemotherapy followed by concurrent hyperfractionated RT and chemotherapy vs. induction chemotherapy alone and adjuvant RT post-operatively for a similar group of NSCLC patients, however only toxicity data have been presented to date (50). Once completed, this trial should help to further define the role of an aggressive induction chemoRT approach.

The role of surgery after chemoRT in patients with pathologically confirmed stage IIIA (N2) bulky or stage IIIB disease remains an important, but as yet unanswered question. Until recently, these patients have been considered non-surgical candidates due to their bulk of disease and are treated with a non-surgical combined modality approach. As noted above however, this patient population has in recent years been included in single

Table 3. Selected phase II trials of concurrent induction chemoradiotherapy in stage III NSCLC

Reference	Number of Patients	IIIA(N2) (%)	T3N0-1/ T4 or N3 (%)	Induction Therapy	Response Rate (%)	Complete Resection Rate (%)	Treatment Mortality (%)	Overall Survival
Faber et al[43]	85	73	21/6	PF/PEF, split RT (40 Gy)	92 (includes SD)	71	4	40% 3-yr.
Albain et al[44,48]	126	60	0/40	EP, concurrent RT (40Gy)	59	71	10	27% IIIA 3-yr. 24% IIIB 3-yr. (20% IIIA 6-yr.) (22% IIIB 6-yr.)
Eberhardt et al[45]	94	49	6/45	EP x 3, then EP x 1 concurrent hfRT (45Gy)	64	53	6	31% IIIA 4-yr. 26% IIIB 4-yr.
Thomas et al[46]	54	46	0/54	ICE x 2, then EC concurrent hfRT (45Gy)	69	63	9	30% 3-yr.
Choi et al[47]	42	100	0/0	PVF x 2 concurrent hfRT (42Gy)	74	81	7	37% 5-yr.

PF = cisplatin, 5-fluorouracil; PEF = cisplatin, etoposide, 5-fluorouracil; EP = etoposide, cisplatin; RT = radiotherapy; SD = stable disease; hfRT = hyperfractionated radiotherapy; ICE = ifosfamide, carboplatin, etoposide; EC = etoposide, carboplatin; PVF = cisplatin, vinblastine, 5-fluorouracil

arm phase II induction feasibility trials. To date though, no randomized study has shown a survival benefit associated with the resection of loco-regional disease after combined modality therapy. An important, National Cancer Institute designated high-priority, ongoing Intergroup trial is attempting to answer this question (51). Patients with histologically confirmed N2 disease are enrolled and randomized to receive induction concurrent chemoRT followed by surgical resection or additional RT. Table 4 outlines this trial as well as other ongoing or planned phase III trials that are attempting to define the optimal combination of modalities for this patient population.

Randomized Induction Trials

Two randomized trials were designed to directly address the value of postinduction surgery versus postinduction RT, one reported by the National Cancer Institute of Canada (52) and the other by the Radiation Therapy Oncology Group (RTOG) (53). Both protocols randomized the study population to induction chemotherapy (cisplatin and vinblastine, with or without mitomycin) followed by either surgical resection or definitive RT. These trials required biopsy-proof of mediastinal nodal involvement and only patients with stage IIIA (N2) disease were eligible. Both studies closed prematurely due to impaired accrual, but were recently reported with mature follow-up. The survival curves overlap in both studies. The 4-year survival was 13% in the surgery

Table 4. Ongoing or planned phase III trials that address the role of surgery for biopsy-proven advanced stage IIIA(N2) NSCLC

Trial	Stage Subsets	Treatment Arms
North American Intergroup 0139[51]	Stage IIIA(N2)	EP x 2 concurrent RT (45Gy) then: Surgery → EP x 2 vs. Complete RT to 61Gy concurrent EP x 2
EORTC-08941 (Intergroup)	Stage IIIA(N2) responding to induction chemotherapy	Any cisplatin containing regimen x 3 then: Surgery vs. RT
Medical Research Council-LU20	Stage IIIA (T3N1 or T1-3N2), unresectable	RT vs. Induction MVP or MIC followed by Surgery or RT
West German Consortium	Stage IIIA(N2) and IIIB (T4 or N3)	Induction PT x 3 then: hfRT (45Gy) concurrent EP then: Surgery vs. Continue RT to 66-75Gy (conformal)

EP = etoposide, cisplatin; RT = radiotherapy; MVP = mitomycin, vinblastine, cisplatin; MIC = mitomycin, ifosfamide, cisplatin; PT = cisplatin, paclitaxel; hfRT = hyperfractionated radiotherapy

arm and 20% for the RT group in the 71 patients enrolled onto the RTOG study (53). Of the 31 patients enrolled onto the Canadian trial, the observed response rates were equivalent, i.e. 50% with induction chemotherapy (cisplatin and vinblastine) vs. 53% with RT. Median survival was 18.7 months for induction chemotherapy followed by surgery and 16.2 months for RT followed by surgical resection (52). These findings are intriguing, but do not answer the question due to lack of statistical power.

A third randomized study conducted by the CALGB tested whether induction chemotherapy versus induction RT was preferred. In this trial patients with surgically staged N2 disease were randomized to preoperative RT, receiving 40 Gy, vs. two cycles of induction chemotherapy with cisplatin and etoposide (54). Two additional cycles of systemic therapy were administered postoperatively to patients in the induction arm, and both arms received RT to a total dose of 54 Gy to 60 Gy. Unfortunately, this trial too was terminated early prior to its anticipated accrual goal due to slow accrual. Only 57 patients were enrolled, 47 of which were evaluable. Although an improvement in response rate was observed in the chemotherapy arm (47% vs. 38%), this did not translate into an overall survival benefit. In fact, there was a non-statistically significant trend toward improvement in median survival in the radiotherapy followed by surgery arm over induction chemotherapy, 23 months vs. 19 months respectively (p=0.64) (54).

ADJUVANT VS. INDUCTION VS. SURGERY ALONE FOR EARLY STAGE OPERABLE NSCLC

Adjuvant Radiation Therapy

Adjuvant RT after surgery in the post-operative setting adds little to the results observed with surgery alone. Most older series show long-term survival between 8% and 20% in patients who successfully underwent surgery for their resectable stage III disease (including those with N2 or T3 N0 disease) (55). In a large Veteran's Administration study, RT given after surgery actually decreased long-term survival (56). Kirsh et al found 5-year survival rates of 30% for squamous cell carcinoma and 13% for adenocarcinoma in patients who were resected and treated with postoperative RT (57). In a report from Kemeny et al, patients who were resected and received postoperative RT had a survival rate at 5 years of 11% (58). Hilaris et al obtained a 5-year survival rate of 22% by combining aggressive resection with intraoperative brachytherapy and postoperative external RT (59). Finally, a recent large meta-analysis of randomized trials evaluating postoperative RT found a 21% increase in the relative risk of dying that was greatest for patients with N0 or N1 disease (60). Therefore, from this data it can be concluded that there is no demonstrable benefit of postoperative RT for patients with stage IIIA NSCLC, including those with N2 disease.

Adjuvant Chemotherapy

Chemotherapy administered in the postoperative setting has been evaluated, but in general, has resulted in no survival benefit at 5 years in most studies (61-63). Some of these reports showed an increase in recurrence-free survival that did not manifest as a prolongation of overall survival. A few other studies showed a survival benefit, although it was of relatively small magnitude (64,65). Due to the unclear nature of the benefits of postoperative chemotherapy, a large meta-analysis of all available randomized trials evaluating postoperative chemotherapy was conducted (66). This analysis suggested that chemotherapy after surgery provided a small benefit of approximately 5% in long-term survival. Given this relatively low magnitude of benefit, the routine use of post-operative adjuvant chemotherapy is not generally recommended.

Adjuvant Radiation Therapy vs. ChemoRT

One randomized phase III Intergroup trial addressed the question of adjuvant post-operative therapy using RT vs. chemoRT in resected stage II and IIIA NSCLC (67). In this trial, 488 patients who had undergone complete resection of their primary NSCLC with thorough mediastinal lymph node sampling or dissection were randomized to receive either four cycles of concurrent cisplatin and etoposide with RT (50.4 Gy – 61.2 Gy) or the same radiation therapy alone in the post-operative setting. All patients must have had pathologically staged T1-3N1-2M0 disease. Treatment related mortality was low, 2.2% - 2.4% in each arm, however the combined modality arm had a significantly higher rate of grade III and IV leukopenia and esophagitis. No survival advantage was observed, in that median survival was equivalent: 41.9 months with RT alone vs. 38.6 months with chemoRT. Relapse rates within the irradiated field were similar in the two arms, as were extrathoracic recurrences. Therefore, it can be concluded that the concomitant administration of adjuvant cisplatin and etoposide with mediastinal RT in the post-operative setting for patients with resected node-positive NSCLC does not improve overall outcome when compared with adjuvant RT alone.

Induction Chemotherapy for Early-Stage Operable NSCLC

Recent investigation has focused on the role of induction chemotherapy in patients with earlier stage, non-bulky, disease (stage IB-IIIA) due to the substantial percentage of these patients who go on to develop recurrent disease following resection. Several recent reports are encouraging and support the concept of proposed or ongoing randomized phase III trials in these patient subgroups (68,69). One trial known as the Bimodality Lung Oncology Trial (BLOT), included 94 patients with T2N0, T1-2N1, T3N0-1 tumors, stages IB, IIA, and IIB respectively (68). Patients enrolled onto this phase II trial received two cycles of induction paclitaxel and carboplatin prior to undergoing surgical resection, followed by three additional cycles postoperatively for completely resected patients. Overall response rate to induction therapy was reported as 54%, but survival data have yet to be reported. Toxicity was felt to be tolerable. de Boer et al, reported similar results in a British pilot randomized phase II study of induction mitomycin, vinblastine and cisplatin in 22 patients with early stage disease (69). Again, toxicity was not excessive.

Randomized Trials of Induction Therapy vs. Surgery Alone in Early Stage NSCLC

To date, there have been five-reported randomized phase III trials designed to assess the effect of induction chemotherapy on survival in patients with stage III NSCLC (Table 5) (70-76). Three of the five trials closed before the target accrual goal was met. The National Cancer Institute (NCI) trial was halted due to slow accrual (70), whereas the Spanish (71,72) and M.D. Anderson (73,74) studies were stopped early due to large survival differences by data monitoring committees. Investigators at the NCI enrolled 27 patients with histologically confirmed N2 NSCLC to a randomized trial comparing immediate surgery with postoperative RT (54 Gy to 60 Gy) or two cycles of induction chemotherapy using cisplatin and etoposide prior to surgery (70). Four additional cycles of this chemotherapy regimen were administered postoperatively to responding patients in the induction arm. A radiographic response rate of 60% was observed to the induction regimen. Although not statistically significant, there was a trend toward improved survival for patients who received induction cisplatin and etoposide (28.7 months vs. 15.6 months, p=0.095) (70).

In the Spanish trial, 60 patients with stage IIIA disease were randomized to either induction chemotherapy using mitomycin, ifosfamide, and cisplatin followed by surgery, vs. surgery alone (71,72). Both treatment arms received postoperative mediastinal RT, receiving 50 Gy. This was not a pure N2 study however, in that 22% of the study population had T3N0 disease and 5% T3N1. Pathologic documentation via mediastinoscopy was used in only 73% of patients. All patients classified as N2 had

Table 5. Randomized phase III trials of induction chemotherapy in operable stage III NSCLC

Reference	Number of patients	Stage subset(s)	Induction Therapy	Median survival (months)	Overall Survival (%)
Pass et al, 1992[70]	27	IIIA(N2) by biopsy	none	16	12
			vs.	p=0.095	(3-yr)
			EP	29	42
Rosell et al, 1999[71,72]	60	IIIA(N2) not required; node biopsy not required	none	10	0
			vs.	p=0.005	(5-yr)
			PIM	22	17
Roth et al, 1998[73,74]	60	IIIA(N2) not required; node biopsy not required; some IIIB	none	14	15
			vs.	p=0.048	(5-yr)
			CEP	21	36
Yoneda et al, 1995[75]	83	Clinical IIIA and IIIB	none	15	40
			vs.	NS	(3-yr)
			VdP	14	37
Depierre et al, 1999[76]	373	Clinical T2N0, II, IIIA	none	26	41
			vs.	p=0.11	(3-yr)
			PIM	36	49

PIM = cisplatin, ifosfamide, mitomycin; CEP = cyclophosphamide, etoposide, cisplatin; VdP = vindesine, cisplatin; NS = not statistically significant

clinically enlarged mediastinal lymph nodes as well as pathologic confirmation by node biopsy. Induction chemotherapy led to a response rate of 60%. After 24 months, enrollment was stopped due to a statistically significant difference in both disease free, 22 months vs. 5 months (p<0.001), and overall survival, 22 months vs. 10 months (p<0.005). Criticisms of this trial include an imbalance in both K-ras mutations and aneuploid tumors favoring the chemotherapy arm. That is, K-ras mutations were observed in 15% of tumors in the chemotherapy arm vs. 42% in the surgery arm (p=0.05). Aneuploid tumors were present in 29% of the chemotherapy treated patients vs. 70% in the surgery arm (p=0.02). Such a discrepancy may be reflected in the fact that the surgery-alone arm had a median survival much less than would be expected for resected stage IIIA disease, especially given that 30% of the patients on this arm had T3N0 tumors.

Roth et al, reported another randomized trial designed for patients with stage IIIA NSCLC and performed at M.D. Anderson Cancer Center (73). This trial too was terminated early due to a significant survival benefit for those patients receiving induction chemotherapy that included cyclophosphamide, etoposide and cisplatin followed by surgery vs. surgery alone. A total of 85% of patients underwent histologic staging by mediastinoscopy or mini-thoracotomy (Chamberlain procedure). All patients classified as N2 had clinically enlarged N2 nodes as well as pathologic confirmation of malignant involvement. However, both T3N0 (23%) and T3N1 (3%) tumors were also included. A total of 60 patients were enrolled onto this study. Responding and completely resected patients in the induction arm received additional chemotherapy after surgery. Postoperative RT was administered to those patients in either arm with unresectable or incompletely resected tumors. A 35% major response rate (complete plus partial response) to induction chemotherapy was reported. Long-term follow-up data have recently been reported (74). The median survival was 21 months in the induction arm and 14 months in the surgery alone arm (p=0.048). The five-year survival was 36% vs. 15% favoring the chemotherapy group. A criticism of this trial is that a postoperative stage imbalance existed, in that 40% stage IIIB and IV patients were identified in the surgery-alone arm compared with 11% in the chemotherapy arm. It is conceivable however, that since preoperative staging was equivalent in both arms, this difference may in fact represent downstaging due to induction therapy. The impact on the survival difference between the two treatment arms remains unclear therefore.

Larger phase III experience is required to more accurately evaluate the impact on long-term survival induction therapy has on early-stage NSCLC. One small-randomized Japanese trial compared induction chemoRT using a combination of vindesine and cisplatin with concurrent RT to surgery alone in this patient population (75). Eighty-three patients were enrolled, but no survival benefit was observed for the induction arm, in fact, survival was identical. However, only clinical staging was required in this phase III trial, resulting in stage and disease bulk imbalances.

Preliminary phase III data have been presented by the French Thoracic Cooperative Group using induction chemotherapy in patients with operable early-stage NSCLC (76). Induction chemotherapy with mitomycin, ifosfamide, and cisplatin followed by surgery was compared with surgery alone in 373 patients with clinical stage IB-IIIA (including N2 disease). Patients responding to induction therapy received additional cycles of chemotherapy in the post-operative setting. Patients with T3 or N2 disease received post-operative RT (60 Gy) as well. Induction therapy led to an overall response rate of 64% with an overall pathologic complete response rate of 11%. A trend toward improved median survival was observed in the chemotherapy arm, 36 months vs. 26 months, although this was not statistically significant, p=0.11. Overall survival rates were similar, with a three-year survival of 49% in the induction arm vs. 41% in the surgery only arm, which again, did not meet statistical significance. A delayed survival advantage was observed in the induction arm after compensation was made for an increased perioperative mortality rate in the induction chemotherapy group. Also, a slight survival advantage was observed but restricted to N0-1 patients after subset analysis (p=0.02). In contrast to the previous two trials discussed, BLOT and the British trial, there was a trend toward increased perioperative toxicity in the chemotherapy induction arm that was related predominantly to the development of bronchopleural fistula. From this, it is clear that additional follow-up is required before definitive conclusions can be drawn. An ongoing phase III trial by the Medical Research Council, as well as a planned randomized phase III study comparing the BLOT regimen to surgery alone, will also be helpful in defining the role of induction therapy in patients with early-stage NSCLC (69).

Unfortunately, some of the same drawbacks ascribed to the phase II trials discussed above may also be applied to the phase III experience. That is, limited sample sizes, and heterogeneity in patient populations and treatment regimens make definitive conclusions nearly impossible. Both the Spanish (71,72)) and M.D. Anderson (73,74) trials are encouraging in that, although stopped early, both reported a significant survival advantage in their respective induction chemotherapy arms. However, possible explanations for these positive results include an imbalance in stage or other poor prognostic factors. Both trials included patients with T3N0 tumors, therefore, it is not possible to attempt to generalize these results to all patients with stage IIIA disease, especially those with histologically confirmed N2 involvement prior to surgery. The last three trials described above were a bit more homogeneous in that all patients were surgically staged and a specific N2 population was evaluated. However, a significant survival advantage was not observed in three of the five trials reported (70,75,76).

Active Phase III Trials Addressing the Role of Chemotherapy in Early Stage NSCLC

Table 6 summarizes ongoing phase III trials considering whether or not chemotherapy is indicated before surgery in patients with early stage, nonbulky disease. These trials are large and include careful restriction of eligible stage subsets, in order that the critiques of the completed trials discussed above can be appropriately addressed (70-76). The German Krebshilfe trial is ongoing for patients with central T3N0-1 or very minimal N2 disease (1 or 2 positive nodes only). The designs of the North American Intergroup (follow-up of the BLOT phase II study (68)), European Organization for Research and Treatment of Cancer (EORTC), and Netherlands trials are similar, differing primarily in the use or not of newer chemotherapy regimens.

PREDICTORS OF LONG-TERM SURVIVAL

Methods of analysis for predictors of long-term survival have varied among phase II induction trials. Univariate versus multivariate analyses have been utilized, and either predictors of overall survival from registration or from time of thoracotomy have been described. Favorable outcome predictors included postinduction pathologic CR, complete resection, T3N0 or T3N1 disease, T4N0 or N1 disease, and pathologic elimination of initial N2 or N3 involvement (nodal downstaging). The significance of these predictive factors varied across studies, but all factors were not uniformly assessed in each study. Nevertheless, a factor related to the efficacy of the induction therapy was important in most trials. Response to induction therapy was not an important predictive factor in some trials, most likely due to the requirement in those studies that patients undergo resection of their disease even if "stable disease" was the best response (44). This observation emphasizes the relative inability of standard CT scanning to detect those patients with major postinduction responses.

In the CALGB 8935 study, tumor downstaging occurred in 22% of the patients (30). These results compare to 39% in the Memorial Sloan-Kettering series (26) and 67% downstaging in the Massachusetts General Hospital (MGH) series (47). The five-year survival from the start of therapy for those patients treated on the MGH trial for postoperative pathologic stage 0 and I, stage II, and stage III was 79%, 42%, and 18%, respectively (p=0.04). In the Memorial series, a complete pathologic response resulted in an estimated five-year survival from the start of therapy of 54% (77). In SWOG 8805, the best predictor for long-term survival in univariate analysis was the presence of negative mediastinal nodes in the post-operative specimen (44). This variable was also the most important univariate discriminant of 6-year survival, although complete resection emerged as a long-term survival predictor as well (48). The survivals 3 and 6 years after thoracotomy for patients with uninvolved nodes at surgery were 41% and 33%, respectively, versus only 11% and 11% if there was persistent mediastinal disease.

Implications of this nodal downstaging observation are that lack of residual disease in the mediastinum may serve as a surrogate marker for eradication of distant chemotherapy-sensitive micrometastases. Such patients may therefore be optimal candidates for additional post-operative chemotherapy. Alternatively, persistent N2 or N3 disease may predict the presence of distant resistant disease. Therefore, the question arises as to whether surgery was necessary for those patients with nodal downstaging – or – were these patients the best candidates for maximal local control with surgery? If post-induction mediastinal lymph node status is of clear prognostic value, then it follows that there would be a critical role for a second mediastinal assessment after induction, although this might be technically difficult in some cases. Whether molecular correlates such as proliferative rate, p53 or K-ras obtained on biopsy material pre- and/or post-induction might improve identification of the optimal patients for surgical resection await the results of ongoing ancillary projects within several of these trials and current phase III studies described above.

TREATMENT RELATED MORBIDITY AND MORTALITY IN COMBINED MODALITY TRIALS INVOLVING SURGERY

The morbidity from combined modality therapy that includes surgery is not insignificant. The morbidity and mortality associated with induction therapy largely depends on the particular treatment regimen in question. The most commonly described toxicities involve hematologic, gastrointestinal, and pulmonary organ systems. Myelosuppression, although relatively common, is typically transient and well tolerated. Serious infectious complications however, have been reported, including occasional treatment related deaths. In the CALGB 8935 phase II trial, 6% of patients experienced a serious grade III infection (30). Investigators at the Memorial Sloan Kettering Cancer Center (26) and the University of Toronto (28) reported rates of febrile neutropenia requiring hospitalization of 15% and 10% respectively, using similar cisplatin-based combination chemotherapy plus mitomycin. With regard to the incidence of significant esophagitis and pneumonitis, these rates are generally higher when radiation is added to induction therapy, especially in those series evaluating the impact of concurrent or accelerated RT schedules. In the SWOG 8805 study (44,48), serious grade III or higher esophagitis was observed in 11% of patients. This compares to 14% grade IV in the MGH series (47), 8% grade III or IV in the German series (46), and 43% serious grade III or higher esophagitis in the West German Cancer Center report (45). The incidence of bronchial-stump insufficiency is of particular concern in those regimens designed to use preoperative hyperfractionated RT. In the trials reported by Eberhardt (45) and Thomas (46) this occurred in 5% and 10% of the patients respectively. Interestingly, in both reports, right-sided resections were more likely to develop this complication, and the incidence decreased after protection of the bronchial-stump was applied by an intercostal muscle flap.

The incidence of perioperative complications as a direct result of induction therapy remains a real concern. Some investigators have been more vocal about this concern. In a retrospective analysis, Roberts et al reported a statistically significant increase in the incidence of life-threatening complications (78). That is, in a cohort of patients treated with preoperative chemotherapy alone compared with a similar cohort of patients taken immediately to surgery, a significant increase in pneumonia, intubation or transfer to the intensive care unit occurred (p=0.0054). It must be noted however, that these two patient populations differed in stage and no multivariate analysis of potential etiologies for this observation was performed.

The randomized phase III experience has for the most part been encouraging in that induction chemotherapy has generally been well tolerated without consistent adverse effects on postoperative morbidity or mortality. Concerns regarding potential impairment in bronchial healing and postoperative pulmonary morbidity are significant, however, the increase in bronchopleural fistula development observed in the French trial reported by Depierre et al (76) may in fact reflect the impact of mitomycin, a known pulmonary toxic agent, rather than an impact of induction chemotherapy in general. In contradistinction, the induction chemotherapy trials reported from Spain (71,72), M.D. Anderson (73,74), and the National Cancer Institute (70) did not reveal any significant increase in postoperative complications or mortality. The question of whether the addition of radiotherapy or newer chemotherapeutic agents will contribute to an increase in postoperative complication rates remains to be answered.

AN OVERALL PERSPECTIVE

Combined-modality approaches are considered standard of care for the majority of patients with advanced NSCLC. Questions remain however, as to which regimen, schedule and combination are optimal. Over the preceding ten years, a number of randomized trials have confirmed a survival advantage associated with combination chemotherapy and RT over RT alone for those patients with unresectable stage IIIA and IIIB disease. Much less data and no definitive randomized trials exist for patients with operable stage III or earlier disease. Several phase II trials in more advanced bulky disease suggest that induction chemotherapy with or without RT may improve survival, particularly in those patients who experience significant downstaging of their disease. Unfortunately, heterogeneous patient populations in most of these studies limit our ability to define the optimal group of patients who would benefit from such an approach. We await the successful completion of ongoing phase III trials in both subsets of patients (Tables 4 and 6).

Aside from these important questions, a number of other areas must be addressed in order to continue to improve the outcome of these patients. One of the most critical areas of investigation requires novel approaches for the treatment of residual microscopic distant disease after completion of induction therapy. Newer chemotherapy regimens are enticing but are not expected to lead to dramatic improvements in overall survival. Novel approaches are actively being tested as "consolidation" including matrix metalloproteinases, angiogenesis inhibitors, antibodies to growth factor receptors, gene therapy and vaccines. As well, newer and better approaches to achieving improved local control are also needed. This area of investigation is left open to optimal use of PET scanning and functional imaging approaches within induction therapy programs, as well as improved use of molecular markers and other variables to better predict which patients will benefit from surgical resection after induction therapy.

Table 6. Randomized phase III trials, ongoing or planned, of induction chemotherapy in early-stage NSCLC

Investigators	Stage Subsets	Treatment
North American Intergroup (Chair: SWOG)	Resectable stage IB, IIA, IIB	Surgery alone vs. Induction CT x 3 → surgery
German Krebshilfe	Resectable Central T3N0-1, Minimal N2 (1 or 2 nodes)	Surgery → RT vs. Induction PE x 3 → hfRT + PE → surgery
EORTC	Resectable stage IB, II	Surgery alone vs. Induction CT, PG, PV x 3 (choice) → surgery
Netherlands	Resectable T2N0, N1, T3N0	Surgery alone vs. PE x 2-4 (to maximum response) → surgery

SWOG = Southwest Oncology Group; CT = carboplatin, paclitaxel; RT = radiotherapy; PE = cisplatin, etoposide; hfRT = hyperfractionated radiotherapy; EORTC = European Organization for Research and Treatment of Cancer; PG = cisplatin, gemcitabine; PV = cisplatin, vinorelbine

Other areas of investigation that require more aggressive input include studies on how to maximize quality of life and functional reserve, especially pulmonary, during combined modality programs and to minimize treatment-related pulmonary morbidity and mortality. Better prevention of brain metastases is required, since this is a major site of first distant relapse in this patient population. Chemoprevention of second primary cancers, active smoking cessation initiatives and treatment of co-morbid conditions will help to lengthen survival of patients who are free of recurrence after completion of combined modality induction programs.

REFERENCES

1.	Strauss GM, Langer MP, Elias AD, Skarin AT, Sugarbaker DJ. Multimodality treatment of stage IIIA non-small cell lung carcinoma: A critical review of the literature and strategies for future research. J Clin Oncol 10:829-838, 1992.
2.	Rusch VW, Benfield JR. Neoadjuvant therapy for lung cancer: A note of caution. Ann Thor Surg 55:820-821, 1993.
3.	Green M, Bordin O, Choi N et al. Pre-operative and post-operative treatments in stage III NSCLC. Lung Cancer 10(suppl.):S15-S17, 1994.
4.	Johnson DH, Piantadosi S. Chemotherapy for resectable stage III non-small cell lung cancer – Can that dog hunt? J Natl Cancer Inst 86:650-651, 1994.
5.	Edelman MJ, Gandara DR, Roach M III, Benfield JR. Multimodality therapy in stage III non-small cell lung cancer. Ann Thorac Surg 61:1564-1572, 1996.
6.	Albain KS. Induction chemotherapy with or without radiation followed by surgery in stage III non-small lung cancer: Update and perspectives. Oncology 11(suppl. 9):51-57, 1997.
7.	Perry MC, Deslauriers J, Albain KS et al. Induction treatment for resectable non-small cell lung cancer: A consensus report. Lung Cancer 17(suppl. 1):15-18, 1997.
8.	Holmes EC, Bleehen NM, Chevalier TL et al. Postoperative adjuvant treatments for non-small lung cancers: A consensus report. Lung Cancer 7:11-13, 1991.
9.	Martini N, Flehinger BJ, Zaman M, Beattie EJ. Results of resection in non-out cell carcinoma of the lung with mediastinal lymph node metastases. Ann Surg 198:386-397, 1983.
10.	Martini N, Flehinger BJ. The role of surgery in N2 lung cancer. Surg Clin North Amer 67:1037-1049, 1987.
11.	Vansteenkiste JF, De Leyn PR, Deneffe GJ, Lerut TE, Demedts MG. Clinical prognostic factors in surgically treated stage IIIAN2 non-small cell lung cancer: Analysis of the literature. Lung Cancer 19:3-13, 1998.
12.	Gordon GS, Vokes EE. Chemoradiation for locally advanced, unresectable NSCLC: New standard of care, emerging strategies. Oncology 13:1075-1088, 1999.
13.	Dillman RO, Seagren SL, Propert KJ et al. A randomized trial of induction chemotherapy plus high-dose radiation versus radiation alone in stage III non-small-cell lung cancer. N Engl J Med 323:940-945, 1990.

14.   Bromley LL, Szur L. Combined radiotherapy and resection for carcinoma of the bronchus: Experience with 66 patients. Lancet 2:937-941, 1955.

15.   Bloedorn RG, Cowley RA, Cuccia CA, Mercado R. Combined therapy with irradiation and surgery in the treatment of bronchogenic carcinoma. Am J Roentgenol 85:875-885, 1961.

16.   Shields T, Higgins G, Lawton KR, Heilbrunn A, Khean RJ. Preoperative x-ray therapy as an adjuvant in the treatment of bronchogenic carcinoma. J Thorac Cardiovasc Surg 59:49-61, 1970.

17.   Warram J. Preoperative irradiation of cancer of the lung: Final report of a therapeutic trial. A collaborative study. Cancer 36:914-923, 1975.

18.   Sherman DM, Neptune WB, Weichselbaum R et al. An aggressive approach to marginally resectable lung cancer. Cancer 41:2040-2045, 1978.

19.   Payne DG. Pre-operative radiation therapy in non-small cell cancer of the lung. Lung Cancer 7:47-56, 1991.

20.   Lad T, Wagner H, Piantadosi S for the Lung Cancer Study Group. Randomized phase II evaluation of pre-operative chemotherapy alone and radiotherapy alone in stage IIIA non-small cell lung cancer. Proc Amer Soc Clin Oncol 10:258, 1991.

21.   Skarin A, Jochelson M, Sheldon T et al. Neoadjuvant chemotherapy in marginally resectable stage III M0 non-small cell lung cancer: Long-term follow-up in 41 patients. J Surg Oncol 40:266-274, 1989.

22.   Eagan RT, Ruud C, Lee RE et al for the Lung Cancer Study Group. Pilot study of induction therapy with cyclophosphamide, doxorubicin and cisplatin (CAP) and chest irradiation prior to thoracotomy in initially inoperable stage III M0 non-small cell lung cancer. Cancer Treat Rep 71:895-900, 1987.

23.   Bitran JD, Golomb HM, Hoffman PC et al. Protochemotherapy in non-small cell lung carcinoma. An attempt to increase surgical respectability and survival. A preliminary report. Cancer 57:44-53, 1986.

24.   Elias AD, Skarin AT, Gonin R et al. Neoadjuvant treatment of stage IIIA non-small cell lung cancer. Am J Clin Oncol (CCT) 17:26-36, 1994.

25.   Darwish S, Minotti V, Crino L et al. Neoadjuvant cisplatin and etoposide for stage IIIA (clinical N2) non-small cell lung cancer. Am J Clin Oncol (CCT) 17:64-67, 1994.

26.   Martini N, Kris MG, Flehinger BJ et al. Preoperative chemotherapy for stage IIIA (N2) lung cancer: The Sloan-Kettering experience with 136 patients. Ann Thorac Surg 55:1365-1374, 1993.

27.   Takita H, Blumenson LE, Raghavan D. Neoadjuvant chemotherapy of stage IIIA and B lung carcinoma using the PACCO regimen. J Surg Oncol 59:147-150, 1995.

28.   Burkes RL, Shepherd FA, Ginsberg RJ et al. Induction chemotherapy with MVP in patients with stage IIIA(N2) unresectable non-small cell lung cancer: The Toronto experience. Proc Amer Soc Clin Oncol 13:327, 1994.

29.   Elias AD, Skarin AT, Leong T et al. Neoadjuvant therapy for surgically staged IIIAN2 non-small cell lung cancer. Lung Cancer 17:147-161, 1997.

30. Sugarbaker DJ, Herndon J, Kohman LJ, Krasna MJ, Green MR. Results of Cancer and Leukemia Group B Protocol 8935: A multi-institutional phase II trimodality trial for stage IIIA(N2) non-small-cell cancer. J Thorac Cardiovasc Surg 109:473-485, 1995.

31. Wagner H Jr, Lad T, Piantadosi S et al. Randomized phase II evaluation of preoperative radiation therapy and preoperative chemotherapy with Mitomycin, vinblastine, and cisplatin in patients with technically unresectable stage IIIA and IIIB non-small cell cancer of the lung: LCSG 881. Chest 106(suppl 6):348S-354S, 1994.

32. Dautzenberg B, Benichou J, Allard P et al. Failure of the perioperative PCV neoadjuvant polychemotherapy in resectable bronchogenic non-small cell carcinoma: Results from a randomized phase II trial. Cancer 65:2435-2441, 1990.

33. Kumar P, Herndon J II, Langer M et al. Patterns of disease failure after trimodality therapy on non-small cell lung carcinoma pathologic stage IIIA(N2): Analysis of Cancer and Leukemia Group B Protocol 8935. Cancer 77:2393-2399, 1996.

34. Shepherd FA. Induction chemotherapy for locally advanced non-small cell lung cancer. Ann Thorac Surg 55:1585-1592, 1993.

35. Sause WT, Scott C, Taylor S et al. Radiation Therapy Oncology Group (RTOG) 88-08 and Eastern Cooperative Oncology Group (ECOG) 4588: Preliminary results of a phase III trial in regionally advanced, unresectable non-small-cell lung cancer. J Natl Cancer Inst 87:198-205, 1995.

36. Le Chevalier T, Arriagada R, Quoix E et al. Radiotherapy alone versus combined chemotherapy and radiotherapy in nonresectable non-small-cell lung cancer: First analysis of a randomized trial in 353 patients. J Natl Cancer Inst 83:417-423, 1991.

37. Tannock IF. Treatment of cancer with radiation and drugs. J Clin Oncol 14:3156-3174, 1996.

38. Arriagada R, Le Chevalier T, Quiox E et al. ASTRO (American Society of Therapeutic Radiology and Oncology) plenary: Effect of chemotherapy on locally advanced non-small cell lung carcinoma. A randomized study of 353 patients. GETCB (Groupe d'Etude et Traitement des Cancers Bronchiques), FNCLCC (Federation Nationale des Centeres de Lutte contre le Cancer) and the CEBI trialists. Intl J Radiat Oncol Biol Phys 20:1183-1190, 1991.

39. Schaake-Koning C, Van Den Bogaert W, Daleisio O et al. Effects of concomitant cisplatin and radiotherapy on inoperable non-small-cell lung cancer. N Engl J Med 326:524-530, 1992.

40. Jeremic R, Shibamoto Y, Acimovic L et al. Hyperfractionated radiation therapy with or without concurrent low-dose daily carboplatin/etoposide for stage III non-small-cell lung cancer: A randomized study. J Clin Oncol 14:1065-1070, 1996.

41. Saunders M, Dische S, Barrett A et al. Continuous hyperfractionated accelerated radiotherapy (CHART) versus conventional radiotherapy in non-small-cell lung cancer: A randomized multicentre trial. CHART Steering Committee. Lancet 350:161-165, 1997.

42. Furuse K, Fukuoka M, Takada Y et al. Phase III study of concurrent vs. sequential thoracic radiotherapy (TRT) in combination with mitomycin (M), vindesine (V) and cisplatin (P) in unresectable stage III non-small cell lung cancer (NSCLC): Five-year median follow-up results. Proc Amer Soc Clin Oncol 18:458a, 1999.

43. Faber LP, Kittle CF, Warren WH et al. Preoperative chemotherapy and irradiation for stage III non-small cell lung cancer. Ann Thorac Surg 47:669-677, 1989.

44. Albain KS, Rusch VW, Crowley JJ et al. Concurrent cisplatin/etoposide plus chest radiotherapy followed by surgery for stages IIIA(N2) and IIIB non-small-cell lung cancer: Mature results of Southwest Oncology Group phase II study 8805. J Clin Oncol 13:1880-1892, 1995.

45. Eberhardt W, Wilke H, Stamatis G et al. Preoperative chemotherapy followed by concurrent chemoradiation therapy based on hyperfractionated accelerated radiotherapy and definitive surgery in locally advanced non-small-cell lung cancer: Mature results of a phase II trial. J Clin Oncol 16:622-634, 1998.

46. Thomas M, Rhbe C, Semik M et al. Impact of preoperative bimodality induction including twice-daily radiation on tumor regression and survival in stage III non-small-cell lung cancer. J Clin Oncol 17:1185-1193, 1999.

47. Choi NC, Carey RW, Daly W et al. Potential impact on survival of improved tumor downstaging and resection rate by preoperative twice-daily radiation and concurrent chemotherapy in stage IIIA non-small-cell lung cancer. J Clin Oncol 15:712-722, 1997.

48. Abain K, Rusch V, Crowley J et al. Long-term survival after concurrent cisplatin/etoposide (PE) plus chest radiotherapy (RT) followed by surgery in bulky, stages IIIA(N2) and IIIB non-small cell lung cancer (NSCLC): 6-year outcomes from Southwest Oncology Group Study 8805. Proc Amer Soc Clin Oncol 18:467a, 1999.

49. Fleck J, Camargo J, Godoy D et al. Chemoradiation therapy (CRT) vs. chemotherapy (CT) alone as neoadjuvant treatment for stage III non-small lung cancer (NSCLC): Preliminary report of a phase III prospective randomized trial. Proc Amer Soc Clin Oncol 12:1108a, 1993.

50. Thomas M, Rhbe C, Semik M et al. Randomized trial of chemotherapy (CT) and twice-daily chemoradiation (hfRT/CT) versus chemotherapy (CT) alone before surgery in stage III non-small cell lung cancer: Interim analysis of toxicity. Proc Amer Soc Clin Oncol 18:1769a, 1999.

51. Albain K, Rusch V, Turrisi A et al. for the Lung Cancer Intergroup. Interim update of the National Cancer Institute High Priority North American Intergroup Trial 0139 (RTOG 9309) for stage III(N2) non-small cell lung cancer: A phase III comparison of concurrent chemotherapy plus standard radiotherapy versus concurrent chemotherapy plus radiotherapy followed by surgical resection. Proc Perugia Internatl Cancer Conf 6:35-37, 1998.

52. Shepherd FA, Johnston MR, Payne D et al. Randomized study of chemotherapy and surgery versus radiotherapy for stage IIIA non-small-cell lung cancer: A

National Cancer Institute of Canada Clinical Trials Group study. Br J Cancer 78:683-685, 1998.

53. Inculet R, Scott C, Dar AR et al. Phase III study comparing chemotherapy and radiation with preoperative chemotherapy and surgical resection in patients with non-small cell lung cancer with spread to mediastinal lymph nodes: A Radiation Therapy Oncology Group study (RTOG 89-01). Lung Cancer 18(Suppl. 1):65, 1997.

54. Elias A, Herndon J, Kumar P et al. A phase III comparison of "best local-regional therapy" with or without chemotherapy for stage IIIA T1-3N2 non-small cell lung cancer (NSCLC): Preliminary results. Proc Amer Soc Clin Oncol 16:448a, 1997.

55. Overholt RH, Neptune WB, Ashraf MM. Primary cancer of the lung: A 42-year experience. Ann Thorac Surg 20:511-519, 1975.

56. Shields TW, Yee J, Conn JH et al. Relationship of cell type and lymph node metastasis to survival after resection of bronchial carcinoma. Ann Thorac Surg 20:501-510, 1975.

57. Kirsh MM, Rotman H, Argenta L et al. Carcinoma of the lung: Results of treatment over ten years. Ann Thorac Surg 21:371-377, 1976.

58. Kemeny MM, Block LR, Braunn DW Jr et al. Results of surgical treatment of carcinoma of the lung by stage and cell type. Surg Gynecol Obstet 147:865-871, 1978.

59. Hilaris BS, Gomez J, Nori D et al. Combined surgery, intraoperative brachytherapy, and postoperative external radiation in stage III non-small cell lung cancer. Cancer 55:1226-1231, 1985.

60. PORT Meta-analysis Trialists Group. Postoperative radiotherapy in non-small-cell lung cancer: Systematic review and meta-analysis of individual patient data from nine randomized controlled trials. Lancet 352:257-263, 1998.

61. Pisters KMW, Kris MG, Gralla RJ et al. Randomized trial comparing postoperative chemotherapy with vindesine and cisplatin plus thoracic irradiation with irradiation alone in stage III (N2) non-small cell lung cancer. J Surg Oncol 56:236-241, 1994.

62. Holmes EC, Gail M, for the Lung Cancer Study Group. Surgical adjuvant therapy for stage II and stage III adenocarcinoma and large-cell undifferentiated carcinoma. J Clin Oncol 4:710-715, 1986.

63. Lad T, Rubinstein L, Sadeghi A, for the Lung Cancer Study Group. The benefit of adjuvant treatment for resected locally advanced non-small-cell lung cancer. J Clin Oncol 6:9-17, 1988.

64. Niiranen A, Niitamo-Korhonen S, Kouri M et al. Adjuvant chemotherapy after radical surgery for non-small-cell lung cancer: A randomized study. J Clin Oncol 10:1927-1932, 1992.

65. Wada H, Hitomi S, Teramatsu T et al. Adjuvant chemotherapy after complete resection in non-small-cell lung cancer. J Clin Oncol 14:1048-1054, 1996.

66. Stewart LA, Pignon JP, Arriagada R et al. A meta-analysis using individual patient data from randomized clinical trials (RCTS) of chemotherapy (CT) in non-small-cell lung cancer (NSCLC): (1) Survival in the surgical setting. Proc Am Soc Clin Oncol 13:336, 1994.

67. Keller SM, Adak S, Wagner HJ et al. Randomized prospective comparison of adjuvant mediastinal radiation (RT) with or without concurrent chemotherapy with cisplatin and etoposide (PE) for patients with completely resected T1-3N1-2M0 non-small cell lung cancer (NSCLC): US. Int J Rad Oncol Biol Phys 45(3)(suppl. 1):145-146, 1999.

68. Pisters KMW, Ginsberg RJ, Putnam JB et al. Induction paclitaxel and carboplatin (PC) in early stage non-small cell lung cancer (NSCLC): Early results of a completed phase II trial. Proc Amer Soc Clin Oncol 18:467a, 1999.

69. de Boer RH, Smith IE, Pastorino U et al. Pre-operative chemotherapy in early stage resectable non-small-cell lung cancer: A randomized feasibility study justifying a multicenter phase III trial. Br J Cancer 79:1514-1518, 1999.

70. Pass HI, Pogrebniak HW, Steinberg SM et al. Randomized trial of neoadjuvant therapy for lung cancer: Interim analysis. Ann Thorac Surg 53:992-998, 1992.

71. Rosell R, Gomez-Codina J, Camps C et al. A randomized trial comparing preoperative chemotherapy plus surgery with surgery alone in patients with non-small-cell lung cancer. N Engl J Med 330:153-158, 1994.

72. Rosell R, Gomez-Codina J, Camps C et al. Preresectional chemotherapy in stage IIIA non-small-cell lung cancer: A 7-year assessment of a randomized controlled trial. Lung Cancer 26:7-14, 1999.

73. Roth JA, Fossela F, Komaki R et al. A randomized trial comparing perioperative chemotherapy and surgery with surgery alone in resectable stage IIIA non-small-cell lung cancer. J Natl Cancer Inst 86:673-680, 1994.

74. Roth JA, Atkinson EN, Fossela F et al. Long-term follow-up of patients enrolled in a randomized trial comparing perioperative chemotherapy and surgery with surgery alone in resectable stage IIIA non-small-cell lung cancer. Lung Cancer 21:1-6, 1998.

75. Yoneda S, Hibino S, Gotoh I et al. A comparative trial of induction chemoradiotherapy followed by surgery (CRS) or immediate surgery (IS) for stage III non-small cell lung cancer (NSCLC). Proc Amer Soc Clin Oncol 14:1128a, 1995.

76. Depierre A, Milleron B, Moro D et al. Phase III trial of neoadjuvant chemotherapy (NCT) in resectable stage I (except T1N0), II, IIIa non-small cell lung cancer (NSCLC): The French experience. Proc Amer Soc Clin Oncol 18:465a, 1999.

77. Pisters KM, Kris MG, Gralla RJ et al. Pathologic complete response in advanced non-small-cell lung cancer following preoperative chemotherapy: Implications for the design of future non-small-cell lung cancer combined modality trials. J Clin Oncol 11:1757-1762, 1993.

78. Roberts JR, DeVore RF, Carbone DP et al. Neoadjuvant chemotherapy increases perioperative complications in patients undergoing resection of NSCLC. Proc Amer Soc Clin Oncol 18:1794a, 1999.

CHEMORADIATION IN LOCALLY ADVANCED NON-SMALL CELL LUNG CANCER

Philip Bonomi, M.D.
Rush Medical Center, Chicago, IL 60612 USA

Wasif Shirazi, M.D.
Rush Medical College, Chicago, IL 60612 USA

INTRODUCTION

It is estimated that approximately 164,000 cases of lung cancer will occur in 2000 (1) with 84% of the patients (138,000 individuals) having non-small cell lung cancer. (NSCLC) (2). The number of deaths due to non-small cell lung is virtually equal to the combined total deaths of breast cancer, prostate cancer, and colon cancer, which are the second, third, and fourth leading causes of deaths in the United States (1). A large percentage, approximately 44%, of non-small cell lung cancer patients will have locally advanced disease (stage IIIa/b) (3). Previously, radiation therapy has been the sole treatment modality for this group of patients. Although this treatment provides palliation of dyspnea, cough, hemoptysis, pain, and other symptoms from locally advanced disease, the overall five year survival is approximately 5% (4-6). The disappointing long term survival in stage III NSCLC is due to both recurrent local regional disease and to the development of distant metastases. The results of efforts to develop more effective local treatment are discussed in chapter ____, while studies in which chest radiation was combined with systemic therapy are reviewed here.

In the mid 1980's it became apparent that platinum containing chemotherapy regimens produce higher response rates in stage III than in stage IV disease (7). Although there was a large amount of data comparing different chemotherapy regimens there was no convincing evidence that stage IV patients treated with chemotherapy survived longer than patients treated with supportive care only.

Despite the inconclusive survival results for chemotherapy in stage IV disease, the relatively high response rates observed in stage III patients raised the possibility that chemotherapy might have a positive survival effect in locally advanced non-small cell lung cancer. Starting in the late 1980's this consideration encouraged a number of investigators to initiate phase III trials comparing radiation therapy alone to a variety of chemotherapy regimens combined with radiation. Subsequent meta-analyses have shown a modest survival improvement for both stage III (8-10) and stage IV (8) patients who were treated with chemotherapy. Phase III trials and selected phase I-II trials which have evaluated sequential chemotherapy and radiation, sensitizing doses of single agent chemotherapy given simultaneously with radiation , sensitizing doses of chemotherapy doublets given concurrently with radiation, full doses of chemotherapy and simultaneous thoracic radiation, and regimens consisting of combination chemotherapy regimens followed by radiation and sensitizing doses of chemotherapy will be discussed in this chapter.

SEQUENTIAL CHEMORADIATION

The largest number of randomized combined modality trials have involved sequential therapy with chemotherapy being followed by radiation (8-10). This approach provides the potential advantages of reducing local-regional disease before starting local therapy, and it allows a full dose of each modality to be used with avoidance of overlapping toxicity.

The results from three (4-6,11-13) positive studies are summarized in table 1. Dillman et al (11) were the first group to report results of a relatively small randomized study conducted by the Cancer Leukemia Group B(CALGB), in which eligibility was limited to stage III patients with good performance status (Eastern Cooperative Group performance status of 0-1) and minimal weight loss (<5% of usual body weight). One hundred and fifty-five patients were randomized to either chemotherapy with cisplatin ($100mg/m^2$ on days 1 and 29) and vinblastine ($5mg/m^2$/wk for weeks 1-5) followed by standard radiation therapy (60 Gy given in daily 2 Gy fractions), or to the same radiation therapy alone. Tumor responses were 56% for the chemoradiotherapy group (36% response to chemotherapy alone) and 43% for the radiotherapy group (p =0.09). A seven year follow up of this study reported median survival of 13.8 months for chemoradiotherapy compared to 9.7 months for the radiation alone with five year survival of 17% versus 6% in favor of chemoradiotherapy. Though the frequency of serious infection, nausea, and severe anemia was greater in the chemoradiotherapy group, there were no treatment related deaths. Additionally, the incidence of severe esophagitis or pneumonitis was only 1% in both treatment arms.

In 1995 Sause et al (12) published the results of a randomized study in which the two treatment arms were identical to those from the CALGB trial. This trial also included a third arm consisting of hyperfractionated radiation alone (total 69.9 Gy given in 1.2 Gy fractions, twice daily). Recently published final results of this trial reported median survival of 13.8 months for induction chemotherapy, 12.3 months for hyperfractionated arm, and 11.4 months for standard radiation.

Table 1. Positive Randomized Trials Comparing Chest Radiation to Sequential Chemoradiation

Investigators	Treatment	Patients	MST	% 2 YR	% 5 YR
Dillman et al [11]	Radiation*	77	9.7 months	13%	6%
	Vinblastine-Cisplatin-Radiation	78	13.8 months	26%	17%
LeChevalier et al [13]	Radiation**	176	10 months	14%	3%
	Vindesine-Lomustine Cyclophosphamide-Radiation**	176	12 months	21%	6%
Sause et al [12]	Radiation once daily*	149	11.4 months	19%	5%
	Radiation twice daily***	152	12.3 months	24%	6%
	Vinblastine-Cisplatin Radiation*	151	13.8 months	32%	8%

*	*Radiation*	-	*60 Gy over 6 weeks*
**	*Radiation*	-	*65 Gy over 45 days*
***	*Radiation*	-	*69 Gy given as 1,2 Gy twice daily 5 days per week.*

Similarly five year survival rates were 8% for chemoradiotherapy, 6% for hyperfractionated radiation, and 5% for conventional radiation (p = 0.04).

A third phase III study from France, reported by LeChevalier et al (13) compared standard radiotherapy (65 Gy) to three courses of induction chemotherapy with cisplatin, lomustine, vindesine, and cyclophosphamide (PCVC) followed by the same radiation. Three additional cycles of PCVC were administered after the completion of radiotherapy to patients whose disease remained stable or had responded to initial chemotherapy. Median survival was 12 months for the combined modality arm versus 10 months for radiation alone with five year survival of 6% for chemoradiotherapy compared to 3% for radiation alone (p = 0.02).

It is somewhat surprising that improved survival was observed with only two courses of chemotherapy in two of the trials (11,12). In the remaining study, patients received three courses of chemotherapy prior to radiation, and 53% of patients received 3 additional courses of chemotherapy after radiation (13). The results observed in these studies suggest the modest survival advantage achieved with chemotherapy occurs early and that additional treatment may only increase toxicity. Although it would be reasonable to conduct a combined modality trial testing more prolonged chemotherapy, it seems more likely that better survival results will result from the development of more effective chemotherapy regimens.

Although there was an absolute 11% improvement in the 5 year survival rate in the CALGB study, (4) this was the smallest of the three trials with approximately 80 patients per treatment arm.

In the larger trials (5-6) (150 and 175 patients per treatment arm) the absolute increase in the five year survival rate was only 3%. It is encouraging that the rate of distant metastases was significantly reduced in chemotherapy treated patients in the French study, (5) but disseminated disease continues to occur in a large percentage of stage III patients emphasizing the need for more effective systemic therapy. In addition, the French investigators maintained long-term follow up, and they found that local disease progression occurred in 92% of their patients at five years (5). Taken together, their insightful observations indicate that more effective treatments for both local and distant disease are needed.

A number of randomized trials comparing induction chemotherapy followed by radiotherapy to radiation alone in stage III NSCLC have failed to show a survival advantage for chemoradiotherapy (14-16). However, a meta-analysis (8) which involved patients treated with induction chemotherapy, post-radiation chemotherapy and, or both induction and post-radiation chemotherapy from January 1, 1965 to December 31, 1991 has shown reduction in the risk of death with chemoradiotherapy. Both published and unpublished trials were included in this study, and updated survival information was sought on each patient. Trials in which chemotherapy was given simultaneously with chest radiation were not included. The results showed a significant overall benefit for chemotherapy with an absolute survival benefit of 2% at five years over radiation alone (8). More specifically, the survival benefit was greatest with cisplatin based induction therapy.

Two additional meta-analyses which were limited to published trials (9,10) trials have shown a modest survival advantage for chemoradiotherapy over chest radiation alone. Trials which involved sequential, as well as simultaneous chemoradiotherapy were included in these analyses. Although the collective results of the meta-analyses have shown that chemoradiotherapy is associated with superior survival, the authors have emphasized that the modest survival improvement should be balanced with toxicity and quality of life (8-10).

RADIATION AND SENSITIZING DOSES OF CHEMOTHERAPY

Daily Cisplatin

Two groups of investigators have tested small frequent doses of cisplatin ($6mg/m^2$ /day) given simultaneously with thoracic radiation (17,18). In the first trial conducted by the European Organization For Research and Treatment Of Cancer (EORTC) (17), patients received split course chest radiation consisting of 30 Gy given as ten fractions over two weeks followed by a three week rest, after which patients received an additional 25 Gy given as ten fractions over two weeks. In an Italian study patients received thoracic radiation given as 3 Gy daily fractions for a total of 15 treatments given over 3 consecutive weeks (18). In each study radiation therapy alone was compared to daily cisplatin and simultaneous radiation. The two year survival rate in the EORTC study was 13% for radiation therapy alone and 26% for daily cisplatin and radiation (p = 0.009) (17).

In contrast in the Italian study median survival was virtually identical for patients who received radiation therapy versus those who received cisplatin and radiation, (median survival about 10 months), and there was no significant difference in overall survival between treatment groups (p = .89) (18).

Both groups of investigators observed increased nausea and vomiting, with the cisplatin regimen but no treatment related deaths were seen in either study (17,18). In addition, severe esophagitis was relatively infrequent, and not significantly different for cisplatin-radiation versus radiation therapy in the EORTC trial. In contrast the Italian study revealed more grade 3 esophagitis in patients treated with cisplatin-radiation therapy.

Analysis of sites of failure in the EORTC trial revealed a significant reduction in the local failure rate for patients who received cisplatin and radiation therapy, suggesting treatment has an impact on survival. While there is no apparent explanation for the conflicting survival results observed in the EORTC (17) and in the Italian trials (18), it is somewhat surprising that superior survival was observed with the less intense EORTC radiation schedule.

Weekly Cisplatin

Weekly doses of cisplatin given concurrently with thoracic radiation were also evaluated in the phase III EORTC trial (17). Although there was a trend for longer survival with weekly cisplatin, 30 mg/m^{2}week in the EORTC trial (two year survival rates of 19% for combined modality versus 13% for radiation alone), the survival difference was not significant.

Similarly, in a smaller randomized study 95 patients were randomized to either standard radiation therapy (50 Gy) versus the same radiation with weekly cisplatin (15mg/m^2 IV week) (19). Although median survival was longer (16 months versus 11 months) and intra-thoracic relapses were lower (48% versus 59%) with cisplatin and radiation, the overall survival difference was not significant (p = 0.18).

Carboplatin Trials

Bishop, et al have reported preliminary results for a randomized trial of concurrent carboplatin and radiotherapy in locally advanced, good performance status NSCLC patients (20). A total of 208 patients were randomized to four treatment arms; standard radiation (60 Gy/30 fractions over 6 weeks) with or without carboplatin 70 mg/m^2 per day, days 1-5 and 29-34; accelerated radiation (60 Gy in 2 Gy fractions twice daily for three weeks) with or without the same dose and schedule of carboplatin. Objective response rates were similar in all four arms. At a median follow up of 39 months, the overall survival was 15.7 months, 2 year survival was 31%, and there were no significant differences between the treatment regimens (20). The carboplatin arms were associated with more hematologic toxicity. Although was no significant difference in the incidence of severe esophagitis, a trend for more severe esophagitis was observed with the accelerated radiation schedule.

Investigators from the Netherlands have evaluated carboplatin given as continuous 6 week intravenous infusion to a total accumulative dose of 840mg/m^2 (21). During this 6 week infusion patients received simultaneous radiotherapy (60 Gy in 30 fractions). One hundred and forty-three stage III NSCLC patients were randomized either to standard radiation therapy or to continuous infusion carboplatin plus radiation. The overall response rate was 41% and the survival duration for the entire group was 11 months with no significant difference between the treatment arms. Additionally, bronchoscopic examination after completion of treatment revealed a similar percentage of persistent local tumor for each treatment arm suggesting no improvement in local control with combined modality therapy.

NEW AGENTS

Despite the improved survival results observed in some of the individual randomized trials (4-6) and in the meta-analyses (8-10), the majority of stage III patients continue to succumb from local and distant metastases. Many researchers have incorporated newer agents including paclitaxel, docetaxel, vinorelbine, gemcitabine, and irinotecan (22) into combined regimen in an attempt to improve survival results. Each of these agents has the potential advantage of enhancing effectiveness of radiation. The results of selected phase I-II trials of these agents combined with chest radiation are summarized in table 2.

Paclitaxel

Choy et al were the first group of investigators to report the results of single agent paclitaxel given currently with a conventional dose of chest radiation (2 Gy daily/60 Gy total) (23). Esophagitis was the dose limiting toxicity, and these investigators concluded that the maximum tolerated dose was 60 mg/m^2 given weekly as a three hour infusion.

In their subsequent phase II trial of paclitaxel (60mg/m^2 weekly administered IV over 3 hours for six weeks) with radiation they observed an overall response rate of 86% with median survival duration and two year survival rate of 20 months and 33%, respectively (24). Significant toxicity included grade 3-4 esophagitis (37%), grade 3-4 pneumonitis (12%), and grade 4 neutropenia (6%).

Table 2. Phase I/II Trials of Sensitizing Doses of Single Agents with Simultaneous Radiation

Investigator	Dose Schedule/MTD	RT Schedule	Toxicity/Doe-Limiting Toxicity
Choy et al[23,24]	Paclitaxel 60 mg/m² weekly X 6 weeks	60 Gy in 2 Gy fx over 6 weeks	Esophagitis pneumonitis
Kaukourakis et al[28]	Docetaxel 30 mg/m² weekly X 6 weeks	64 Gy in 2 Gy fx over 6.5 weeks	Esophagitis
Scalliet et et*[29]	Gemcitabine 1000mg/m² weekly X 6 weeks	60 Gy in 2 Gy fx over 6 weeks	Pulmonary toxicity Severe esophagitis
Kudoh et al[31]	Irinotecan 60 mg/m² weekly X 6 weeks	60 Gy in 2 Gy fx over 6 weeks	Esophagitis Pneumonitis Diarrhea
Saka et al[32]	Irinotecan 60 mg/m² weekly X 6 weeks	60 Gy in 2 Gy fx over 6 weeks	Pneumonitis

*   *Study closed early due to treatment related deaths. Excessive toxicity*
FX = fractions

*   -   *radiation – 60 Gy 6 weeks*
**   -   *radiation – 64 Gy in 2 Gy fractions over approximately 6 weeks*

In another phase I trial which tested twice weekly paclitaxel, given over 1 hour for 6 weeks, with concurrent radiation (61 Gy in 1.8-2 Gy/d) the maximum tolerated dose of paclitaxel was at 35mg/m², and dose-limiting toxicity was esophagitis (25). The overall response rate and the median survival time were 80% and 20 months, respectively. The 3 year survival rate was 20%.

Docetaxel

A weekly schedule of docetaxel and simultaneous thoracic chest radiation has been studied in two phase I trials (26,27). Esophagitis was the dose limiting toxicity in each trial with one group concluding that MTD was 20mg/m² week , while the other group observed a MTD of 30 mg/m²/week. A phase I/II study from Greece by Koukourakis et al evaluated docetaxel 30 mg/m² weekly for six weeks with concurrent radiation (total dose 64 Gy over 6.5 weeks) (28). The main toxicity observed was esophagitis with approximately 50% of patients experiencing treatment delay. Though marked lymphocytopenia was seen in all patients, overall hematologic toxicity was minimal with grade 2 neutropenia being observed in two of thirty-five patients.

Gemcitabine

Gemcitabine, a nucleoside analogue that inhibits cellular repair and repopulation, has significant activity in metastatic non-small cell lung cancer and has been shown to be potent radiosensitizer (22). A phase II trial testing full doses of gemcitabine (weekly, gemcitabine at 1000mg/m^2 for six weeks) with concurrent standard radiation therapy (60 Gy in 2 Gy fractions) in stage III NSCLC was associated with unacceptable toxicity (29). The study was closed after enrolling only 8 patients because there were 3 treatment related deaths. Lethal pulmonary toxicity occurred in 3 of 8 patients. Severe esophagitis or pneumonitis was observed in three additional patients.   More recently gemcitabine has been given with weekly continuous radiation 63 Gy/35 fractions) (30). Dose limiting esophagitis was observed with a gemcitabine dose of 125mg/m^2/week for 7 doses, two dimensional radiation. However, when gemcitabine was combined with three dimensional radiation, the maximum tolerated dose had not been reached at 150mg/m^2/week (30).

Irinotecan

Kudoh, et al reported a maximum tolerated dose of 45 to 60 mg/m^2 for irinotecan given weekly with concurrent radiation (60 Gy) (31).   The dose-limiting toxicities were esophagitis, pneumonitis and diarrhea. A phase II study by the Japan Clinical Oncology Goup evaluated weekly CPT-11 (60 mg/m^2 weekly for 6 doses) with concurrent thoracic radiotherapy (60 Gy in 30 fractions) (32).

Vinorelbine

Vinorelbine, a semi-synthetic vinca alkaloid, is a potent inhibitor of mitotic microtubule polymerization. This results in blockade of cells in the G2/M phase of the cell cycle allowing subsequent radiation to effectively kill these cells. Single agent Vinorelbine has also been combined with conventional doses of chest radiation (2 Gy daily/60 Gy total) and the dose limiting toxicity was 15 mg/m^2/week (33).

CARBOPLATIN-ETOPOSIDE

Jeremic and his colleagues have conducted two relatively small randomized trials comparing hyper-fractionated chest radiation alone to sensitizing doses of carboplatin and etoposide given simultaneously with the same dose and schedule of radiation (34-35).

In the first trial 61 (34), patients received thoracic radiation consisting of 1.2 Gy twice daily to a total dose of 64.8 Gy; 52 patients were treated with same dose and schedule of radiation combined with carboplatin 100 mg on first and second days and etoposide 100 mg on the first three days of each week; 56 patients received the same dose and schedule of radiation plus carboplatin 200 mg on the first two days of each week and etoposide 100 mg on each day of radiation. Chemotherapy doses were not determined by body surface area or by area under the curve. In addition, the route of administration for etoposide (oral versus intravenous) was not stated.

Survival for the lower dose chemotherapy regimen (weekly carboplatin 100 mg for 2 days and weekly etoposide 100 mg for 3 days) was significantly better than survival for radiation alone – median survival of 18 versus 8 months and 3 year survival rates of

23% versus 6%, p = .0027 (34). Similar rates of acute and late grade 3-4 toxicities were observed with radiation alone and with the lower dose chemoradiation regimen.

In a subsequent trial Jeremic et al (35), treated 131 patients with either hyperfractionated chest radiation alone or with the same radiation and simultaneous carboplatin 50 mg and etoposide 50 given on each day of radiation. Like their earlier trial fixed chemotherapy doses were used and the route of administration for etoposide was not defined. Again significantly, superior survival was observed in patients treated with modest, frequent doses of carboplatin and etoposide and radiation – median survival duration 22 months versus 14 months and 4 year survival rates of 23% versus 9%, p = .021 (35). There were no significant differences in acute and late severe toxicities treatment related complications.

NEW DRUG DOUBLETS

Each of the new drugs combined with a platinum compound has been given concurrently with thoracic irradiation. The results of these phase I-II trials are summarized in table 3.

Table 3. Phase I/II Trials with Sensitizing Doses of Doublets with Radiation

Investigator	Recommended Dose Schedule	Radiation Schedule	Toxicity
Choy et al [24]	Paclitaxel 50 mg/ (1 hr infusion) and Carboplatin (AUC 2) weekly x 7 then TRT followed by consolidation With Paclitaxel 200mg/m^2 and Carboplatin (ACU 6) every 21 Days x 2 cycles.	66 Gy in 2 Gy fx over 7 weeks	Esophagitis Pneumonitis
Choy et al [38]	Same doses/regimen as Above given weekly for 6 weeks	69.6 Gy in 1.2 Gy fx twice daily	Esophagitis Pneumonitis.
Lau et al [39]	Paclitaxel 35mg/m^2 (1 hr infusion), twice weekly and Carboplatin (AUC 1.5) weekly for 6 weeks then TRT followed by consolidation with Paclitaxel 200 mg/m^2 and Carboplatin (AUC 6) every 21 days x 2 cycles.	61 Gy in 1.8-2 Gy fx over 6-7 weeks.	Esophagitis Neutropenia
Masters et al [40]	Cisplatin 80 mg/m^2 day 1 and Vinorelbine 15mg/m^2 days 1,8 both every 21 days x 2 cycles	60 Gy in 2 Gy fx over 6 weeks	Esophagitis Myelosupression

CARBOPLATIN - PACLITAXEL

Choy et. al. evaluated paclitaxel 50 mg/m² over one hour and carboplatin (AUC of 2) weekly for seven weeks with concomitant radiation to a total dose of 66 Gy which was followed by paclitaxel 200 mg/m² and carboplatin (AUC of 6) every 3 weeks for two cycles (36).

In 39 patients survival time was 20.5 months with a two year survival of 38%. Grade 3-4 esophagitis was observed in 46% of the patients with two of them developing late esophageal toxicity in the form of strictures which required esophageal dilatation. Additionally, grade 3 pulmonary toxicity in the form of pneumonitis was experienced by 22% of patients. Pneumonitis improved rapidly with corticosteroid administration. Other significant toxicities included neutropenia (37%) and anemia (14%).

In a study of 38 patients Belani et al reported the results of weekly paclitaxel 45mg/m² (3 hour infusion) and carboplatin 100 mg/m² with concurrent standard radiation given in 1.8 Gy daily fractions over 6-7 weeks (total 60-65Gy). Median survival time had not been reached at the time of abstract publication and a two year actuarial survival was reported at 54%. This regimen was well tolerated with an 8% incidence of grade 3 esophagitis. The relatively low rates of severe esophagitis in this trial compared to the study reported by Choy et al maybe explained by the lower doses of paclitaxel (45mg/m² versus 50mg/m² and radiation (1.8 Gy 1 day versus 2 Gy/day.

Choy et al, have (38) also reported results for a trial with carboplatin and paclitaxel (same doses over 6 weeks) with concurrent hyperfractionated radiation therapy (69.6 Gy/1.2 Gy twice daily fractions). The response rate in 43 patients was 78.6% with a one year survival of 63% and the median survival not reached at the time of reporting. The incidence of grade 3-4 esophagitis and pulmonary toxicity was 26% and 16.5%, respectively. The toxicity and survival are similar to the results observed with paclitaxel-carboplatin and conventional radiation.

Lau et al, (39) have evaluated twice weekly paclitaxel (30-35 mg/m² over 1 hour for 6 weeks) plus carboplatin (AUC 1.5 weekly for 6 weeks) and concurrent thoracic radiation (61 Gy in 1.8-2 Gy daily fractions) followed three weeks later by two cycles of paclitaxel (200 mg/m² over 3 hours) and carboplatin (AUC 6) in patients whose tumor response was classified as stable disease, partial remission or complete remission. Grade 3-4 esophagitis occurred in 35% of patients, and grade 4 neutropenia was observed in 29% of patients. Grade 3 or 4 pneumonitis was not observed in this group of patients.

Vinorelbine Platinum Compounds

Several studies have evaluated vinorelbine in combination with platinum agents and concurrent radiation. A phase I trial by Masters et al, (40) identified cisplatin 80 mg/m² on day 1 , and vinorelbine 15 mg/m² on days 1 and 8 every three weeks for two cycles with concurrent standard radiotherapy (60 Gy in 2 Gy daily fractions), as the maximum tolerated doses with this chemoradiotherapy regimen. Myelosuppression and esophagitis were the dose-limiting toxicities. They reported an overall response rate of 47%.

A phase II trial by Zatloukal et al, (41) reported on the feasibility of combining vinorelbine/cisplatin with concurrent radiotherapy. In this study, chemotherapy consisted of four cycles of cisplatin (80 mg/m^2 every 28 days) and vinorelbine 25 mg/m^2 on days 1,8,15 with the dose reduced to 12.5 mg/m^2 during concurrent radiation therapy which was started on day 4 of cycle 2(60 Gy in 2 Gy fractions over 6 weeks). A response rate of 62.5% was reported. Grade 3-4 toxicity included neutropenia (26%), nausea/vomiting (16%), esophagitis (5%) and anemia (5%).

Irinotecan – Platinum compounds

While one dose-escalation study with combination cisplatin/Irinotecan with concurrent radiotherapy was discontinued early because of excessive diarrhea and myelosuppression, subsequent studies have demonstrated feasibility of this regimen. A phase I dose-escalating study by Fukuda et al, (42) evaluated cisplatin (60-80 mg/m^2 every 28 days) with Irinotecan (40-60 mg/m^2 days 1,8,15) and concurrent radiation (split course schedule with 24 Gy given beginning day 2 of cycle one as 2 Gy daily fractions and then 26-36 Gy in 2 Gy fractions beginning day 2 of cycle two, again in 2 Gy fractions). Cisplatin 80 mg/m^2 and Irinotecan 60 mg/m^2 were recommended for further investigation. Esophagitis and pneumonitis were the dose limiting toxicities. The overall response rate in 23 patients entered onto this phase I trial was 65%.

Another small phase I /II Japanese trial evaluated escalating weekly doses of Irinotecan(CPT-11) with Carboplatin 20 mg/m^2 daily for four weeks with concurrent standard radiation therapy to a total of 60 Gy in 2 Gy fractions and reported tolerable toxicity at a CPT-11 dose of 50 mg/m^2/week for four weeks. The dose limiting toxicity was pneumonitis (43). Their overall response rate was 69.6%.

RADIATION AND CONCURRENT CYTOTOXIC DOSES OF CHEMOTHERAPY: PHASE III TRIALS

The Hoosier Oncology Group has evaluated the addition of single agent cisplatin to radiation therapy for unresectable NSCLC (44). In this study 215 patients were randomized to conventional chest radiation alone (total dose-60 to 65 Gy, daily fractions 1.8 to 2 Gy) versus the same radiation with simultaneous cisplatin 70 mg/m^2 every three weeks for three cycles. There were no significant differences in response rates or survival results. There was more nausea, vomiting, leukopenia and mild renal toxicity with the combined modality treatment regimen. There were two deaths felt to be clearly related to therapy, both in the combination arm.

So far there is only one report of a mature randomized which compared sequential to concurrent chemoradiotherapy using full doses of a combination chemotherapy. Furuse et al, (45) treated 320 in a trial in which each patient received MVP chemotherapy which included two cycles of cisplatin 80 mg/m^2 on day 1, vindesine 3 mg/m^2 on days 1, 8 and mitomycin 8 mg/m^2 on day 1. Patients were randomized to receive chemotherapy and concurrent chest radiation consisting of 28 Gy (2 Gy fraction/5 fractions per week/a total of 14 fractions), followed by a 10 day rest period and then an additional 28 Gy of radiation versus sequential chemotherapy which consisted of two courses of MVP chemotherapy followed by continuous thoracic irradiation (56 Gy total). Survival was significantly superior in the patients receiving concurrent therapy (median = 16.5 months, 5 years = 16%) compared to those receiving sequential therapy (median survival = 13.3 months, 5 year rate – 9%,) (p = 0.04) (45).

Although esophagitis and myelosuppression were slightly more common in the concurrent arm, overall toxicity profiles for both arms were similar.

The Radiation Therapy Oncology Group (RTOG) has reported preliminary results for a phase III trial in sequential vinblastine-cisplatin radiation versus simultaneous vinblastine-cisplatin – radiation versus simultaneous etoposide cisplatin-hyperfractionated radiation (46). They observed a trend for superior survival with simultaneous vinblastine-cisplatin-radiation compared to sequential chemoradiation (median survival for simultaneous = 17 months versus 14.6 months for sequential = 0.08). There was no apparent survival advantage for chemotherapy and simultaneous hyper-fractionated radiation (median survival 15.6 versus 14.6 (46) months p =.31). There was more acute toxicity with concurrent chemoradiotherapy.

CHEMOTHERAPY FOLLOWED BY CHEMORADIO-THERAPY

The CALGB and ECOG have compared sequential chemoradiotherapy to sequential and concurrent chemoradiotherapy in a large randomized trial (47). All patients received induction chemotherapy with vinblastine and cisplatin given as in the land-mark Dillman et al trial, and then were randomized to subsequent standard radiation therapy (60 Gy/6 week), or to concurrent therapy with carboplatin 100 mg/m^2 /wk for six weeks with simultaneous standard radiation therapy. The overall response to induction chemotherapy was 37%. The overall response rate in both arms was similar at 63%, as were the median survival and three year survival, 13 months and 19% respectively. Patients who received carboplatin suffered more neutropenia, thrombocytopenia, and esophagitis. However, no patients died of neutropenic infection.

CALGB has also evaluated the same treatment strategy using new drugs in combination with cisplatin. In a recent randomized phase II trial patients were assigned to one of the following regimens: gemcitabine/cisplatin, paclitaxel/cisplatin or vinorelbine/cisplatin (48).

All patients received four cycles of cisplatin at 80 mg/m^2 on days 1,22, 43, 64. The doses of the other agents were gemcitabine 1,250 mg/m^2 on days 1, 8, 22, 29, and 600 mg/m^2 on days 43, 50, 64, and 71. paclitaxel 225 mg/m^2 over three hours on days 1, 22, and 135 mg/m^2 on days 43, 64, vinorelbine 25 mg/m^2 on days 1, 8, 15, 22, 29, and 15 mg/m^2 on days 43, 50, 64, and 71. Radiation, a total of 66 Gy given in 2 Gy daily fractions, was initiated on day 43. The dominant toxicities during radiation were grade 3-4 neutropenia which occurred in approximately 50% of the patients and esophagitis which was observed in 25 to 49% of the patients median survival for entire group in 18 months (48).

SUMMARY AND FUTURE DIRECTIONS

Based on the results of meta-analyses (8-10) and several relatively large randomized trials (4-6) treatment with chemotherapy followed by radiation has produced superior survival compared to radiation alone. However, the long term survival benefit is modest with a 2-3% improvement in the 5 years survival rate (5,6,8). More recent observations from a single phase III study suggest that cytotoxic doses of chemotherapy and concurrent radiation are superior to sequential chemoradiotherapy (45), and preliminary results from another randomized trial comparing simultaneous versus sequential chemoradiotherapy also shows a trend for superior survival with concurrent treatment (46).

In contrast most trials which have tested radiation and simultaneous treatment with low doses of single agent cisplatin or carboplatin have not shown significant survival differences (18-21). However, superior survival has been observed with radiation and concurrent sensitizing doses of a two drug chemotherapy regimen consisting of carboplatin and etoposide, versus radiation alone (34,35).

In some randomized chemotherapy trials the newer drugs have produced superior survival results compared to older regimens (49-51), and it appears that the magnitude of the survival advantage is greater in stage IIIb compared to stage IV patients (50,51). At present many randomized studies have incorporated the new agents, but it appears that most investigators have made the assumption that the newer treatments are superior to the older regimens because direct comparison of the new versus the older agents is not being done. Instead, investigators are carrying out the following studies: chemotherapy (paclitaxel-carboplatin) followed by conventional radiation versus hyper-accelerated radiation therapy (E2597); sequential chemoradiotherapy (paclitaxel-carboplatin) with or without thalidomide, an anti-angeogenesis agent (E3598); sensitizing doses of a chemotherapy doublet (weekly paclitaxel-carboplatin) and simultaneous chest radiation with or without amifostine, a radiation protecting agent (RTOG 9801); and sensitizing doses of a chemotherapy doublet (weekly paclitaxel carboplatin) with or without two courses of the same chemotherapy given as induction treatment (CLB39801).

In addition there is a phase III trial in stage III NSCLC comparing marimastat, a matrix metalloproteinase inhibitor, versus placebo following initial anti-neoplastic therapy which is given at the investigators discretion.

Currently, investigators face a dilemma with respect to the design of phase III trials in stage III NSCLC. There are many interesting questions but there are a limited number of patients. Should efforts be directed towards attempting to identify the optimal chemoradiotherapy regimen – choice of chemotherapy agents, radiation dose and schedule, chemoradiation schedule? Or, should new studies incorporate new biologic treatments – inhibition of angiogenesis, (52) enhancement of apoptosis, (53) inhibition of autocrine growth factors (54,55)? It is likely that there will be considerable controversy regarding the design of phase III NSCLC trials in the next ten years.

Tables 4. Summary CT Schedule/Toxicity of Phase I/II Trials with Sensitizing Doses of Doublets with Papiation

Investigator	Dose Schedule	RT Schedule	Toxicity
Zatloukal et al [41]	Cisplatin 80 mg/^{2} Every 28 days and Vinorelbine 25mg/m^2 days 1,8,15 (12.5 mg/m^2 given for cycles 2 and 3) both given for 4 cycles	60 Gy in 2 Gy fx over 6 weeks (beginning day #4 of cycle #2)	Neutropenia
Fukuda et al [42]	Cisplatin 80 mg/m^2 Above given weekly for 6 weeks Irinotecan 60mg/m^2 Days 1,8,15	24 Gy in Gy fx beginning with cycle #1 then rest period then 26-36 Gy in 2 Gy fx beginning day 2 cycle #2.	Esophagitis diarrhea

REFERENCES

1. American Cancer Society. Cancer Facts and Figures 2000: Pages 11-12.
2. Travis WD, Travis LB, Devessa SS. Lung Cancer. Cancer 75:191-202, 1995.
3. Bulzebruck H, Bopp R, Drings P, et al. New aspects of the staging of lung cancer. Prospective validation of the International Union Against Cancer TNM classification. Cancer 70: 1102-1110, 1992.
4. Dillman RP, Herndon J, Seagren SL, et al. Improved survival in stage III NSCLC: Seven year follow-up of CALGB 8433. J Natl Cancer Inst 88:1210-1215, 1996.
5. Arriagada R, LeChevalier et al. Cisplatin-based chemotherapy (CT) in patients with locally advanced non-small cell lung cancer (NSCLC): late analysis of the French randomized trial. Proc Am Soc Clin Oncol 16:446a (abstr 1601), 1997.
6. Sause WT, Kolesar P, Taylor SG et al. Final results of phase III trial in regionally advanced unresectable non-small cell lung cancer. Chest 17 (2): 212-223, 2000.
7. Bonomi P. Brief overview of combination chemotherapy in non-small cell lung cancer. Semin Oncol 13(suppl 3): 89-9, 1986.
8. Non-small cell lung cancer collaborative group. Chemotherapy in non-small cell lung cancer: A meta-analysis using updated data on individual patients from 52 randomized clinical trials. Br. Med J 311: 899-909, 1995.

9.   Marino P, Preatoni A, Cantoni A. Randomized trials for radiotherapy alone versus combined chemotherapy and radiotherapy in stages IIIa and IIIb non-small cell lung cancer. A meta-analysis. Cancer 76:593-60, 1995.

10. Pritchard RS, Anthony SP. Chemotherapy plus radiotherapy compared with radiotherapy alone in the treatment of locally advanced, unresectable, non-small cell lung cancer. Ann Intern Med 125:723-729, 1996.

11. Dillman R, Seagren SL, Propert K, et al. A randomized trial of induction chemotherapy plus high-dose radiatin versus radiation alone in stage III non-small cell lung cancer. N Engl J Med 323:940-945, 1990.

12. Sause WT, Scott C, Taylor S, et al. RTOG 8808 and ECOG 4588. Preliminary results of a phase III trial in regionally advanced unresectable non-small cell lung cancer. J Natl Cancer Inst 87:198-205, 1995.

13. LeChevalier T, Arriagada R, Quoix E, et al. Radiotherapy alone versus combined chemotherapy and radiotherapy in non-resectable non-small cell lung cancer: first analyses of a randomized trial in 353 patients. J Natl Cancer Inst 83:417-422, 1991.

14. Mattson K, Holsti LR, Holsti P, et al. Inoperable non-small cell lung cancer: Radiation with or without chemotherapy. Eur J Cancer Clin Oncol 24:477-482, 1988.

15. Morton RF, Jett JR, McGinnis WL, et al. Thoracic radiation therapy alone compared with combined chemoradiotherapy for locally advanced unresectable non-small cell lung cancer. A randomized phase III trial. Ann Intern Med 1151:681-686, 1991.

16. Crino L, Latini P, Meacci M, et al. Induction chemotherapy plus high-dose radiotherapy versus radiotherapy alone in locally advanced unresectable non-small cell lung cancer. Ann Oncol 4:847-851, 1993.

17. Schaake-Koning C, Vanden Bogaert W, Dalesio O, et al. Effects of concomitant cisplatin and radiotherapy on inoperable non-small cell lung cancer. N Engl J Med 326:524-530, 1992.

18. Trovo MG, Minatel E, Franchin G, et al. Radiotherapy versus radiotherapy enhanced by cisplatin in stage III non-small cell lung cancer: Int J Rad Oncol Biol Phys 24(1):11-15, 1992.

19. Soresi E, Clerici M et al. A randomized clinical trial comparing radiation therapy, radiation therapy plus cis-Dichlorodiammine platinum (II) in the treatment of locally advanced non-small cell lung cancer. Sem Oncol 15(6) (Suppl 7): 20-25, 1988.

20. Bishop JF, Ball DL, Smith JG, et al. A randomized phase III trial of concurrent carboplatin and twice daily radiotherapy (RT) in locally advanced non-small cell lung cancer. (NSCLC). Proc Am Soc Clin Oncol 17:464a, 1998.

21. Groen HJM, VanderLeest AHW, Snoek WJ, et al. Phase III study of continuous carboplatin over 6 weeks with radiation versus radiation alone in stage III on-small cell lung cancer (NSCLC). Proc Am Soc Clin Oncol 18:466a (abstr 1797), 1999.

22. Lilenbaum RC, Green MR. Novel chemotherapeutic agents in the treatment of non-small cell lung cancer. J Clin Oncol 11:1391-1402, 1993.

23. Choy H, Akerley W, Safran H, et al. Phase I trial of outpatient weekly paclitaxel and concurrent radiation therapy for advanced non-small cell lung cancer. J Clin Oncol 12:2682-2686, 1994.

24. Choy H, Safran H, Akerley W, et al. Phase II trial of weekly paclitaxel and concurrent radiation therapy for locally advanced non-small cell lung cancer. Clin Can Res 4:1931-1936, 1998.

25. Lau D, Ryu J, Grandara D. Concurrent twice–weekly paclitaxel and thoracic irradiation for stage III non-small cell lung cancer. Seminar Radiat Oncol 9 (2 Suppl 1):117-120, 1999.

26. Amdal S, Wibe E, Hallen M, et al. Phase I study of concomitant docetaxel (Taxotere) and radiation in locally advanced non-small cell lung cancer (NSCLC). Proc Am Soc Clin Oncol 1997; 16:460a, 1997.

27. Teng M. Choy H, DeVore KR, et al. Phase I trial of outpatient weekly docetaxel and concurrent radiation therapy for stage III unresectable non-small cell lung cancer: A Vanderbilt Cancer Center affiliate network (VCCAN). Proc Am Soc Clin Oncol 17:503a, 1998.

28. Koukourakis M, Bahlitzanakis N, Froudarakis M,   et al.   Concurrent conventionally fractionated radiotherapy and weekly docetaxel in the treatment of stage IIIb non-small cell lung cancer. British Journal of Cancer 80 (11): 1792-1796, 1999.

29. Scalliet P, Goor C, Galdermans D, et al. Gemzar (gemcitabine) with thoracic radiotherapy – a phase II pilot study in chemonaive patients with advanced non-small cell lung cancer (NSCLC). Proc Am Soc Clin Oncol 17:499a , 1998.

30. Zinner RG, Fossella FV, Komaki R, et al. Gemcitabine with concurrent 3D conformal radiation followed by consolidation gemcitabine plus cisplatin: a phase I trial for patients with stage III non-small cell lung cancer. Proc Amer Soc Clin Oncol 19:510a, 2000.

31. Kudoh S, Kuriharan, Akishio K, et al. A phase I-II study of weekly irinotecan (CPT-11) and simultaneous thoracic radiotherapy (TRT) for unresectable locally advanced non-small cell lung cancer (NSCLC). Proc Am Soc Clin Oncol 15: 372, 1996.

32. Saka H, Shimokata K, Yoshida S, Shimokata K, Yoshida S, et al. Irinotecan (CPT-11) and concurrent radiotherapy in locally advanced non-small cell lung cancer (NSCLC): a phase II study of Japan Clinical Oncology Group (JCOG 9504). Proc Am Soc Clin Oncol 16: 447a, 1997.

33. Edelstein MP. Wolfe LA, Duch DS. Potentiation of radiation radiation therapy by vinorelbine (navelbine) in non-small cell lung cancer. Semin Oncol 23 (Suppl 5): 41-47, 1996.

34. Jeremic B, Shabamoto Y, Acimovic L. et al.   Randomized trial of hyperfractionated radiation therapy with or without concurrent chemotherapy for stage III non-small cell lung cancer. J Clin Oncol 13:452-458, 1995.

35. Jeremic B, Shibamoto Y, Acimovic L, et al. Hyperfractionated radiation therapy with or without concurrent low-dose daily carboplatin etoposide for stage III non-small cell lung cancer: A randomized study. J Clin Oncol 14 (14): 1065-1070, 1996.

36. Choy H, Akerley W, Safran H, et al. Multi-institutional phase II trial of paclitaxel, carboplatin and concurrent radiation therapy for locally advanced non-small cell lung cancer. J Clin Oncol 16 (10): 3316-3322, 1998.

37. Belani CP. Aisner J, Day R. Weekly paclitaxel and carboplatin with simultaneous thoracic radiotherapy (TRT) for locally advanced non-small cell lung cancer (NSCLC): three year follow-up. Proc Am Soc Clin Oncol 16:448a (abstr 1608), 1997.

38. Choy H, DeVore RD, Hande JR, et al. Phase II study of paclitaxel, carboplatin and hyperfractionated radiation therapy for locally advanced inoperable non-small cell lung cancer. A Vanderbilt cancer center affiliate network (VCCAN) trial (Proc Am Soc Clin Oncol 17:467a (abstr 1794), 1998.

39. Lau D, Leigh B, Gandova DR, et al. Weekly carboplatin twice weekly, paclitaxel, and thoracic radiation followed by carboplatin/paclitaxel for stage III non-small cell lung cancer. Semin Oncol 26 (suppl 2): 70, 1999.

40. Masters GA, Havat DJ, Hoffman PC, et al. Phase I study of vinorelbine, cisplatin and concomitant thoracic radiation in the treatment of advanced chest malignancies. J Clin Oncol 16: 2157-2163, 1998.

41. Zatloukal P, Petruzelka L, Zowanova M, et al. Vinorelbine (VRL) plus cuisplatin (CODP) and concurrent radiotherapy in advanced non-small cell lung cancer. Proc Am Soc Clin Oncol 17:505a, 1998.

42. Fukuda M, Soda H, Ichiki M, et al. Phase I study of irinotecan (CPT-11) and cisplatin (CDDP) with concurrent thoracic radiotherapy (TRT) in locally advanced non-small cell lung cancer (NSCLC) Proc Am Soc Clin Oncol 18: 466a, 1999.

43. Yokoyama A, Kurita Y, Saijo N, et al. Dose-finding study of irinotecan and cisplatin plus concurrent radiotherapy for unresectable stage III non-small cell lung cancer. Br. J Cancer 78(2): 257-262, 1998.

44. Blanke C, Ansari R, Mantravadi R, et al. Phase III trial of thoracic irradiation with or without cisplatin for locally advanced unresectable non-small cell lung cancer: a Hoosier Oncology Group protocol. J Clin Oncol 13:1425-1429, 1995.

45. Furuse K, Fukuoka M, Kowahara M, et al. Phase III study of concurrent versus sequential thoracic radiotherapy in combination with mitomycin, vindesine, and cisplatin in unresectable stage III non-small cell lung cancer. J Clin Oncol 17:2692-2699, 1999.

46. Curran WJ Jr, Scott C, Langer C, et al. Phase III comparison of sequential versus concurrent chemoradiation for patients with unresectable stage III non-small cell lung cancer: initial report of radiation therapy oncology group (RTOG) 9410. Proc Amer Soc Clin Oncol 19:484a, 2000.

47. Clamon G, Herndon J, Cooper R, et al. Radiosensitization with carboplatin for patients with unresectable stage III non-small cell lung cancer: A phase III trial of the Cancer and Leukemia Group B and the Eastern Cooperative Oncology Group. J Clin Oncol 17:4-11, 1999.

48. Vokes E, Leopold KA, Herndori JE, et al. A randomized phase II study of gemcitabine or paclitaxel or vinorelbine with cisplatin as induction chemotherapy

and concomitant chemoradiotherapy for unresectable stage III non-small cell lung cancer. (CCALGB study 9431). Proc Amer Soc Clin Oncol 18:459a, 1999.

49. LeChevalier T, Brisgand D, Douillard J, et al. Randomized study of vinorelbine and cisplatin versus vindesine and cisplatin and vindesine alone in advanced non-small cell lung cancer: results of a European multicenter trial including 612 patients. J Clin Oncol 12-360-367, 1994.

50. Sandler AB, Nemunaitis J, Denhem C, et al. Phase III trial of gemicitabine plus cisplatin versus cisplatin alone in patients with locally advanced or metastatic non-small cell lung cancer. J Clin Oncol 18:122-130, 2000.

51. Bonomi P, Kim K, Fairclough D, et al. Comparison of survival and quality of life in advanced non-small cell lung cancer patients treated with two dose levels of paclitaxel combined with cisplatin versus etoposide with cisplatin results of Eastern Cooperative group trial. J Clin Oncol 18:623-631, 2000.

52. Zhu Z, Witte L, Inhibition of tumor growth and metastasis by targeting tumor-associated angiogenesis with antagonists to the receptors of vascular endothelial growth factor. Invest New Drugs 17:195-212, 1999.

53. Reed JC. Dysregulation of apoptosis in cancer. J Clin Oncol 17:2941-2953, 1999.

54. Rowinsky EK, Winoele JJ, Von Hoff DD. Ras protein farnesy/transferase: a strategic target for anticancer therapeutic development. J Clin Oncol 17:3631-3652, 1999.

55. Levitt ML, Koty PP. Tyrosine Kimase inhibitors in preclinical development. Inves New Drugs 17:215-226, 1999.

LUNG CANCER: THERAPEUTIC OPTIONS FOR STAGE IV AND RECURRENT NSCLC

Alejandro R. Calvo, M.D.
University of Pittsburgh School of Medicine, Pittsburgh, PA USA

Chandra P. Belani, MD
University of Pittsburgh School of Medicine, Pittsburgh, PA USA

INTRODUCTION

In the year 2000 the American Cancer Society estimates there will be 164,100 new cases of lung cancer in the United States and approximately 157,000 deaths, making it the leader in cancer-related deaths (1). More than 50% of cases will be unresectable at diagnosis, a substantial number of these could be potential candidates for systemic chemotherapy at some time during the course of their disease (2,3).

Almost all patients with advanced lung cancer have symptoms due to the disease at the time of presentation. Weight loss, associated with poor prognosis, fatigue, and cachexia are common. Local-regional signs and symptoms such as dyspnea, chest pain, cough, hemoptysis, Horner's syndrome and superior vena-cava syndrome arise primarily from involvement of the mediastinum and associated structures. In some patients the symptoms are due to metastatic involvement of the central nervous system, bones and/or solid organs such as the liver and adrenal glands. Occasionally humoral hypercalcemia or hypertrophic pulmonary osteoarthropathy, often with finger clubbing, may be seen at presentation (3).

The outcome of untreated patients with advanced non-small cell lung cancer (NSCLC) is predictable with a median survival time of 4 months, and a 1-year survival rate of 10% to 15% (4,5). Chemotherapy has demonstrated benefits for patients with prolongation of disease free survival and improvement in quality of life (6-10). The 1-year survival of patients with advanced and metastatic NSCLC has gradually increased in the last 2 decades to approximately 40-50% with the use of novel chemotherapeutic agents in selected patient groups (4,11).

In the 1970s and 1980s the role of chemotherapy was marginal at best. Chemotherapeutic intervention was found to be effective and consisted of cisplatin (6), mitomycin-C (12), ifosfamide (13), vindesine (14) and vinblastine (15). Other agents that established a place in the management of NSCLC include etoposide (16) and carboplatin (17). Combination chemotherapy was tested in phase II and III trials in metastatic NSCLC. It became evident that the cisplatin-containing regimens were associated with higher response rates, and phase III studies using these first-generation regimens reported median survival of 6 months and 1-year survival rates in the range of 15% to 20% (18-20).

Newer drugs such as vinorelbine, paclitaxel, docetaxel, gemcitabine and irinotecan in combination with a platinum agent have provided 1-year survival rates ranging from 33% to 50%, nearly double those observed with traditional first generation cisplatin-based regimens (9). In 1997 the American Society of Clinical Oncology adopted clinical practice guidelines for the treatment of unresectable NSCLC (21). Combination chemotherapy with cisplatin and a new agent such as vinorelbine, paclitaxel or gemcitabine was recommended as the standard of care for advanced NSCLC patients with Eastern Cooperative Oncology Group (ECOG) performance status 0 or 1 and possibly 2. However, the best platinum-based doublet regimen was not defined.

Performance status is the single most important prognostic factor in advanced NSCLC (Table 1). Patients with ECOG performance status of 0 and 1 are more likely to tolerate combination chemotherapy better and have a prolonged survival compared to those with ECOG performance status equal or greater than 2 (18). Thus, we need to exercise caution when we treat patients with poor performance status. The cisplatin-based regimens appear to be associated with significant adverse effects in these patients. (7,19,20,22). The use of "kinder-gentler" regimens may be of benefit but their role in survival of those patients with poor performance status requires further investigation.

Table 1.   Prognostic Factors for Survival in Patients with Advanced NSCLC

FAVORABLE
• ECOG performance status 0-1
• Single metastasis
• Weight loss less than 10 lb.
• Normal LDH
• Normal alkaline phosphatase
• Hemoglobin >11 g/dl

UNFAVORABLE
• ECOG performance status ≥ 2
• Disseminated disease
• Elevated WBC
• Elevated calcium level
• Age > 60 years old
• Weight loss > 10 lb.

CHEMOTHERAPY VERSUS BEST SUPPORTIVE CARE

The therapeutic nihilism surrounding the use of chemotherapy in advanced NSCLC prompted several prospective studies in the early 1980s that compared chemotherapy to best supportive care (BSC) (23). A meta-analysis of trials providing BSC only to patients with advanced NSCLC (patients fit enough for chemotherapy) showed a uniform median survival of 4 months and a 1-year survival rate of 10%, compared to median survival of approximately 7 months and 1-year survival rate of 25% following cisplatin-based combination therapy (5). This study reflected a 27% reduction in risk of death and an absolute increase in survival rate of 10% at one year in patients with advanced disease who received chemotherapy (24). These results were affirmed in a large randomized trial in Great Britain in which chemotherapy with mitomycin-C, ifosfamide and cisplatin (MIC) was compared to BSC in patients with advanced NSCLC. Patients treated with MIC chemotherapy survived an average of 6.7 months compared to just 4.8 months in the group managed with BSC (25). In addition to improvement in survival, there was an associated significant improvement in quality of life in patients receiving MIC chemotherapy (26). More recently, Roszkowski's trial (27) of docetaxel 100 mg/m^2 every 21 days versus BSC in untreated patients with advanced NSCLC also demonstrated significant benefit in terms of pain improvement (68% vs 10%). One- and two- year survival rates for single agent docetaxel versus BSC were found to favor docetaxel (25% vs 16% and 12% vs 0%, respectively). From here on it will be difficult to accrue patients to trials where BSC is the control arm. There is almost universal acceptance that chemotherapeutic intervention in advanced NSCLC is beneficial.

Cisplatin versus Carboplatin

Cisplatin is a water soluble, platinum-containing complex. Intracellularly, it reacts with DNA strands, forming both intrastrand and interstrand cross-links. DNA adducts formed by cisplatin inhibit replication and transcription and lead to breaks and miscoding. The effects of cisplatin are most pronounced during the S-phase (28).

Carboplatin's mechanism of action and spectrum of clinical activity are similar to those of cisplatin. However, the drug is not bound to proteins to a significant extent and is excreted primarily by the kidney. There is less nausea, neurotoxicity, ototoxicity and nephrotoxicity than with cisplatin. Moreover, there is no need for aggressive, resource-consuming hydration. The dose-limiting toxicity is myelosuppression, primarily evident as thrombocytopenia (29,30).

Carboplatin and cisplatin have not been compared directly as single agents for the treatment of NSCLC; therefore the selection of a platinum compound has traditionally been left to the treating physician. There is data that support the preferential use of carboplatin in NSCLC, however it has recently been challenged by results of a pan-European trial presented by Gatzemeier et al (31). This randomized study compared paclitaxel 200 mg/m^2 with either carboplatin AUC=6 mg/ml.min or cisplatin 80 mg/m^2 as first-line therapy for advanced NSCLC. Preliminary results show response rates of

25% and 28% and median survival times of 8.5 months and 9.8 months for the carboplatin and cisplatin arms respectively. One-year survival rates were 33% on the carboplatin arm and 38% on the cisplatin arm. The incidence of grade 3/4 neutropenia was similar in both arms. As expected, grade 3/4 thrombocytopenia was observed more commonly in patients receiving carboplatin (8%), compared to patients receiving cisplatin (2%). Renal and gastrointestinal toxicity occurred more often in the paclitaxel/cisplatin arm. A quality-of-life analysis showed similar scores in terms of physical, emotional, cognitive, or social functioning. Patients reported a possible advantage for the cisplatin-containing arm in controlling pain.

In a randomized study conducted by ECOG (18) single agent carboplatin was compared with single agent iproplatin and three regimens of cisplatin-containing combination chemotherapy, MVP (mitomycin-C, vincristine, cisplatin) VP (vincristine and cisplatin) and MVP alternating with CAMP (cyclophosphamide, doxorubicin, methotrexate and procarbazine). Single agent carboplatin had the longest median survival (32 weeks) and led to a significant improvement in median time to progression (29 weeks). Patients who received carboplatin experienced less life-threatening and lethal toxicity than those who received combination chemotherapy.

A prospective randomized trial (32) by the European Organization for Research and Treatment of Cancer (EORTC) compared carboplatin/etoposide against cisplatin/etoposide in patients with unresectable NSCLC. Even though response rates were higher in the cisplatin arm (27% vs 16%), both arms had similar efficacy (median survival 27 vs 30 weeks respectively) with less toxicity for the carboplatin containing regimen. Since carboplatin does not require the aggressive hydration necessitated by cisplatin therapy, patients receiving carboplatin/etoposide were treated as outpatients whereas those receiving cisplatin/etoposide required hospitalization. Carboplatin causes much less non-hematological toxicity than cisplatin, and in combination regimens yields equivalent survival in advanced NSCLC, despite a lower overall response rate (33). Ongoing randomized trials by ECOG and other cooperative groups will provide more data on the relative benefits of these two platinum compounds in NSCLC.

Conventional body surface area dosing of carboplatin results in unpredictable myelosuppression. As carboplatin is primarily excreted by the kidneys, Calvert et al (34) and Egorin et al (35) incorporated such parameters as baseline glomerular filtration rate (GFR) or creatinine clearance, body surface area and desired percent change in platelet count into carboplatin dosing formulas (Table 2). These were developed by correlating the pharmacokinetic parameters to pharmacodynamic effects. Later, Chatelut et al (36) reported a formula to predict carboplatin clearance using body weight, age, gender and serum creatinine without the need for measurement of GFR. Calvert's formula uses a target area under the curve (AUC) and GFR to calculate a carboplatin dose that would cause a predictable degree of thrombocytopenia. Because of the ease of calculation of the carboplatin dose with the Calvert's formula, it has been utilized widely both in clinical trials and in the community.

Table 2. Carboplatin, Dose Calculations Formulas

Calvert et al (34)	Dose (mg) = (target AUC mg/ml.min) x (GFR ml/min+25)
Egorin et al (35)	Dose (mg/m^2) = (0.91) x (creatinine clearance/BSA)x (desired % change in platelet count) + 86
Chatelut et al (36)	Dose (mg) = (0.134 x weight) + (218 x weight x(1-0.00457 x age) x (1-0.314 x sex) (creatinine) x (target AUC)

Weight in kg, age in years, and sex = 0 if male and sex = 1 if female, creatinine expressed in micromolar concentration.

CHEMOTHERAPY OPTIONS FOR ADVANCED NSCLC

Prior to 1990 the most popular regimens used were cisplatin plus an epipodophyllotoxin or a vinca alkaloid. Recently, platinum-based regimens that include newer agents with demonstrated activity against NSCLC, such as paclitaxel, vinorelbine, gemcitabine, irinotecan, and docetaxel have been extensively evaluated (Table 3) (9). In several randomized trials the combination of the newer agent with cisplatin proved superior to single agent cisplatin (Table 4). Based on these data, single-agent cisplatin has been discarded as the standard of comparison for all future trials.

Table 3. First-line therapy for patients with advanced NSCLC, commonly used doublets

Regimen	Drug 1	Drug 2	Schedule
Paclitaxel/carboplatin (56,58)	Paclitaxel 175-225 mg/m^2 (3 hr)	Carboplatin AUC=6 mg/ml. min over 3 min.	every 21 days
Paclitaxel/cisplatin (49)	Paclitaxel 175 mg/m^2 (3 hr)	Cisplatin 80 mg/m^2	every 21 days
Vinorelbine/cisplatin (99)	Vinorelbine 25 mg/m^2/ days 1, 8, 15	Cisplatin 100 mg/m^2/ day 1	every 28 days
Gemcitabine/cisplatin (109, 115)	Gemcitabine 1,000 mg/m^2 on days 1, 8, 15	Cisplatin 100 mg/m^2 on day 1 or 15	every 28 days
Gemcitabine/carboplatin (121)	Gemcitabine 1,000 mg/m^2 on days 1 and 8	Carboplatin AUC=5.5 mg/ml. min day 1	every 21 days
Docetaxel/cisplatin (169)	Docetaxel 75 mg/m^2 day 1	Cisplatin 75 mg/m^2 day 1	every 21 days
Irinotecan/cisplatin (128, 129)	Irinotecan 60 mg/m^2 on days 1, 8, 15	Cisplatin 80 mg/m^2 day 1	every 28 days

Table 4. Single agent Cisplatin versus Cisplatin-based Combination Regimens in Advanced NSCLC

Lead Author	Dose and Schedule (mg/m^2 q 21 d)	Response Rate (%)	Median Survival (months)	1-yr Survival (%)
Sandler (115)	C100 C100/G 1g/m²/w	11 30	7.6 8.7	30 36
Gatzemeier (167)	C100 C80/P175 3 hr.	17 26	8.6 8.1	35 30
Von Pawel (168)	C75 C75/T390	13.7 27.5	6.4 8.0	21 33
Wozniak (99)	C100 C100/V25	12 26	6.0 8.0	20 36

E – etoposide, G – gemcitabine, P – paclitaxel, T – teniposide, V - vinorelbine

Paclitaxel-Based Regimens

Paclitaxel is an antimicrotubule agent that shifts the equilibrium towards microtubule assembly from tubulin polymers by preventing depolymerization. This disrupts the normal dynamic reorganization of the microtubule network leading to arrest in mitosis. Paclitaxel initially identified as the active constituent in the bark of the western yew tree (Taxus Brevifolia) is now obtained via a semisynthetic process (37). Myelosuppresion is the principal toxicity. The onset of neutropenia is usually on days 8 to 10 with complete recovery by days 15 to 21. Severe thrombocytopenia or anemia is unusual (37). Cardiac arrhythmias are rare and usually asymptomatic. Arthralgias and myalgias are reported in over 50% of patients (38). Severe peripheral neuropathy due to axonal degeneration and demyelinization is uncommon when paclitaxel is given at doses below 200 mg/m². Peripheral neuropathy is due to axonal degeneration and demyelinization, it usually occurs after the third or fourth cycle. Grade 3 neuropathy occurs in less than 15% of patients receiving short infusions of paclitaxel. (39).

Phase II results from NSCLC studies conducted by MDACC (40) and ECOG (41) have shown that paclitaxel has single agent activity with response rates of 24% and 21% respectively and 1 year survival rates of approximately 40%. ECOG investigators concluded that paclitaxel was the most active new agent evaluated in the previous 10 years. In these trials paclitaxel was administered by 24-hour infusion at doses of 250 mg/m² (ECOG) and 200 mg/m² (MDACC), mainly due to concerns of hypersensitivity reactions, which have been substantially reduced with pre-medications such as dexamethasone, antihistamines and H2 blockers (42).

Gatzemeier et al (38) studied a 3-hour paclitaxel infusion at 225 mg/m² in patients with stage IIIB/IV NSCLC. Hematological toxicities were minor with only one patient developing grade 3 neutropenia. 56% of patients had grade 1 to 2 neuropathy, and 63% developed grade 1 to 2 myalgia/arthralgia syndrome. The overall response rate was

24 %. Median time to response was 8.7 weeks, median survival was 10 months. The 1-hour infusion schedule has also shown a similar degree of activity in metastatic NSCLC (43).

A sequence dependent drug interaction leading to increased myelotoxicity when cisplatin is administered before paclitaxel has been described (44,45). This is thought to be due to modulating effects of cisplatin on cytochrome P-450 enzymes resulting in decreased plasma clearance of paclitaxel. Thus, it is recommended that paclitaxel be administered before cisplatin. This combination has shown response rates ranging from 35% to 47% (9,46,47).

Several phase III trials compared paclitaxel/cisplatin with other standard regimens (Table 5). ECOG 5592, a randomized study, compared paclitaxel/cisplatin against etoposide/cisplatin in a 3-arm study (48). Paclitaxel 24-hour infusion was given at 2 different dose levels (135 mg/m^2 and 250 mg/m^2) with etoposide 100 mg/m^2 was given on days 1, 2 and to 3. Each regimen included cisplatin at a dose of 75 mg/m^2 and was repeated every 21 days. Response rates for the moderate-dose and high-dose arms were 25.3% and 27.7%, respectively; whereas the etoposide/cisplatin arm had a response rate of 12.4%. One-year survival was 37.4% for the moderate-dose paclitaxel arm and 40.3% for the high-dose arm; the cisplatin/etoposide regimen achieved 31.8% for one-year survival. When both paclitaxel arms are combined in comparison to the reference regimen, there is significant improvement using paclitaxel. Progression-free survival with paclitaxel is 4.8 mos. vs 2.8 mos with etoposide/cisplatin (p=0.0048), and overall survival is 9.8 vs 2.8 mos (p=0.0048). Thus, the moderate-dose paclitaxel/cisplatin regimen was chosen as the new ECOG standard in a subsequent randomized study (ECOG 1594), which has recently completed accrual (Table 6).

The EORTC conducted another randomized trial where paclitaxel/cisplatin was compared to teniposide/cisplatin (49). Progression-free survival was 5.4 and 4.9 months, and 1-year survival rates were 43% and 41%, respectively. Selected centers participated in a quality-of-life (QoL) assessment, which was performed by the EORTC QLQ-C30 and LC-13 administered at baseline and every 6 weeks thereafter. Patients receiving paclitaxel/cisplatin achieved a better score at week 6 for emotional, cognitive and social functioning, global health status, fatigue, and appetite loss (at 12 weeks).

Carboplatin, the less toxic analog of cisplatin, has an improved therapeutic index over cisplatin and can be administered with ease in the outpatient setting. Thus, it was combined with paclitaxel to assess the efficacy and toxicity of the combination in patients with NSCLC. In phase II studies response rates ranged from 30% up to 60%, median survival time from 10 to 12 months, and 1-year-survival from 30% to 50% (50,51). Initial studies used a carboplatin dose to achieve an area under the curve of 6 mg/ml.min with varying doses and schedules of paclitaxel.

Table 5. Paclitaxel-based doublets, Phase III trials in Patients with Advanced NSCLC

Lead Author	Schedule	Overall Response Rate (%)	Survival (months)	1-Year Survival (%)
Bonomi (182) ECOG 5592	E100/C75	12	7.7	31
	P135/C75	25	9.5	37
	P250/C75 + G-CSF	28	10	40
Belani (55)	E100/C75	14	9.9	NR
	P225/Cb AUC6	22	9.5	NR
Giaconne(49)	P175/C80	44	9.9	41
	T100/C80	28	9.7	43
Gatzemeier (167)	C100	17	8.6	8.1
	P175/C80	26	8.1	30
Kelly (56)	P225/Cb AUC6	28	8.0	36
	V25/C100	25	8.0	38

E – etoposide, P – paclitaxel, T – teniposide, V – vinorelbine, C – cisplatin, Cb - carboplatin
(mg/m^2) $mg/m^2)$ (mg/m^2) (mg/m^2) (mg/m^2) (mg/ml.min)

Table 6. ECOG 1594

<table>
<tr>
<td rowspan="4">R
A
N
D
O
M
I
Z
E</td>
<td>➡ Paclitaxel (135 mg/m²) 24-hr IV
Cisplatin (75 mg/m²)   (every 21 days)</td>
</tr>
<tr>
<td>➡ Docetaxel (75 mg/m²) 1-hr IV
Cisplatin (75 mg/m²)   (every 21 days)</td>
</tr>
<tr>
<td>➡ Gemcitabine (1,000 mg/m²) days 1, 8, 15
Cisplatin (100 mg/m2)   (every 21 days)</td>
</tr>
<tr>
<td>➡ Paclitaxel (225 mg/m²) 3-hour IV
Carboplatin dose AUC 6 mg/mL.min
(every 21 days)</td>
</tr>
</table>

Short infusion schedules of paclitaxel (3-hour and 1-hour) have similar degrees of efficacy as compared to 24-hour infusion regimens when combined with carboplatin. (9,51-53). The dose-limiting toxicity found with 24-hour infusions of paclitaxel/carboplatin is myelosuppression. Shorter infusions cause less myelosuppression, but neuropathy becomes dose-limiting. Severe thrombocytopenia has not been observed with this combination suggesting a myeloprotective effect of paclitaxel on carboplatin-associated thrombocytopenia (54).

Another phase III trial by Belani et al (55) compared paclitaxel/carboplatin to etoposide/cisplatin. Response rates were better in the paclitaxel/carboplatin group (23% versus 14%), but median survival rates were 9.5 months vs 9.9 months), respectively, and 1-year survival rates were not significantly different (32% vs 37%). A phase III trial by South West Oncology Group (SWOG) (56) compared paclitaxel/carboplatin with vinorelbine/cisplatin showing equal efficacy with response rates of 25% and 28%, respectively. Median and 1-year survival rates were similar as well. Quality of life was reported as improved or maintained by 60% of patients receiving either combination. However, paclitaxel/carboplatin had less toxicity, and twice as many patients were removed from the vinorelbine/cisplatin arm because of severe toxicity. Peripheral neuropathy was increased in the paclitaxel/carboplatin arm compared to vinorelbine/cisplatin (13% vs 3%). Because of the favorable toxicity profile and patient convenience, paclitaxel/carboplatin was selected as the SWOG reference chemotherapy regimen for future comparisons.

Several reasons have been proposed for the lack of survival benefit in these randomized studies. The most common one suggests that patients who failed in the control arms of the studies subsequently received second-line therapy with a taxane, which may have lead to better survival, obscuring any survival difference that might have emerged. Another hypothesis to explain the lack of survival advantage in some of the studies relates to the schedule of paclitaxel administration. ECOG 5592 employed a 24-hour infusion, whereas the remaining studies used shorter infusion times (57).

ECOG 1594 (ref below) was designed to compare the reference regimen of cisplatin/ paclitaxel to the three investigational regimens - cisplatin/gemcitabine, cisplatin/ docetaxel and carboplatin/paclitaxel (see table 6). Of the 1207 patients entered, 1163 were eligible. There was no significant difference in response rates and survival between the reference arm and each of the three investigational arms. The cisplatin/gemcitabine arm was associated with a higher median time to progression but this difference may have been confounded by the fact that this regimen was administered every 4 weeks while the other 3 were repeated at 3 week intervals causing a difference in the time points where patients were evaluated for response (6 vs 8 wks). Nausea and vomiting was significantly lower on the carboplatin/paclitaxel arm as expected. It appears that all four regimens are effective options for treatment of advanced NSCLC. It will be difficult to demonstrate substantial differences between various doublets as demonstrated by this study. This may be due to the effect of "salvage" or "second-line" therapies which also have an effect on survival and thus overall total therapy may be the same.

ECOG 1594: Results

	Cisplatin Paclitaxel	Cisplatin Gemcitabine	Cisplatin Docetaxel	Carboplatin Paclitaxel
Anemia Grade 3/4	13%	29%	16%	10%
Thrombocytopenia Grade 3/4	5%	48%	3%	10%
Overall Response Rate	21%	20%	17%	15%
Median Time to Progression	3.5 mos	4.5 mos	3.6 mos	3.3 mos
1 Year Survival	31%	36%	31%	35%
Median Survival Time	7.8 mos	8.1 mos	7.4	8.2 mos

Schiller JH, Harrington D, Sandler A et al. A randomized Phase III trial of four chemotherapy regimens in advanced non-small cell lung cancer (NSCLC). Proc Am Soc Clin Oncol 19:1a (Abstract #2), 2000

To test the dose-response effect of paclitaxel, Kosmidis (58) conducted another phase III study comparing paclitaxel, 3-hour infusion at two doses - 175 mg/m^2 and 225 mg/m^2 - plus carboplatin AUC=6 mg/ml.min in patients with advanced NSCLC. Both groups received 94% of their planned doses. There was a trend for a higher response rate in favor of the higher dose arm (31.8% vs 25.6%), although not statistically significant. Time to disease progression was also in favor of the higher dose paclitaxel arm (6.4 months vs 4.3 months). There was a trend for higher survival rate in this group of patients as well (median survival 11.4 months vs 9.5 months; 1-year survival 44% vs 37 %). Neurotoxicity was more prominent in patients receiving high dose paclitaxel (22% vs 10 %), but neuropathy symptoms were reversible in almost all patients who lived more than 6 months. These results emphasize the concept that higher doses of paclitaxel in combination with carboplatin are well tolerated. There is a trend for higher response rates and survival in favor of higher doses of paclitaxel combined with carboplatin for the treatment of advanced NSCLC.

Taxane therapy is phase-specific, and prolonged or enhanced exposure to paclitaxel may improve cytotoxic activity (59). Administering paclitaxel on a weekly regimen has been studied in several tumor types, including breast (60), prostate (61), ovarian (62), and NSCLC (63), and has shown promising results.

Reducing the interval between doses of paclitaxel from 3 weeks to 1 week increases the dose intensity of treatment. This may limit the emergence of malignant cell populations resistant to chemotherapy and may inhibit tumor regrowth between cycles. In addition to improving cytotoxic activity, preliminary data suggest that more frequent exposure to paclitaxel may also enhance its apoptotic antiangiogenic effects (64).

Akerley et al, for the Cancer and Leukemia Group B (CALGB), studied weekly paclitaxel 150 mg/m^2 over 3 hours given for 6 weeks in an 8-week cycle in 39 patients. The response rate was 40%, median survival 10.5 months and 1-year survival 42%. Grade 3/4 neutropenia was acceptable at 8%. Neuropathy was common, with 31% of patients having grade 2 and 30% having grade 3 neurotoxicity. However, the investigators found that if the dose was decreased by 50%, there was no progression of neuropathy and in some patients it actually regressed (65).

Chang et al studied weekly paclitaxel in advanced NSCLC patients with fair performance status (50% of patients had ECOG PS 2). The dose was 80 mg/m^2 on days 1, 8 and 15 every 28 days. The response rate was 32%, median survival 8 months and the 1-year survival rate was 35%. This regimen was well tolerated, even among patients with poor performance status and/or advanced age (66).

The tolerability and efficacy of this delivery strategy creates an alternative treatment option that may be well suited for impaired patients. Responses have been seen in heavily pretreated patients and in those who have failed platinum or anthracycline therapy. Activity has also been documented in patients who did not respond to standard treatment schedules of paclitaxel (67). There is a large ongoing randomized trial testing the efficacy of various weekly schedules of paclitaxel in combination with carboplatin. A recent survey of U.S. medical oncologists showed paclitaxel to be the preferred chemotherapy agent for use in combination with platinum agents in advanced NSCLC (68).

Docetaxel-based therapy

Docetaxel is a compound partially synthesized from 10-deacetylbaccatin III, which is isolated from the needles of the European yew tree (Taxus Baccata). A semi-synthetic analog of paclitaxel, docetaxel is a promoter of microtubule polymerization leading to cell cycle arrest at G2/M, apoptosis and cytotoxicity. Docetaxel has significant activity in breast, non-small-cell lung, ovarian and head and neck cancers (69).

In four phase II trials involving 160 previously untreated patients with advanced NSCLC single agent docetaxel was administered as 100 mg/m^2 1-hour intravenous infusion every 21 days. Of the 141 patients evaluable for response, 31% had an objective response (70-73). Median duration of response, median time to progression, and median survival were 6 months, 3 months and 9.2 months respectively. The 1-year survival was 39% (74). In a subset of 88 platinum-refractory patients with advanced NSCLC, 17% achieved an objective response rate with docetaxel monotherapy, median survival was 9 months (75).

The docetaxel dose used in most phase II trials to date is 100 mg/m^2 every 21 days but similar response rates may be seen with doses of 60 or 75 mg/m^2 (76). The dose limiting toxicity of this drug is neutropenia (9,77). Abnormal liver function increases the risk of docetaxel myelosuppression (78). Other toxicities include nail changes, skin rash, acral erythema, fatigue, peripheral edema and effusions (79,80). Fluid retention with administration of docetaxel is dose related (81). In a study at Memorial Sloan Kettering Cancer center (MSKCC) (82), six of eight patients who received a cumulative dose of >500 mg/m^2 developed symptomatic pleural effusions. The introduction of prophylactic steroids has significantly reduced the incidence and severity of fluid retention possibly associated with docetaxel administration (83-85).

Phase II studies in advanced NSCLC using docetaxel in combination with cisplatin (Table 7) showed response rates ranging from 32% to 45% with median overall survival duration of 8 to 13 months (86). In all studies, myelosuppression was the most frequent toxicity; the incidence of febrile neutropenia fluctuated between 9% and 26%, and peripheral neuropathy with this regimen was predominantly sensory and dose-dependent (87,88).

This combination is an active regimen for patients with advanced NSCLC, but hematological toxicity remains high despite the prophylactic use of G-CSF (89).

Table 7. Docetaxel plus Platinum Studies in Advanced NSCLC

Lead Author	# of Patients	Dose and Schedule (q21 days)	Overall Response Rate (%)	Median Survival (mo)	1-Year survival (%)
Belani (170)	47	D75/C75	32	11.5	NR
Millward (171)	47	D75/C75	39	10	NR
Le Chevalier (172)	51	D75/C100	33	8	NR
Androulakis (173)*	53	D100/C80	45	13	48
Millward (93)	45	D75/Cb AUC 6	37	NR	NR
Arcenas (92)	15	D65/Cb AUC 6	30	NR	NR
Belani (90)	33	D80/Cb AUC 6	48	NR	52

G-CSF support given upfront C - cisplatin, Cb - carboplatin, D - docetaxel
mg/m^2 AUC=mg/ml.min mg/m^2

As noted earlier, carboplatin has activity similar to cisplatin, but with a superior toxicity profile. The carboplatin/docetaxel combination was developed because of the prospect of lower toxicity and therefore a higher therapeutic index. A phase I trial (90) using carboplatin AUC=6 mg/ml.min with escalating doses of docetaxel as a 1 hour infusion every three weeks found that the maximum tolerated dose (MTD) was 90 mg/m^2 without growth factor support, and 100 mg/m^2 with growth factor support. A multicenter phase II trial of docetaxel 80 mg/m^2 and carboplatin AUC=6 mg/ml.min every 21 days was instituted in patients with advanced NSCLC. An objective response rate was seen in 48%. (91) Other phase II trials have shown response rates of 30% (92) and 37%. (93) A large randomized trial is ongoing to compare the efficacy of each of two docetaxel/platinum regimens (docetaxel/cisplatin and docetaxel/carboplatin) with the reference combination of vinorelbine/cisplatin in patients with advanced and metastatic NSCLC (86,89).

The possibility of reducing myelosuppression with weekly administration of docetaxel has become a focus of clinical investigation, based on positive recent experiences with weekly paclitaxel (79,94). A phase I study (95) showed evidence that the toxicity profile of docetaxel can be markedly changed when administered on a weekly schedule. At doses of up to 40 mg/m^2/wk myelosuppression is mild, peripheral neuropathy and other non-hematological toxicities are less common as well. Phase II studies on this regimen are ongoing. Preliminary results of a study of weekly docetaxel 36 mg/m^2 weekly for 6 weeks with 2 weeks rest period in medically unfit elderly patients with advanced NSCLC are encouraging. Among the first 15 patients, three partial responses (21%) have been observed and six patients (43%) have stable disease (94). Though the concept of docetaxel weekly administration is interesting, further investigation is needed to evaluate its efficacy in advanced NSCLC.

Vinorelbine-based therapy

This synthetic analogue of vinblastine is a vinca alkaloid whose cytotoxicity results from the disruption of microtubule assembly and resultant metaphase arrest (96). It has greater specificity for the mitotic spindle microtubule than for the axonal microtubule and this accounts for its decreased neurotoxicity compared with vinblastine (97). During the 1980s, single agent cisplatin became a common therapy for advanced NSCLC, particularly when randomized trials did not show any advantages for cisplatin/mitomycin-C or high-dose cisplatin (98).

When vinorelbine was established as an active agent in advanced NSCLC, SWOG instituted a randomized trial comparing the standard single agent cisplatin with the combination vinorelbine/cisplatin (99). The response rate was higher with the combination (26% vs 12%), along with a significantly longer median survival (8 months vs 6 months) and 1-year survival rate (36% vs 20%). Thus, the vinorelbine/cisplatin combination became SWOG's standard therapy for its next phase III trial.

In 1999 Kelly et al (56) compared the standard vinorelbine/cisplatin to paclitaxel/carboplatin (Table 8). Both treatment regimens demonstrated equal efficacy, with response rates of 28% and 25%, respectively, median survival (both arms 8 months) and one-year survival (36 % and 38%) were also similar in both arms of the study. However, nausea, vomiting, hematological toxicity and grade 4 neutropenia were significantly higher in the vinorelbine/cisplatin arm causing a higher drop out rate (28% vs 14%), while the rate of neuropathy was four times higher in the paclitaxel/carboplatin arm of the trial. Despite cost issues, because of its lower toxicity profile and more convenient dosing schedule, the paclitaxel/carboplatin combination was selected as the control regimen for future phase III trials.

Gemcitabine-based therapy

Gemcitabine is an analog of the pyrimidine antimetabolite cytosine arabinoside. It has been proven effective as a single agent in the first-line treatment of advanced NSCLC. Response rates of 20% or more with a median survival of 40 weeks and 1-year survival rates of 40% have been reported (100,101). Toxicity has been manageable (102), and, in many cases, the patient's performance status has improved by its use (103).

Two randomized studies (104,105) showed that single agent gemcitabine is just as effective as the traditionally recommended combination of etoposide and cisplatin. There were no statistical differences in median survival or median time to disease progression. Hematological and non-hematological toxicity were lower in the gemcitabine arm, and 5-HT$_3$ antagonists were only seldom required for nausea/vomiting. Alopecia was minimal. Anemia and thrombocytopenia were mild and febrile neutropenia occurred exclusively in the etoposide/cisplatin arm. Moreover, a separate cost comparison study between gemcitabine versus cisplatin/etoposide demonstrated a cost-reduction of $264 per cycle in favor of gemcitabine (106).

Table 8. Vinorelbine in Patients with Advanced NSCLC

Author	Schedule	Overall Response Rate (%)	Median Survival (months)	1-Year Survival (%)
Le Chevalier (179)	C/Vnd	14	7.2	35
	C/V	30	9.3	40
	V	14	7.2	35
DePierre (180)	C/V	43	7.7	26
	V	16	7.4	22
Crawford (181)	5-FU/Lv	3	5.1	16
	V	12	7.0	25
Wozniak (99)	C/V	26	8.0	36
	C	12	6.0	20
ELVIS (161)	BSC	-	4.9	14
	V	20	6.5	32
Kelly (56)	P/Cb	28	8.0	36
	C/V	25	8.0	38

P – paclitaxel, V – vinorelbine, Vnd – vindesine, C – cisplatin, Cb – carboplatin, 5-FU – 5-fluorouracil, Lv – leucovorin,

Gemcitabine and cisplatin have the potential for synergistic interaction. This synergism is dependent on exposure time to the drugs, and is schedule-dependent. (107) Cisplatin exerts its cytotoxic action by binding to DNA and producing DNA-DNA cross-links and DNA-protein cross-links. Resistance to cisplatin occurs when the damaged DNA undergoes excision repair. Gemcitabine appears to inhibit this repair process. (107)

Most phase II studies have been aimed at giving both agents at full dose (gemcitabine 1000 mg/m^2; cisplatin 80 mg/m^2) administering gemcitabine on days 1,8 and 15 within a 28-day cycle; cisplatin was given in different schedules. Weekly cisplatin was intended to increase the possibility of synergism between the two agents (108). Cisplatin given on day 2 (17) allowed for the possibility of increased renal toxicity with the simultaneous administration of both drugs. Cisplatin given on day 15 schedule (109,110) was based on the cytokinetic theory that the initial fractionated administration of a phase-specific agent be followed by a cycle-specific agent. There was no evidence of increased renal toxicity when the drugs were administered on the same day (111). The regimen in which cisplatin is given on day 15 followed by a 2 week rest period until the beginning of the next 28 day cycle is associated with the best dose intensity and the longest median duration of exposure to gemcitabine. Thrombocytopenia was dose limiting for those studies in which the administration of cisplatin was not followed by a rest period of at least 14 days (111).

Ricci (112) conducted a phase II study looking at the toxicity profile of the gemcitabine/cisplatin combination utilizing different sequence schedules (Table 9).
Based on these data, cisplatin on day 15 was associated with a significant reduction in

the degree of thrombocytopenia. Phase II trials of gemcitabine and cisplatin in patients with inoperable stage III and stage IV NSCLC have shown response rates ranging from 28% to 54% (113).

Three randomized phase III trials (Table 10) compared gemcitabine/cisplatin to cisplatin alone, to etoposide/cisplatin and to mitomycin-C/ifosfamide/cisplatin (MIC) respectively. (114-116) Response rates were significantly higher for the gemcitabine/cisplatin doublet. These results provide evidence that the gemcitabine/cisplatin combination has high response rates and acceptable toxicity in patients with advanced or metastatic NSCLC, as well as offers considerable advantages over first generation cisplatin-based regimens or cisplatin alone (117).

Table 9. Gemcitabine plus Cisplatin: Day 2 versus Day 15 Schedules

Lead Author	Study Arm	Dose and Schedule	Overall Response Rate (%)	Anemia	Thrombocytopenia
Ricci (112)	ARM A N=45	G 1 g/m^2 d1, 8 and 15 C 80 mg/m^2 d 2 q28 d	35%	8.4%	15.6%
	ARM B N=43	G 1 g/m^2 d1, 8 and 15 C 80 mg/m^2 d 15 q28 d	54%	0%	1.5%

G – gemcitabine; C - cisplatin

Thrombocytopenia continues to be observed with gemcitabine based combinations, is dose-limiting (118) and usually occurs after 2 weeks of treatment (119).

Table 10. Gemcitabine with Cisplatin, Phase III Trials in Patients with Advanced NSCLC

Lead Author	Schedule	Overall Response Rate (%)	Median Survival (%)	1-Year Survival (mos.)
SLCG (114)	G/C	40	8.7	NR
	E/C	22	7.2	NR
HOG (115)	G/C	30	8.9	9.1
	C	11	7.6	7.6
ILCP (183)	G/C	38	8.6	NR
	MIC	26	9.6	NR

MIC – mitomicyn-C/ifosfamide/cisplatin, G – gemcitabine, E – etoposide, C – cisplatin, HOG – Hoosier Oncology group, SLCG – Spanish Lung Cancer Group, ILCP – Italian Lung Cancer Project

Based on the advantages of carboplatin over cisplatin, as mentioned earlier, investigators conducted phase I and II trials using gemcitabine combined with carboplatin. Carmichael (120) used gemcitabine 1000 mg/m² on days 1,8 and 15. The MTD of carboplatin was AUC 5.5 mg/ml.min, and the sequence iteration did not show any difference in toxicity. Phase II studies (33) of gemcitabine/carboplatin combination have shown response rates of approximately 50% with good tolerance. More recently Edelman et al described a novel 21-day schedule of carboplatin AUC=5.5 mg/ml.min on day 1 and gemcitabine 1,000 mg/m² on days 1 and 8. This regimen was well tolerated and not associated with the severe thrombocytopenia reported with the 28-day regimen (121). Moreover, the every-three-week regimen maintains a response rate similar to the monthly regimen (122). The combination of gemcitabine and carboplatin is being compared with paclitaxel/carboplatin and paclitaxel/gemcitabine in a recently initiated multicenter randomized trial.

Irinotecan-based therapy

Irinotecan, a semisynthetic derivative of the plant alkaloid camptothecin, is bioactivated by carboxylesterases to the topoisomerase I inhibitor SN-38.(123) Irinotecan weekly (100 mg/m² on days 1,8 and 15 every 28 days) was found to be active against NSCLC (124) with single-agent activity similar to that reported for other newer agents.

The combination of irinotecan and cisplatin has shown marked synergism (125), with response rates of up to 75% (126). Dose limiting toxicities are neutropenia and severe diarrhea. The latter is not dose-limiting when cisplatin is given in divided doses. Oral alkalinization and bowel habit regulation seem to decrease the incidence of late diarrhea, vomiting and leukopenia without a decrease in effectiveness (127). This is thought to be mediated by a decrease in reabsorption of the active metabolites of irinotecan in the intestinal mucosa and by avoiding stasis of stool containing these metabolites.

Phase III studies (Table 11) indicate that irinotecan/cisplatin is a more effective regimen than vindesine/cisplatin. Kunitoh et al (128) reported a randomized study comparing these two regimens showing response rates of 29% in the irinotecan arm and 22% in the vindesine arm. Masuda et al (129) reported another randomized trial with response rates of 43% versus 31% favoring the irinotecan-containing arm. Overall, there was little difference in the toxicity profile. Grade 3/4 diarrhea was more common with irinotecan whereas grade 3/4 neutropenia was higher with vindesine. Quality of life data are not yet available. The combination of irinotecan/cisplatin was superior to irinotecan alone with response rates of 43% for the combination versus 21% for irinotecan alone (129). The irinotecan/cisplatin regimen has become the new reference regimen for studies by the Japanese cooperative groups.

Non-Platinum Combinations

Non-platinum combinations may prove to be reasonable alternatives for NSCLC patients who cannot tolerate cisplatin, and for relapsed patients and patients with compromised performance status. Docetaxel and vinorelbine are active agents in NSCLC. Although they have different effects on tubulins, both phosphorylate and inactivate the protooncogene bcl-2, thus promoting apoptosis through a common mechanism. (130) The combination has been tested in different schedules, every 21 days (131) and every 28 days. (119,132) In two phase II studies the combination of docetaxel 60-100 mg/m^2 and vinorelbine 25 mg/m^2 every 21 days usually required G-CSF support. The main toxicities were neutropenia, dyspnea/infiltrates, alopecia, onycholysis and lacrimation (130,133).

The combination of gemcitabine and docetaxel has been shown to be feasible (134) and active (135), without prohibitive toxicity at doses of 1000 mg/m^2 and 30-40 mg/m^2, respectively, administered on day 1, 8 and 15. The overall incidence of neutropenia in a phase I trial (136) was 27%, and there were no cases of febrile neutropenia. In this study patients received primary prophylaxis with G-CSF.

Gemcitabine and docetaxel has been compared to docetaxel and cisplatin in a randomized phase II trial in chemo-naive patients with advanced NSCLC(137). The probability of response to docetaxel/cisplatin was higher in patients with non-adenocarcinoma, while the opposite was observed in patients with adenocarcinoma. Response rates were 34% for docetaxel/gemcitabine and 32% for docetaxel/cisplatin. Mean survival times were 9 and 10 months, respectively. Toxicities were also comparable, except for diarrhea, which was more common in the cisplatin-treated group. Despite the use of G-CSF primary prophylaxis there was a higher incidence of febrile neutropenia with the docetaxel/gemcitabine arm. These new combinations of docetaxel with non-platinum agents are promising, however new data from phase III studies are needed. It is too early to discard the continued role of platinum compounds in advanced NSCLC.

The combination of gemcitabine with a taxane is attractive because of non-overlapping toxicity profiles, their proven activity as single agents in NSCLC and the convenience of outpatient administration. Gemcitabine has been used with paclitaxel in different schedules in both first and second line therapy with success. Martin et al (138) tested the safety and response rate of biweekly gemcitabine with paclitaxel in previously untreated patients with advanced NSCLC. In 88 evaluable patients the response rate was 35%. The incidence of grade 3/4 neutropenia, thrombocytopenia and arthralgia/myalgia was 2%, 1% and 8% respectively. Grade 2/3 neutropenia occurred in 15% of patients. Giaccone et al (139) used this combination in chemotherapy-naïve patients. Out of 23 patients evaluable for response, 7 had a partial response (30%) with minimal toxicity.

Weekly gemcitabine combined with vinorelbine has shown response rates as high as 70% in phase II studies, especially when vinorelbine was given first, followed by gemcitabine. (140) Initial studies with this combination aimed at giving full doses of gemcitabine and vinorelbine, however hematological toxicity proved to be substantial and required dose reduction of both drugs. Pirker et al (141) conducted a phase II study in 70 previously untreated patients with advanced NSCLC. Patients received vinorelbine 25 mg/m^2 followed by gemcitabine 1200 mg/m^2 on days 1,8 and 15 every 28 days up to a total of 8 cycles. Response rate was 19%. Kaplan-Meier analysis revealed a median survival of 9 months. Grade 3/4 neutropenia and thrombocytopenia, respectively, occurred in 55% and 15% of patients. respectively. Other non-hematological toxicities include thrombophlebitis and elevated liver enzymes.

Table 11. Phase III trials of Irinotecan plus Cisplatin in advanced NSCLC

Lead Author	Dose and Schedule	Response Rate (%)	Median Survival (wks)	1-Year Survival (%)	Diarrhea Grade > 3 (%)	Leukopenia Grade > 3 (%)
Kunitoh (128)	**ARM A** C 80 mg/m² d 1 CPT-11 60 mg/m² d 1, 8, 15 q28d	29	45	NR	13	39
	Arm B C 80 mg/m² d 1 VDS 3 mg/m² d 1, 8, 15 q28d	22	49	NR	1	58
Masuda (129)	**Arm A** C 80 mg/m² d 1 CPT-11 60 mg/m² d 1, 8, 15 q28d	43	52	49	12.6	36
	Arm B C 80 mg/m2 d 1 VDS 3 mg/m² d 1, 8, 15 q28d	31	47	40	4	53
	Arm C CPT-11 100 mg/m² d 1, 8, 15 q28d	21	47	43.5	15	7.9

VDS – Vindesine, C – Cisplatin, CPT11 – irinotecan

Barr et al (142) tested gemcitabine/vinorelbine as salvage chemotherapy for taxane-resistant NSCLC. The treatment regimen consisted of vinorelbine 30 mg/m² on days 1 and 15 alternated with 15 mg/m² on day 8 along with gemcitabine 750 mg/m² on days 1,8 and 15, every 28 days. The response rate in these taxane-resistant patients was 20%. The combination was well tolerated with manageable hematological toxicity. Toxicity in this combination is mainly hematological; up to 40% of patients complained of flu-like syndrome (140).

Other agents that have been combined with gemcitabine, include vincristine (143), high dose epirubicin (144), topotecan and irinotecan (145). In addition, irinotecan is being studied in combination with other new agents. In particular, its combination with oral uracil/tegafur (UFT) looks promising in lung cancer (146).

RECURRENT DISEASE

With 1-year survival rates of approximately 40-50% with current chemotherapy regimens, second-line treatment has become an important issue for patients whose disease progresses after receiving platinum combinations. To date, there is no established second-line therapy.

First-line chemotherapy failure is predictive of the development of resistant clones. (74) The question of non-cross resistance between novel agents and cisplatin has not been fully answered. However, there is a possibility of response in platinum refractory and resistant patients using taxanes, since these two groups of agents have different mechanisms of action. (74) In previously treated patients, response rates to single agent vindesine, etoposide, epirubucin and cisplatin have not exceeded 10%. With the advent of novel agents the scenario of second-line therapy must be reconsidered.

Studies with paclitaxel, (43,147,148,149) vinorelbine (150), irinotecan (151) and gemcitabine (152) do not appear to have consistent response rates in the second-line setting (Table 12). One study showed that patients receiving taxanes after cisplatin/etoposide had a significantly improved survival when compared with patients who received no further chemotherapy, highlighting the need for sequential combination regimens with non-cross resistance in advanced NSCLC. (55) In a study by Hainsworth et al (43), 30 previously treated patients received either 200 mg/m^2 or 135 mg/m^2 of paclitaxel by 1-hour infusion. The response rate was 38% in the subset of previously treated NSCLC patients who received paclitaxel at the dose of 200 mg/m^2. None of the patients treated at the lower dose experienced objective response.

Of the second-generation agents with activity against previously treated NSCLC, docetaxel appears promising with response rates of approximately 20%. (75,153) Early studies with this agent showed some activity against platinum-resistant or refractory NSCLC. These data led to two large phase III randomized trials (Table 13): docetaxel at 100 mg/m^2 compared to BSC, and docetaxel at two different doses - 100 mg/m^2 or 75 mg/m^2 – compared with either vinorelbine or ifosfamide in patients previously treated with platinum based therapy. (154,155) Survival was the primary end point for both studies. In the docetaxel versus BSC trial (155), the treatment group had a longer median survival and statistically better quality of life assessments (pain, fatigue and use of cancer-related medications) compared to BSC patients. While it should be noted that a third of patients in the second study had received paclitaxel in the first-line setting, the trial confirmed the statistical advantage of docetaxel in the second line setting. When docetaxel 100 mg/m^2 was compared to 75 mg/m^2, the survival for the lower dose was

Table 12. Single Agents in Second-line Therapy for Advanced NSCLC

Lead Author	Dose and Schedule	# of Patients	Overall Response Rate (%)	Median Survival (wks)
Murphy (148)	P 175mg/m^2 24 hr q21d	40	3	18
Ruckdeschel (147)	P 200-225 mg/m^2 24 hr q21d	14	17	
Socinski (149)	P 140 mg/m^2 96 hr q21d	11	0	NR
Hainsworth (43)	P 200 mg/m^2 1 hr q21d	26	23	NR
Fossella (75)	D 100 mg/m^2 q2d	42	21	11
Burris (70)	D 100 mg/m^2 q21d	35	17	NR
Gandara (174)	D 100 mg/m^2 q21d	80	16	7
Rinaldi (150)	V 20 mg/m^2/wk	18	0	NR
Nakai (151)	CPT-11 200 mg/m^2 q21-28d	22	14	NR
Negoro (175)	CPT-11 100 mg/m^2/wk	26	0	NS
Crino (152)	G 1000 mg/m^2/wk q 28d	83	19	NR
Rosvold (176)	G 1000 mg/m^2/wk	43	17	NR
Gridelli (177)	G 1000 mg/m^2 q 28d	30	20	22
Postmus (156)	MTA 500 mg/m^2 q21d	22 PT 22 NP	8 35	NR NR

P - paclitaxel, D – docetaxel, V – vinorelbine, CPT-11 – irinotecan, G – gemcitabine, PT - failed prior platinum containing regimen, NP - failed prior non-platinum

notably superior. This probably stems from higher rates of toxicity, mainly neutropenia, in patients receiving 100 mg/m^2 as second-line therapy. From these two trials we can conclude that docetaxel at 75 mg/m^2 clearly outweighs the risks, is superior to BSC and should be an option for selected patients who need second-line therapy. With recent approval by the Food and Drug Administration for docetaxel in this setting it will be the standard reference for second-line chemotherapy trials. The role of docetaxel in patients who failed front-line therapy with paclitaxel needs to be further confirmed and vice-versa. In addition, multitargeted antifolate (MTA) has recently shown activity in the second-line setting as a single agent. Its impact seems to be more significant in patients who failed non-platinum containing regimens. (156)

Table 13. Second-line Chemotherapy in Advanced NSCLC, Phase III trials

Lead Author	Dose and Schedule	# of Patients	Response Rate (%)	Median Survival (mos.)	1-Year Survival (%)
Fosella (154)	**Arm A** D 100 mg/m^2 q 21 d	121	12	5.5	21
	Arm B D 75 mg/m^2 q 21 d	121	6	5.7	32
	Arm C V or I	119	1	5.6	19
Shepherd (155)	**Arm A** D 100 mg/m^2 q 21 d	49	6.1	5.9	19
	Arm B D 75 mg/m^2 q 21 d	54	5.5	9	40
	Arm C BSC	100	0	4.7	

D – docetaxel, V – vinorelbine, I – ifosfamide, BSC – best supportive care

Recently, resistance to taxane-based therapy was linked to β-tubulin gene mutations. In a study by Martin et al (138), tumors of 16 out of 49 patients checked for the abnormality were found to have point mutations within exon four of β-tubulin. All of the patients with tubulin mutations failed to respond to paclitaxel and had rapidly progressive disease. On the other hand, 13 of 33 patients with wild type β-tubulin had an objective response to paclitaxel. (138,157) Another study evaluated the effects of β-tubulin mutations in a group of patients receiving docetaxel and vinorelbine in three different dosing schedules. Four of 13 patients with mutations in exon four of β-tubulin developed progressive disease, presumably due to docetaxel-resistance (158). Thus pharmacogenomics may allow us to individualize therapies and improve the overall outcome.

NSCLC IN POOR PERFORMANCE STATUS AND ELDERLY PATIENTS

Advanced age has been considered an unfavorable prognostic factor in patients with NSCLC. Physicians tend to associate advanced age with declining performance status and therefore inability to tolerate the toxicities of aggressive chemotherapy, particularly cisplatin-based therapy. However, recent studies in this population demonstrate that elderly patients with good performance status do as well as their younger counterparts (Table 14). In fact, some studies even showed a positive association between older age and objective response rates (159,160), which is thought to be due to earlier disease stage at diagnosis in this group of patients. (160) Quality of life scores, cancer related symptoms and performance status were improved with chemotherapy in patients older than 70 years. (159,161,162) Chemotherapy also offers survival advantage over BSC for elderly patients (161), and demonstrates similar median and 1-year survival rates as younger counterparts with similar performance status. (163) Several studies noted that the most significant toxicities occurred in patients with performance status ECOG 2 or higher. (19) Toxicity was not exacerbated in elderly patients simply because of age. (164) As discussed earlier, weekly paclitaxel at 80 mg/m^2 on days 1,8 and 15 every 28 days provided a potential for response in both elderly and poor performance status NSCLC patients. (66) This gentler chemotherapy has an improved therapeutic index with decreased toxicity and a modest degree of efficacy (165).

ECOG 1594 is a phase III randomized study comparing the activity and toxicity of four platinum-based doublets in patients with advanced NSCLC (Table 6). Accrual of ECOG performance status 2 (PS 2) patients was halted after an increased number of adverse effects in this patient group were noted. Only 64 PS 2 patients had been randomized at the time accrual was stopped. Analysis of the data showed an overall response rate of 13%. The toxicity profile for the paclitaxel/carboplatin combination was the most favorable among the regimens studied (Table 15). Rosvold and Langer reported that while advanced age is associated with lower response rates to paclitaxel/carboplatin, toxicity and survival are comparable for equally fit older and younger patients (163). This reiterates again the fact that performance status, irrespective of age, is the most important prognostic factor in deciding which patients to treat aggressively and in predicting response and survival for patients receiving chemotherapy (166).

Table 14. Response to Treatment for Advanced NSCLC in Elderly Patients

Lead Author	Age	Schedule	Overall Response Rate (%)	Median Survival (mos.)	1-Year Survival (%)	Comment
ELVIS (161)	>70	BSC	-	4.9	14	Improved QOL
		V	-	6.5	36	
Shepherd (101)	< 65	G	16	8.1	27	
	> 65	G	24	9.1	36	
Frasci (159)	>70	Oral E/Cb	24	11	NR	Improved QOL 41% Improved PS 33%
Gridelli (162)	>70	V	23	8.4	36	Improved PS 26% Improved symptoms 40%
Martin (ASCO 99)	-	V/C	54	7.2	37	
Nguyen (164)	< 70	G/C	29	9.4	NR	Similar toxicity
	> 70	G/C	15	7.7	NR	
Rosvold (163)	> 70	P/Cb	32	9.8	44	Increase fatigue in > 70 Similar toxicity otherwise
	All Patients	P/Cb	50	12.1	50	
Frasci (178)	> 70	G/V	22	6.5	NR	Increased toxicity with combination
		V	15	4.4	NR	

BSC – best supportive care, V – vinorelbine, G – gemcitabine, E – etoposide, Cb – carboplatin, C – cisplatin, P - paclitaxel

Table 15.   ECOG 1594 - Outcome of PS 2 NSCLC Patients

Regimen	# of Patients	Response Rate (%)	Median Survival (mos)	Toxicities Grade 3/4/5 (%)
P/C	19	16	7.4	22/66/0
G/C	12	33	7.9	7/62/15
D/C	18	4	2.1	11/56/17
P/Cb	15	13	4.6	27/28/0
Overall	64	17	4.1	

P/C - paclitaxel and cisplatin, G/C – gemcitabine and cisplatin, D/C – docetaxel and cisplatin, P/Cb – paclitaxel and carboplatin

CONCLUSION (Table 16)

There is no clear winner among the newer first-line doublet regimens used for the treatment of advanced or metastatic NSCLC. Elderly patients ($\geq$ 70 years) with a good performance status tolerate chemotherapy comparable to younger patients. We have exploited the role of chemotherapy to the maximum possible extent and the addition of a third chemotherapeutic agent to the doublet regimens will only add to the toxicity rather than extend the survival benefit. On the other hand, we are encouraged to see the activity of selective and biologic agents such as signal transduction inhibitors, epidermal growth factor receptor blockers, farnesyltransferase inhibitors and antisense molecules. These novel agents have the potential of taking the management of NSCLC to the next level, especially when used in combination with chemotherapy. In the new millennium we are not only talking about the impact on survival with first-line chemotherapy in advanced NSCLC, but it is definite that there is a clear benefit of second-line chemotherapy in recurrent NSCLC, both on survival as well as on quality of life. We are also heading towards individualized therapy, e.g., tubulin point mutations appear to predict chemoresistance; therefore, patients without tubulin point mutations may benefit more from taxane therapy. Finally, NSCLC is a systemic disease, so treatment strategies, especially chemotherapeutic interventions, should move beyond metastatic disease into management of early stage disease.

Table 16. Non-Small Cell Lung Cancer

- Survival benefit for second-line chemotherapy
- Lack of efficacy differences among new first-line combinations
- Tolerability of combination regimens in elderly patients with good performance status
- Individualized therapy, especially with taxanes
- Need for early treatment of NSCLC because disease is systemic
- Role of combination therapy (versus single agents), including biologic agents
- Role of multi-modality therapy

REFERENCES

1. Greenlee RT, Murray T, Bolden S, Wingo S. Cancer Statistics, 2000. CA Cancer J Clin 2000;50:7-11, 2000.

2. Le Chevalier T. [Chemotherapy of non-small-cell lung cancers]. Presse Med. 25:1699-1703, 1996.

3. Feld R, Ginsberg RJ, Payne DG, Shepherd FA. Lung Cancer, in: Abeloff M, Armitage JO, Lichter AS, Niederhuber JE (eds): Clinical Oncology. Philadelphia, Churchill Livingstone 1398-1477, 2000.

4. Grilli R, Oxman AD, Julian JA. Chemotherapy for advanced non-small cell lung cancer: How much benefit is enough? J Clin Oncol 11:1866-1872, 1993.

5. Non-Small Cell Lung Cancer Collaborative Group. Chemotherapy in non-small cell lung cancer: a meta-analysis using updated data on individual patients from 52 randomised clinical trials. Br Med J 311:899-909, 1995.

6. Vogl SE, Berenzweig M, Camacho F, et al. Efficacy study of intensive cisplatin therapy in advanced non-small cell broncho-genic carcinoma. Cancer 50:24-26, 1982.

7. Klastersky J, Sculier JP, Bureau G, et al. Cisplatin versus cisplatin plus etoposide in the treatment of advanced non-small-cell lung cancer. Lung Cancer Working Party, Belgium. J Clin Oncol 7:1087-1092, 1989.

8. Frei E III. Non-small cell lung cancer: novel treatment strategies. Chest 112:266S-268S, 1997.

9. Ramanathan RK, Belani CP. Chemotherapy for advanced non-small cell lung cancer: past, present, and future. Semin.Oncol 24:440-454, 1997.

10. Greco FA, Hainsworth JD. Multidisciplinary approach to potentially curable non-small cell carcinoma of the lung. Oncology 11:27-36, 1997.

11.   Carney DN. Management (chemotherapy/best supportive care) of advanced stage non-small cell lung cancer. Semin Oncol 22:58-62, 1996.

12.   Samson MK, Comis RL, Baker LH, et al.   Mitomycin C in advanced adenocarcinoma and large cell carcinoma of the lung. Cancer Treat Rep 62:163-165, 1978.

13.   Costanzi JJ, Morgan LR, Hokanson J.   Ifosfamide in the treatment of extensive non-oat cell carcinoma of the lung. Semin Oncol 9:61-65, 1982.

14.   Furnas BE, Williams SD, Einhorn LH, et al. Vindesine: An effective agent in the treatment of non-small cell lung cancer. Cancer Treat Rep 66:1709-1711, 1982.

15.   Schulman P, Budman DR, Vinciguerra V, et al. Phase II study of divided-dose vinblastine in non-small cell bronchogenic carcinoma. Cancer Treat Rep 66:171-172, 1982.

16.   Anderson G, Peel ET, Cheong CM, et al. Etoposide - An effective single drug for treating bronchogenic carcinioma. Clin Oncol 8:215-218, 1982.

17.   Crino L, Scagliotti G, Marangolo M, et al.   Cisplatin-gemcitabine combination in advanced non-small-cell lung cancer: a phase II study. J Clin Oncol 15:297-303, 1997.

18.   Bonomi PD, Finkelstein DM, Ruckdeschel JC, et al. Combination chemotherapy versus single agents followed by combination chemotherapy in stage IV non-small cell lung cancer: A study of the Eastern Cooperative Oncology Group. J Clin Oncol 7:1602-1613, 1989.

19.   Ruckdeschel JC, Finkelstein DM, Ettinger DS, et al. A randomized trial of the four most active regimens for metastatic non- small-cell lung cancer. J Clin Oncol 4:14-22, 1986.

20.   Einhorn LH, Loehrer PJ, Williams SD, et al. Phase III randomized study of vindesine v cisplatin ($120\ mg/m^2$) plus vindesine v cisplatin ($60\ mg/m^2$) plus vindesine plus mitomycin C. J Clin Oncol 4:1037-1043, 1986.

21.   Clinical practice guidelines for the treatment of unresectable non- small-cell lung cancer. Adopted on May 16, 1997 by the American Society of Clinical Oncology. J Clin Oncol 15:2996-3018, 1997.

22.   Johnson D, Zhu J, Schiller J, et al. A randomized phase III trial in metastatic NSCLC- outcome of PS 2 patients: An Eastern Cooperative Group Trial E1594. Proc Am Soc Clin Oncol 18(abstract 1779), 1999.

23.   Splinter TA. Chemotherapy in advanced non-small cell lung cancer. Eur J Cancer 26:1093-1099, 1990.

24.   Lopez PG, Stewart DJ, Newman TE, Evans WK. Chemotherapy in stage IV (metastatic) non-small-cell lung cancer. Provincial Lung Disease Site Group. Cancer Prev Control 1:18-27, 1997.

25. Cullen MH, Billingham LJ, Woodroffe CM, et al. Mitomycin, ifosfamide, and cisplatin in unresectable non-small-cell lung cancer: effects on survival and quality of life. J Clin Oncol 17:3188-3194, 1999.

26. Han JY, Kim HK, Choi BG, et al. Quality of life (QOL) assessment of MIP (mitomycin, ifosfamide and cisplatin) chemotherapy in advanced non-small cell lung cancer (NSCLC). Jpn J Clin Oncol 28:749-753, 1998.

27. Roszkowski, K. Taxotere (TXT) versus best supportive care (BSC) in chemonaive patients with unresectable NSCLC: Final results of the phase III study. Abstracts and Proceedings of ECCO 10 Vienna, Austria 1999(abstr).

28. Bunn PA, Jr. The expanding role of cisplatin in the treatment of non-small-cell lung cancer. Semin Oncol 16:10-21, 1989.

29. Budd GT, Ganapathi R, Bauer L, et al. Phase I study of WR-2721 and carboplatin. Eur.J.Cancer 29A:1122-1127, 1993.

30. Rapp E, Pater JL, Willan A, et al. Chemotherapy can prolong survival in patients with advanced non-small cell lung cancer - Report of a Canadian multicenter randomized trial. J Clin Oncol 6:633-641, 1988.

31. Gatzemeier U, Rosell R, Belticher D, et al. Randomized Pan-European trial comparing paclitaxel/carboplatin versus paclitaxel/cisplatin in advanced NSCLC. Abstracts and Proceedings of ECCO 10 Vienna, Austria 1999(abstr 973).

32. Klastersky J, Sculier JP, Lacroix H, et al. A randomized study comparing cisplatin or carboplatin with etoposide in patients with advanced non-small cell lung cancer: European organization for research and treatment of cancer protocol 07861. J Clin Oncol 8:1556-1562, 1990.

33. Langer CJ, Gandara DR, Calvert P, et al. Gemcitabine and carboplatin in combination: an update of phase I and phase II studies in non-small cell lung cancer. Semin Oncol 26:12-18, 1999.

34. Calvert AH, Newell DR, Grumbrell LA, et al. Carboplatin dosage: Prospective evaluation of a simple formula based on renal function. J Clin Oncol 7:1748-1756, 1989.

35. Egorin MJ, Van Echo DA, Olman EA, et al. Prospective validation of a pharmacologically based dosing scheme for the cis-diamminedichloro-platinum(II) analogue diamminecyclobutanedicarboxylatoplatinum. Cancer Res 45:6502-6506, 1985.

36. Chatelut E, Canal P, Brunner V, et al. Prediction of carboplatin clearance from standard morphological and biological patient characteristics. J Natl Cancer Inst 87:573-580, 1995

37. Rowinsky EK. Paclitaxel pharmacology and other tumor types. Semin Oncol 24:S19-S19, 1997.

38. Gatzemeier U, Heckmayer M, Neuhauss R, et al. Chemotherapy of advanced inoperable non-small cell lung cancer with paclitaxel: a phase II trial. Semin Oncol 22:24-28, 1995.

39. Hainsworth JD, Urba WJ, Hon JK, et al. One-hour paclitaxel plus carboplatin in the treatment of advanced non- small cell lung cancer: results of a multicentre, phase II trial. Eur J Cancer 34:654-658, 1998.

40. Murphy WK, Fossella FV, Winn RJ, et al. Phase II study of taxol in patients with untreated advanced non-small cell lung cancer. J Natl Cancer Inst 85:384-388, 1993.

41. Chang AY, Kim K, Glick J, et al. Phase II study of taxol, merbarone, and piroxantrone in Stage IV non-small cell lung cancer: The Eastern Cooperative Oncology Group Results. J Natl Cancer Inst 85:388-394, 1993.

42. Rowinsky RK, Donehower RC. Paclitaxel (taxol). N Engl J Med 332:1004-1014, 1995.

43. Hainsworth JD, Thompson DS, Greco FA. Paclitaxel by 1-hour infusion: an active drug in metastatic non-small cell lung cancer. J Clin Oncol 13:1609-1614, 1995.

44. Rowinsky EK, Gilbert MR, McGuire WP, et al. Sequences of taxol and cisplatin: A phase I and pharmacologic study. J Clin Oncol 9:1692-1703, 1991.

45. Rowinsky EK, Citardi MJ, Noe DA, et al. Sequence-dependent cytotoxic effects due to combinations of cisplatin and the antimicrotubule agents Taxol and vincristine. J Cancer Res Clin Oncol 119:727-733, 1993.

46. Klastersky J, Sculier JP. Cisplatin plus taxol in non-small cell lung cancer: A dose finding trial. Proc Am Soc Clin Oncol 36:A1423, 1995(abstr).

47. Belli L, Le Chevalier T, Gottfried M, et al. Phase I-II trial of paclitaxel (Taxol) and cisplatin in previously untreated advanced non-small cell lung cancer (NSCLC). Proc Am Soc Clin Oncol 14:A1058, 1995(abstr).

48. Bonomi P, Kim K, Fairclough D, et al. Comparison of survival and quality of life in advanced non-small-cell lung cancer patients treated with two dose levels of paclitaxel combined with cisplatin versus etoposide with cisplatin: results of an Eastern Cooperative Oncology Group trial. J Clin Oncol 18:623, 2000.

49. Giaccone G, Splinter TA, Debruyne C, et al. Randomized study of paclitaxel-cisplatin versus cisplatin-teniposide in patients with advanced non-small-cell lung cancer. The European Organization for Research and Treatment of Cancer Lung Cancer Cooperative Group. J Clin Oncol 16:2133-2141, 1998.

50. Kosmidis PA, Mylonakis N, Fountzilas G, et al. Paclitaxel and carboplatin in inoperable non-small-cell lung cancer: a phase II study. Ann Oncol 8:697-699, 1997.

51. Belani CP, Aisner J, Hiponia D, et al. Paclitaxel and carboplatin with and without filgrastim support in patients with metastatic non-small cell lung cancer. Semin Oncol 1995;22:7-12, 1995.

52. Langer C, Rosvold E, Millenson M, et al. Paclitaxel (P) by 1 hour or 24 hour (HR) infusion combined with carboplatin (C) in advanced non-small cell lung carcinoma (NSCLC): a comparative analysis. Proc Am Soc Clin Oncol 16:452a, 1997.

53. Roa V, Conner A, Mitchell RB. Carboplatin and paclitaxel for chemotherapy-naive patients with advanced non-small cell lung cancer. Proc Am Soc Clin Oncol 15:A1231(abstr), 1996.

54. Belani CP, Kearns CM, Zuhowski EG, et al. Phase I trial, including pharmacokinetic and pharmacodynamic correlations, of combination paclitaxel and carboplatin in patients with metastatic non-small-cell lung cancer. J Clin Oncol 17:676-684, 1999.

55. Belani CP, Natale RB, Lee JS, et al. Randomized Phase III Trial Comparing Cisplatin/Etoposide Versus Carboplatin/Paclitaxel in Advanced and Metastatic Non-Small Cell Lung Cancer (NSCLC). Proc Am Soc Clin Oncol 17:455a, 1998.

56. Kelly K, Crowley J, Bunn PA Jr, et al. A randomized phase III trial of paclitaxel plus carboplatin versus vinorelbine plus cisplatin in untreated advanced NSCLC. A Southwest Oncology Group trial. Proc Am Soc Clin Oncol 18:461a, 1999.

57. Johnson DH. Treatment Strategies for Metastatic Non-Small-Cell Lung Cancer. Clin Lung Cancer 1:34-41, 1999.

58. Kosmidis P, Mylonakis N, Fountzilas G, et al. Paclitaxel (175 mg/m^2) plus carboplatin versus paclitaxel (225 mg/m^2) plus carboplatin in non-small cell lung cancer: a randomized study. Semin Oncol 24:S12-S12, 1997.

59. Lopes NM, Adams EG, Pitts TW, Bhuyan BK. Cell kill kinetics and cell cycle effects of taxol on human and hamster ovarian cell lines. Cancer Chemother Pharmacol 32:235-242, 1993.

60. Seidman AD. One-hour paclitaxel via weekly infusion: dose-density with enhanced therapeutic index. Oncology 12:19-22, 1998.

61. Aggarwal L, Akerley W, Wingate P, et al. Weekly paclitaxel effect on platelets inp atients with NSCLC and in patients with prostate cancer and thrombocytopenia. Proc Am Soc Clin Oncol 17(abstr 202), 1998.

62. Fennelly D, Aghajanian C, Shapiro F, et al. Phase I and pharmacologic study of paclitaxel administered weekly in patients with relapsed ovarian cancer. J Clin Oncol 15:187-192, 1997.

63. Akerley W, Glantz M, Choy H, et al. Phase I trial of weekly paclitaxel in advanced lung cancer. J Clin Oncol 16:153-158, 1998.

64. Belotti D, Vergani V, Drudis T, et al. The microtubule-affecting drug paclitaxel has antiangiogenic activity. Clin Cancer Res 2:1843-1849, 1996.

65. Akerley W, Herndon J, Egorin M J, et al. Phase II trial of weekly paclitaxel for advanced non-small cell lung cancer. Proc Am Soc Clin Oncol 18(abstr 1783), 1999.

66. Chang AY, Asbury RF, Boros L, et al. Stage IV NSCLC: weekly Taxol and beyond. The Fox Chase Cancer Center and Free University Hospital 1999 Investigators' Workshop and Consensus Conference on Paclitaxel, Lana'i, Hawai.

67. Loffler TM, Freund W, Lipke J, Hausamen TU. Schedule and dose-intensified paclitaxel as weekly 1-hour infusion in pretreated solid tumors: results of a phase I/II trial. Semin.Oncol 23:32-34, 1996.

68. Shyr Y, Choy H, Cmelak A, et al. Pattern of Practice Survey: Non-small Cell Lung Cancer (NSCLC) in US. Proc Am Soc Clin Oncol 17:463a, 1998.

69. Clarke SJ, Rivory LP. Clinical pharmacokinetics of docetaxel. Clin Pharmacokinet 36:99-114, 1999.

70. Burris H, Eckardt J, Fields S. Phase II trials of Taxotere in patients with non-small cell lung cancer. Proc Am Soc Clin Oncol 12:A116, 1993 (abstr).

71. Cerny T, Kaplan S, Pavlidis N, et al. Docetaxel (Taxotere) is active in non-small-cell lung cancer: a phase II trial of the EORTC Early Clinical Trials Group (ECTG). Br J Cancer 70:384-387, 1994.

72. Fossella FV, Lee JS, Murphy WK, et al. Phase II study of docetaxel for recurrent or metastatic non-small cell lung cancer. J Clin Oncol 12:1238-1244, 1994.

73. Francis PA, Rigas JR, Kris MG, et al. Phase II trial of docetaxel in patients with stage III and IV non-small cell lung cancer. J Clin Oncol 12:1232-1237, 1994.

74. Belani CP. Single agents in the second-line treatment of non-small cell lung cancer. Semin Oncol 25:10-14, 1998.

75. Fossella FU, Lee JS, Shin DM, et al. Phase II study of docetaxel for advanced or metastatic platinum refractory non-small cell lung cancer. J Clin Oncol 13:651, 1995.

76. Kunitoh H, Watanabe K, Onoshi T, et al. Phase II trial of docetaxel in previously untreated advanced non-small-cell lung cancer: a Japanese cooperative study. J Clin Oncol 14:1649-1655, 1996.

77. Fossella FV. Overview of docetaxel (Taxotere) in the treatment of non-small cell lung cancer. Semin Oncol 1999;26:4-8, 1999.

78. Klink-Alakl M, Riva A, Bruno R, et al. Taxotere safety profile in patients with liver metastases with or without impaired liver function. Proc Am Soc Clin Oncol 16:220a, 1997.

79. Hainsworth JD, Burris HA III, Greco FA. Weekly administration of docetaxel (Taxotere): summary of clinical data. Semin Oncol 1999;26:19-24.

80. Bissett D, Setanoians A, Cassidy J, et al. Phase I and pharmacokinetic study of taxotere (RP 56976) administered as a 24-hour infusion. Cancer Res 53:523-527, 1993.

81. Behar A, Pujade-Lauraine E, Maurel A, et al. The pathophysiological mechanism of fluid retention in advanced cancer patients treated with docetaxel, but not receiving corticosteroid comedication. Br J Clin Pharmacol 43:653-658, 1997.

82. Miller VA, Rigas JR, Francis PA, et al. Phase II trial of a 75 mg/m^2 dose of docetaxel with prednisone premedication for patients with advanced non-small cell lung cancer. Cancer 75:968-972, 1995.

83. Ravdin PM, Valero V. Review of docetaxel (Taxotere), a highly active new agent for the treatment of metastatic breast cancer. Semin Oncol 22:17-21, 1995.

84. Latreille J, Gelmon KA, Hirsh V, et al. Phase II trial of docetaxel with dexamethasone premedication in patients with advanced non-small cell lung cancer: the Canadian experience. Invest New Drugs 16:265-270, 1998.

85. Piccart MJ, Klijn J, Paridaens R, et al. Corticosteroids significantly delay the onset of docetaxel-induced fluid retention: final results of a randomized study of the European Organization for Research and Treatment of Cancer Investigational Drug Branch for Breast Cancer. J Clin Oncol 15:3149-3155, 1997.

86. Belani CP. Docetaxel (Taxotere) in combination with platinum-based regimens in non- small cell lung cancer: results and future developments. Semin Oncol 26:15-18, 1999.

87. Hilkens PH, Verweij J, Vecht CJ, et al. Clinical characteristics of severe peripheral neuropathy induced by docetaxel (Taxotere). Ann Oncol 8:187-190, 1997.

88. Pace A, Bove L, Pietrangeli A, et al. Docetaxel neuropathy [letter]. Neurology 1996;47:615.

89. Georgoulias V, Androulakis N, Dimopoulos AM, et al. First-line treatment of advanced non-small-cell lung cancer with docetaxel and cisplatin: a multicenter phase II study. Ann Oncol 9:331-334, 1998.

90. Belani CP, Hadeed V, Ramananthan RK, et al. Docetaxel and carboplatin: A phase I and pharmacokinetic trial for advanced non-hematologic malignancies. Proc Am Soc Clin Oncol 16(abstract 771):220a, 1997.

91. Capozzoli MJ, Belani CP, Eizing A, et al. Multi-institutional phase II trial of docetaxel and carboplatin combination in patients with stage IIIB and IV NSCLC. Proc Am Soc Clin Oncol 17(abstr 1845):479a, 1998.

92.   Arcenas A, Anderson A and Krasnow S. Docetaxel/Carboplatin combination therapy for stage IIIB/IV NSCLC. Proc Am Soc Clin Oncol 18(abstr 1910): 495a, 1999.

93.   Millward M J, Bishop J, Lehnert M. Phase II trial of docetaxel and carboplatin in advanced NSCLC. Proc Am Soc Clin Oncol 18(abstr 1994): 517a, 1999.

94.   Greco FA. Docetaxel (Taxotere) administered in weekly schedules. Semin Oncol 26:28-31, 1999.

95.   Hainsworth JD, Burris HA III, Erland JB, et al. Phase I trial of docetaxel administered by weekly infusion in patients with advanced refractory cancer. J Clin Oncol 16:2164-2168, 1998.

96.   Niitani H. Navelbine (vinorelbine): a review of its antitumor activity and toxicity in clinical studies. Gan To Kagaku Ryoho 26:1495-1507, 1999.

97.   Binet S, Chaineau E, Fellous A, et al. Immunofluorescence study of the action of navelbine, vincristine and vinblastine on mitotic and axonal microtubules. Int J Cancer 46:262-266, 1990.

98.   Gandara DR, Crowley J, Livingston RB, et al. Evaluation of cisplatin intensity in metastatic non-small-cell lung cancer: a phase III study of the Southwest Oncology Group. J Clin Oncol 11:873-878, 1993.

99.   Wozniak AJ, Crowley JJ, Balcerzak SP, et al. Randomized Phase III Trial of Cisplatin (CDDP) versus CDDP Plus Navelbine (NVB) in Treatment of Advanced Non-Small Cell Lung Cancer (NSCLC): An Update of a Southwest Oncology Group Study (SWOG-9308). Proc Am Soc Clin Oncol 17:453a, 1998.

100.   Abratt RP, Bezwoda WR, Falkson G, et al. Efficacy and safety profile of gemcitabine in non-small cell lung cancer: A phase II study. J Clin Oncol 12:1535-1540, 1994.

101.   Gatzemeier U, Shepherd FA, Le Chevalier T, et al Activity of gemcitabine in patients with non-small cell lung cancer: A multicentre, extended phase II study. Eur J Cancer 32A:243-248, 1996.

102.   Aapro MS, Martin C, Hatty S. Gemcitabine--a safety review. Anticancer Drugs 9:191-201, 1998.

103.   Thatcher N, Jayson G, Bradley B, et al. Gemcitabine: symptomatic benefit in advanced non-small cell lung cancer. Semin Oncol 24:S8-S8, 1997.

104.   Manegold C, Bergman B, Chemaissani A, et al. Single-agent gemcitabine versus cisplatin-etoposide: early results of a randomised phase II study in locally advanced or metastatic non-small- cell lung cancer. Ann Oncol 8:525-529, 1997.

105.   Perng RP, Chen YM, Ming-Liu J, et al. Gemcitabine versus the combination of cisplatin and etoposide in patients with inoperable non-small-cell lung cancer in a phase II randomized study. J Clin Oncol 15:2097-2102, 1997.

106. Ulsperger E, Puganigg K, Thaler J, et al. A cost-comparison study of gemcitabine versus cisplatin plus etoposide in NSCLC. Proc Am Soc Clin Oncol 18:526a, 1999.

107. Peters GJ, Ruiz vH, V, Bergman AM, et al. Preclinical combination therapy with gemcitabine and mechanisms of resistance. Semin Oncol 23:16-24, 1996.

108. Shepherd FA, Burkes R, Cormier Y, et al. Phase I dose-escalation trial of gemcitabine and cisplatin for advanced non-small-cell lung cancer: usefulness of mathematic modeling to determine maximum-tolerable dose. J Clin Oncol 14:1656-1662, 1996.

109. Abratt RP, Hacking DJ, Goedhals L, Bezwoda WR. Weekly gemcitabine and monthly cisplatin for advanced non-small cell lung carcinoma. Semin Oncol 24:S8-S8, 1997.

110. Anton A, Diaz-Fernandez N, Gonzalez Larriba JL, et al. Phase II trial assessing the combination of gemcitabine and cisplatin in advanced non-small cell lung cancer (NSCLC). Lung Cancer 22:139-148, 1998.

111. Abratt RP, Sandler A, Crino L, et al. Combined cisplatin and gemcitabine for non-small cell lung cancer: influence of scheduling on toxicity and drug delivery. Semin Oncol 25:35-43, 1998.

112. Ricci S, Antonuzzo A, Galli L, et al. Combination chemotherapy with two different schedules of gemcitabine plus cisplatin in patinets with stage IIIB-IV NSCLC: A multicentric Randomized phase II study. Proc Am Soc Clin Oncol 18:480a, 1999.

113. Sandler A, Ettinger DS. Gemcitabine: single-agent and combination therapy in non-small cell lung cancer. Oncologist 4:241-251, 1999.

114. Cardenal F, Lopez-Cabrerizo MP, Anton A, et al. Randomized phase III study of gemcitabine-cisplatin versus etoposide- cisplatin in the treatment of locally advanced or metastatic non-small- cell lung cancer. J Clin Oncol 17:12-18, 1999.

115. Sandler AB, Nemunaitis J, Denham C, et al. Phase III Trial of Gemcitabine Plus Cisplatin Versus Cisplatin Alone in Patients With Locally Advanced or Metastatic Non-Small-Cell Lung Cancer. J Clin Oncol 18:122, 2000.

116. Crino L, Conte P, DeMarinis F, et al. A Randomised Trial of Gemcitabine Cisplatin (GP) Versus Mitomycin, Ifosfamide and Cisplatin (MIC) in Advanced Non-Small Cell Lung Cancer (NSCLC): A Multicenter Phase III Study. Proc Am Soc Clin Oncol 17:455a, 1998.

117. Rosell R, Tonato M, Sandler A. The activity of gemcitabine plus cisplatin in randomized trials in untreated patients with advanced non-small cell lung cancer. Semin Oncol 25:27-34, 1998.

118. Gross G, Holiday D, Hampton J, Kieman H. A combination therapy of gemcitabine and carboplatin in advanced stage NSCLC. Proc Am Soc Clin Oncol 18:507a, 1999.

119. Masotti A, Morandini G. Phase II trial of gemcitabine and carboplatin in advanced NSCLC. Proc Am Soc Clin Oncol 18:517a. 1999.

120. Carmichael J, Allerheiligen S, Walling J. A phase I study of gemcitabine and carboplatin in non-small cell lung cancer. Semin Oncol 23:55-59, 1996.

121. Edelman M J, Gandara D R, Lau D, et al. Sequential carboplatin/gemcitabine-paclitaxel in advanced NSCLC: An effective and well-tolerated regimen. Proc Am Soc Clin Oncol 18(abstr 1936):476a, 1999.

122. Carrato A, Garcia-Gomez J, Alberola VMBJ, et al. Carboplatin in combination with gemcitabine in advanced NSCLC. Comparison of two consecutive phase II trials using different schedules. Proc Am Soc Clin Oncol 18:498a, 1999.

123. Kuhn JG. Pharmacology of irinotecan. Oncology 12:39-42, 1998.

124. Fukuoka M, Niitani H, Suzuki A, et al. A phase II study of CPT-11, a new derivative of camptothecin, for previously untreated non-small-cell lung cancer. J Clin Oncol 10:16-20, 1992.

125. Fukuoka M, Masuda N. Clinical studies of irinotecan alone and in combination with cisplatin. Cancer Chemother.Pharmacol. 34 Suppl:S105-S111, 1994.

126. Sandler A, van Oosterom AT. Irinotecan in cancers of the lung and cervix. Anticancer Drugs 10 Suppl 1:S13-S17, 1999.

127. Kobayashi K, Takeda Y, Akiyama Y, et al. Reduced irinotecan-induced side-effects by oral alkalinization. Proc Am Soc Clin Oncol 18(abstract 1900): 492a, 1999.

128. Kunitoh H, Sailo N, Nagao K, et al. Cisplatin and irinotecan versus cisplatin and vindesine in advanced stage IIIB/IV NSCLC: A multicentric phase II study. Abstracts and Proceedings of ECCO 10 1999.

129. Masuda N, Fukuoka M, Negoro S, et al. Randomized trial comparing cisplatin and irinotecan versus cisplatin and vindesine versus irinotecan alone in advanced NSCLC: A multicenter phase II study. Proc Am Soc Clin Oncol 18:459a, 1999.

130. Krug LM, Kris MG, Grant SC, et al. Phase II trial of dose dense docetaxel plus vinorelbine with prophylactic G-CSF in advanced NSCLC. Proc Am Soc Clin Oncol 18:460a, 1999.

131. Miller V. Docetaxel (Taxotere) in combination with vinorelbine in non-small cell lung cancer. Semin Oncol 26:12-14, 1999.

132. Sederholm C. A phase II study of gemcitabine plus carboplatin in chemonaive patients with advanced NSCLC. Proc Am Soc Clin Oncol 18:490a, 1999.

133. Levin M and Novetsky A. A phase II study of docetaxel, vinorelbine, G-CSF chemotherapy in patients with unresectable or metastatic NSCLC. Proc Am Soc Clin Oncol 18:514a, 1999.

134. Spiridonidis CH, Laufman LR, Jones J, et al. Phase I study of docetaxel dose escalation in combination with fixed weekly gemcitabine in patients with advanced malignancies. J Clin Oncol 16:3866-3873, 1998.

135. Bildat S, Harstrick A, Gatzemeier U, et al. Phase I study of docetaxel in combination with gemcitabine as first line chemotherapy in patients with metastatic NSCLC. Proc Am Soc Clin Oncol 18:497a, 1999.

136. Rizvi NA. Docetaxel (Taxotere) and gemcitabine in combination therapy. Semin Oncol 26:19-22, 1999.

137. Georgoulias V, Papadakis E, Alexopoulos A, et al. Docetaxel plus cisplatin versus docetaxel plus gemcitabine chemotherapy in advanced NSCLC: A preliminary analysis of a multicenter randomized phase II trial. Proc Am Soc Clin Oncol 18:461a, 1999.

138. Martin C, Isla D, Gonzalez-Larriba JL, et al. A phase II study of bi-weekly gemcitabine plus paclitaxel in advanced NSCLC. Proc Am Soc Clin Oncol 18:462a, 1999.

139. Giaccone G, Smit E, Laan D, and et al. Phase I/II study of paclitaxel and gemcitabine in advanced non-small cell lung cancer (NSCLC). Proc Am Soc Clin Oncol 17(abstract 1869), 1998.

140. Chen YM, Whang-Peng J, Perng RP, et al. A multi-center phase II study of gemcitabine and vinorelbine in patients with advanced stage IIIB/IV NSCLC. Proc Am Soc Clin Oncol 18:481a, 1999.

141. Pirker R, Krajnic G, Mohn-Staudner A, et al. Vinorelbine/gemcitabine in advanced NSCLC, an AASLC phase II trial. Proc Am Soc Clin Oncol 18 (abstract 1849):479a. 1999.

142. Barr F., Mirsky H., Clinthorne D, et al. Phase III study of gemcitabine and vinorelbine salvage chemotherapy for taxane-resistant NSCLC. Proc Am Soc Clin Oncol 18(abstract 1914):496a, 1999.

143. Zwitte M, Cufer T, Wein W. Phase II trial of gemcitabine and vincristine for stage IV NSCLC. Proc Am Soc Clin Oncol 18:529a, 1999.

144. Van Putten JWG, Fokkema E, Smeets J, Groen HJM. Phase II study of high-dose epirubicin and gemcitabine in patients with advanced NSCLC. Proc Am Soc Clin Oncol 18:487a, 1999.

145. Cole JL, Rinaldi DA, Lormand NA, et al. A phase I-II trial of topotecn and gemcitabine for patients with previously treated advanced NSCLC. Proc Am Soc Clin Oncol 18:499a, 1999.

146. Yamazaki H, Funakoshi S, Hirano A, et al. Phase I and pharmacokinetic study of irinotecan given by 24 hours infusion plus oral uracil/tegafur in patients with lung cancer. Proc Am Soc Clin Oncol 18:528a, 1999.

147. Ruckdeschel J, Wagner HJr, Williams C, et al. Second-line chemotherapy for resistant, metastatic, non-small cell lung cancer (NSCLC): The role of Taxol (TAX). Proc Am Soc Clin Oncol 13:357a, 1994.

148. Murphy WK, Winn RJ, Huber M, et al. Phase II study of taxol (T) in patients (pts) with non-small cell lung cancer (NSCLC) who have failed platinum (P) containing chemotherapy (Ctx). Proc Am Soc Clin Oncol 13:A1224 (abstr), 1994.

149. Socinski MA and Steagal A. Phase II trial of 96 hour paclitaxel infusion in patients with non-small cell lung cancer failing previous platinum based or short duration paclitaxel therapy. Proc Am Soc Clin Oncol 16:1735, 1997.

150. Rinaldi M, Della GM, Venturo I, et al. Vinorelbine as single agent in the treatment of advanced NSCLC. Proc Am Soc Clin Oncol 13:360, 1994.

151. Nakai H, Fukuoka M, Furuse K, et al. An early phase II study of CPT-11 for primary lung cancer. Jpn J Cancer Chemother 1991;18:607-612, 1991.

152. Crino L, Mosconi AM, Scagliotti G, DeMarinis F, Darwish S, Calandri C, Adamo V, Scarcella L, Pucci F, Tonato M. Salvage therapy with gemcitabine (GEM) in pretreated, advanced non-small cell lung cancer (NSCLC). Proc Am Soc Clin Oncol 16:446a, 1997.

153. Fossella FV, Lee JS, Berille J, et al. Summary of phase II data of docetaxel (Taxotere), an active agent in the first- and second-line treatment of advanced non-small cell lung cancer. Semin Oncol 22:22-29, 1995.

154. Fossella FU, De Vore R, Kerr Rea. Phase III trial of docetaxel 100 mg/sqm or 75 mg/sqm versus vinorelbine/ifosfamide for NSCLC previously treated with platinum-based chemotherapy. Proc Am Soc Clin Oncol 18:460a, 1999.

155. Shepherd FA, Ramlau R, Mattson K, et al. Randomized study of taxotere versus best supportive care (BSC) in NSCLC patients previously treated with platinum-based chemotherapy. Proc Am Soc Clin Oncol 18:463a, 1999.

156. Postmus PE, Mattson K, von Pawel C, et al. Phase II trial of MTA (LY231514) in patients with NSCLC who relapsed after previous platinum or non-platinum therapy. Abstracts and Proceedings of ECCO 10 Sept 12-16, Vienna, Austria, 1999.

157. Monzo M, Rosell R, Sanchez J, et al. Paclitaxel resistance in non-small-cell lung cancer associated with beta-tubulin gene mutations. J Clin Oncol 17:1786-1793, 1999.

158. Balana C, Barnadas A, Martin C, et al. A phase II study of sequence-dependent docetaxel-vinorelbine DNA damage-induced apoptosis in patients with NSCLC. Proc Am Soc Clin Oncol 18 (abstract 1786):476a, 1999.

159. Frasci G, Comella P, Panza N, et al. Carboplatin-oral etoposide personalized dosing in elderly non-small cell lung cancer patients. Gruppo Oncologico Cooperativo Sud-Italia. Eur J Cancer 34:1710-1714, 1998.

160. Kubota K, Furuse K, Kawahara M, et al. Cisplatin-based combination chemotherapy for elderly patients with non- small-cell lung cancer. Cancer Chemother.Pharmacol. 40:469-474, 1997.

161. Effects of vinorelbine on quality of life and survival of elderly patients with advanced non-small-cell lung cancer. The Elderly Lung Cancer Vinorelbine Italian Study Group. J Natl Cancer Inst 91:66-72, 1999.

162. Gridelli C, Perrone F, Gallo C, et al. Vinorelbine is well tolerated and active in the treatment of elderly patients with advanced non-small cell lung cancer. A two-stage phase II study. Eur J Cancer 33:392-397, 1997.

163. Rosvold E, Langer C J, McAleer C A, et al. Advancing age does not exacerbate toxicity or compromise outcome in non-small cell lung cancer patients receiving paclitaxel-carboplatin. Proc Am Soc Clin Oncol 18(abstract 1846), 478a.

164. Nguyen, B., Sandler, A. and Denham, C. The safety and efficacy of gemcitabine plus cisplatin in the elderly chemonaive patient (age > 70 years) as compared to those with age < 70 years. Proc Am Soc Clin Oncol 18 (abstract 1818), 471a. 5-15, 1999.

165. Chang A, Hui L, Boros L, et al. Phase I Study of Weekly One-Hour Paclitaxel Treatment in Advanced Malignant Diseases. Proc Am Soc Clin Oncol 16:817, 1997.

166. Kris MG. What does chemotherapy have to offer patients with advanced-stage non- small cell lung cancer? Semin Oncol. 25:1-4, 1998.

167. Gatzemeier U, von Pawel J, Gottfried Met al. Phase III Comparative Study of High-Dose Cisplatin (HD-CIS) Versus a Combination of Paclitaxel (TAX) and Cisplatin (CIS) in Patients with Advanced Non-Small Cell Lung Cancer (NSCLC). Proc Am Soc Clin Oncol 17:454a, 1998.

168. von Pawel J, von Roemeling R. Survival Benefit from Tirazone™ (Tirapazamine) and Cisplatin in Advanced Non-Small Cell Lung Cancer (NSCLC) Patients: Final Results from the International Phase III Catapult I Trial. Proc Am Soc Clin Oncol 1998;17:454a, 1998.

169. Le Chevalier T, Berille J, Zalcberg JR, et al. Overview of docetaxel (Taxotere)/cisplatin combination in non-small cell lung cancer. Semin Oncol 26:13-18, 1999.

170. Belani CP, Bonomi PD, Dobbs T, et al. Multicenter phase II trial of docetaxel and cisplatin combination in patients with non-small cell lung cancer. Proc Am Soc Clin Oncol 16:221a, 1997.

171. Zalcberg JR, Bishop JF, Millward MJ, et al. Preliminary results of the first phase II trial of docetaxel in combination with cisplatin in patients with metastatic or locally advanced non-small cell lung cancer (NSCLC). Proc Am Soc Clin Oncol 14:A1062 (abstr), 1995.

172. Le Chevalier T, Belli L, Monnier A, et al. Phase II study of docetaxel (Taxotere) and cisplatin in advanced non-small cell lung cancer (NSCLC): An interim analysis. Proc Am Soc Clin Oncol 14:A1059 (abstr), 1995.

173. Androulakis N, Dimopoulos AM, Kourousis C. First-line treatment of advanced non-small cell lung cancer (NSCLC) with docetaxel and cisplatin: A multicenter phase II study. Proc Am Soc Clin Oncol 16, 1997.

174. Gandara DR, Vokes E, Green M, et al. Activity of Docetaxel in Platinum-Treated Non-Small-Cell Lung Cancer: Results of a Phase II Multicenter Trial. J Clin Oncol 18:131, 2000.

175. Negoro S, Fukuoka M, Niitani H, et al. A phase II study of CPT-11, a camptothecin derivative, in patients with primary lung cancer. CPT-11 cooperative study group. [Japanese]. Gan to Kagaku Ryoho 18:1013-1019, 1991.

176. Rosvold E, Langer CJ, Schilder R, et al. Salvage Therapy with Gemcitabine in Advanced Non-Small Cell Lung Cancer (NSCLC) Progressing after Prior Carboplatin-Paclitaxel (C-P). Proc Am Soc Clin Oncol 17:467a, 1998.

177. Gridelli C, Perrone F, Gallo C, et al. Single-agent gemcitabine as second-line treatment in patients with advanced non small cell lung cancer (NSCLC): a phase II trial [In Process Citation]. Anticancer Res 19:4535-4538, 1999.

178. Lorusso V, Mancarella S, Carpagnano F, et al. Gemcitabine Plus Vinorelbine in Patients with Stage IIIB-IV Non-small Cell Lung Cancer (NSCLC): A Phase II Study. Proc Am Soc Clin Oncol 17:470a, 1998.

179. Le Chevalier T, Brisgand D, Douillard JY, et al. Randomized study of vinorelbine and cisplatin versus vindesine and cisplatin versus vinorelbine alone in advanced non-small cell lung cancer: Results of a European multicenter trial including 612 patients. J Clin Oncol 12:360-367, 1994.

180. Depierre A, Chastang C, Quoix E, et al. Vinorelbine versus vinorelbine plus cisplatin in advanced non-small cell lung cancer: a randomized trial. Ann Oncol 5:37-42, 1994.

181. Crawford J, O'Rourke M, Schiller JH, et al. Randomized trial of vinorelbine compared with fluorouracil plus leucovorin in patients with stage IV non-small-cell lung cancer. [published erratum appears in J Clin Oncol 14(12):3175, 1996] J Clin Oncol 14:2774-2784, 1996.

182. Bonomi PD, Kim K, Chang A, et al. Phase III trial comparing etoposide (E) cisplatin versus Taxol (T) with cisplatin-G-CSF (G) versus cisplatin in advanced non-small cell lung cancer: Eastern Cooperative Oncology Group (ECOG). Proc Am Soc Clin Oncol 15:A1145, 1996 (abstr).

183. Crino L, Scagliotti GV, Ricci S, et al. Gemcitabine and cisplatin versus mitomycin, ifosfamide, and cisplatin in advanced non-small-cell lung cancer: A randomized phase III study of the Italian Lung Cancer Project. J Clin Oncol 17:3522-3530, 1999.

THERAPY OF LIMITED STAGE SMALL CELL LUNG CANCER

Walter J. Curran, Jr., M.D.

Kimmel Cancer Center of Jefferson Medical College, Philadelphia, PA 19107 USA

INTRODUCTION

Bronchogenic carcinoma is divided into two distinct entities, small cell lung cancer (SCLC) and non-small cell lung cancer (NSCLC) and these categories have distinguishing clinical, biologic, and histologic features. SCLC accounts for approximately 20% of the 164,000 cases of bronchogenic carcinoma expected to be diagnosed in the United States in 2000 (1). Until the late 1960's, physicians did not differentiate the management of SCLC from NSCLC; in fact, clinical trials for lung cancer until the early 1970's sometimes included both patient categories. It was recognized at that time, however, that most patients with SCLC had poor survival outcome with surgery and/or radiation and had little apparent survival benefit from either therapy. The breakthrough which occurred in the late 1960's was the recognition that SCLC tumors were relatively more responsive to the available chemotherapeutic agents than NSCLC tumors (2). Since that time, it has been recognized that the standard of care for most SCLC patients has included systemic therapy in addition to locoregional therapy, if appropriate.

Pathology and Pathways of Spread

There are two commonly used systems for classifying SCLC histology. The 1981 World Health Organization (WHO) system described these three subtypes: (1) the classic "oat cell" type; (2) the intermediate type, characterized by larger cells with more pleomorphic nuclei and more abundant cytoplasm; and (3) the combined type, which included tumors with squamous cell or adenocarcinoma-like features. The International Association for the Study of Lung Cancer (IASLC) presented a new system in 1988, in which those tumors with clearly NSCLC features are excluded. The three IASLC categories are: (1) the classic small cell type; (2) a small cell/large cell cancer, in which a population of larger cell with more abundant cytoplasm can be identified; and (3) a combined small cell carcinoma, in which squamous or glandular elements are present (3).

The majority of patients with SCLC have either International Union Against Cancer (IUCC) Stage III or IV disease. It is uncommon for small cell tumors to be confined to the lung alone. While the nodal extension tends to follow established patterns of lymphatic drainage within the thorax, there are fewer anatomic staging data available for SCLC as opposed to NSCLC.

Biologic Characteristics/Molecular Biology

There are a number of genetic mutations observed in SCLC tumors. The most common are: (1) a deletion in the short arm of chromosome 3 in the 3p14-23 region (over 80% of SCLC cases); (2) inactivation of the retinoblastoma (Rb) gene on chromosome 13 (90%); (3) mutations of the p53 tumor suppressor gene on the short arm of chromosome 17 (over 80%); and (4) overexpression of the myc family of oncogenes (over 50%). There has been tremendous progress in recent years in understanding the relationship of these mutations and the possible events leading bronchial epithelium from a preneoplastic lesion to an invasive carcinoma.

The chromosome 3 genetic deletions have been observed in both dysplastic and pre-neoplastic changes and have been most convincingly demonstrated as the known genetic mutation associated with the transformation of pre-cancerous changes into carcinoma. There has recently emerged evidence that the critical deletion in SCLC and many other malignancies may be in a fragile portion of chromosome 3 known as the FHIT gene deletion (4,5). Inactivation of the retinoblastoma gene most likely results in a loss of control of growth. It is thought that a functional Rb gene will keep the G1/S cell cycle boundary in check and that its inactivation will result in uncontrolled growth. It is of interest that the Rb gene is less frequently inactivated in NSCLC (20%) and that uncontrolled growth of that disease may relate to other genetic alterations, in particular in the regulation of cyclin D1 and cyclin-dependent kinases (6). The p53 mutations specific to SCLC have also been observed in preneoplastic lesions and appear to most closely resemble p53 mutations observed in other malignancies for which tobacco is a known carcinogen. It is likely that the mutation of p53 in SCLC tumors impairs the ability of tumor cells to undergo apoptosis in response to anti-cancer therapy (7). Another growth regulator, which is over expressed in 65-75% of SCLC tumors, is bcl-2. It is believed that this overexpression also interferes with the tumor's apoptotic response to therapy (8). There are ongoing research efforts to develop therapies, which could target these tumor-specific biologic lesions.

In many NSCLC specimens studied, point mutations in the *ras* family of oncogenes has been observed (9). These mutations are rarely observed in SCLC specimens, but commonly, amplification or overexpression of the *myc* family of oncogenes is observed, most notably, c-*myc*, N-*myc*, and L-*myc*. It appears that abnormalities are more often observed in recurrent tumors, tumors with variant rather than classic SCLC histology, or tumors with a more aggressive and unfavorable prognosis. This has led to the hypothesis that the overexpression of the *myc* oncogenes is a relatively late event in the pathogenesis of SCLC (10).

Table 1. Syndromes Associated with SCLC

Syndrome	Manifestation(s)	Frequency	Correctable with Therapy
SIADH (Syndrome of Inappropriate ADH Secretion)	Hyponatremia, Hypo-osmality	11-46%	Yes
ANP Syndrome (Atrial Natriurectic Peptide Syndrome)	Hyponatremia, Hypotension, Natriuresis	15%	Yes
Etopic ACTH Production	Cushinoid Symptoms	<5%	Rarely
Lambert-Eaton Syndrome	Myasthenia Gravis-Like Symptoms	<5%	Yes
Cerebellar Degeneration Syndrome	Cerebellar Symptoms	<5%	Rarely
Cancer-Associated Retinopathy (CAR)	Visual Loss	<5%	Rarely

Another distinguishing biologic feature of SCLC versus NSCLC is the more common expression of neuro-endocrine markers. These markers include such enzymes as neuron-specific enolase and L-dopa decarboxylase, peptide hormones including gastrin-relasing peptide and arginine vasopressin, and surface markers, such as neural cell adhesion molecule (NCAM). The two peptide hormones mentioned here meet the criteria of autocrine growth factor, which requires the cellular production of a growth-promoting protein for which the producing cell has functional receptors. In the case of gastrin-releasing peptide, there is clear evidence that it is produced and secreted by many SCLC cells and then attaches to its cellular membrane receptors, thereby stimulating further cellular growth (11). There are murine monoclonal antibodies which have been developed against the gastrin-releasing peptide and which are undergoing clinical testing at this time (12). Such an antibody could potentially block this autocrine growth cycle function. A murine monoclonal antibody against NCAM which was linked with a toxin has also undergone early clinical testing for patients with recurrent SCLC and has been found to be feasible and worthy of further development (12).

Clinical Manifestations/Patient Evaluation/Staging

The presentation of patients with SCLC differs somewhat from those with NSCLC. These differences include: (1) fewer cases of SCLC diagnosed by imaging of asymptomatic patients; (2) a shorter time from first thoracic symptoms to life threatening symptoms; and (3) the occasional presentation of SCLC with paraneoplastic symptoms. Signs and symptoms from either SCLC or NSCLC depend on the location and bulk of the primary tumor, its nodal extension, and/or its metastatic disease. Because of the high frequency of nodal involvement with SCLC cases, patients frequently present with such symptoms as dyspnea, dysphagia, horseness, and superior vena cava syndrome. As with NSCLC, many SCLC patients present with other thoracic symptoms, including cough, hemoptysis, chest pain, as well as weight loss.

SCLC is the most common solid tumor to have a number of associated paraneoplastic syndromes. Several of these are endrocrinologic, and several are neurologic. The most common endrocrinologic syndrome is the syndrome associated with inappropriate secretion of antidiuretic hormone (SIADH). This condition results from the excessive secretion of ADH from tumor tissue, leading to severe hyponatremia with resultant hypo-osmality. SIADH occurs in 11-46% of SCLC patients and typically resolves after response to anti-cancer therapy (13). Two less common endrocrinologic syndromes are the atrial natriuretic peptide (ANP) syndrome, which can produce hyponatremia, natriuresis, and hypotension, and the ectopic ACTH production syndrome resulting in Cushingoid symptoms. The former occurs in about 15% of SCLC cases and responds to therapy, while the latter occurs in 5% of cases and is associated with a poor prognosis (14).

The neurologic syndromes associated with SCLC include the Lambert-Eaton syndrome, the cerebellar degeneration syndrome, encephalomyelitis, sensory neuropathy, and cancer-associated retinopathy. Each of these is observed in well under 5% of all SCLC patients. Patients with Lambert-Eaton syndrome present with myasthenia gravis-like symptoms of proximal myopathy, autonomic dysfunction and hyporeflexia. Like many paraneoplastic syndromes, this condition is improved with response to anti-cancer therapy, although there can be symptomatic responses to anti-myasthenia therapies (15). The other neurologic syndromes are thought to be primarily autoimmune phenomena and respond poorly to cancer therapy (16,17). Table 1 summarizes these SCLC-associated syndromes.

SCLC can be diagnosed via histology or cytology. In most cases, a diagnosis can be obtained via sputum expectoration or bronchoscopic technique. Occasionally, transthoracic fine aspiration is required, and less frequently, mediastinoscopy or thoracotomy. Cytologic techniques have improved sufficiently that bronchoscopic brush technique can usually distinguish SCLC from NSCLC, as can the needle aspirate from a transthoracic needle. Once the diagnosis of SCLC is established, there is not the need for additional invasive mediastinal staging as there sometimes is for NSCLC. There is due to the limited role of surgical resection in management.

The IUCC/American Joint Commission on Cancer (AJCC) has modified its staging system for bronchogenic cancer in 1996 (18). This system has been universally adopted for staging patients with NSCLC but is less frequently employed for SCLC. Instead, the 1973 Veterans Administration Lung Cancer Study Group's recommended staging of "limited" versus "extensive" is more commonly used, despite its considerable imprecision (19). The initial definition of limited disease was an extent of intrathoracic disease emcompassable within a "reasonable" radiation field. Such a vague definition allows for many interpretations, which have ranged from patients with ipsilateral pleural effusions and contralateral mediastinal, supraclavicular, and hilar adenopathy to only those without effusions and with ipsilateral adenopathy. Investigators in recent years have recognized the dangers of variable interpretations, and recent North American cooperative group trials require staging of all SCLC patients with the standard UICC TNM system prior to study entry.

Approximately two-thirds of SCLC patients have "extensive" stage or Stage IV disease at presentation. This figure is increased from approximately 50% in the 1970's and 1980's, in part due to the greater sensitivity of screening techniques for metastatic disease. One of the principal goals of staging is to distinguish Stage III from Stage IV patients. This evaluation would typically include a contrast-enhanced CT of the thorax and upper abdomen, a bone scan, and either a CT or MRI scan of the brain. In addition, serum studies would include a complete blood count with differential and a complete chemistry screening panel. If all of the above studies reveal no metastatic disease beyond regional nodal sites, then bilateral bone marrow aspirates and biopsies should be performed. If all of these investigations confirm that the patient has locally advanced or limited-stage SCLC (L-SCLC), the patient should also undergo pulmonary function testing to confirm his/her ability to tolerate aggressive thoracic radiotherapy (TRT).

Investigators need to be cautioned regarding the influence of better staging on the interpretation of survival results. If, for example, many patients previously thought to have L-SCLC are "upstaged" to the extensive disease category because of more sensitive screening, it is likely that their inclusion in the extensive disease group and their exclusion from the L-SCLC category will improve survival rates in both groups. This effect is known as the "Will Rogers phenomenon" and was first described in oncology among patients with SCLC. One method of reducing the statistical distortions of the "Will Rogers" phenomenon is to compare survival outcome of entire populations rather than on a stage-by-stage basis. The best method of controlling for this effect is to conduct randomized trials, as has been successfully done for this disease many times.

There have been several efforts to identify other prognostic factors than staging as a means to better select patients for specific therapies. As with many malignancies, good performance status, young age, and female gender are associated with better prognosis, and these have been verified in most large multivariate analyses (20-22). Among available laboratory tests, elevated lactate dehydrogenase (LDH) serum levels were most commonly associated with a poor prognosis, and hyponatremia and low albumin were found in several studies to be independent adverse prognostic factors. The metastatic site found to be most unfavorable was the liver. While such studies are valuable in understanding a disease, such analyses are confounded by the extent and quality of imaging evaluation, the available therapies, and the selection of variables tested. Risk categories have been created by two different British groups in which prognostic factors such as performance status and several laboratory tests such as LDH, alkaline phosphatase, and sodium level have pretreatment prognostic significan (21,22). Currently, these categories are infrequently used at this time in clinical trial design.

Primary Therapy of Limited Stage SCLC

Decisions regarding optimal therapy of patients with limited stage-SCLC must consider a patient's pulmonary and cardiac fitness, ability to tolerate specific chemotherapeutic agents, prior history of malignancies and their treatment, as well as patient age and performance status. Since the diagnosis of limited stage disease by definition implies the potential ability to receive an aggressive course of thoracic radiotherapy, such treatment should by definition be feasible as a component of therapy. The issues discussed below have generally been studied in trials involving patients with an ambulatory performance status, no prior anti-cancer therapy, and acceptable pulmonary, cardiac, renal, and hepatic function. How these principles can be applied to patients not meeting those criteria should be determined on an individual basis.

While performance status is an important prognostic factor among SCLC patients, it is important to recognize that a decline in performance status may be related other factors than the malignancy. With the help of pulmonary physicians or other caregiviers, a patient suffering from treatable conditions such as tracheobronchitis, pneumonia, or an exacerbation of chronic obstructive lung disease can improve his or her performance status prior to the initiation of therapy. Such an improvement may in turn increase the likelihood of tolerating and benefitting from aggressive multi-modality therapy. Recent weight loss among patients with a lung malignancy is usually considered a symptom of cancer-related cachexia and thought to be only reversible with a response to anti-cancer therapy. However, there can be more easily reversible causes of weight loss among these patients, including problems with dentition or dentures, oral candidiasis, thoracic pain requiring analgesia, or gastro-esophageal reflux. Management of these problems is also likely to improve a patient's tolerance of therapy.

Use of Thoracic Radiation

After the demonstration in the late 1960's of activity of several chemotherapeutic agents and the poor prognosis of patients treated with surgery and/or radiation, multi-agent chemotherapy became the primary therapy for all stages of SCLC (23,24). After the recognition that recurrences inevitably occurred after response to chemotherapy and most commonly at sites of initial bulk disease, the use of thoracic RT during or following chemotherapy particularly for patients with limited stage disease regained favor (25,26). A series of randomized trials have now been completed comparing chemotherapy alone to chemotherapy with thoracic RT (27-30). Two meta-analysis of these and other trials published in 1992 demonstrated a statistically significant survival advantage associated with the use of thoracic RT (30-31). In the analysis published by Pignon et al (30), a total of thirteen randomized trials testing chemotherapy with versus without thoracic radiation were evaluated among 2,140 patients. There was a 3-year survival rate of 8.9% for chemotherapy alone versus 14.3% for those receiving both chemotherapy and radiation (p=0.001). This 5.4 % difference in relatively long-term survival results in more than 50% increase in survivorship at 3 years. The benefit of thoracic radiotherapy for younger patients (less than age 55) was even more substantial. In addition, the intrathoracic tumor control rate was nearly 30% less in the radiotherapy-containing arms as opposed to chemotherapy alone arms. This benefit occurred despite a variable quality of radiotherapy and radiotherapy quality control in many of these trials, inadequate total RT doses in many trials, and the use of earlier and less effective chemotherapy regimens than are presently available.

Sequencing and Timing of Thoracic RT and Chemotherapy

Chemotherapy and thoracic RT have been delivered either concurrently, sequentially, or in an alternating manner. The advantages of concurrent delivery include the shorter overall treatment time, an increase in overall treatment intensity, and potential anti-cancer syngerism between the various therapies. Disadvantages include the heightened risk of toxicity, particularly esophagitis, pneumonitis, and myelosuppression and the inability to assess the anti-tumor response rate of the chemotherapy alone. Since the majority of trials testing TRT with chemotherapy cited in the meta-analysis listed above employed concurrent chemotherapy and radiation, there has been motivation to test the optimal timing of TRT when administered during chemotherapy.

There have been at least six randomized trials addressing the issue of timing of concurrent thoracic RT (27,32-36). Three of these trials employed older alkylator- or doxorubicin-based chemotherapy, and the three more recent studies involved etoposide and cisplatin or etoposide and carboplatin. In an older trial conducted by the Cancer and Leukemia Group B from 1981 to 1984, 426 L-SCLC patients were treated with cyclophosphamide (C), etoposide (E) or doxorubicin (A), and vincristine (V) and randomized to: (1) no radiotherapy; (2) RT starting during cycle 1 of chemotherapy; or (3) RT starting during cycle 4 (27). Total thoracic RT dose in both arms was 50 Gy delivered over 6 weeks. There was a survival advantage favoring arms 2 and 3 over the no radiotherapy arm, with the best results achieved in arm 3. The 5-year survival rates were 3% for chemotherapy alone, 7% for early radiation, and 13% for delayed RT. One criticism of this trial is that the doses of chemotherapy in arm 2 are intentionally reduced to lessen the risk of heightened toxicity during concurrent TRT early in a chemotherapy program. In the other two older trials, no significant survival differences were noted between patients receiving TRT beginning day 1 or day 120 (35) or week 1 or week 18 (34).

All three of the trials employing etoposide and a platinating agent demonstrated a survival advantage to earlier versus delayed concurrent thoracic RT. A National Cancer Institute of Canada trial compared thoracic RT (40 Gy/15 fractions/3 weeks) applied during cycle 2 versus during cycle 6 of an alternating chemotherapy regimen of CAV and cisplatin-etoposide (32). A survival advantage was noted for the patients randomized to cycle 2 radiotherapy, with MST's of 16 versus 12 months and four-year survival rates of 25 versus 15%. The Japanese Clinical Oncology Group randomized L-SCLC patients to either TRT beginning with cycle 1 versus 4 of cisplatin and etoposide chemotherapy (33). There was a significant survival advantage favoring the earlier TRT, with MST's of 31 versus 21 months, respectively. These two trials and the Yugoslavian study from Jeremic, et al (36) employing carboplatin and etoposide support the concept that the current standard of care for patients with limited stage SCLC involves etoposide, a platinum compound, and the early application of concurrent thoracic RT.

There have also been at least three trials comparing post-chemotherapy TRT to no TRT for L-SCLC patients who have experienced a complete or partial response to chemotherapy. One of these trials, conducted by the Northern California Oncology Group, compared TRT versus no TRT among responders to a non-cisplatin containing regimen of alternating chemotherapy (37). There was a statistically significant difference in intrathoracic failure patterns (58% versus 29%) favoring the TRT-containing arm but no difference in survival results. The two other trials, conducted by the Southwest Oncology Group and the French "Petite Cellules" failed to demonstrate a survival benefit with the use of consolidative TRT following achievement of a complete response to chemotherapy (38,39).

Alternating chemotherapy with TRT has been tested in a series of French trials, in which induction chemotherapy precedes the temporal alternation between chemotherapy cycles and portions of a split course TRT course (38,43). The appeal of this approach is the potential reduction in toxicity due to the concurrent delivery of therapies. Despite escalating of the total RT dose from 45 to 55 and to 65 Gy, there does not appear to be an advantage to this approach in terms of either tumor control or treatment-related toxicity. Many investigators have objected to the treatment interruptions in radiotherapy delivery inherent in any alternating therapy regimen.

In summary, there is no evidence to support delaying TRT until after the completion of an L-SCLC patient's chemotherapy program. Based on available evidence, it would appear that the "therapeutic window" of opportunity for the thoracic radiotherapy to improve survival includes the period of chemotherapy administration. There is less certainty regarding the optimal timing of TRT during chemotherapy. Evidence favors its earlier use based on the Canadian and Japanese trials demonstrating a survival benefit of earlier over delayed concurrent TRT and the confounding factor of unequal chemotherapy doses in one trial (CALGB) favoring delayed over earlier concurrent TRT. A review by Murray of all randomized and non-randomized trials investigating concurrent TRT and chemotherapy for L-SCLC concluded that the optimal time to begin TRT is within six weeks of the start of chemotherapy (40). He postulated that a greater delay than this might increase the risk of accelerated tumor repopulation and the development of a treatment-resistant tumor clone. Early concurrent RT, meaning starting during the first two cycles of chemotherapy, has been adopted as the standard approach in most currently active institutional and multi-institutional trials within North America. There may be reason to delay the initiation of concurrent TRT beyond the second chemotherapy cycle for patients with a large tumor and/or impaired pulmonary function or those with post-obstructive atelectasis, for whom the margins of tumor definition are difficult to determine. A response to two cycles of chemotherapy may allow such patients to receive a more appropriate course of TRT than would have been possible prior to chemotherapy.

Thoracic RT Dose

Small cell lung cancer is considered a relatively radioresponsive malignancy. Because of that, relatively low total doses of TRT have previously been employed and produced encouraging tumor responses. Total TRT doses for L-SCLC have ranged from 25-30 Gy in 10 fractions in the 1970's to up to 60 Gy in 30-33 fractions in recent years. While doses in the lower end of this range may have been acceptable at a time when chemotherapy was more inadequate and progressive disseminated disease occurred early in most patient's disease course, the improvement in systemic therapy has increased the need for more aggressive TRT regimens. This is mainly due to the longer period of time in which patients are at risk for loco-regional relapse and the need to more effectively reduce the risk of progression and/or relapse at the site of initial bulky disease. It was estimated by Choi, et al that the risk of intrathoracic tumor recurrence at total doses $\leq$ 40 Gy is 80% (41), and this was confirmed in an NCIC L-SCLC trial in which patients were randomized between 25 Gy in 10 fractions and 37.5 Gy in 15 fractions (40). The 2-year actuarial rates of local tumor failure in that study were 80 and 69%, respectively. Such estimates depend on how local tumor failure is defined, particularly in a disease where complete imaging clearance is rare and in which post-treatment imaging changes can be confused with progressive disease.

The most commonly administered total TRT dose currently ranges from 45 to 54 Gy in 1.8 to 2.0 Gy daily fractions. While a RT dose response can be well demonstrated for tumor control below 40 Gy, it is difficult to conclusively establish an RT dose to tumor control relationship between 40 to 60 Gy in standard fractionation. Most randomized and non-randomized trials estimate the local tumor control rates in that dose range as between 58 and 85% (43-46). A single institution trial from Yale New Haven Hospital reported a local tumor control rate of 96% with a total RT dose in excess of 60 Gy (47). The CALGB conducted a phase I dose escalation of standard fractionation and found that a dose of over 70 Gy was the maximal tolerated dose (48). That trial was not designed to detect a difference in tumor control rates but demonstrated that total doses above the usual range of L-SCLC doses could be tested in subsequent trials. In summary, there is currently inadequate information available to recommend that total RT doses in excess of 54-56 Gy in once-daily fractionation be administered outside of a clinical trial. However, the Intergroup randomized trial summarized below clearly illustrates the inadequate tumor control achieved with intermediate total RT doses in once-daily fractionation.

Altered Fractionation RT

Another means of intensifying therapy for this disease is via altered radiation fractionation. For L-SCLC patients, most altered fractionation strategies have employed twice-daily fractionation with fraction sizes varying from 1.1 to 1.8 Gy, with total doses ranging from 40 to 54 Gy. Most regimens have tested the principle of accelerated hyperfractionation (AHF), in which a twice-daily regimen allows the delivery of a standard total RT dose over a shortened time period. Such a regimen should be benefit patients with rapidly growing tumors with a small shoulder and a steep slope on its radiobiologic cell survival curve. Such is clearly the case for SCLC. In addition, AHF

TRT may increase the response of less radioresponsive variant histology cell lines than standard fractionation RT. A potential disadvantage of this approach is the likelihood of increased esophageal and pulmonary toxicity.

Several encouraging pilot studies led to the development of a national Intergroup trial (0096) testing the concept that accelerated hyperfractionated RT will contribute to improved tumor control for L-SCLC patients. The tested regimen was 45.0 Gy in 1.5 Gy BID fractionation beginning on day 1 of a four-cycle regimen of cisplatin and etoposide. The interfraction interval was 6-8 hours and the number of elapsed days of thoracic RT delivery was 19 to 21. This regimen was piloted by Turrisi et al at the University of Pennsylvania, in which 23 patients received this treatment resulting in a median survival time of 25 months and 5-year survival rate of 36% (49). A subsequent multi-institution phase II trial of the same regimen conducted by ECOG resulted in a 2-year survival rate of 36% (50). These results were considered sufficiently promising to launch a phase III trial in 1988. A total of 419 patients were randomized on Intergroup Trial 0096 between TRT regimens of 45.0 Gy in 1.8 Gy standard fractionation and 45.0 Gy in 30 1.5 Gy twice-daily fractions. In both arms the TRT began on day 1 of a four-cycle course of cisplatin and etoposide. With a minimum follow-up time of 5 years, there is a statistically significant survival advantage among all randomized patients favoring the AHF-RT arm, with 5-year survival rates of 26% versus 16%, respectively (p=0.04 by the log-rank test). The intrathoracic tumor failure rate was 36% for the AHF-RT arm and 52% for the standard RT arm (p=0.06). The principal difference in toxicity was a higher grade 3 esophagitis rate in the AHF-RT arm: 27% versus 11%, respectively (p<0.001) (51). These results are summarized in Table 2. This study confirms the important principle that an intensification of thoracic radiotherapy beyond standard RT can both improve intrathoracic tumor control rates and patient survival. In addition, it has altered the standard of care of L-SCLC patients in the United States and challenges the adequacy of intermediate dose once-daily RT in this disease.

It is of interest that a randomized trial conducted by the North Central Cancer Treatment Group (NCCTG) failed to demonstrate any benefit of a hyperfractionated thoracic RT regimen as compared with standard RT when delivered during the fourth cycle of cisplatin and etoposide chemotherapy (52). This hyperfractionated regimen included a 2.5 week break, resulting in a similar elapsed treatment time as the once-daily regimen. The lack of thoracic RT treatment intensity present in Intergroup trial 0096 may explain the lack of benefit of this regimen.

Thoracic RT Volume

The ability of an L-SCLC patient to tolerate increasing aggressive RT regimens and higher total doses during concurrent chemotherapy is in part related to RT target volume selection (43). In the early 1980's, both CALGB and SWOG authors demonstrated poorer survival when patients were not treated with the recommended large fields employing elective nodal RT (53,54). Mira and Livingston also demonstrated that tumor failures just beyond the margins of the TRT fields when the fields were designed following a response to chemotherapy (55). These reports lend further support for the

Table 2. Summary of Intergroup 0096 Comparing Once- with Twice-daily Thoraic Rt for L-sclc Patients Treated with Concurrent Cisplatin and Etoposide

	Arm 1 (Once-Daily)	*Arm 2 (Twice-Daily)*	*P Value*
Patient Number	206	211	
Med Surv Time (months)	19	23	
2-Yr Survival Rate	41%	47%	
5-Yr Survival Rate	16%	26%	0.04
Failure-Free Survival Rate	24%	29%	0.10
Local Failure Rate	52%	36%	0.06
Simultaneous Local & Distant Failure Rate	23%	6%	0.005
Grade 3 Esophagitis Rate	11%	27%	<0.001

need for generous TRT fields. An example of such a field would be that the RT target volume for a patient with a tumor in the left upper lobe with ipsilateral hilar and mediastinal adenopathy only might include the tumor itself with a 2.0 cm margin, the left and right hilar regions, the mediastinum from the thoracic inlet to at least the subcarinal region, and both supraclavicular regions. Such large fields were in part responsible for the acceptance of a moderate total RT dose as appropriate for SCLC, since the volume irradiated might preclude a substantial increase in dose.

In the 1980-1990's evidence emerged that smaller radiation target volume definition did not adversely influence tumor control among patients receiving concurrent cisplatin-containing chemotherapy. Liengswangwong et al. from the Mayo Clinic studied L-SCLC patients from the Mayo Clinic and the NCCTG with intrathoracic recurrence and found the recurrences to all be contained within the TRT high dose volume, regardless of whether patients were irradiated to the pre-chemotherapy or post-chemotherapy volume (56). A similar conclusion was made by Kies et al from SWOG, who noted no recurrence rate difference between patients randomized to receive wide field (pre-chemotherapy target volume) or reduced field (post-chemotherapy target volume) TRT (57). Brodin et al. from Uppsala also found that most (86%) intrathoracic recurrences occurred "in-field", suggesting inadequate total dose rather than inadequate fields (58). All of these reports support the concept advocated by Lichter and Turissi that reductions in target volumes do not compromise patient outcome and may allow for higher TRT doses to be delivered (43).

The fields employed in the Intergroup trial 0096 for such a patient confined the high dose radiation volume to the tumor with a 1.5 cm. margin, the ipsilateral hilum, and the mediastinum from the thoracic inlet to the subcarinal region. The contralateral hilum and both supraclavicular regions were excluded, and the regions requiring therapy were treated with a smaller margin than defined in previous national trials. These treatment recommendations have been widely adopted in subsequent clinical trials conducted in both North America and Europe.

Chemotherapy Selection and Dosing

The selection of chemotherapeutic agents to combine with TRT for patients with L-SCLC is largely based on trials of multi-agent regimens for E-SCLC. The first generation of therapies for E-SCLC included such alkylating agents as cyclophosphamide. Subsequently the anthracycline doxorubicin was added to multi-agent regimens with improved results. The currently accepted standard chemotherapeutic regimen for both E-SCLC and L-SCLC in the United States is the two drug regimen of etoposide and cisplatin (EP). This regimen was first studied in SCLC in the late 1970's (59), and its efficacy in E-SCLC is comparable to the previously used standard of cyclophosphamide, doxorubicin, and vincristine (CAV) (60). The wide acceptance for this regimen over CAV was initially due to its more manageable toxicity and the ability to stop therapy after four rather than six cycles. The concept of alternating cycles of such regimens as EP and CAV was conceptually attractive and at least one randomized trial demonstrated a survival benefit for E-SCLC patients with alternating regimens as opposed to either regimen alone (61). Despite this, etoposide and cisplatin alone are the standard American chemotherapeutic agents for both E-SCLC and L-SCLC patients. It is worth noting that a particularly popular regimen in Europe is cyclophosphamide, doxorubicin, and etoposide, in part because of its ease of outpatient administration and its lack of platinum-related nephrotoxicity (62).

SWOG was the first group to report a completed trial of concurrent TRT with etoposide and cisplatin for L-SCLC. This trial reported a MST of 17.5 months and 4-year survival rate of 30%, which appeared substantially superior to the previously reported results with TRT combined with CAV and other non-platinum containing regimens (63). In addition, the pulmonary, cardiac, and cutaneous risks of combining EP with TRT were believed to be lower than with CAV or other anthracycline-containing regimens. Additional promising results were subsequently reported from groups at the University of Pennsylvania (49), the National Cancer Institute (64), and ECOG (50) with TRT and EP and were confirmed in the previously discuss Intergroup Trial 0096 (61). It is important to note that no randomized trial has ever demonstrated the superiority of TRT and EP over any other regimen for L-SCLC, including CAV and TRT. It remains uncertain to what to extent stage migration played in the apparent improvement in survival of L-SCLC patients from the early 1980's to the early to mid 1990's.

There have also been a series of clinical trials evaluating chemotherapy dose intensity and its influence on survival and response rate for SCLC. Most standard chemotherapeutic regimens employ doses ranging from 75-90% of the maximum tolerated dose. A meta-analysis of survival of both L-SCLC and E-SCLC patients treated in this dose range with EP, CAV, and CAV with etoposide failed to demonstrate an overall dose response in this range (65). One small trial in which patients were randomized to 50% dose levels of CCNU and cyclophosphamide (with methotrexate) versus standard doses of all three agents did establish a detrimental effect on survival of such a dose reduction (66). While no benefit has been observed when higher chemotherapy doses are employed against E-SCLC, two randomized trials for L-SCLC have demonstrated a survival benefit to higher chemotherapy doses. One of these trials was conducted by ECOG and has only been published in abstract form without information on the use of TRT (67), while the other trial is a French multi-center trial which randomized patients to standard versus higher doses of cisplatin and cyclophosphamide in cycle 1 in addition to fixed does of doxorubicin and etoposide (68). Chemotherapy and TRT were delivered in an alternating fashion, and the overall survival was superior for those patients who received the higher cisplatin and cyclophosphamide doses in cycle 1 (p=0.01). Based on these L-SCLC studies, physicians usually deliver chemotherapy, with early concurrent TRT, at doses close to the maximal tolerated dose as feasible.

New Agents

Because standard doses of EP chemotherapy are less myelosuppressive as CAV or other SCLC regimens, investigators have tested the addition of a third agent to this regimen. The alkalating agent ifosfamide has been added to EP and was demonstrated in one randomized trial to improve survival among E-SCLC (69). This was not the case in an RTOG phase II study (93-12) of L-SCLC patients in which ifosphamide was added to the established Intergroup 0096 EP and AHF-RT regimen (70). In that trial the median survival time was quite similar to the Intergroup 0096 results, however the 2-year locoregional regional tumor control rate of 80% was enocuraging. Paclitaxel, a tubulin toxin, has also been added to EP for E-SCLC with encouraging phase II results (72). Results from a recently completed phase II RTOG trial evaluating the addition of paclitaxel to EP and AHF-RT for L-SCLC demonstrated a promising estimated one-year survival rate of 83%, with further follow-up necessary (71). In addition paclitaxel and carboplatin have been evaluated in phase II trials and are currently being tested against EP in a phase III trial for E-SCLC (73). A phase II trial of paclitaxel, oral etoposide, carboplatin and concurrent TRT for 41 patients with limited stage SCLC demonstrated a response rate of 98%, with further follow-up needed (74).

There are several other chemotherapeutic agents with demonstrated activity against SCLC for which further investigation is warranted. These include the vinca alkaloid vinorelbine, the topoisomerase I inhibitors topotecan and irinotecan, the nucleotide analogue gemcitabine, and other taxane derivatives, including docetaxel (75-79). There has been acceptance in the United States that it is both ethical and appropriate that regimens containing new agents be tested in newly diagnosed E-SCLC patients (80). Agents are typically tested with TRT for L-SCLC only after promising results are obtained among E-SCLC patients. A phase III trial demonstrating a survival benefit of the addition of irinotecan to cisplatin and etoposide for ES-SCLC has heightened interest in testing this agent among L-SCLC patients (81).

Role of Surgery

The use of surgical resection as primary management of SCLC was abandoned by the 1970's when poor survival rates were reported and few complete resections were achieved (82). There have been several indications for surgical intervention evaluated since that time, including: the management of patients with N0 or N1 lesions with surgical resection followed by chemotherapy or chemoradiation, the resection of residual disease following chemotherapy or chemoradiation, and the role of surgical salvage of intrathoracic recurrences of SCLC. This section will briefly review each of those issues.

In a report by the Veterans Administration Surgical Oncology Group published in 1982, 5-year survival rates for patients with resected T1N0, T1 N1, and T2N0 SCLC lesions were 60%, 31%, and 28%, respectively (83). All of these patients received chemotherapy as available in the 1970's post-operatively. A SWOG protocol enrolled fifteen SCLC patients to undergo surgical resection followed by chemoradiation and found this group to have a better 2-year survival rate than a cohort of matched patients treated non-operatively in other SWOG trials (45% versus14%) (84). Ichinose et al reported on 112 SCLC patients who underwent surgical resection and were then randomized between two chemotherapy regimens (85). While the chemotherapy regimens produced comparable outcomes, the 3-year survival rates were encouraging for all enrolled patients: 65% for N0 disease, 52% for N1 disease, and 29% for N2 disease. Each of these three reports suggests that for the rare SCLC patients with N0 or N1 disease, surgical resection followed by chemotherapy produces survival results which may be superior to any available non-operative approaches. The role of post-operative TRT in addition to chemotherapy in this setting remains uncertain. A pattern of failure study of patients with completely resected SCLC receiving post-operative chemotherapy alone may clarify this issue.

There are at least 4 studies evaluating the role of surgical resection of patients with L-SCLC following initial chemotherapy. In the three phase II trials conducted at Vanderbilt, University of Toronto, and on a multi-institutional basis, a post-chemotherapy pathologic N0 status or a pathologic complete response was associated with long-term survival (86-88). A randomized trial was conducted by the Lung Cancer Study Group in which L-SCLC patients achieving a partial or complete response to chemotherapy were randomized between resection and no resection (89). There was no survival difference between the arms, with a two-year survival rate of 20% in both arms (p=0.55). Based on this trial and on the clear survival benefit of concurrent TRT given early in a patient's course, adjuvant surgery following chemotherapy is not recommended.

There is limited information regarding the role of surgical resection of intrathoracic recurrences. Shepherd et al. from the University of Toronto reported on 28 L-SCLC patients who underwent salvage surgery following either a partial response to chemotherapy or subsequent progressive disease (90). Ten of these 28 had NSCLC elements in their specimen. Their five-year survival rate from the date of surgical salvage was 23%. There is only anecdotal information of surgical salvage of patients initially treated with both chemotherapy and TRT.

Prophylactic Cranial Irradiation

Prophylactic cranial irradiation (PCI) was initially introduced into practice in the 1960's for patients with acute lymphoblastic leukemia and a high risk of leukemic failure in the central nervous system (CNS) (91). It was first tested for patients with SCLC in the 1970's following the recognition that both asymptomatic and symptomatic brain metastases are frequent and that the CNS is a relative sanctuary for most chemotherapeutic agents. The first trials demonstrated a substantial reduction in subsequent disease relapse in the brain, with one randomized trial of over 200 patients conducted by ECOG noting a decrease from 22 to 5% (92). Unfortunately, at the same time, a number of long-term survivors of SCLC were noted to have various neurologic abnormalities, including dementia, and many of these patients had had PCI (93,94). The lack of prospective evidence linking PCI to these changes as well as the uncertainty as to the optimal total PCI dose and fractionation and its optimal time of delivery contributed to a confused and controversial status for PCI.

There have now been two large randomized trials evaluating both the therapeutic benefit and neurotoxicity of PCI for SCLC patients following response to initial therapy. In two French trials jointly coordinated to run parallel (PCI 85 and PCI 88), a total of 505 patients were randomized between PCI and no PCI following a complete response to chemotherapy (95). The majority of patients received 24.0 Gy in eight 3.0 Gy fractions. There was a highly significant reduction in overall and isolated brain relapse rates favoring the PCI-containing arms (40% vs 59% and 39% vs 57%, respectively, p<0.0001) and a non-significant trend toward improved survival at 2 years (31% vs 27%, p=.10). There was a slight increase in clinical asymptomatic imaging abnormalities but no significant CNS morbidity reported.

Gregor et al. reported on a 314 patient multi-center trial conducted in the United Kingdom (UK02) which randomized L-SCLC patients in remission after completion of chemotherapy between PCI and no PCI (96). Forty percent of the PCI patients received 30.0 Gy in ten fractions , and other regimens ranged from 8 Gy in one fraction to 36.0 Gy in eighteen fractions. At two-year follow-up, a reduction in brain relapse was seen for the PCI arm from 52% to 29% (p=0.0002). The advantage was strongest for the patients receiving the higher PCI doses, particularly 36.0 Gy in eighteen fractions. There was also a non-significant trend in overall survival outcome favoring the PCI arm (p=0.14). Detailed neuropsychometric testing of both PCI patients and controls failed to demonstrate a substantial treatment-related deficit. There was, however, substantial impairment of function in up to 40% of patients prior to PCI, suggesting that factors other than PCI may contribute to neurologic dysfunction among some SCLC patients. Table 3 summarizes both the French and United Kingdom trials.

Table 3. Summary of Recent Randomized Trials of Prophylactic Cranial Irradiation for Sclc Patients

Trial	PCI Dose	Outcome		
PCI 85 & 88	24 Gy/8 Fractions	Less Brain Metastases with PCI:	41 vs 59%	P<0.0001
(Arriagada Ref 88)	(Most)	Less Isolated Brain Metastases with PCI:	39 vs 57%	P<0.0001
		2-Yr Survival Rate Not Different	31 vs 27%	P=0.1
UK02 (Gregor)	36 Gy/18 Fractions	Less Brain Metastases with PCI	29 vs 52%	P=0.0002
	24 Gy/12 Fractions	PCI Dose Response between 24 and 36 Gy		
	30 Gy/10 Fractions	No Neuropsychometric Testing Differences		
	8 Gy/ 1 Fraction			

In addition, a meta-analysis was conducted evaluating 987 SCLC patients entered into seven randomized trials comparing PCI to observation among complete responders to initial therapy (97). There was a 16% reduction in mortality and a 5.4 % increase in 3-year survival rate favoring the PCI arm. A statistically significant PCI dose response was noted for the risk of intracranial tumor recurrence but not survival. Neurotoxicity was not evaluated in this analysis.

Based on the currently available data, it is recommended that SCLC patients achieving a complete or near-complete response to initial therapy should be evaluated for prophylactic cranial irradiation. While further definition of optimal dose is required, there is emerging evidence that total PCI doses above the commonly administered 25.0 Gy in ten fractions may yield the best therapeutic ratio.

Management of Recurrent SCLC

The prognosis of any patient suffering a recurrence of SCLC is grave, regardless of the site(s) of relapse. While there are responses noted to second line chemotherapy such as topotecan, paclitaxel, and re-treatment with platinum-based therapy, these responses are usually short-lived and often precede rapid tumor progression. Palliative or salvage radiation or re-irradiation can be of substantial benefit to such patients, with a higher likelihood of palliative benefit than observed with most solid tumors.

TREATMENT ALGORITHM/CONTROVERSIES/ CLINICAL TRIALS

Limited Stage Disease, Good Performance Status

Management of patients with small cell lung cancer is highly dependent on patient stage and medical fitness. For patients with good performance status and limited stage disease (clinical stages I-IIIB, excluding those with a malignant pleural effusion), the recommended management would be concurrent thoracic RT with platinum-based chemotherapy. Specifically, the most widely accepted management in the United States in 1999 would include 4 cycles of cisplatin and etoposide chemotherapy with twice-daily thoracic RT beginning on day 1. The twice-daily RT would be delivered in 1.5 Gy fractions with an interfraction interval of 6-8 hours to a total dose of 45.0 Gy, with ten of the thirty fractions sparing the spinal cord. This recommendation is based on the recently published Intergroup 0096 trial. For patients with post-obstructive pneumonia or atelectasis, there may be value in delaying the initiation of thoracic RT until the second or third cycle of chemotherapy.

Limited Stage Disease, Lower Performance Status

Lower PS patients tolerate the aggressive twice-daily thoracic RT and platinum-based therapy more poorly than better PS patients. However, there is still a likely benefit to concurrent chemoradiation for these patients, particularly if their reduced functional status is primarily due to their tumor burden. One reasonable option would be to deliver once-daily thoracic RT in 1.8 Gy fractions to 50-54 Gy, while sparing the spinal cord above 45 Gy. This could be delivered beginning with the first or second cycle of platinum-based chemotherapy.

Prophylactic Cranial Irradiation

PCI should be considered for any SCLC patient who has achieved a complete response or >90% response of all evaluable disease following initial management with chemotherapy or chemoradiation and without evidence of disease progression elsewhere. The recommended dose is currently 25 Gy in ten 2.5 Gy fractions.

Controversies/Clinical Trials

Several issues likely to be the subject of clinical trials over the next several years include: the benefit of accelerated hyperfractionated thoracic RT versus higher total dose RT with standard fractionation; the value of new chemotherapeutic agents in the management of limited stage SCLC; and the optimal dose-fraction regimen for PCI.

While the benefit of accelerated hyperfractionated RT versus standard RT to 45 Gy is now established, there may be no advantage of this regimen as compared with a higher total dose of once-daily RT. Such regimens are now under pilot study within the CALGB, and SWOG. Results from the recently completed ECOG phase II study evaluating the addition of paclitaxel to EP as well as increasing the dose of TRT to 63 Gy with fractions given once daily, did not appear to demonstrate superior results to that of the AHF-RT regimen in the Intergroup 0096 study (98).

There are now several new agents under evaluation in both extensive disease and limited disease patients as substitutes for cisplatin and etoposide. These include irinotecan, carboplatin, paclitaxel, and topotecan. There is one active phase III trial comparing carboplatin and paclitaxel to cisplatin and etoposide, and there is an ongoing Intergroup trial comparing cisplatin and etoposide with versus without paclitaxel. Both of these trials are studying these agents without thoracic RT for extensive stage patients. While it is likely that carboplatin will substitute in future trials for cisplatin, the additional benefit of taxane and/or topoisomerase-inhibiting chemotherapy in this disease remains uncertain.

REFERENCES

1.   Greenlee RT, Murray T, Bolden S, Wingo PA. Cancer statistics, 2000. CA: A Cancer Journal for Clinicians 50:7-33, 2000.
2.   Green, RA, Humprey, E, Close, H, et al. Alkylating agents in bronchogenic carcinoma. Am J Med 49:360-367, 1969.
3.   Hirsch, FR, Matthews, MJ, Aisner, S, et al. Histopathologic classification of small cell lung cancer: Changing concepts and terminology. Cancer 62:973-977, 1988.
4.   Hibi, K, Takahashi, T, Yamakawa, K, et al. Three distinct regions involved in 3p deletion in human lung cancer. Oncogene 7:445-449, 1992.
5.   Sozzi, G, Veroneses, ML, Negrini, M, et al. The FHIT gene at 3p14.2 is abnormal in lung cancer. Cell 85:17-26, 1996.
6.   Harbour, JW, Lai, SL, Whang-Peng, J, et al. Abnormalities in structure and expression of the human retinoblastoma gene in SCLC. Science 241:353-357, 1988.
7.   Gazdar, AF. Molecular markers for the diagnosis and prognosis of lung cancer. Cancer 69:1592-1599, 1992.
8.   Ben-Ezra, JM, Kornstein, MJ, Grimes, MM, et al. Small cell carcinomas of the lung express Bcl-2 protein. Am J pathol 145:1036-1040, 1994.
9.   Slebos, RJO, Kribbalaar, RE, Dadesic, O, et al. K-ras oncogene activation as a prognostic marker in adenocarcinoma of the lung. N Engl J Med 323:561-565, 1990.
10. Gazdar, A. The molecular and cellular basis of human lung cancer. Anticancer Res 13:261-268, 1994.
11. Kelly, MJ, Linnoila, RI, Avis, IL, et al. Antitumor activity of a monoclonal antibody directed against gastrin-releasing peptide in patients with small cell lung cancer. Chest 112:256-261, 1997.
12. Johnson, BE, Kelly, MJ. Autocrine growth factors and neuroendocrine markers in the development of small cell lung cancer. Oncology 12:11-14 (S1), 1998.
13. List, AF, Hainsworth, JD, Devis, BV, et al. The syndrome of inappropriate secretion of antidiuretic hormone (SIADH) in small cell lung cancer. J Clin Oncol 4:1191-1198, 1986.
14. Dimopoulos, MA, Fernandez, JF, Samaan, NA, et al. Paraneoplastic Cushing's syndrome as an adverse prognostic factor in patients who die early with small cell carcinoma of the lung. Am J Med 77:851-857, 1984.
15. Patel, AM, Davila, DG, Peters, SG. Paraneoplastic syndromes associated with lung cancer. Mayo Clin Proc 68:278-287, 1993.
16. De La Monte, SM, Hutchins, GM, Moore, GW. Paraneoplastic syndromes and constitutional symptoms in prediction of metastatic behavior of small cell carcinoma of the lung. Am J Med 77:851-857, 1984.
17. Marchioli, CC, Graziano, SL. Paraneoplastic syndromes associated with small cell lung cancer. Chest Surg Clin North Am 7:65-80, 1997.
18. American Joint Committee on Cancer (AJCC). Manual for staging of cancer, 4th ed., pp127-137, Philadelphia, JB Lippincott, 1997.

19. Stahel, RA, Ginsberg, R, Havermann, K, et al. Staging and prognostic factors in small cell lung cancer: A consensus. Lung Cancer 5:119-126, 1989.

20. Albain, KS, Crowley, JJ, LeBlanc, M, et al. Determinants of improved outcome in small cell lung cancer: An analysis of the 2,580-patient Southwest Oncology Group database. J Clin Oncol 8:1563-1574, 1990.

21. Souhami, RL, Bradbury, I, Geddes, OM, et al. Prognostic significance of laboratory parameters measured at diagnosis in small cell carcinoma of the lung. Cancer Res 45:2878-2882, 1985.

22. Cerny, T, Blair, V, Anderson, H, et al. Pretreatment prognostic factors and scoring system in 407 small cell lung cancer patients. Int J Cancer 39:146-149, 1987.

23. Edmondson, JH, Lagakos, SW, Selawry, OS, et al. Cyclophosphamide and CCNU in the treatment of inoperable small cell carcinoma and adenocarcinoma of the lung. Cancer Treatment Rep 60:925-932, 1976.

24. Lowenbraun, S, Bartolucci, A, Smalley, RV, et al. The superiority of combination chemotherapy over single agent chemotherapy in small cell lung carcinoma. Cancer 44:406-413, 1979.

25. Souhami, RI, Geddes, DM, Spiro, SG, et al. Radiotherapy in small cell cancer of the lung treated with combination chemotherapy: A controlled trial. Br J Med 288:1643-1646, 1984.

26. Byhardt, RW, Cox, JD, Holoye, PY, et al. The role of consolidation irradiation in combined modality therapy of small cell carcinoma of the lung. Int J Radiat Oncol Biol Phys 8:1271-1276,1982.

27. Perry, M, Eaton, WC, Propert, KJ, et al. Chemotherapy with or without radiation therapy in limited small-cell lung cancer. N Eng J Med 316:912-918, 1987.

28. Bunn, PA, Lichter, AS, Makuch, RW, et al. Chemotherapy alone or chemotherapy with chest radiation therapy in limited-stage small-cell lung cancer. Ann Intern Med 106:655-662, 1987.

29. Perez, CA, Krauss, S, Bartolucci, AA, et al. Thoracic and elective brain irradiation with concomitant or delayed multiagent chemotherapy in the treatment of localized small cell carcinoma of the lung: a randomized prospective study by the Southeastern Cancer Study Group. Cancer 47:2407-2413, 1981.

30. Pignon, JP, Arrigada, R, Ihde, D. Meta-analysis of small-cell lung cancer. N Eng J Med 327:1618-1624, 1992.

31. Warde, P, Payne, D. Does thoracic irradiation improve survival and local control in limited-stage small cell carcinoma of the lung? A meta-analysis. J Clin Oncol 10:890-895, 1992.

32. Murray, N, Coy, P, Pater, JL, et al. The importance of timing of thoracic irradiation in the combined modality treatment of limited-stage small-cell lung cancer. J Clin Oncol 11:336-344, 1993.

33. Goto, K, Nishiwaki, Y, Takada, M, et al. Final results of a phase III study of concurrent vs sequential thoracic radiotherapy in combination with cisplatin and etoposide for limited stage small-cell lung cancer: The Japan Clinical Oncology Group Study. Proc Am Soc Clin Oncol 18:468a, 1999 (Abstr).

34. Work, E, Nielson, O, Bentzen, S, et al. Randomized study of initial versus late chest irradiation combined with chemotherapy in limited-stage small cell lung cancer. J Clin Oncol 15:3030-3037, 1997.

35. Schultz, HP, Neilson, OS, Sell, A, et al. Timing of chest radiation with respect to combination chemotherapy in small cell lung cancer, limited disease. Lung Cancer 4:153, 1988 (Abstr).

36. Jeremic, B, Shibamoto, Y, Acimovic, L, et al. Initial versus delayed accelerated hyperfractionated radiation therapy and concurrent chemotherapy in limited stage small cell lung cancer: A randomized study. J Clin Oncol 15:893-900, 1997.

37. Carlson, RW, Sikic, BI, Gandara, DR et al. Late consolidative radiation therapy in the treatment of limited-stage small cell lung cancer. Cancer 68;948-958, 1991.

38. Kies, MS, Mira, JG, Crowley, JJ, et al. Multimodal therapy for limited small cell lung cancer: A randomized trial of induction combination chemotherapy with or without thoracic irradiation in complete responders: and with wide field versus reduced field in partial responders: A Southwest Oncology Group Trial. J Clin Oncol 5:592-600, 1987.

39. Lebeau, B, Chastang, C, Brechot, JM, et al. A randomized trial of delayed radiotherapy in complete responder patients with small cell lung cancer. Chest 104:726-733, 1993.

40. Murray, N. Treatment of small cell lung cancer: the state of the art. Lung Cancer 17 Suppl.1:75-89, 1997.

41. Choi, N, Carey, R. Importance of radiation dose in achieving improved loco-regional tumor control in limited stage small cell lung carcinoma: An update. Int J Radiat Oncol Biol Phys 17:307-310, 1989.

42. Coy, P, Hodson, I, Payne, D, et al. The effect of dose of thoracic irradiation on recurrence in patients with limited stage small cell lung cancer. Initial results of a Candian multicenter randomized trial. . Int J Radiat Oncol Biol Phys 14:219-226, 1988.

43. Lichter, AS, Turrisi, AT. Small-cell lung cancer: The influence of dose and treatment volume on outcome. Semin Radiat Oncol 5:44-49, 1995.

44. Papac, RJ, Son, Y, Bien, R, et al. Improved local control of thoracic disease in small cell lung cancer with higher dose thoracic irradiation and cyclic chemotherapy. Int J Radiat Oncol Biol Phys 13:993-998, 1987.

45. Shank, B, Scher, H, Hilaris, BS, et al. Increased survival with high-dose multifield radiotherapy and intensive chemotherapy in limited small cell carcinoma of the lung. Cancer 56:2771-2778, 1985.

46. Komaki, R, Shin, DM, Glisson, BS, et al. Interdigitating versus concurrent chemotherapy and radiotherapy for limited small cell lung cancer/ Int J Radiat Oncol Biol Phys 31:807-811, 1995.

47. Armstrong, J, Shank, B, Scher, H, et al. Limited small cell lung cancer: Do favorable short-term results predict ultimate outcome? Am J Clin Oncol 14:285-290, 1991.

48. Choi, N, Herndon, J, Rosenman, J, et al. Phase I study to determine the maximum tolerated dose of radiation in standard daily and accelerated twice daily

radiotherapy schedules with concurrent chemotherapy for limited stage small lung cancer: CALGB 8837. J Clin Oncol16:3528-3536, 1998.

49. Turrisi, AT, Glover, DJ, Mason, B, et al. Concurrent twice-daily multi-field radiotherapy and platinum-etoposide chemotherapy for limited small-cell lung cancer: Update 1987 (Abstract). Proc Am Soc Clin Oncol 6:172, 1987.

50. Johnson, DH, Turrisi, AT, Chang, AY, et al. Alternating chemotherapy and twice-daily thoracic radiotherapy in limited small cell lung cancer: A pilot study of the Eastern Cooperative Oncology Group. J Clin Oncol 11:879-884, 1993.

51. Turrisi, A, Kim, K, Blum, R, et al. Twice-daily compared with once-daily thoracic radiotherapy in limited small-cell lung cancer treated concurrently with cisplatin and etoposide. N Engl J Med 340:265-71, 1999.

52. Bonner, JA, Slaon, JA, Shanahan, TG, et al. Phase III comparison of twice-daily split-course irradiation versus once-daily irradiation for patients with limited stage small-cell lung cancer. J Clin Oncol 17:2681-2691, 1999.

53. Eaton, W, Maurer, H, Glicksman, A, et al. The relationship of infield recurrences to prescribed tumor dose in small cell carcinoma of the lung. Int J Radiat Oncol Biol Phys 7:1223, 1981 (Abstr).

54. White, J, Chen, R, McCracken, J, et al. The influence of radiation therapy quality control on survival, response, and sites of relapse in oat cell carcinoma of the lung: Preliminary report of a SWOG study. Cancer 50:1084-1090, 1982.

55. Mira, JG, Livingston: Evaluation and radiotherapy implications of chest relapse patterns in small cell lung carcinoma treated with radiotherapy-chemotherapy: Study of 34 cases and review of the literature. Cancer 46:2557-2565, 1980.

56. Liengswangwong, V, Bonner, JA, Shaw, EG, et al. Limited-stage small cell lung cancer: Patterns of intrathoracic recurrence and the implications for thoracic radiotherapy. J Clin Oncol 12:496-502, 1994.

57. Kies, MS, Mira, JG, Crowley, JJ, et al. Multimodal therapy for limited small cell lung cancer: A randomized study of induction combination chemotherapy with or without thoracic radiation in complete responders; and with wide-field versus reduced-field radiation in partial responders: A Southwest Oncology Group study. J Clin Oncol 5:592-600, 1987.

58. Brodin, O, Rikner, G, Steinholtz, L, et al. Local failure in patients treated with radiotherapy and multidrug chemotherapy for small cell lung cancer. Acta Oncol 29:739-746, 1990.

59. Sierocki, JS, Hilaris, BS, Hopfan, S, et al. Cis-dichlorodiammineplatinum (II) and VP-16-213: An active induction regimen for small cell carcinoma of the lung. Cancer Treat Rep 63:1593-1597, 1979.

60. Roth , BJ, Johnson, DH, Einhorn, LH. Randomized study of cyclohosphamide plus doxorubicin plus vincristine versus etoposide plus cisplatin versus alternation of these two regimens in extensive small cell lung cancer: a phase II study of the Southeastern Cancer Study Group. J Clin Oncol 10:282-291, 1992.

61. Fukuoka, M, Furuse, K, Saijo, N. Randomized trial of cyclophosphamide, doxorubicin, and vincristine versus cisplatin and etoposide versus alternation of these regimens in small cell lung cancer. J Nat Cancer Inst 83:855-861, 1991.

62.   Postmus, P, Smit, EF. Small cell lung cancer: Is there a standard therapy? Oncology 12(S2):25-30, 1998.

63.   MacCracken, JD, Janaki, LM, Crowley, JJ, et al. Concurrent chemotherapy/radiotherapy for limited small-cell lung carcinoma: A Southwest Oncology Group study. J Clin Oncol 8:892-898, 1990.

64.   Johnson, BE, Salem, C, Nesbitt, J, et al. Limited stage small cell lung cancer treated with concurrent BID chest radiotherpy and etoposide/cisplatin followed by chemotherapy selected by in vitro drug sensitivity testing. Proc Amer Assoc Clin Oncol 10:240, 1991.

65.   Murray, N. Treatment of small cell lung cancer: the state of the art. Lung Cancer 17 (S1) S75-89, 1997.

66.   Cohen, MH, Creaven, PJ, Fossiak, BE. Intensive chemotherapy of small cell bronchogenic carcinoma. Cancer Treat Rep 9:499-508, 1997.

67.   Mehta, C, Vogl, SE, et al. High-dose cyclophosphamide, doxorubicin, and vincristine for extensive-stage small cell lung cancer: minor improvements in the rate of remission and survival. Proc Am Assoc Cancer Res 23:155, 1982 (Abstr).

68.   LeChevalier, T, Arrigada, R, Pignon, J. Initial chemotherapy doses have a significant impact on survival iin limited small cell lung cancer: Results of a multicentre prospective randomized study in 105 patients. N Engl J Med 329:1848-1852, 1993.

69.   Loehrer, P, Ansari, R, Gonin, R, et al. Cisplatin plus etoposide with and without ifosfamide in extensive stage small cell lung cancer: a Hoosier Oncology Group study. J Clin Oncol 13:2494-2499, 1995.

70.   Glisson, B, Scott, C, Komaki, R, et al. Cisplatin, ifosfamide, prolonged oral etoposide, and concurrent accelerated hyperfractionated thoracic radiotherapy for patients with limited small cell lung cancer: Proc Am Soc Clin Oncol 11:336-344, 1998.

71.   Ettinger, DS, Seiferheld, WF, Abrams, R, et al. Cisplatin, etoposide, paclitaxel, and concurrent hyperfractionated thoracic radiotherapy for patients with limited disease small cell lung cancer: Preliminary results of RTOG 96-09. Proc Am Soc Clin Oncol 19:490a, 2000 (Abstr).

72.   Ettinger, DS, Finkelstein, DM, Sarma, RP, et al. Phase II study of paclitaxel in patients with extensive stage small cell lung cancer: An Eastern Cooperative Oncology Group study. J Clin Oncol 13:1430-1435, 1995.

73.   Hainsworth, JD, Hopkins, LG, Thomas, M, et al. Paclitaxel, carboplatin, and extended-schedule oral etoposide for small cell lung cancer. Oncology 12(S2):31-35, 1998.

74.   Hainsworth, J,Gray, J,Stroup, S, et al. Paclitaxel, carboplatin, and extended-schedule etoposide in the treatment of small-cell lung cancer: Comparison of sequential phase II trials using different dose levels. J Clin Oncol 15:3464-3470, 1997.

75.   Ardizzoni, A, Hansen, H, Dombernowsky, P et al. Topotecan, a new active drug in the second-line treatment of small cell lung cancer: A phase II study in patients with refractory and sensitive disease. J Clin Oncol 15:2090-2096, 1997.

76. Masuda, N, Fukuka, M, Kusunoki, Y, et al. CPT-11: A new derivative of camptothecin for the treatment of refractory or relapsed small cell lung cancer. J Clin Oncol 10:1225-1229, 1992.

77. Smyth, JF, Smith, IE, Seesa, C, et al. Activity of docetaxel (Taxotere) in small cell lung cancer. Eur J Cancer 30A:1058-1060, 1994.

78. Abratt, R, Bezwoda, WR, Goedhals, W, et al. Weekly gemcitabine with monthly cisplatin: Effective chemotherapy for advanced non-small cell lung cancer. J Clin Oncol 15:744-749, 1997.

79. Evans, WK, Radwi, J, Tomiak, E, et al. Oral etoposide and carboplatin: Effective therapy for elderly patients with small cell lung cancer. Am J Clin Oncol 18:149-155, 1995.

80. Ettinger, DS. Evaluation of new drugs in untreated patients with small-cell lung cancer: Its time has come (Comment). J Clin Oncol 8:374-377, 1990.

81. Noda, K, Nishiwaki, Y, Kawahara, S, et al. Randomized phase III study of irinotecan and cisplatin versus etoposide and cisplatin in extensive-disease small-cell lung cancer: Japan Clinical Oncology Group Study (JCOG 9511). Proc Am Soc Clin Oncol 19:482a, 2000 (Abstr).

82. Fox, W, Scadding, JG. Medical Research Council comparative trial of surgery and radiotherapy for primary treatment of small-celled or oat-celled carcinoma of the bronchus: Ten year follow-up. Lancet 2:63-5, 1973.

83. Shields, TW, Higgins, GA, Matthews, MJ, et al. Surgical resection in the management of small cell lung cancer. J Thorac Cardiovas Surg 84:481-488, 1982.

84. Friess, GG, McCracken, JD, Troxell, MJ, et al. Effect of initial resection of small cell carcinoma of the lung: A review of Southwest Oncology Group study 7628. J Clin Oncol 3:9644-968, 1985.

85. Ichonose, Y, Hara, N, Ohta, M, et al. Comparison between resected and irradiated small cell lung cancer in patients in stage I through IIIa. Ann Thorac Surg 53:95-100, 1992.

86. Prager, RL, Foster, JM, Hainsworth, JM, et al. The feasibility of adjuvant surgery in limited stage small cell carcinoma: a prospective evaluation. Ann Thorac Surg 38:622-625, 1984.

87. Shepherd, FA, Ginsberg, RJ, Patterson, GA, et al. A prospective study of adjuvant surgical resection after chemotherapy for limited small cell lung cancer: A University of Toronto Lung Oncology Group study. J Thorac Cardiovasc Surg 97:177-186, 1989.

88. Baker, RR, Ettinger, DS, Ruckdeschel, JD. The role of surgery in the management of selected patients with small cell cancer of the lung. J Clin Oncol 5:697-702, 1987.

89. Lad, T, Piantadosi, S, Thomas, P, et al. A prospective randomized trial to determine the benefit of surgical resection of residual disease following response of small cell llung cancer to combination chemotherapy. Chest 106:320-323, 1994.

90. Shepherd, FA, Ginsberg, R, Patterson, GA, et al. Is there ever a role for salvage operations in limited small cell lung cancer? J Thorac Cardiovasc Surg 101:196-200, 1991.

91. Bleyer, WA, Poplack, DG, et al. Prophylaxis and treatment of leukemia in the central nervous system and other sanctuaries. Semin Oncol 12:131-148, 1985.

92. Gregor, A. Prophylactic cranial irradiation in small cell lung cancer: Is it ever indicated? Oncology 12:19-24, 1998.

93. Johnson, BE, Becker, B, Geoff, WB, et al. Neurologic, neuropsychologic, and computed cranial tomography scan abnormalities in 2 to 10 year survivors of small cell lung cancer. J Clin Oncol 3:1659-1667, 1985.

94. Catane, R, Schwade, JG, Varr, I, et al. Follow-up neurologic evaluation in patients with small cell lung carcinoma treated with prophylactic cranial irradiation and chemotherapy. Int J Radiat Oncol Biol Phys 7:105-109, 1981.

95. Arriagada, R, LeCahvalier, T, Borie, F, et al. Prophlactic cranial irradiation for patients with small cell lung cancer in complete remission. J Nat Cancer Inst 87:183-190, 1995.

96. Gregor, A, Cull, A,Stephens, RJ, et al. Prophylactic cranial irradiation as indicated following complete response to induction therapy in small cell lung cancer: Results of a multicentre randomised trial. Eur J Cancer 33:1752-1758, 1997 (supp 11).

97. Auperin, A, Arriagada, R, Pignon, JP, et al. Prophylactic cranial irradiation in patients with small cell lung cancer in complete remission. N Engl J Med 341:476-484, 1999.

98. Sandler A, Declerck L, Wagner H, et al. A phase II study of cisplatin plus etoposide plus paclitaxel and concurrent radiation therapy for previously untreated limited stage small cell lung cancer (E2596): An Eastern Cooperative Oncology Group Trial. Proc Am Soc Clin Oncol 19:491a, 2000 (Abstr).

TREATMENT OF EXTENSIVE STAGE SMALL CELL LUNG CANCER

Karen Kelly, M.D.
University of Colorado Cancer Center, Denver, CO 80220 USA

INTRODUCTION

Small cell lung cancer (SCLC) is one of the most aggressive and lethal cancers in man (1). In 1999, approximately 40,000 new cases of SCLC were diagnosed in the United States (2). Two-thirds of these patients will have extensive stage disease for which combination chemotherapy is the treatment of choice. Combination chemotherapy has been the cornerstone of treatment for these patients since the 1970's when it was demonstrated that regimens containing multiple agents improved responses and survival as compared to single agents (1).

CURRENT COMBINATION CHEMOTHERAPY REGIMENS

Recent randomized trials in extensive stage SCLC are summarized in Table 1. The most extensively evaluated regimens are CAV (cyclophosphamide, adriamycin, vincristine) and PE (cisplatin and etoposide). Three randomized trials compared CAV to PE or to an alternating sequence of CAV/PE. Evans and his Canadian colleagues enrolled 289 patients with extensive stage SCLC to receive CAV or CAV alternating with PE for 6 cycles (3). Response rates were 63.2% versus 80%, (p<.002) and median survival was 8.0 months versus 9.6 months, (p=.03), respectively favoring the alternating regimen. Survival differences failed to achieve significance when patients with locoregional - only disease were excluded. Roth and the Southeastern Cooperative Study Group (SECSG) completed a trial comparing CAV(6 cycles) versus PE (4 cycles) versus CAV/PE (3cycles each) (4). Approximately 140 extensive stage patients were entered into each arm. The overall response rates were not statistically different at 51%, 61% and 59%, respectively. The median survivals were comparable at 8.3, 8.6, and 8.1 months respectively. Fukuoka et al., completed a similar trial to that of the SECSG but allowed patients with limited stage disease to participate (5). Approximately 97 patients were accrued to each arm. Patients with limited stage SCLC received thoracic radiotherapy after completing the chemotherapy. The objective response rates were superior for PE (78%) and CAV/PE (76%) as compared to 55% for CAV. Median survival was 9.9 months for the CAV, 9.9 months for PE and 11.8 months for CAV/PE (P = .027 compared to CAV and p=.056 compared to PE). When analyzed by stage there was no difference in survival for the patients with extensive stage disease with a median survival of 8-9 months.   Differences in toxicity were apparent in all trials with more frequent myelosuppression, neurotoxicity and cardiac toxicity observed in patients receiving CAV while considerable nausea and vomiting occurred in patients receiving PE (6). Overall, 4 – 6 cycles of PE were as efficacious as CAV or CAV/PE with less toxicity.

Building upon these results, investigators became interested in determining whether higher doses of chemotherapy could overcome drug resistance and further improve survival. Ihde et al., randomized 90 extensive stage patients to receive standard dose cisplatin (80 mg/m^2, day 1) plus etoposide (80 mg/m^2, day 1-3) or high dose cisplatin (27.5 mg/m^2, day 1-5) with etoposide (80 mg/m^2, day 1-5) for 1-2 cycles (7). All patients received standard doses in cycles 3 and 4. There was no difference in response rate (60% vs 61%) or median survival (10.7 vs 11.4 months) respectively (Table 1). However there was statistically more leukopenia, febrile neutropenia, thrombocytopenia and weight loss in the high-dose arm.   Another dose intense regimen that has been commonly used is CAE (cyclophosphamide, adriamycin, and etoposide). In light of the greater myelosuppression produced by this regimen a randomized trial with the addition of G-CSF was conducted. Two hundred and seven patients were randomized to receive either CAE alone ((104 patients) or CAE plus G-CSF (95 patients) (8). The incidence of febrile neutropenia, the incidence, duration and severity of neutropenia, days of intravenous antibiotics and days of hospital stay were all decreased in the arm receiving G-CSF. Outcome was similar between the two arms. The response rate and median survival was 80% and 12.2 months respectively for patients in the CAE group and 72% and 11.4 months, respectively for patients in the CAE plus G-CSF group. Even with G-CSF the dose-intense CAE regimen was considerably more toxic but no more efficacious than PE. Most recently NCI-Canada published their results comparing a dose intense weekly regimen CODE (cisplatin, vincristine, doxorubicin, and etoposide) to CAV/EP (9). One hundred and ten patients received CODE, (cisplatin 25mg/m^2 weekly for 8 weeks, vincristine 1mg/m^2 weeks 1,2,4,6,8, doxorubicin 40 mg/m^2 weeks 1,3,5,7,9 and etoposide 80 mg/m2 IV, day 1 and 80 mg/m^2 PO days 2 and 3, week 1,3,5,7,9 plus supportive drugs including steroids and antibiotics) and 109 patient received the standard CAV/EP regimen. The trial was terminated early due to the higher incidence of toxic deaths in the CODE arm, 8.2% as compared to 0.9% on the CAV/EP arm. Response rates were higher with CODE 87% versus 70% with CAV/EP (p=.006) but overall survival was similar, 11.8 months on the CODE arm and 10.9 months on the CAV/EP arm. The Japanese randomized phase III trial of CODE versus CAV/EP also failed to show a survival advantage for CODE (10). In this study 228 patients with extensive stage SCLC were randomized to CODE with G-CSF or CAV/PE. The objective response rate was 84% for the CODE arm and 77% the CAV/PE arm with median survivals of 11.6 months for CODE and 10.9 months for CAV/PE. Leukopenia was similar in both arms but febrile neutropenia was significantly greater in the CODE group 18.8% versus 8.8% in the CAV/PE group (p=.031). In summary, dose intense regimens do not improve survival over standard therapy but are clearly more toxic. Thus, PE has become the most commonly used regimen to treat patients with SCLC.

Table 1. Randomized Phase III Trials in Extensive Stage SCLC

Author (Ref)	Regimen	# Eval Pts	RR (%)	MS (Months)
Evans	CAV	144	63	8.0
(3)	CAV/PE	145	80[a]	9.6[b]
Roth	CAV	140	51	8.3
(4)	PE	140	61	8.6
	CAV/PE	138	59	8.1
Fukuoka	CAV	97[c]	55	9.9
(5)	PE	97	78	9.9
	CAV/PE	92	76	11.8[d]
Ihde	PE (std)	42	60	10.7
(7)	PE (hd)	39	61	11.4
Crawford	CAE	104	80	12.2
(8)	CAE + G-CSF	95	72	11.4
Murray	CODE	110	87[e]	11.8
(9)	CAV/PE	109	70	10.9
Furuse	CODE + G-CSF	114	84	11.6
(10)	CAV/PE	113	77	10.9
Skarlos	PE	30	60	12.5[f]
(12)	CE	31	69	11.8
Loehrer	PE	84	67	7.3
(13)	VIP	87	73	9.1[g]

Abbreviations: Ref = References; # Eval Pts = Number of evaluable patients; RR = Response rate; MS = Median survival; CAV = Cyclophosphamide, adriamycin, vincristine; PE = cisplatin, etoposide; Std = standard dose; hd = high dose; CAE = cyclophosphamide, adriamycin, etoposide; CODE = cisplatin, vincristine, doxorubicin, etoposide; VIP = etoposide, ifosfamide, cisplatin

a = $p<.002$
b = $p=.03$
c = Includes patients with limited disease
d = CAV/PE vs CAV $p=.027$; CAV/PE vs PE $p=.056$
e = $p=.006$
f = includes 82 patients with limited disease
g = $p=.045$

Carboplatin is highly active in this disease and is less toxic than cisplatin, therefore it was logical to compare cisplatin/etoposide to carboplatin/etoposide (CE) (11). Skarlos et al., randomized 143 patients (82 patients had limited stage disease and 61 patients had extensive stage disease) to cisplatin plus etopside or carboplatin plus etoposide (12). Preliminary data revealed the response rate for patients with extensive stage disease were comparable, 60% for patients receiving cisplatin and 69% for patients receiving carboplatin. Overall survival for the entire group (including the patients with limited disease) was 12.5 months for the PE arm and 11.8 months for the CE arm. Leukopenia, neutropenic infections, nausea, vomiting, neurotoxicity and hypersensitivity reactions were more frequent in the PE group. CE is an active regimen and associated with less toxicity than PE. It is now often employed to treat patients with SCLC.

Ifosfamide is a highly active agent in SCLC. The Hoosier Oncology Group examined the addition of ifosfamide to PE (VIP) in a randomized trial (13). One hundred seventy one extensive stage patients were randomized to receive PE or VIP for 4 cycles. Objective responses were observed in 67% of patients on the PE arm and 73% of patients receiving VIP. The median survival was statistically superior for patients on the VIP arm, 9.1 months versus 7.3 months for PE (p=.045). Myelosuppression was greater on the VIP arm. Although this trial suggests a benefit for VIP, survival in the PE arm was surprisingly low.

MAINTENANCE THERAPY

Several randomized trials have been performed to determine the value of maintenance chemotherapy in patients who respond to 4-6 cycles of chemotherapy. Most trials have included both limited and extensive stage patients but 3 trials were conducted in patients with only extensive stage disease. Ettinger and the Eastern Oncology Cooperative Group (ECOG) randomized 577 evaluable patients to CAV or CAV alternating with hexamethylmelanime, etoposide and methotrexate (HEM) (14). Eighty six patients with a complete response continued to receive the same chemotherapy or observation. Survival was not altered with maintenance therapy although remission duration was prolonged for patients receiving CAV but not CAV-HEM. A smaller randomized trial of four or eight cycles of EVI (etoposide, vincristine, ifosfamide) in 122 patients revealed no survival difference with a median survival of 9 months for patients receiving four cycles versus 7.7 months with eight cycles (15). Most recently a trial was conducted by the Hoosier Oncology Group (HOG). Two hundred twenty eight patients received VIP and 149 nonprogressing patients were randomized to oral etoposide 50 mg/m^2/day for 21 of 28 days for 3 cycles or observation (16). There was a significant improvement in progression-free survival for the patients who received the oral etoposide 5.6 months as compared to 4.5 months for the observation arm (p=.0097) however there was no difference in median survival 11.6 months versus 11.1 months respectively. Toxicity from the maintenance regimen included grade 3 / 4 neutropenia (43%), febrile neutropenia (4%), and thrombocytopenia (21%). These trials do not support the routine use of maintenance chemotherapy for patients with extensive stage SCLC.

In total, 21 phase III trials employing combination chemotherapy have been conducted in patients with extensive stage SCLC during the last two decades. An analysis of these trials revealed a median survival of 7 months during 1972 –1981 which increased to 8.9 months during the time period from 1982 –1990(17). Although we are encouraged by this trend, continued improvement in survival will require evaluation of new chemotherapeutic agents as well evaluating other strategies.

NEW CHEMOTHERAPEUTIC AGENTS FOR SCLC

Today there are several new cytotoxic agents with activity in SCLC as shown in Table 2. The list includes the taxanes (paclitaxel and docetaxel), the topoisomerase I inhibitors (topotecan and irinotecan), gemcitabine and vinorelbine. The current status of these agents in the treatment of SCLC is described below.

Table 2. Phase II Trials of New Cytotoxic Agents in SCLC

<u>Agent</u>	<u># of Studies (Ref)</u>	<u># Eval Pts</u>	<u>RR (%)</u>	<u>MS (Months)</u>
Topotecan	2 (19,20)	6/ 48	33/39	NR/10
	3[S] (21-23)	57/45/96 17/38/26	NR/6.9/NR	
	3[R] (21,22,24)	41/47/25	2/6/12	NR/4.7/NR
Paclitaxel	2 (31,32)	32/37	34/68	11/7.3
Docetaxel	1 (45)	46	26	9
	1* (46)	28	25	NR
Vinorelbine	2 (48,49)	30/6	27/0	NR
	3[S] (50,51,52)	24/25/31	13/16/15	NR
Irinotecan	2 (55,56)	15/8	47/50	6.8/NR
	2* (56,57)	27/32	33/16	NR/4.5
Gemcitabine	1 (61)	25	27	12
	1[R] (62)	36	14	NR

*Abbreviations: # of Studies = Number of studies; Ref = References; # Eval Pts = Number of evaluable patients; RR = Response rate; MS = Median survival; NR = Not reported; R = Resistant relapse; S = Sensitive relapse; * = Previously treated*

Topotecan

Single agent topotecan was the first agent for which two phase III studies have been completed. In Phase I trials myelosuppression was dose-limiting and the recommended dose was 1.5 mg/m^2 IV over 30 minutes for 5 days every 21 days (18). Table II reveals the results from several phase II trials of topotecan. The first trial in 48 untreated patients revealed a partial response (PR) rate of 39% and a median survival of 10 months (19). A smaller trial of only 6 untreated patients reported a response rate of 33% (20). Three trials have been conducted in patients with a sensitive relapse (patients who have relapsed greater than 3 months for their last treatment) (21-23). The response rates varied between 17% and 38% with one trial reporting a median survival of 6.9 months. Three trials have been performed in patients with resistant disease (patients who relapse within 3 months from their last chemotherapy). Response rates ranged from 2 - 12% with one trial observing a 4.7 month median survival time (21,22,24). These encouraging results lead to a randomized phase III comparative trial of topotecan versus CAV in patients who relapsed 60 days or more after completion of first line therapy (25). One hundred seven patients received topotecan and 104 patients received CAV. Response rates, median time to progression and median survival were similar between the two groups (24%, 3.3 months and 6.3 months for the topotecan arm and 18%, 3 months and 6.2 months for the CAV arm, respectively). The incidence of febrile neutropenia was also similar in both arms but more neutropenia, thrombocytopenia and anemia were observed in the topotecan arm (p<0.001). No difference in nonhematological toxicities were noted between the two groups. Symptom relief was greater with topotecan than CAV (p< or =.043). Based on these results the FDA approved topotecan for second-line treatment of patients with sensitive relapse. Meanwhile, topotecan was being evaluated as front line therapy. ECOG recently completed a phase III trial of 4 cycles of PE with subsequent randomization of nonprogressing patients to 4 cycles of topotecan or observation. The oral derivative of topotecan as been studied in patients with extensive stage SCLC ineligible for standard therapy (26). Twenty-eight patients received 1.7 – 2.0 mg/m^2/day for 5 days every 21 days. Responses were seen in 9/25 patients (36%) with 1 complete response (CR). Grade 4 neutropenia developed in 58% of patients and grade 4 thrombocytopenia in 25% of patients. The regimen was active with less myelosuppression than the intravenous formulation. Additional trials are ongoing.

Ardizzoni in his trial of topotecan for second line therapy, documented responses in the brain in 5/7 patients (70%) suggesting that topotecan may be valuable for the treatment of brain metastases (22). A phase II study to further evaluate this observation was performed in 15 patients with symptomatic brain metastases, 8 who had previous whole brain irradiation (27). Six patients (40%) responded with 2 patients achieving a CR (13%). The median duration of response was 75 days. No neurological deterioration was seen. This promising result requires further evaluation.

Trials combining topotecan with other agents are underway (Table 3). An exciting combination is paclitaxel plus topotecan. Jacobs et al., administered toptoecan at 1.0 – 1.25 mg/m^2 for 5 days with paclitaxel 135 mg/m^2 intravenously over 24 hours on day 5 with G-CSF to 28 evaluable patients with extensive disease (28). Seventeen patients responded (60%) with 21% of patients having a complete response (CR). The median survival time was 13.5 months. Hematological toxicity was severe with grade 4 neutropenia occurring in greater than 90% of cycles and 27/28 patients (96%). Neutropenic fever developed in 21% of cycles given. Grade 4 thrombocytopenia occurred in 18% of cycles. A similar trial design by Tweedy et al., evaluated 15 untreated patients with extensive SCLC with topotecan at 1 mg/m^2, d 1-5 with paclitaxel at 135 mg/m^2 over 3 hours on day 5 with growth factor support (29). All 15 patients have responded with ten patients (67%) achieving a CR. Survival was not reported nor was grade 4 leukopenia. Grade 3 leukopenia was observed in 12/15 patients and no patient was hospitalized for neutropenic fever. These impressive efficacy results with topotecan plus paclitaxel are being further explored in a randomized trial. Panza and the Southern Italy Cooperative Oncology Group added cisplatin to the toptoecan/paclitaxel regimen. Twenty-nine untreated and 6 previously treated patients received topotecan

(2.25 mg/m^2), cisplatin (40 mg/m^2) and paclitaxel (85 mg/m^2) weekly with G-CSF (30). The objective response rate was 72% (13/18 chemonaive patients) with 17% CRs (3 patients) and 60% (3/5 previously treated patients) with 20% CRs (1 patient). Survival was not reported. Grade 4 neutropenia occurred in 12% of patients. This regimen was well tolerated and accrual to the trial is continuing. Other combination being pursued are: topotecan, paclitaxel and carboplatin, topotecan, carboplatin plus etoposide, and topotecan with etoposide.

Table 3. Topotecan Combination Regimens in Extensive Stage SCLC

Author (Ref)	Regimen	# Eval Pts	RR (%)	CR (%)	MS (Months)	% G4 ANC
Jacobs (28)	TOPO/PAC/G-CSF	28	60	21	13.5	96
Tweedy (29)	TOPO/PAC/G-CSF	15	100	67	NR	NR
Panza (30)	TOPO/PAC/CDDP/G-CSF	18	72	17	NR	12
		5*		60	20	NR

Abbreviations: Ref = Referneces; # Eval Pts = Number of evaluable patients; RR = Response rate; CR = Complete response; MS = Median survival, G4 ANC = Grade 4 absolute neutrophil count; TOPO = Topotecan; PAC = Paclitaxel; CDDP = Cisplatin;
** = Previously treated*

Taxanes

Two phase II studies established the efficacy of paclitaxel in SCLC (Table 2). The ECOG study administered paclitaxel at 250 mg/m^2 by a 24 hour infusion and reported a 34% response rate in 11/32 untreated patients with an 11 month median survival (31). Using a similar study design the North Central Cancer Treatment Group (NCCTG) reported a 68% response rate in 37 patients and a median survival of 7.3 months (32). Grade 4 leukopenia was the major toxicity seen in both studies.

To improve upon the results with single agent paclitaxel, several combination trials with platinum agents were performed (Table 4). Nair et al., enrolled patients with untreated extensive stage SCLC to either 135 mg/m^2 or 175 mg/m^2 of paclitaxel with 75 mg/m^2 of cisplatin on day 1 (33). Fifteen of 21 patients (71%) on the low dose arm (LDA) responded and 39/44 patients (89%) on the high dose arm (HDA) had an objective response. Median survival was 8.5 months on the LDA versus 9.5 months on the HDA. The one year survival rate was 24% versus 38%, respectively. Only 1 patient (2%) on the HDA experienced grade 4 neutropenia. The CALGB completed a trial with paclitaxel (230 mg/m^2) plus cisplatin (75 mg/m^2) and G-CSF in 34 patients (34). The objective response rate was 71% (24/34 patients) with a 9% CR rate (3 patients). The median survival was 7.6 months, similar to standard therapy. Four studies have been conducted adding paclitaxel to the active regimen of cisplatin and etoposide (PET). Glisson et al., treated 38 assessable patients with 110 –130 mg/m^2 of paclitaxel over 3 hours with cisplatin 75 mg/m^2 on day 1 and etoposide 80 mg/m2, IV on days 2-4 (35). The overall response was 90% with 6 complete responders (16%) and a median survival of 11.8 months. Grade 4 neutopenia developed in 47% of courses. Kelly et al., performed a phase I trial of escalating doses of paclitaxel ($135 - 200$ mg/m^2, IV over 3 hours) with cisplatin 80 mg/m^2 and etoposide $50 - 80$ mg/m^2 IV day 1 with $100 - 160$ mg/m2 PO, days 2 and 3 (36). Objective responses were seen in 19/23 patients (61%) with 5 CRs (22%) and a median survival of 10 months. Grade 4 neutropenia occurred in 82% of patients but febrile neutropenia was uncommon (14% of patients). Dose limiting peripheral neuropathy developed with 200 mg/m^2 of paclitaxel. Based on these results, SWOG investigated the PET regimen using paclitaxel at 175 mg/m^2, IV over 3 hours, with cisplatin 80 mg/m^2 and etoposide 80 mg/m^2 on day 1 and etoposide 160 mg/m^2 orally, on days 2 and 3 with prophylactic G-CSF (37). Eighty-eight patients were evaluable for response. Objective responses were observed in 36/82 patients (56%) with 10 patients (12%) achieving a complete response. The median survival was 11 months with a 1 year survival of 43%. Six patients (7%) died from toxicity and 29 additional patients (35%) developed grade 4 neutropenia but no patient developed grade 4 febrile neutropenia. Meanwhile, the Cancer and Leukemia Group B (CALGB) has launched a randomized phase III trial of PE (cisplatin 80 mg/m^2, day 1and etoposide 80 mg/m^2 day 1-3) versus PET (same doses of PE with paclitaxel 175 mg/m^2 over 3 hours on day 1) with growth factor support in untreated patients with a good performance status. The Greek Lung Cancer Cooperative Group (GLCCG) has completed a similar randomized trial (38). One hundred thirty eight untreated patients were randomized to PE (cisplatin 80 mg/m^2, day 1 plus etopside 120 mg/m^2, day 2-4) or PET (cisplatin 80 mg/^{2} day 2, etoposide 80 mg/m^2, day 2-4 and paclitaxel 175 mg/m^2, IV over 3 hours, day 1) with G-CSF. The overall response rates were 45% with 4% CRs for PE and 57% with 9% CRs for PET. Median survival was 10 months and 11 months, respectively. No difference in grade 3 and 4 neutropenia was seen, 40% and 41% but there were 7 toxic deaths in the PET arm versus 0 in the PE arm (p =.005). Due to the significant difference in toxic deaths the trial was terminated. No detailed information regarding the toxic deaths were reported.

Two additional trials substituting carboplatin for cisplatin in the PET regimen have been completed. Hainsworth and colleagues administered paclitaxel at a dose of 135mg/m^2, IV over 1 hour with carboplatin at an AUC = 5 and etoposide 50 mg alternating with 100 mg orally for 10 days (39). The response rate was 65% for the 15 patients with extensive stage disease with a CR rate of 17%. The median survival was 7 months. The regimen was extremely well tolerated therefore the paclitaxel dose was escalated to 200 mg/m^2 and an additional 38 patients with extensive stage disease were treated. The response rate was 84% (32/38 patients) with CRs achieved in 21% (8 patients). The median survival was 10 months for this cohort of patients. Grade 3 and 4 neutropenia increased to 38% of courses for all patients (including patients with limited stage). A phase III trial comparing paclitaxel, carboplatin and etoposide to carboplatin plus etoposide has completed accrual. Niell reported results of a trial with paclitaxel 200 mg/m^2, IV over 3 hours, carboplatin AUC = 6, and etoposide 80-100 mg/m^2, IV day 1-3 with G-CSF in patients with advanced lung cancer (40). Of the 22 patients treated objective responses were seen in 91% and CRs in 18% (4 patients). Survival was not documented. Forty one percent of patients developed grade 4 neutropenia.

Table 4. Paclitaxel Combination Regimens in Extensive Stage SCLC

Author (Ref)		Regimen	# Eval Pts	RR(%)	CR(%)	MS(Months)	% G4 ANC
Nair	(33)	PAC/CDDP (Low)	21	71	NR	8.5	0
		PAC/CDDP (High)	44	89	NR	9.5	2
Lyss	(34)	PAC/CDDP/G-CSF	34	71	9	7.6	18
Glisson	(35)	PAC/CDDP/VP-16	38	90	16	11.8	47
Kelly	(36)	PAC/CDDP/VP-16	23	61	22	10	82
Kelly	(37)	PAC/CDDP/VP-16/G-CSF	88	56	12	11	35
Mavroudis	(38)	CDDP/VP-16/PAC/G-CSF	62	57	9	11	40
		CDDP/VP-16	64	45	4	10	41
Hainsworth	(39)	PAC/Carbo/VP-16	23	65	17	7	0
			38	84	21	10	38[a]
Neill	(40)	PAC/Carbo/VP-16/G-CSF	22	91	18	NR	41
Thomas	(41)	PAC/Carbo	33	67	10	8	27[a]
Depperman	(42)	PAC/Carbo	69	61	7	12	43[a]
Agelcki	(43)	PAC/Carbo	18[R]	17	0	7	28
Lad	(44)	PAC/Adria	15	27	6	12	44

Abbreviations: Ref = References; # Eval Pts = Number of evaluable patients; RR = Response rate; CR = Complete response; MS = Median survival, G4 ANC = Grade 4 absolute neutrophil count; PAC = Paclitaxel; CDDP = Cisplatin; Carbo = Carboplatin; Adria = Adriamycin; NR = Not reported
a = % of courses
R = Refractory

Most recently preliminary reports of trials with paclitaxel plus carboplatin have been published. Thomas et al., gave paclitaxel 200 mg/m^2, 3 hour infusion with carboplatin AUC = 6 to 33 evalauble patients (41). The overall response rate was 67% with 10% (3 patients) having a CR. Median survival was 8 months. Grade 3 and 4 neutropenia was observed in 27% of courses and Grade 1 and 2 neuropathy occurred in 13% of patients. A phase II trial by Depperman et al., administered the identical regimen to 75 patients with metastatic SCLC (42). Of the 69 assessable patients, 61% (42 patients) responded. Five patients achieved a CR (7%). The median survival was 12 months. Grade 3 / 4 neutropenia was observed in 43% of courses and grade 2/3 neuropathy in 29% of courses. The GLCCG has also evaluated this doublet in patients with refractory SCLC (43). Twenty-one patients were accrued to the study. Partial responses were seen in 3 patients (17%). Time to progression was 5.5 months with a median survival was 7 months. Significant neutropenia developed in 28% of patients and grade 3 neuropathy in 14% of patients.   Paclitaxel plus carboplatin appears to be an effective regimen as first line and second line treatment for patients with SCLC, additional trials are being pursed.

One study combining paclitaxel plus adriamycin has been performed (44). Sixteen patients were treated with paclitaxel (175 mg/m^2, IV over 3 hours) with adriamycin 50 mg/m^2. Patients who had stable or progressing disease after 2 cycles were given platinum-based therapy. Four patients responded (27%) and 1 patient achieved a complete remission. The median survival for the entire group was 12 months. Forty-four percent of patients had grade 4 neutropenia. The low response rate observed after 2 cycles was disappointing. Future trials with this regimen should be pursued with caution.

A limited number of studies have employed docetaxel (Table 2). SWOG conducted a phase II trial in 47 chemonaive patients with 100 mg/m^2 of docetaxel (45). They reported a response rate of 26% (12/46 patients) and a median survival of 9 months. Grade 4 neutropenia occurred in 52% of patients. Smyth et al., administered the same regimen to 28 previously treated patients with SCLC and saw a 25% response rate (46). Grade 4 neutropenia developed in 71% of patients. One phase II trial with cisplatin is ongoing in Spain. Currently twenty two patients received docetaxel 75 mg/m^2 with cisplatin 75 mg/m^2. Eleven of twenty patients have had a PR (55%). Grade 3/4 neutropenia was seen in 55% of patients (47).

Vinorelbine

Vinorelbine has been evaluated in SCLC by several investigators as shown in Table 2. Two trials were carried out in untreated patients. Depierre et al, adminstered vinorelbine weekly at 30 mg/m^2 to 30 patients (48). Eight of 30 patients acheived a PR (27%). Myelosuppression was dose limiting and developed in 12 patients (40%). Three patient experienced grade 3/4 constipation. No responses were seen in a small trial of 6 patients (49). Furuse et al., gave 25 mg/m^2 of vinorelbine to 24 patients in sensitive relapse (50). Responses were reported in 3 patients (13%) and 60% of patients developed grade 3 or 4 leukopenia. Jassem studied a similar population (51). Twenty six patients with a sensitive relapse received 30 mg/m^2, weekly. Four of 25 evaluable patients (16%) achieved an objective response. Significant leukopenia occurred in 32% of patients. Lake et al., also conducted a trial in 34 sensitive relapsed patients but gave the vinorelbine 3 out of 4 weeks (52). He documented PR's in 5/31 patients (15%) and reported a median survival of 5 months. Grade 4 neutropenia was noted in 40% of patients. One small phase II trial combining vinorelbine with cisplatin and etoposide has been reported from investigators in Argentina (53). Fourteen untreated patients including 5 patients with extensive stage disease received this triplet. Two of the 5 patients (40%) with achieved a response with a median survival of 7 months. Neutropenia was observed in 7% of patients. The Italians conducted a phase II trial of carboplatin plus vinorelbine in advanced SCLC (54). Twenty three of the 33 evaluable patients (70%) had an objective response with 24% having a CR. The treatment was well tolerated with 4% grade 4 neutropenia.

Irinotecan

Irinotecan is a camptothecian derivative similar to toptotecan. Two very small studies have evaluated the single agent activity of irinotecan in untreated patients with SCLC (Table 2). Masuda et al administered 100 mg/m2 of irinotecan weekly to 16 patients (55). Seven of 15 patients (47%) had PRs with a median survival of 6.8 months. Using the same dose and schedule, Negoro treated 33 patients including 8 chemonaive patients

(56). Nine of 27 previously treated patients (33%) and 4/8 (50%) untreated patients achieved a response. Two previously treated patients (7%) obtained a CR. Le Chevalier et al., examined a 3 week schedule of 350 mg/m^2 of irinotecan in this relapsed population (57). The overall response rate was 16% (5/32 patients) and the median survival was 4.5 months. The major toxicities in all trials were neutropenia and diarrhea. A retrospective analysis of 134 patients with SCLC treated in Japan between 1980 and 1997 revealed the median survival time for patients with extensive stage disease who received second line treatment with irinotecan was 14.7 months versus 7.8 months for patients receiving alternative therapy (p<.05) (58). This survival advantage is provocative but needs to be confirmed in prospective trials.

One phase II combination trial with irinotecan (80 mg/m^2, day 1,8,15) and cisplatin (60 mg/m^2, day) every 28 days was administered to 75 untreated patients with SCLC. In the 35 patients with extensive disease the objective response rate was 86% (30/35 patients) with 10 patients (29%) having CRs (59). The median duration of response was 13 months. Toxicity was as follows: grade 3 or 4 neutropenia 77%, anemia 39% and diarrhea 19%. A randomized phase trial III comparing irinotecan plus cisplatin to cisplatin plus etoposide is reported to show a statistical survival benefit for the irinotecan arm (Gandara, DR, personal communication). Irinotecan has also been combined with etoposide. Fifty one untreated patients with metastatic disease were treated with irinotecan 60 mg/m^2, day 1,8,15 and etoposide 80 mg/m^2, IV days 2-4 every 4 weeks (60). The overall response rate was 66% with a 10% CR rate. Median survival was 12 months. Grade 3/4 neutropenia occurred in 72% of patients and diarrhea in 2% of patients. Trials incorporating irinotecan need to be conducted in the United States.

Gemcitabine

Gemcitabine is a new potent antimetabolite with activity in SCLC (Table 2). Cormier studied gemcitabine in 29 untreated patients with SCLC (61). Doses of 1000 -1250 mg/m^2 were administered weekly for 3 out of 4 weeks. Seven of 25 evaluable patients (27%) responded and the median survival was 12 months. Toxicities were mild with only 18% of courses reporting grade 3/4 myelosuppression. One additional trial has been performed in resistant patients given 1000 mg/m^2 of gemcitabine on days 1, 8, and 15 (62). Partial responses were observed in 5/36 patients (14%). Grade 3/4 thrombocytopenia was the major toxicites occurring in 32% of patients. The SWOG recently completed a phase II trial of the gemcitabine (1250 mg/m^2, day 1 and 8) plus cisplatin (75 mg/m^2, day 1). No results are available.

HIGH DOSE CHEMOTHERAPY

Chemotherapy regimens incorporating bone marrow or peripheral stem cell support as late intensification therapy have been conducted in patients with SCLC. To date, one, multicenter randomized trial was completed in 1987 (63). Patients with limited or extensive stage SCLC who were less than 65 years old with a PS greater than 50% and no serious organ dysfunction were eligible. All 101 patients received 3 cycles of methotrexate, vincristine, cyclophosphamide, and doxorubicin plus prophylactic cranial irradiation. Two additional cycles of PE were given and then the patients were restaged. Patients with limited disease in CR or PR and patients with extensive stage disease in CR were randomly assigned to receive a final cycle of chemotherapy with carmustine, cyclophosphamide, and etoposide at standard doses or high doses. Forty five patients were randomized. The relapse-free survival favored the high dose arm, 28 weeks versus 10 weeks, p =.002 but the median overall survival was not statistically different, 68 weeks for the high dose group and 55 weeks for the standard dose group. There were 4 toxic deaths in the high dose arm.

More recent trials have selected only patients with limited stage disease for transplant. SWOG carried out a phase II study in 58 patients with limited stage disease (64). Patients received induction cisplatin/etoposdie and radiotherapy followed by high dose cyclophosphamide (150 mg/kg) with autologous bone marrow rescue. Twenty-one patients completed the treatment as planned. There were 4 toxic deaths during the high dose consolidation phase. Median survival was 11 months for all patients. Nine of 21 patients in CR had a median survival of 27 months. Elias et al., conducted a similar phase II trial in this population (65). Nineteen responding patients received high dose consolidaton therapy with cyclophosphamide (5625 mg/m^2), cisplatin (165 mg/m^2) and carmustine (480 mg/m^2) with autologous bone marrow transplantation followed by thoracic and prophylactic brain irradiation. Fourteen patients (74%) were in CR or near CR prior to receiving the high dose regimem. After all treatment there were 15 patients (79%) with CRs. The 2 year overall survival rate was 53%. Morbidity was low. These results are intriguing but were obtained in a highly selected population. The CALGB is currently performing a randomized trial in which high dose chemotherapy is the experimental arm.

A review of the data with autologous stem cell transplantation for SCLC from 1989 - 97 at 23 centers was recently reported (66). One hundred three cases were examined. The median age at transplant was 50 years. Patients received bone marrow alone (17%), peripheral blood stem cells alone (42%) or both (41%). Most patients were transplanted in PR (61%) or CR (35%). The 100 day mortality was 14% and the 2 year survival rate was 37%. The 2 year survival rate was higher if the transplant was performed within 6 months of diagnosis and for complete responders receiving a stem cell transplant. Overall, the data for high dose chemotherapy with bone marrow or peripheral stem cell rescue is not better than results obtained with conventional therapies and is associated with more toxicity. This approach remains experimental.

PALLIATIVE CHEMOTHERAPY

Elderly patients and/or patients with a poor performance status (PS) with SCLC are believed to be unable to tolerate chemotherapy leading to investigation with milder chemotherapy regimens such as oral etoposide to palliate symptoms (67,68). However, two randomized trials comparing oral etoposide to combination chemotherapy surprisingly favored the combination arm. The Medical Research Council administered oral etoposide (50 mg twice daily for 10 days) or intravenous etoposide with vincristine

(EV) or CAV to 399 patients with a poor PS (69). The interim analysis showed no difference in palliation of symptoms (41% vs 46%) or response rates (45% vs 51%) between the oral and IV chemotherapy arms respectively but median survival favored the combination regimens (130 days vs 183 days; p = .03 respectively). A second trial performed in 155 patients with poor prognostic factors: elderly (> 75 years), poor PS or high alkaline phosphatase (> 1.5 times normal) randomized patients to oral etoposide (100 mg twice daily for 5 days) or CAV/PE (70). The response rate in the patients receiving oral etoposide was 39% as compared to 61% for CAV/PE (P < .01). Median survival was 5.2 months versus 6.8 months respectively (P = .051). Quality of life favored the combination regimen except in the category of nausea and vomiting. Thus, oral etoposide is inferior to combination chemotherapy which can be safely administered to this compromised population resulting not only palliation of symptoms but improved survival. Newer agents which are characterized as having milder toxicity profiles are excellent candidates for evaluation in this cohort.

SALVAGE CHEMOTHERAPY

The majority of patients with SCLC will ultimately relapse. The decision to administer salvage chemotherapy should be guided by several factors, 1) the duration of time between treatment and relapse, 2) responsiveness to previous therapy and 3) the composition of the first regimen. Today, with several new and active chemotherapy agents available more patients are receiving second-line chemotherapy as discussed above. Another option in this setting is oral etoposide. Vanderbilt showed a 64% response in 9/14 patients with a sensitive relapse and HOG reported a 25% response rate in patients who had received prior CAV or EP (71,72). Remissions however were short lived, approximately 4 months. For patients who relapse after a durable response (≥ 6 months) reinduction with the previous regimen is reasonable.

NEWER CHEMOTHERAPY AGENTS

There are several newer chemotherapy agents are in development for both NSCLC and SCLC and as listed in Table 5. Tirapazamine is a hypoxic cell sensitizer which has been shown to have activity when combined with cisplatin in advanced stage NSCLC (73). In SCLC, tirapazamine with concurrent radiotherapy will be examined in patients with limited stage disease in SWOG. Multi-targeted antifolate (MTA) and oxaliplatin are in early clinical trials in NSCLC but deserve evaluation in SCLC. Decitabine, a nonselective demethylating agent which can reverse DNA hypermethylation is currently in phase I testing in NSCLC and SCLC.

BIOLOGICAL AGENTS FOR THE TREATMENT OF SCLC

Major strides in understanding the biology of SCLC has provided us with numerous therapeutic targets (74). Table 5 provides a preliminary list of potential biological agents which are being explored in SCLC.

Table 5. New Treatments for Small Cell Lung Cancer

1. New Chemotherapeutic Agents -- Tirapazamine -- MTA -- Oxaliplatin -- Decitabine	4. Signal Transduction Inhibitors -- ISIS 2503
2. MMP Inhibitors -- Marimistat -- Bayer 12-9566	5. Dominant Oncogene Inhibitor -- All transretinoic acid -- Antisense bcl-2 -- Dolastatin 10
3. Growth Factor Inhibitors -- SR 49059 -- Antagonist G	6. Suppressor Oncogenes Replacement Therapy -- p53, 3p, 9p, RB 7. Vaccines -- BEC2 + BCG

Abbreviations: MTA = Multi-targeted antifolate, MMP = Matrix metalloprotease, BCG = Bacillus Calmette-Guerin, RB = Retinoblastoma

Matrix Metalloproetease Inhibitors (MMPIs)

Invasion of cancer cells into the underlying stroma is mediated by various degradative enzymes called matrix metalloproteases (MMPs) (75). MMP*s allow migrating tumor cells to move through the extracellular matrix. Secondarily, they facilitate new capillary formation, proliferation and movement into a growing tumor (75). MMPs are a family of 16 enzymes which share common structural and functional features (76). In SCLC, MMP expression was recently evaluated by Michael and colleagues (77). Immunohistochemistry and in situ hybridization of a panel of 7 MMPs were performed on 46 SCLC tumor samples, 29 samples were from patients with limited stage disease. Positive staining was seen with 6/7 MMPs. No tumor tissue expressed MMP - 2. Furthermore, MMP - 11 and MMP - 14 were found to be independent negative predicators for survival in the multi-variate analysis. These data suggests that inhibitors of MMPs known as MMPI's could be beneficial for treating SCLC. Several MMPIs are under study. In animal models, all MMPIs have demonstrated activity in reducing and preventiong tumor growth, invasion, angiogenesis and metastasis (78). MMPIs are oral agents that in phase I trials have demonstrated miminal nonhematological toxicity (79). Two MMPIs, marimistat and Bay 12-9566 have entered into double blind phase III trials as maintenance therapy for responding patients with SCLC. Marimastat is a broad specturm compound capable of inhibiting many MMPs. The study conducted in the United States has completed accrual and the Canadian trial is ongoing. No results are available. The major toxicity with marimastat is myalgias and arthralgias (79). The second agent BAY 12-9566, is a selective MMP inhibitor. Using the same trial design, this agent was found to be ineffective in an interim analysis of 245 patients.

Growth Factor and Signal Transduction Inhibitors

SCLC unlike NSCLC express and respond to many different neuropeptides (74). Binding of neuropeptides to its receptor activates a cascade of proteins resulting in cell proliferation. Prevention of the binding of neuropeptides to their receptors with a peptide or a receptor antagonist is one strategy to decrease cellular prolifieration. For example, SR 49059 is an oral vasopressin receptor antagonist in phase II testing in Canada in patients with refractory SCLC. Antagonist G is a broad spectrum neuropeptide growth factor antagonist which has been shown to inhibit SCLC growth in vitro and in vivo and is about to enter phase II testing in the United Kingdom (80,81)

A second focus for attack is the multiple enzymes that comprise the signal transduction pathway. Using antisense oligonucleotide technology, several enzyme inhibitors have been developed. IS2503 is an antisense oligonucleotide inhibitor of c-raf kinase currently in phase II testing in SCLC and NSCLC in Europe. The agent is administered as a 14 day continuous infusion. Toxicity is mild and includes fatigue, transient fever and thrombocytopenia.

Dominant oncogene inhibitors

Dominant oncogenes identified in SCLC include genes that encode for tyrosine kinase receptors and proteins and serine kinases, the myc gene family and bcl-2. Inhibitors of dominant oncogenes are aimed at their protein product. For example, preclinical work with all trans retinoic acid (ATRA) revealed that ATRA could inhibit c-myc gene protein expression and cellular proliferation (82). Additional evidence suggested that c-myc expression made SCLC cells less sensitive to chemotherapy (82). A phase II trial was performed administering 150 mg/m^2/d of ATRA with PE chemotherapy to patients with extensive stage SCLC (83). The efficacy of ATRA was unable to be determined in this study due to its toxicity. The majority of the 22 patients discontinued treatment because of headaches or mucocutaneous reactions. However, retinoids should not be abandoned but alternative doses and schedules or different retinoids deserve investigation.

Two promising new agents targeting bcl-2 are dolastatin 10 and antisense bcl-2. Kalemkerian et al., has shown that dolastatin 10 induces apoptosis associated with bcl-2 phosphorylation in SCLC cancer cell lines and xenografts while Zeilger and colleagues have demonstrated that an antisense bcl-2 oligonucleotide induces apoptosis in SCLC cell lines by reducing bcl-2 levels (84,85). Thus, these agents warrant clinical evaluation. A trial with antisense bcl-2 oligonucleotide is planned.

Suppressor Oncogene Replacement Therapy

Tumor suppressor genes which are mutated or deleted in high frequency in SCLC are 3p, retinoblastoma gene (RB), p53 and 9p (74). Introducing the normal gene back into the cell to suppress tumor growth has been the focus of several investigators in NSCLC. Roth et al., has demonstrated the feasibility of injecting adenoviral wild type p53 (Ad-p53) into the tumors of patients with NSCLC (86). Twenty eight patients received monthly injections of Ad-p53 by CT guidance or bronchoscopy. The virus was well tolerated, resulted in expression of wild-type p53 and mediated an antitumor response with 2 patients achieving a PR and 16 patients had disease stablization for 2 –14 months. Tumor suppressor replacement therapy has not been attempted in SCLC patients but is worthy of pursuit. Besides p53 an excellent candidate suppressor gene to target for SCLC is RB. Ookawa et a., has shown that reconstitution of the RB gene suppresses the growth of SCLC cell lines carrying multiple genetic alterations (87). Numerous biological agents targeting angiogenesis and the cell cycle are also in early development in solid tumors but not specifically in SCLC.

Immune modulators

Attempts to enhance tumor killing by manipulating the immune system is not a new strategy. Bacillus Calmette-Guerin (BCG) was evaluated in the early 1980's in SCLC. Two randomized trials in patients with limited disease were treated with chemoradiation with or without BCG (88,89). There was no difference in response rates or median survival between the arms in either study. However, one trial showed that for patients who lived longer than a year and continued to receive BCG had a survival advantage of 93 weeks compared to 81 weeks for the control arm (p=.03) (88).

Several trials have been conducted with alfa interferon. Mattson et al., was the first to show a possible role for alfa interferon as maintenace therapy in responding patients with limited stage SCLC (90). A recent update of this randomized trial continued to show a survival advantage for the alfa interferon arm with 10% of patients alive at 5 years versus 2% for patients on the maintenance chemotherapy or observation arm. SWOG attempted to confirm these results in a randomized phase III trial of alfa interferon versus observation for patients with limited disease but was unsuccessful due to the toxicity of interferon (92). More recently Lebeau et al., reported no survival benefit with maintenance interferon (93). Finally, Mattson and colleagues conducted a randomized trial of chemotherapy with or without concurrent alfa interferon and showed no survival difference (94). Overall, it does not appear that there is a role for alfa interferon in SCLC.

Active immunization is an alternative modality. Selecting the appropriate antigenic target has hindered this approach. Carbohydrate antigens such as the gangliosides which are abundant on tumor surfaces but have limited expression in normal tissue are potential targets in development. For example, the ganglioside GD 3 is expressed on the surface of most SCLCs and melanomas but rarely on normal cells. Preliminary work revealed that immunization with the anti-idiotypic antibody BEC2 illicited an immune response by producing anti-GD3 antibodies (95). Furthermore, this response was enhanced with BCG. A trial perfomed in melanoma patients produced encouraging results and lead to a phase II trial in SCLC patients (96,97). Fifteen patients including 7 patients with limited disease and 8 patients with extensive stage disease who had responded to chemotherapy or chemoradiotherapy were given 5 intradermal injections every 2 weeks with BEC2 plus BCG. The median overall survival for all patients was 20.5 months.

The median time to relapse for patients with extensive stage disease was 10.6 months and has not been reached for patients with limited disease with a median follow up of 47 months. The major toxicity from the BEC2 was grade 3 local skin toxicity which occurred in 14 patients and resolved without any treatment. These exciting results have lead to a randomized phase III trial entitled "Survival in an International Phase III Prospective Randomized Limited Disease SCLC Vaccination Study with Adjuvant BEC2 and BCG (SILVA)". The trial is ongoing and is estimated to complete accrual in 1 year. Meanwhile other ganglioside vaccines are being developed and are planning to enter clinical trials within the year in SCLC.

SUMMARY

Over the past twenty years combination chemotherapy has continued to produce small survival gains for patients with SCLC. We enter the next century enthusiastic about the array of new chemotherapeutic agents to evaluate and fascinated by the biological agents with the hope of achieving dramatic improvements in survival for our patients with SCLC.

REFERENCES

1. Cook RM, Miller YE, Bunn PA Jr. Small cell lung cancer: Etiology, biology, clinical features, staging and treatment. Current Problems in Cancer 17(2):69-144, 1993.
2. Greenlee RT, Murray T, Bolden S, Wingo PA. Cancer statistics, 2000. CA: A Cancer Journal for Clinicians 50:7-33, 2000.
3. Evans WK, Feld R, Murray N, et al. Superiority of alternating non-cross-resistant chemotherapy in extensive small cell lung cancer. A multicenter, randomized clinical trial by the National Cancer Institute of Canada. Annals of Internal Medicine 107(4):451-458, 1987.
4. Roth BJ, Johnson DH, Einhorn LH, et al. Randomized study of cyclophosphamide, doxorubicin, and vincristine versus etoposide and cisplatin versus alternation of these two regimens in extensive small-cell lung cancer: A phase III trial of the Southeastern Cancer Study Group. J Clin Oncol 10:282-291, 1992.
5. Fukuoka M, Furuse K, Saijo N, et al. Randomized trial of cyclophosphamide, doxorubicin, and vincristine versus cisplatin and etoposide versus alternation of these regimens in small-cell lung cancer. J Natl Cancer Inst 83:855-861, 1991.
6. Bunn PA Jr and Carney DN. Overview of chemotherapy for small cell lung cancer. Seminars in Oncology 24(2, Suppl 7):S7-69-S7-74, 1997.
7. Ihde DC, Mulshine JL, Kramer BS, et al. Prospective randomized comparison of high-dose and standard-dose etoposide and cisplatin chemotherapy in patients with extensive-stage small-cell lung cancer. J Clin Oncol 12:2022-2034, 1994.
8. Crawford J, Ozer H, Stoller R, et al. Reduction by granulocyte colony-stimulating factor of fever and neutropenia induced by chemotherapy in patients with small-cell lung cancer. N Engl J Med 326(4):269-270, 1992.

9.   Murray N, Livingston RB, Shepherd FA, et al. Randomized study of CODE versus alternating CAV/EP for extensive-stage small-cell lung cancer: An intergroup study of the National Cancer Institute of Canada Clinical Trials Group and the Southwest Oncology Group. J Clin Oncol 17:2300-2308, 1999.

10. Furuse K, Fukuoka M, Nishiwaki Y, et al. Phase III study of intensive weekly chemotherapy with recombinant human granulocyte colony-stimulating factor versus standard chemotherapy in extensive-disease small-cell lung cancer. J Clin Oncol 16:2126-2132, 1998.

11. Bunn PA Jr. Review of therapeutic trials of carboplatin in lung cancer. Semin Oncol 16:27-33, 1989.

12. Skarlos DV, Samantas E, Kosmidis P, et al. Randomized comparison of etoposide-cisplatin versus etoposide-carboplatin and irradiation in small cell lung cancer. A Hellenic Co-operative Oncology Group Study. Ann Oncol 5:601-607, 1994.

13. Loehrer PJ Sr, Ansari R, Gonin R, et al. Cisplatin plus etoposide with and without ifosfamide in extensive small-cell lung cancer: A Hoosier Oncology Group study. J Clin Oncol 13:2594-2599, 1995.

14. Ettinger DS, Finkelstein DM, Abeloff MD, et al. A randomized comparison of standard chemotherapy versus alternating chemotherapy and maintenance versus no maintenance therapy for extensive-stage small-cell lung cancer: A phase III study of the Eastern Cooperative Oncology Group. J Clin Oncol 8(2):230-240, 1990.

15. Jarry O, Fournel P. A randomised trial of 4 versus 8 courses of chemotherapy with ifosfamide, epirubicin and etoposide (EVI) in extensive small cell lung cancer (SCLC). IASLC-SCLC: Denver CO, 1994 (abstr).

16. Sandler AB, Ansari R, Saxman S, et al. Phase III trial of maintenance daily oral VP-16 versus no further therapy following induction chemotherapy with VP-16 (V) plus ifosfamide (I) plus cisplatin (P) (VIP) in extensive small cell lung cancer (SCLC): A Hoosier Oncology Group (HOG) trial (LUN93-2). Proc Am Soc Clin Oncol 18:470a, 1999 (abstr 1813).

17. Chute JP, Chen T, Feigal E, et al. Twenty years of phase III trials for patients with extensive-stage small-cell lung cancer: Perceptible progress. J Clin Oncol 17(6):1794-1801, 1999.

18. Rowinsky EK, Grochow LB, Hendricks CB, et al. Phase I and pharmacologic study of topotecan: A novel topoisomerase I inhibitor. J Clin Oncol 10(4):647-656, 1992.

19. Schiller JH, Kim KM, Hufson P, et al. Phase II study of topotecan in patients with extensive-stage small cell carcinoma of the lung: An Eastern Cooperative Oncology Group trial. J Clin Oncol 14(8):2345-2352, 1996.

20. Watanabe K, Fukuoka M, Niitani H for the Topotecan Lung Cancer Cooperative Study Group, Japan. Phase II trial of topotecan for small cell lung cancer (SCLC). Lung Cancer 1997:18:58 (abstract).

21. Depierre A, von Pawel J, Hans K, et al, international study collaborators, SmithKline Beecham, UK. Evaluation of topotecan (Hycamtin™) in relapsed small cell lung cancer (SCLC). A multicentre phase II study. Lung Cancer 18:35, 1997 (abstract).

22. Ardizzoni A, Hansen H, Dombernowsky P, et al for the European Organization for Research and Treatment of Cancer Early Clinical Studies Group and New Drug Development Office, and the Lung Cancer Cooperative Group. Topotecan, a new active drug in the second-line treatment of small-cell lung cancer: A phase II study in patients with refractory and sensitive disease. J Clin Oncol 1997: 15(5):2090-2096.

23. Nishiwaki Y, Negoro S, Watanabe K, et al. Late phase II trials of topotecan (T) for relapsed small cell lung cancer (SCLC). European Journal of Cancer 35(Suppl 4) S253, 1999 (abstract 1004).

24. Perez-Soler R, Glisson BS, Lee JS, et al. Phase II study of topotecan in patients with small cell lung cancer (SCLC) refractory to etoposide. Proc Am Soc Clin Oncol 14:355 (abstract) 1995.

25. von Pawel J, Schiller JH, Shepherd FA. Topotecan versus cyclophosphamide, doxorubicin, and vincristine for the treatment of recurrent small-cell lung cancer. J Clin Oncol 17(2):658-667, 1999.

26. Eckardt J, Palmer MC, Fanucchi M, et al. Oral topotecan (T) as single-agent first-line treatment for patients (pts) with extensive disease (ED) small cell lung cancer (SCLC) ineligible for standard IV therapy: A phase II study. Proc Am Soc Clin Oncol 18:501a, 1999 (abstract 1925).

27. Korfel A, von Pawel J, Oehm E, et al. Response of symptomatic brain metastases of small cell lung cancer (SCLC) to topotecan also after preceeding whole-brain radiation (WBI). European Journal of Cancer 35(Suppl 4) S251, 1999 (abstract 997).

28. Jacobs SA, Jett JR, Belani CP, et al. Topotecan and paclitaxel, an active couplet, in untreated extensive disease small cell lung cancer. Proc Am Soc Clin Oncol 18:470a, 1999 (abstract 1814).

29. Tweedy CR, Andrews DF, Ball T. Topotecan and paclitaxel in extensive stage small cell lung cancer as initial therapy. Proc Am Soc Clin Oncol 18:525a, 1999 (abstract 2025).

30. Panza N, Frasci G, Comella P, et al. Cisplatin-paclitaxel-topotecan (CPT) weekly administration in chemo-naïve or pretreated extensive disease small cell lung cancer (ED-SCLC). A SICOG phase II study. European Journal of Cancer 35(Suppl 4) S252, 1999 (abstract 1001).

31. Ettinger DS, Finkelstein DM, Sarma RP, Johnson DH. Phase II study of paclitaxel in patients with extensive disease small cell lung cancer: An Eastern Cooperative Oncology Group study. J Clin Oncol 13:1430-1435, 1995.

32. Kirschling RJ, Jung SH, Jett JR for the North Central Cancer Treatment Group. A phase II trial of taxol and G-CSF in previously untreated patients with extensive-stage small cell lung cancer (SCLC). Proc Am Soc Clin Oncol 13:326, 1994 (abstract).

33. Nair S, Marschke R, Grill J, et al. A phase II study of paclitaxel (Taxol®) and cisplatin (CDDP) in the treatment of extensive stage small cell lung cancer (ESSCLC). Proc Am Soc Clin Oncol 16:454a (abstract), 1997.

34. Lyss AP, Herndon JE, Lynch TC, et al. Paclitaxel (P) + Cisplatin (C) + G-CSF (G) in patients with previously untreated extensive stage small cell lung cancer (E-SCLC): Preliminary analysis of Cancer and Leukemia Group B (CALGB) 9430.

Proc Am Soc Clin Oncol 18:468a, 1999 (abstract 1806).

35. Glisson BS, Kurie JM, Perez-Soler R, et al. Cisplatin, etoposide, and paclitaxel in the treatment of patients with extensive small-cell lung carcinoma. J Clin Oncol 17:2309-2315, 1999.

36. Kelly K, Pan Z, Wood ME, et al. A phase I study of paclitaxel, etoposide, and cisplatin in extensive stage small cell lung cancer. Clinical Cancer Research 5:3419-3424, 1999.

37. Bunn PA, Kelly K, Crowley J, et al. Preliminary toxicity results from Southwest Oncology Group trial (SWOG) 9705: A phase II trial of cisplatin, etoposide and paclitaxel (PET) with G-CSF in untreated patients (pts) with extensive small cell lung cancer (SCLC). Proc Am Soc Clin Oncol 18:468a, 1999 (abstract 1807).

38. Mavroudis D, Papadakis E, Veselemes M, et al. Paclitaxel-cisplatin-etoposide (TEP) versus cisplatin-etoposide (EP) as first line treatment in small cell lung cancer (SCLC): A preliminary analysis of a multicenter randomized phase III trial. European Journal of Cancer 35(Suppl 4) S247, 1999 (abstract 980).

39. Hainsworth JD, Gray JR, Stroup SL, et al. Paclitaxel, carboplatin, and extended-schedule etoposide in the treatment of small-cell lung cancer: Comparison of sequential phase II trials using different dose-intensities. J Clin Oncol 15:3464-3470, 1997.

40. Hainsworth JD, Niell HB. Taxol (paclitaxel) injection, carboplatin and etoposide in the management of small cell lung cancer: Clinical update. Princeton, NJ, Bristol-Myers Squibb, 1999.

41. Thomas P, Lena H, Robinet, et al. Preliminary report on paclitaxel/carboplatin phase II multicentric trial in patients with metastatic small cell lung cancer (SCLC). Proc Am Soc Clin Oncol 18:519a, 1999 (abstract 2000).

42. Depperman KM, Serke M, Oehm C, et al. Paclitaxel (TAX) and carboplatin (CBDA) in advanced SCLC: A phase II study. Proc Am Soc Clin Oncol 18:482a, 1999 (abstract 1860).

43. Agelaki S, Agelidou M, Blazogiannakis G, et al. A phase II study of paclitaxel (P) and carboplatin (C) as second-line treatment in patients (PTS) with small-cell lung cancer (SCLC). European Journal of Cancer 35(Suppl 4) S258, 1999 (abstract 1027).

44. Lad T, Mauer A, Hoffman P, et al. Phase II trial of paclitaxel and doxorubicin in small cell lung cancer. Proc Am Soc Clin Oncol 18:513a, 1999 (abstract 1980).

45. Burris HA, Crowley JJ, Williamson SK, et al. Docetaxel (taxotere) in extensive stage small cell lung cancer (SCLC): A phase II trial of the Southwest Oncology Group (SWOG). Proc Am Soc Clin Oncol 17:451a, 1998 (abstract 1737).

46. Smyth JF, Smith IE, Sessa C, et al. Activity of docetaxel (taxotere) in small cell lung cancer. Eur J Cancer (suppl):30A:1058-1060, 1994.

47. Lianes P, Moreno JA, Sevilla I, et al. Phase II study of docetaxel and cisplatin in first line treatment of disseminated small cell lung cancer (SCLC): Preliminary results. Proc Am Soc Clin Oncol 18:514a, 1999 (abstract 1983).

48. Depierre A, LeChevalier T, Quoix E, et al. Phase II trial of navelbine (NVB) in small cell lung cancer (SCLC). Lung Cancer 18 (Suppl 1):3, 1997 (abstract).

49. Tummarello D, Graziano F, Giodani P. A phase II study of vinorelbine (VNB) in small cell lung cancer (SCLC) patients (PTS) unsuitable for standard

chemotherapy (CHT). Proc Am Soc Clin Oncol 14:369, 1995 (abstract).

50. Furuse K, Fukuoka M, Kimura I, et al. Early phase II study of vinorebine (VRB) in small cell lung cancer (SCLC). Proc Am Soc Clin Oncol 14:371, 1995 (abstract).

51. Jassem J, Karnicka-Mlodkowska H, van Pottelsberghe C, et al. Phase II study of vinorelbine (Navelbine) in previously treated small cell lung cancer patients. Eur J Cancer 29A(12):1720-1722, 1993.

52. Lake D, Johnson E, Herndon J, Green M. Phase II trial of Navelbine® (NVB) in relapsed small cell lung cancer (SCLC). Proc Am Soc Clin Oncol 16:473a, 1997 (abstract).

53. Richardet E, Carranza L, Uribe A, et al. Phase II study: Cisplatin (C) + etoposide (E) + navelbine (N) in small cell lung cancer (SCLC). Proc Am Soc Clin Oncol 14:373, 1995 (abstract 1151).

54. Gridelli C, Ianniello G, Brancaccio L, et al. Carboplatin plus vinorelbine: A new active regimen in extensive small cell lung cancer. Results of a multicenter phase II study. Lung Cancer 18 (suppl):55, 1997 (abstract 212).

55. Masuda N, Fukuoka M, Kusunoki Y, et al. CPT-11: A new derivative of camptothecin for the treatment of refractory or relapsed small-cell lung cancer. J Clin Oncol 10(8):1225-1229, 1992.

56. Negoro S, Fukuoka M, Niitani H, et al. A phase II study of CPT-11, a campothecin derivative in patients with primary lung cancer. Gan to Kagaku Ryoho (Japanese Journal of Cancer and Chemotherapy) 18(6):1013-1019, 1991.

57. LeChevalier T, Ibrahim N, Chorny P, et al. A phase II study of irinotecan (CPT-11) in patients (pts) with small cell lung cancer (SCLC) progressing after initial response to first-line chemotherapy (CT). Proc Am Soc Clin Oncol 16:450a, 1997 (abstract).

58. Nishio M, Karato A, Okumura S, et al. Second-line CPT-11 may improve survival in small cell lung cancer. European Journal of Cancer 35(Suppl 4) S261, 1999 (abstract 1038).

59. Kudoh S, Fujiwara Y, Takada Y, et al. Phase II study of irinotecan combined with cisplatin in patients with previously untreated small-cell lung cancer. West Japan Lung Cancer Group. J Clin Oncol 16(3):1068-1074, 1998.

60. Nakamura S, Kudoh S, Komuta K, et al. Phase II study of irinotecan (CPT-11) combined with etoposide (VP-16) for previously untreated extensive-disease small-cell lung cancer (ED-SCLC): A study of the West Japan Lung Cancer Group. Proc Am Soc Clin Oncol 18:470a, 1999 (abstract 1815).

61. Cormier Y, Eisenhauer E, Muldal A, et al. Gemcitabine is an active new agent in previously untreated extensive small cell lung cancer (SCLC): National Cancer Institute of Canada Clinical Trials Group. Ann Oncol 5:283-285, 1994.

62. Van der Lee I, Postmus P, Smit E, et al. The activity of gemcitabine in patients with resistant small cell lung cancer (SCLC): A phase II study. Proc Am Soc Clin Oncol 18:476a, 1999 (abstract 1835).

63. Humblet Y, Symann M, Bosly A, et al. Late intensification chemotherapy with autologous bone marrow transplantation in selected small-cell carcinoma of the lung: A randomized study. J Clin Oncol 5(12):1864-1873, 1987.

64. Goodman GE, Crowley J, Livingston RB, et al. Treatment of limited small-cell

lung cancer with concurrent etoposide/cisplatin and radiotherapy followed by intensification with high-dose cyclophosphamide: A Southwest Oncology Group study. J Clin Oncol 9(3):453-457, 1991.

65. Elias AD, Avash L, Frei E 3d, et al. Intensive combined modality therapy for limited-stage small-cell lung cancer. J National Cancer Institute 85(7):559-566, 1993.

66. Rizzo D, Stiff P, Elias A. Autologous stem cell transplantation for small cell lung cancer. Proc Am Soc Clin Oncol 18:469a, 1999 (abstract 1811).

67. Smit EF, Postmus PE. A phase II study of oral etoposide 100 mg/day for 21 days every 4 weeks in untreated elderly and poor performance status small cell lung cancer patients. Cancer Treat Res 7:136, 1991 (abstract).

68. Doward AJ. A prospective study of low dose oral etoposide in poor prognosis small cell lung cancer. Cancer Treat Res 7:111, 1991 (abstract).

69. Medical Reserch Council Lung Cancer Working Party. Comparison of oral etoposide and standard intravenous multidrug chemotherapy for small-cell lung cancer: A stopped multicentre randomised trial. Lancet 348:563-566, 1996.

70. Harper P, Underhill C, Ruiz de Elvira MC, et al. A randomized study of oral etoposide versus combination chemotherapy in poor prognosis small cell lung cancer. Proc Am Soc Clin Oncol 15:27, 1996 (abstract).

71. Johnson DH, Greco FA, Strupp J, et al. Prolonged administration of oral etoposide in patients with relapsed or refractory small cell lung cancer: A phase II trial. J Clin Oncol 8:1613, 1990.

72. Einhorn LH, Bond WH, Hornback N, et al. Phase II trial of oral VP-16 in refractory small cell lung cancer: A Hoosier Oncology Group study. Semin Oncol 17:32, 1990.

73. von Pawel J and von Roemeling R. Survival benefit from tirazone™ (tirapazamine) and cisplatin in advanced non-small cell lung cancer (NSCLC) patients: Final results from the international phase III Catapult I trial. Proc Am Soc Clin Oncol 17:454A, 1998 (abstract 1749).

74. Kane MA and Bunn PA Jr (eds). Biology of lung cancer. Marcel Dekker Inc, New York, 1998.

75. Stetler-Stevenson W, Aznavovoorian S, Liotta LA. Tumour cell interactions with the extracellular matrix during invasion and metastasis. Cell Biol 9:541-573, 1993.

76. Chambers AF, Matrisian LM. Changing views of the role of metalloproteinases in metastasis. J Natl Cancer Inst 89:1260-1270, 1997.

77. Michael M, Babic B, Khokha R, et al. Expression and prognostic significance of metalloproteinases and their tissue inhibitors in patients with small-cell lung cancer. J Clin Oncol 17(6):1802-1808, 1999.

78. Wojtowicz-Praga SM, Dickson RB, Hawkins MJ. Matrix metalloproteinase inhibitors. Invest New Drugs 15:62-75, 1997.

79. Wojtowicz-Praga S, Torri J, Johnson M, et al. Phase I trial of marimastat, a novel matrix metalloproteinase inhibitor, administered orally to patients with advanced lung cancer. J Clin Oncol 16(6):2150-2156, 1998.

80. Jones DA, Cummings J, Langdon SP and Smyth JF. Preclinical studies on the broad-spectrum neuropeptide growth factor antagonist G. Gen Pharmac

28(2):183-189, 1997.

81. MacKinnon AC, Armstrong RA, Waters CM, et al. [Arg^6,D-Trp^{7,9},N^{me}Phe^8]-substance P (6-11) activates JNK and induces apoptosis in small cell lung cancer cells via an oxidant-dependent mechanism. Br J Cancer 80(7):1026-1034, 1999.

82. Kalemkerian GP, Jasti RK, Celano P, et al. All-trans-retinoic acid alters myc gene expression and inhibits in vitro progression in small cell lung cancer. Cell Growth & Differentiation 5(1):55-60, 1994.

83. Kalemkerian GP, Jiroutek M, Ettinger DS, et al. A phase II study of all-trans-retinoic acid plus cisplatin and etoposide in patients with extensive stage small cell lung cacrincoma: An Eastern Cooperative Oncology Group study. Cancer 83(6):1102-1108, 1998.

84. Kalemkerian GP, Ou X, Adil MR, et al. Activity of dolastatin 10 against small-cell lung cancer in vitro and in vivo: Induction of apoptosis and bcl-2 modification. Cancer Chemotherapy & Pharmacology 43(6):507-515, 1999.

85. Ziegler A, Luedke GH, Fabbro D, et al. Induction of apoptosis in small-cell lung cancer cells by an antisense oligodeoxynucleotide targeting the bcl-2 coding sequence. J Natl Cancer Inst 89(14):1027-1036, 1997.

86. Swisher SG, Roth JA, Nemunaitis J, et al. Adenovirus-mediated p53 gene transfer in advanced non-small-cell lung cancer. J Natl Cancer Inst 91(9):763-771, 1999.

87. Ookawa K, Shiseki M, Takahashi R, et al. Reconstitution of the RB gene suppresses the growth of small-cell lung carcinoma cells carrying multiple genetic alterations. Oncogene 8(8):2175-2181, 1993.

88. McCracken JD, Chen T, White J, et al. Combination chemotherapy, radiotherapy, and BCG immunotherapy in limited small-cell carcinoma of the lung: A Southwest Oncology Group study. Cancer 49(11):2252-2258, 1982.

89. Jackson DV Jr, Paschal BR, Ferree C, et al: Combination chemotherapy-radiotherapy with and without the methanol-extraction residue of Bacillus Calmette-Guerin (MER) in small cell carcinoma of the lung: A prospective randomized trial of the Piedmont Oncology Association. Cancer 50(1):48-52, 1982.

90. Mattson K, Niiranen A, Pryhonen S, et al. Natural interferon alfa as maintenance therapy for small cell lung cancer. European J Cancer 28A(8-9):1387-1391, 1992.

91. Mattson K, Niiranen A, Ruotsalainen T, et al. Interferon maintenance therapy for small cell lung cancer: Improvement in long-term survival. J Interferon & Cytokine Research 17(2):103-105, 1997.

92. Kelly K, Bunn PA Jr, Crowley J, et al. The role of alfa interferon (r-IFN 2a) maintenance in patients with limited stage SCLC responding to concurrent chemoradiation: A Southwest Oncology Group study (SWOG). J Clin Oncol 13:2924-2930, 1995.

93. LeBeau B, de la Salmoniere P, Ozenne G, et al. αInterferon (αIFN) as maintenance therapy for small cell lung cancer (SCLC). Proc Am Soc Clin Oncol 18:475a, 1999 (abstract 1832).

94. Ruotsalainen TM, Halme M, Tamminen K, et al. Concomitant chemotherapy and IFN-alpha for small cell lung cancer: A randomized multicenter phase III study. Journal of Interferon & Cytokine Research 19(3):253-259, 1999.

95. Chapman PB, Houghton AN. Induction of IgG antibodies against GD3

ganglioside in rabbits by an anti-idiotypic monoclonal antibody. J Clinical Investigation 88(1):186-192, 1991.

96.   McCaffery M, Yao TJ, Williams L, et al. Immunization of melanoma patients with BEC2 anti-idiotypic monoclonal antibody that mimics GD3 ganglioside: Enhanced immunogenicity when combined with adjuvant. Clinical Cancer Research 2(4):679-686, 1996.

97.   Grant SC, Kris MG, Houghton AN, Chapman PB. Long survival of patients with small cell lung cancer after adjuvant treatment with the anti-idiotypic antibody BEC2 plus Bacillus Calmette-Guerin. Clinical Cancer Resarch 5(6):1319-1323, 1999.

THYMIC MALIGNANCIES

Patrick J. Loehrer, Sr., M.D.
Indiana University School of Medicine, Indianapolis, IN 46202 USA

Mark R. Wick, M.D.
Washington University Medical Center, Indianapolis, IN 46202 USA

INTRODUCTION

Thymus is derived from the Greek word, Θυμος (thymos), meaning life-force or soul (1). For centuries, the thymus gland has been enigmatic, described by many as a "vestigial structure filled with incompetent cells, and a graveyard for dying lymphocytes" (2). Only within the last several decades has the critical function of the thymus been recognized. The thymus serves a critical role in the maturation and differentiation of lymphocytes. Congenital absence or hypoplasia of the thymus is associated with severe and often fatal disorders of immunologic incompetence such as DiGeorge Syndrome, Nezelof's Syndrome, and severe combined immunodeficiency (3,4).

The thymus consists of a complex microenvironment of specialized epithelial cells, derived from endoderm, which interact with lymphocytes during fetal development (5). The thymus arises mainly from the third (and less consistently the fourth) pharyngeal pouch in close association with the inferior parathyroid glands during the first trimester. By week 8, the primitive thymus grows and descends into the anterior-superior mediastinum. Precursor lymphocytes then migrate to the thymus where they closely approximate the epithelial cells, separated only by perivascular spaces (6). At least 6 different types of thymic epithelium have been identified to date and ultrastructural studies demonstrate a close association with these different epithelial cells and the various steps in the maturation process of the lymphocyte (5,6,7). With the migration of the lymphocytes, the structure of the thymus gland becomes better defined (figure 1), now composed of the outer cortex (site of lymphoblastogenesis), the inner cortex (which contains more mature thymocytes) and the medulla (which contains the mature T-cells which migrate to the peripheral blood) (7). The relative size of the thymus is greatest during the neonatal period but it reaches its maximal absolute weight of about 35 grams during puberty. During adulthood, the gland gradually involutes to a smaller structure which is largely replaced by adipocytes (6).

Thymomas are the most common tumor of the anterior mediastinum, representing approximately 50% of cases described. Other neoplasms which arise in this anatomic location include lymphomas, endocrine tumors (thyroid, parathyroid), and germ cell malignancies (9,10). Several malignant and benign tumors arise within the thymus, but thymoma and thymic carcinoma are the prototypical tumors derived from the thymic epithelium. Thymic carcinoid is also a separate and important entity. Metastatic tumors to the thymus gland occur only rarely.

Thymoma is a unique neoplasm which is often characterized by indolent growth and frequent association with a myriad of paraneoplastic syndromes. Most patients present with a well encapsulated mass detected on a routine chest radiograph. In such cases, complete surgical resection is usually curative. In the 30-40% of patients with invasive or metastatic disease, the prognosis is less favorable. During the past 15 years novel treatment approaches for invasive or metastatic disease have been evaluated. This review will discuss the clinical and pathologic aspects of thymoma and thymic carcinoma.

EPIDEMIOLOGY

The exact incidence of thymoma is unclear because many cases are not included in tumor registries as they may be coded as benign tumors. The Surveillance, Epidemiology and End Results (SEER) section of the National Cancer Institute reported the incidence to be 0.13 cases per 100,000 (11). From the Cancer Registry of England and Wales, an incidence rate of 0.72 and 0.64 per million was reported for men and women, respectively (12). Thymomas and thymic carcinomas most commonly occur between the ages of 40 and 60, but also have been reported in patients in their first and ninth decades of life. There is no gender predominance, but the peak age incidence is approximately one decade later in life for women (13,20).

The risk factors for developing thymic tumors are elusive. Several investigators have reported a relationship of Epstein-Barr viral infection with lymphoepithelioma-like thymic carcinoma including isolation of defective viral genomes in the tumor (21,25). Others have both suggested and discounted this association which is more frequently seen in far-eastern countries (26). Childhood irradiation of the thymus may also be a risk factor (27).

Several cases of familial thymoma have been reported, including the occurrence of the tumor in a sibling as young as nine months old (29,30,31). In the few reported cases of cytogenetic abnormalities in thymic carcinoma, a recurrent pattern of reciprocal translocations involving chromosomes 15 and 19 has been noted by some authors (11), but no consistent abnormalities have emerged making the significance of these findings uncertain (34,35).

HISTOLOGY

Non-Neoplastic Thymus

The fetal thymus attains maturity during the first trimester of pregnancy where it has a multilobated appearance; each lobule is composed of a cortex and a medulla. The cortex has a high lymphocyte:epithelial cell ratio, while the medulla contains nearly an equal number of such elements. Clusters of epithelial cells in both subcompartments commonly undergo keratinization and microcystification, yielding the structures known as "Hassall's corpuscles." Mast cells, found in abundance throughout both the cortex and medulla, become more notable with aging as the lymphocyte content of the gland decreases. Indeed, the postpubertal thymus contains relatively few thymocytes, and instead is represented by a large amount of mature adipose tissue in which residual epithelial cells are embedded (33,34).

Thymic epithelium demonstrates some degree of morphologic variation. Cortical epithelial cells have round to oval nuclear contours with vesicular chromatin and distinct small nucleoli, whereas epithelial cells in the medulla more commonly assume a fusiform shape, contain dispersed chromatin, and manifest few if any nucleoli (figure 2). In prepubescent individuals, thymocytes throughout the gland differ from the appearance of peripheral mature lymphocytes. The latter cells exhibit relatively enlarged nuclei with open chromatin patterns, discernible chromocenters, and folding of the nuclear membranes (36). The structural relationship between intrathymic lymphocytes and the thymic epithelium is an intimate one, wherein elongated and branched cytoplasmic processes of epithelial cells are closely apposed to the plasmalemmae of resident thymocytes (figure 1). Because of the overall constituency of the cortex, there are relatively more epithelial cell extensions than karyons, with the reverse of that statement pertaining to the thymic medulla.

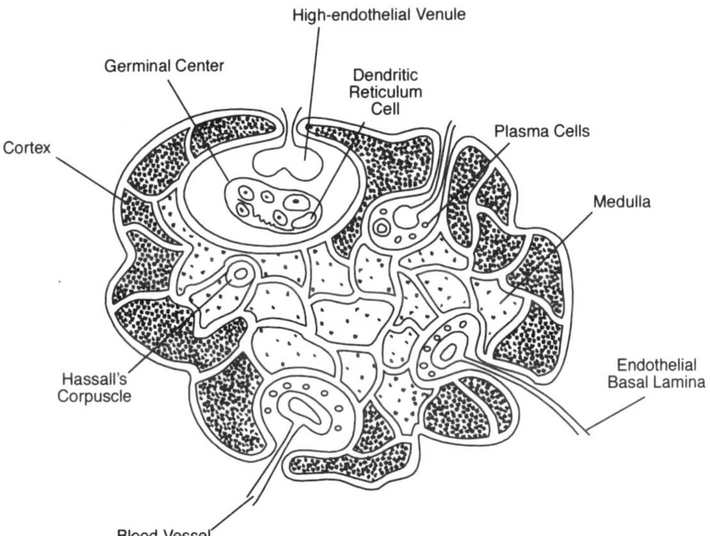

Figure 1: Histologic Structure of Thymoma. *The thymus gland demonstrates a close structural relationship between the elongated and branching epithelial cells with the lymphocytes. Lymphoblastogenesis occurs in the cortex of the thymus from which lymphocytes migrate to the inner cortex and finally to the medulla before exiting the thymus to the peripheral blood.*

Non-neoplastic morphologic abnormalities in the thymus principally are represented by hyperplasia, which almost always involves proliferation of intrathymic lymphocytes but not epithelial cells, and by dysplasia, where one observes only sparse thymocytes and abnormal aggregations of epithelium into rosettes or arborizing cords. The first of these two conditions—which also features the formation of lymphoid germinal centers—is closely associated with myasthenia gravis or Graves' disease, and the second is linked to congenital immunodeficiency states (37).

Thymoma

Thymomas are usually well-localized, nodular, multilobated masses in the anterosuperior mediastinum, often with at least-partial fibrous encapsulation. The cut surfaces of thymomas demonstrate "fleshy tissue" divided by fibrous bands, which generally intersect one another at acute angles. Spontaneous intralesional hemorrhage or necrosis are not usually apparent, but cystic change may be prominent in selected examples (38). Probably secondary to aberrant migration of the thymus during embryogenesis, ectopic thymus tissue has been described in a variety of locations including the middle and posterior mediastinal compartments, the intrapulmonary or extrapulmonary pleura, and the neck (39,40,41).

The neoplastic cells of the thymus are the epithelial cells and not the lymphocytes. These epithelial cells are cytologically-bland. Thus, most of the cytoarchitectural features previously described for the non-neoplastic thymus apply to thymoma as well, which has prompted some investigators to characterize thymoma by presumed cellular origins (3). For example, those thymomas that are composed of epithelium resembling non-neoplastic thymic cortex have been termed by some as "cortical" thymomas. Other tumors comprised of spindle cells which have the attributes of epithelium in the medulla of the thymus (i.e., fusiform nuclei and dispersed chromatin) are called "medullary" thymomas. Another subset of thymoma which exhibits a mixture of these two cytologic morphotypes has been classified as "mixed" thymomas (figure 2).

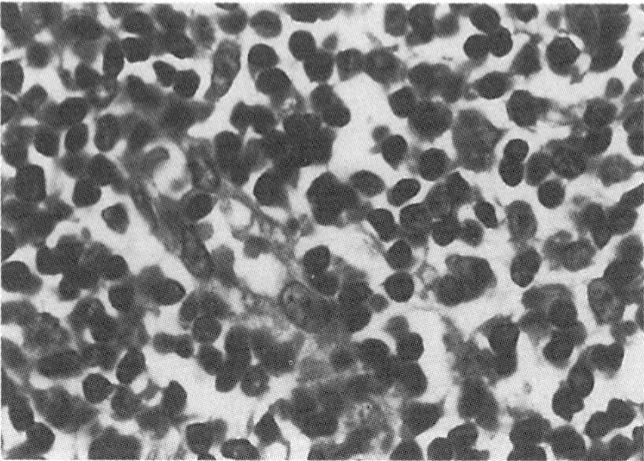

Figure 2a: Histology of Thymic Carcinoma. The normal thymus is composed of the cortex (a), the medulla (b), the epithelial network of the thymus (c) and Hassal's Corpuscle (d). Malignant tumors of the thymus can be classified by structural similarities of the benign counterparts: thymomas labeled as cortical (e), medullary (f) or mixed, cortical-medullary (g).

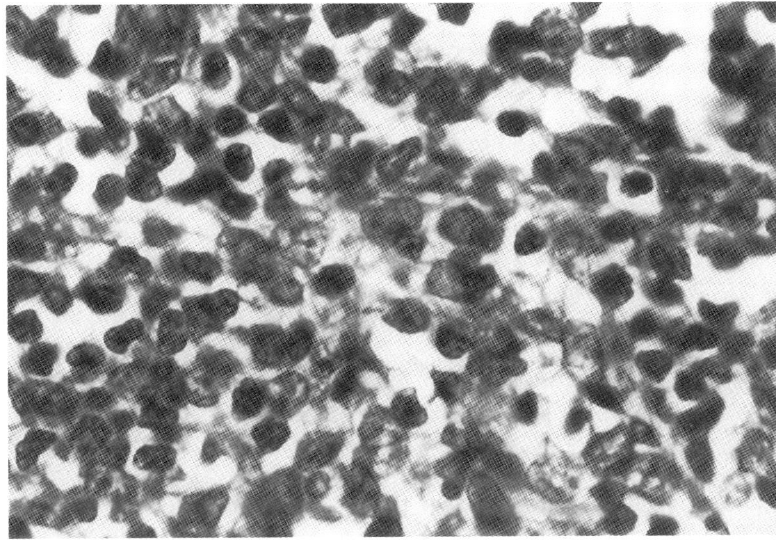

Figure 2b: **Histology of Thymic Carcinoma.** *The normal thymus is composed of the cortex (a), the medulla (b), the epithelial network of the thymus (c) and Hassal's Corpuscle (d). Malignant tumors of the thymus can be classified by structural similarities of the benign counterparts: thymomas labeled as cortical (e), medullary (f) or mixed, cortical-medullary (g).*

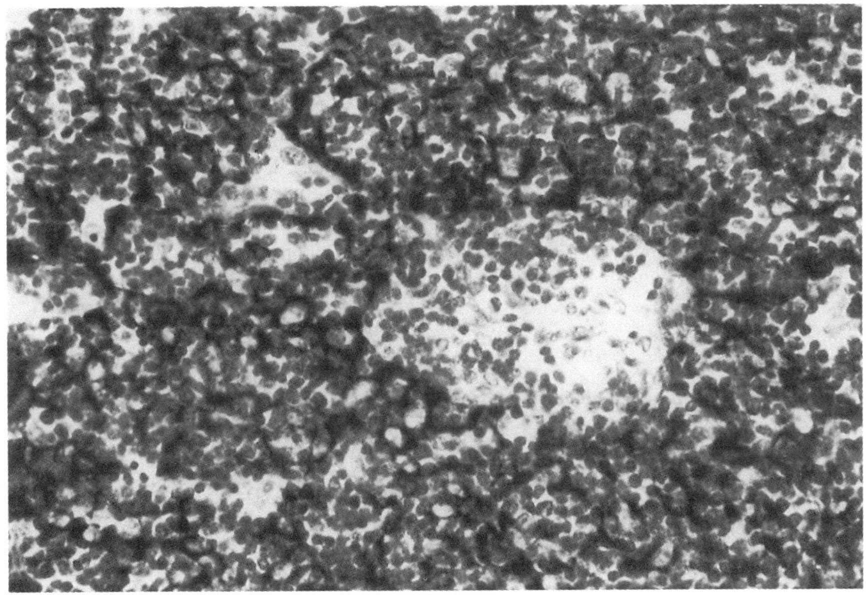

Figure 2c: **Histology of Thymic Carcinoma.** *The normal thymus is composed of the cortex (a), the medulla (b), the epithelial network of the thymus (c) and Hassal's Corpuscle (d). Malignant tumors of the thymus can be classified by structural similarities of the benign counterparts: thymomas labeled as cortical (e), medullary (f) or mixed, cortical-medullary (g).*

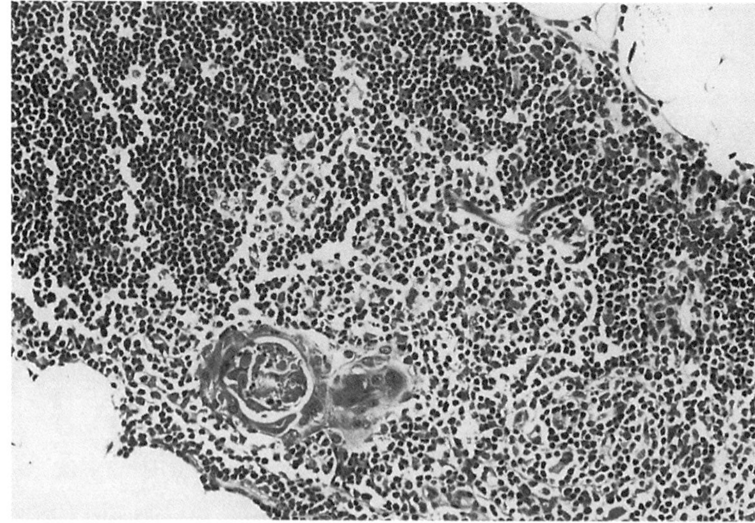

Figure 2d: **Histology of Thymic Carcinoma.** *The normal thymus is composed of the cortex (a), the medulla (b), the epithelial network of the thymus (c) and Hassal's Corpuscle (d). Malignant tumors of the thymus can be classified by structural similarities of the benign counterparts: thymomas labeled as cortical (e), medullary (f) or mixed, cortical-medullary (g).*

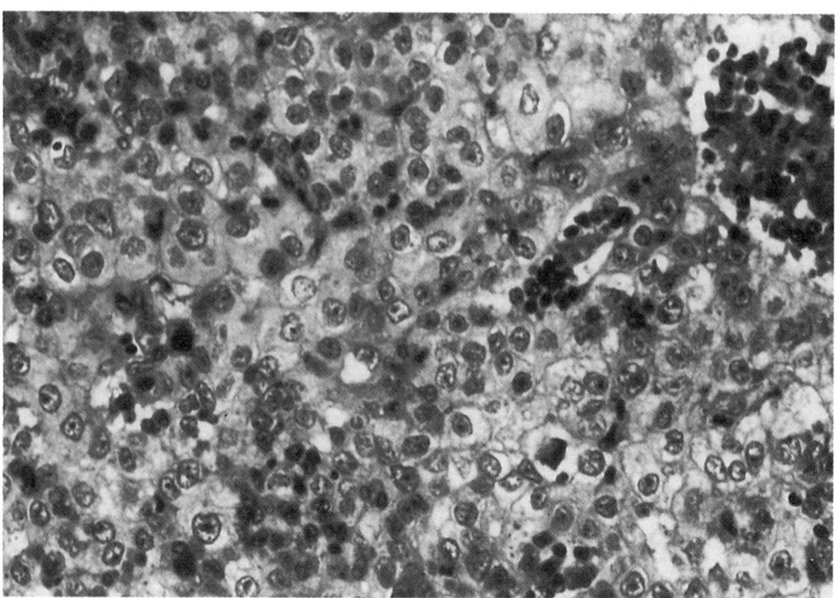

Figure 2e: **Histology of Thymic Carcinoma.** *The normal thymus is composed of the cortex (a), the medulla (b), the epithelial network of the thymus (c) and Hassal's Corpuscle (d). Malignant tumors of the thymus can be classified by structural similarities of the benign counterparts: thymomas labeled as cortical (e), medullary (f) or mixed, cortical-medullary (g).*

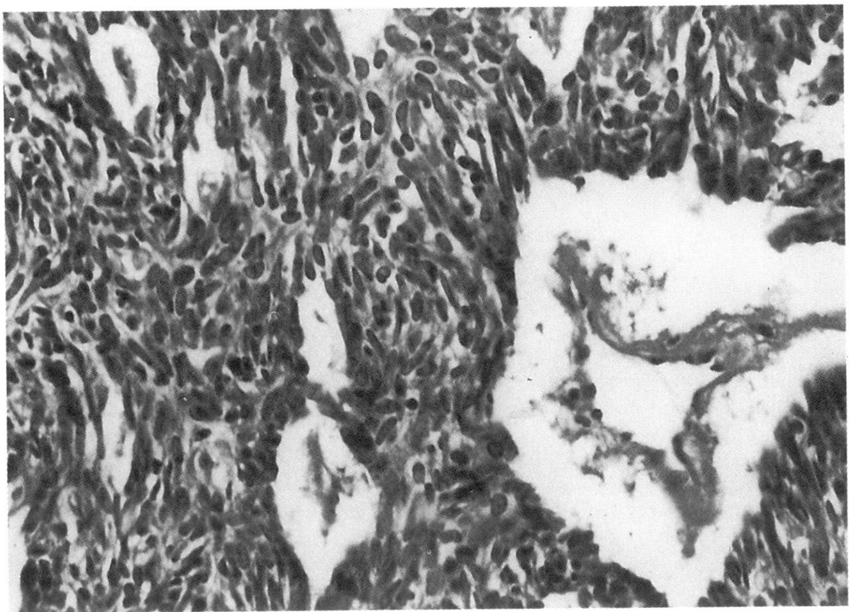

Figure 2f: **Histology of Thymic Carcinoma.** *The normal thymus is composed of the cortex (a), the medulla (b), the epithelial network of the thymus (c) and Hassal's Corpuscle (d). Malignant tumors of the thymus can be classified by structural similarities of the benign counterparts: thymomas labeled as cortical (e), medullary (f) or mixed, cortical-medullary (g).*

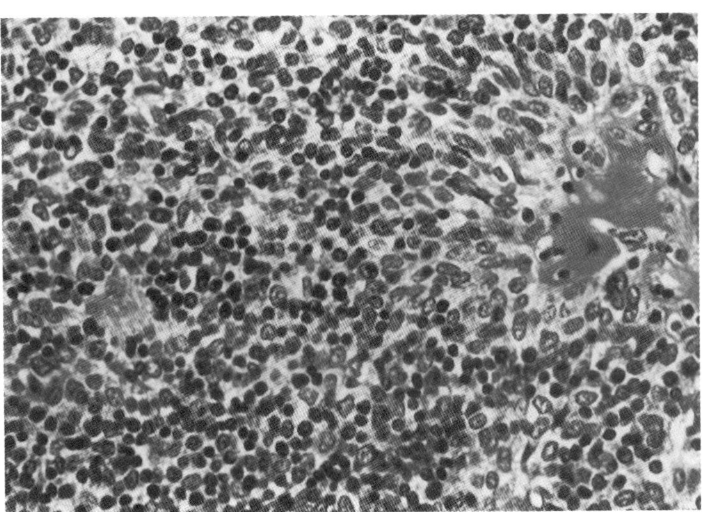

Figure 2g: **Histology of Thymic Carcinoma.** *The normal thymus is composed of the cortex (a), the medulla (b), the epithelial network of the thymus (c) and Hassal's Corpuscle (d). Malignant tumors of the thymus can be classified by structural similarities of the benign counterparts: thymomas labeled as cortical (e), medullary (f) or mixed, cortical-medullary (g).*

Other epithelial thymic tumors which manifest more malignant cytologic characteristics than those of thymoma are classified as thymic carcinomas. Sometimes tumors may strain the morphologic boundary between thymomas and thymic carcinomas suggesting a theoretical continuum between those entities. For example, "well-differentiated thymic carcinoma" described by Kirchner, et al (42), is classified by many other pathologists as a form of thymoma with limited nuclear atypia (37).

HISTOLOGIC SUBCLASSIFICATIONS OF THYMOMA (TABLE 1)

Several histologic classifications for thymoma (Table 1) have been proposed but unfortunately none correlates perfectly with biology. Until recently, the histologic subclassification of thymomas in widest use was that devised by Bernatz & colleagues (48). The Bernatz classification divides thymomas into four groups based on their microscopic features: lymphocyte-predominant (>66% lymphocytes), epithelial-predominant (>66% epithelial cells), mixed lymphoepithelial (34-66% epithelial cells), and spindle cell. The latter category pertains to epithelial-predominant thymoma featuring a virtually-pure population of fusiform cells.

Table 1. ***Histologic Staging Systems of Thymoma***

Authors	No of Patients	Subgroups (proportion)	Clinical Correlation
			15-year survival (%)*
Bernatz, et al (48,17)	283	Predominantly lymphocytic (25%)	90
		Mixed Lymphoepithelial (43%)	80
		Predominantly epithelial (25%)	50
		Spindle cell (6%)	100
			10 year survival (%)
Verley/Hollman (18)	200	Type I: spindle and oval cell (30%)	75
		Type II: lymphocyte-rich (30%)	75
		Type III: differentiated epithelial rich (33%)	50
		Type IV: undifferentiated epithelial-rich (equivalent to thymic carcinoma) (7%)	0
Muller-Hermelink (118)	58	Cortical (43%)	
		Mixed: predominantly cortical (8%)	
		Mixed: (36%)	
		Medullary (5%)	
		Mixed: predominantly medullary (8%)	

disease specific survival

A more recent construct by Marino and Muller-Hermelink (MMH) presupposes that "medullary" thymomas carry a favorable prognosis, while "cortical" lesions have a relatively adverse evolution and "mixed cortical/medullary" thymomas have an intermediary behavior (7). Subsets of cortical thymoma, proposed by some investigators, include "organoid thymoma" and "well differentiated thymic carcinoma" (see above) which behave in a fashion similar to that of conventional cortical thymoma and thus probably do not benefit from a separate terminology (50). Several investigators have debated the uniqueness of the MMH classification because spindle-cell ("medullary") thymomas have long been known to behave innocuously, regardless of what specific adjectives are attached to them (49,51,52,53).

PATHOLOGY OF PRIMARY THYMIC CARCINOMAS

Thymic carcinoma has been well recognized and only recently described as a separate entity (43,44,45). Indeed, the presence of invasion or metastasis alone does not fulfill the criteria for classifying a thymic epithelial tumor as a carcinoma. The histologic appearance of thymic carcinoma is distinctly different from thymoma although both tumors are believed to arise from the epithelial cells of the thymus. Thymic carcinomas commonly lack the encapsulation or fibrous septation of thymomas. Their parenchyma is firm to hard and has a white-gray appearance with frequent necrosis and hemorrhage.

There are several microscopic subtypes of thymic carcinoma (46,47). These variants include the following: small-cell neuroendocrine (oat-cell) carcinoma, basaloid squamous cell carcinoma, keratinizing squamous cell carcinoma, non-keratinizing squamous cell carcinoma, lymphoepithelioma-like squamous carcinoma, adenosquamous and mucoepidermoid carcinomas, clear-cell carcinoma, primary adenocarcinoma (not further specified), and sarcomatoid carcinoma. All cells of thymic carcinoma should stain positively for keratin and often express epithelial membrane antigen as well. Electron microscopy may be needed for specific characterization of the tumors. Because of the many morphologic differential diagnoses that are called to mind by the variations just cited, the pathologist also may want to employ other adjunctive diagnostic studies to solidify an interpretation of thymic carcinoma. These typically center on the use of immunohistochemistry, the results of which serve, in the case of thymoma, to define the presence of a tumor which lacks the features of germ cell malignancies, hematopoietic neoplasms and extrathymic carcinomas.

Levine and Rosai have classified thymic carcinoma into two groups: high and low grade (117). High grade lesions include lymphoepithelioma-like carcinoma, anaplastic large cell carcinoma , small cell carcinoma, clear cell carcinoma and sarcomatoid carcinoma. Low grade lesions include mucoepidermoid carcinoma, keratinizing-squamous, and basiloid-squamous carcinomas. Prognosis is variable in these groups with a median survival time of 11.3 months and 25.4 months, respectively (43,117).

CLINICAL FINDINGS

Signs and symptoms of thymoma are related to local growth and paraneoplastic syndromes. Up to one-third of patients with this lesion present with asymptomatic masses noted on routine chest radiograph (15,16,17). Most patients, however, have some chest symptoms which may include pain, cough, dyspnea and hoarseness. Physical examination may reveal signs of superior vena cava syndrome (dilated chest and neck veins, head swelling or a neck mass). Diminished breath sounds and a respiratory lag may be noted because of intrathoracic spread and pleural involvement. Approximately 50-60% of patients with thymoma will have one or more paraneoplastic disorders during their lifetime (10,17,54). The clinical findings associated with paraneoplastic syndromes vary greatly and are discussed separately.

Myasthenia Gravis

Over a century ago, a neuropathologist, Hermann Hopper, first reported the association of myasthenias gravis with a mediastinal mass (56). Today, myasthenia gravis is the most frequent observed paraneoplastic syndrome linked with thymoma. A concise review of the former condition was recently published (55). Thymic abnormalities occur in at three-quarters of patients with myasthenia gravis, but most of these abnormalities represent thymic hyperplasia (85%) rather than thymoma (15%). Approximately one-third of patients with thymoma have myasthenia gravis, whereas only 10-15% of patients with myasthenia gravis have thymoma.

Several distinctions between myasthenia gravis associated with thymoma and that accompanying thymic hyperplasia are worth noting (59) (Table 2). Patients with thymomas and myasthenia gravis often have more severe neurologic symptoms which may require long term immunosuppressive therapy. Thymectomy is not as useful in reversing the neurologic symptoms in patients with thymoma compared to those with thymic hyperplasia (55,57,58,59). Patients with thymoma have higher acetylcholene receptor activity and titers of anti-striated muscle antibodies. Anti-straited muscle and anti-titin antibodies are found in 80-90% of patients with thymoma and myasthenia gravis (60). Individuals with thymic hyperplasia and myasthenia gravis are more frequently female (by a factor of 3:1) and they have an HLA association with D8:DR3.

Table 2. Myasthenia Gravis and Thymic Pathology(58,61)

Feature of Myasthenia Gravis	Thymic Pathology		
	Atrophy	Hyperplasa	Thymoma/WDTC
Age of Symptom Onset (Yrs)	>40	10-20	15-80
Male:Female	2:1	1:3	1:1
HLA Association	B7; DR2	B8; DR3	None
Elevated Auto Antibodies			
	AchR >90%	90%	30-80%
	Striated Muscle >90%	30-60%	10-20%
	Titin >90%	30-40%	<5%
Aggressive Clinical Course	Less Common	Less Common	Common
Improvement of Symptoms with Thymectomy	?	75-80%	10-15%

Ptosis and extraocular muscular weakness is usually one of the early symptoms of myasthenia gravis associated with thymoma. Other neurologic syndromes occurring in patients with thymoma include the Lambert-Eaton syndrome, peripheral neuropathy, limbic encephalopathy, and Isaac's syndrome (fasciculations, painful myalgia) (62). The symptoms of myasthenia gravis in patients with thymoma can be very severe with rapid progression from minor ocular paresis to generalized weakness and respiratory collapse. The presence of other concurrent paraneoplastic syndromes in patients with thymoma and myasthenia gravis is not uncommon (58,63).

The etiology of the autoimmune response of myasthenia gravis is controversial. A leading theory supports the role of the myoid (muscle-like) cells that are cellular constituents of the thymus gland and which contain a high concentration of surface acetylcholene receptors (55). The close proximity of myoid cells to antigen-presenting cells and T-cells supports the hypothesis of an autoimmune response leading to the development of acetylcholine receptor antibodies (5,61).

Red Cell Aplasia

Pure red cell aplasia is an autoimmune disorder seen in approximately 5% of patients with thymoma (64,65). Two-thirds of such patients have spindle cell histology. In contrast, about 33-50% of patients with pure red cell aplasia have thymoma. Virtually all patients are over the age of 40. Approximately one-third of patients will also have multi-lineage hematologic abnormalities represented by concordant thrombocytopenia and/or leukopenia. One-third of patients with pure red cell aplasia and thymoma also have hypogammaglobulinemia. Bone marrow examination will reveal the absence of erythroid precursors. Thymectomy is associated with reversal of pure red cell aplasia in approximately 40% of patients (66). The mechanism behind this association is unclear, but autoantibodies against erythroid cell progenitors, erythropoietin as well as a proliferation of CD8 + T-cells with monoclonal rearrangement of the T-cell receptor gene has been reported.

Acquired Hypogammaglobulinemia

Approximately 5-10% of patients with thymoma have decreased serum gamma globulins. The majority of patients with this tumor and hypogammaglobulinemia have spindle cell histology. This association of hypogammaglobulinemia with thymoma was first reported by Good in 1954 (54). Patients usually present with symptoms of repeated infections, diarrhea, and lymphadenopathy. Thymectomy is not generally useful in reversing this syndrome (17,54).

Secondary Malignancies

Malignancies of non-thymic origin have been reported in up to 20% of patients with thymoma (54). In many cases, the other malignancy precedes the diagnosis of thymoma. Lymphocytosis, usually of T-cell origin has also been observed by several authors. The spectrum of second malignancies is wide, including tumors of the aerodigestive system, leukemia and lymphoma with no predominant anatomic sites noted (54,61).

Autoimmune Diseases

A variety of rheumatologic and autoimmune diseases have been linked to thymoma. These include rheumatoid arthritis, systemic lupus erythematosis, dermatomyositis, progressive systemic sclerosis, and giant cell myocarditis (54,63). Not uncommonly, patients present with dermatologic lesions such as non-blanching maculopapular rash, purpura or generalized vasculitis.

Unusual infections are also associated with thymoma. Examples include progressive multifocal leukoencepholopathy, disseminated herpes, listeria and cryptococcal meningitis, and candidiasis which may occur in the absence of corticosteroid therapy (69,70).

DIAGNOSTIC TESTS

Posterior-anterior (PA) and lateral chest radiographs will demonstrate a mass in the anterior mediastinum in 45-80% of patients imaged. On the PA film, a portion of the tumor usually projects over one of the hila of the lung, which may be mistaken as part of the heart border or pulmonary outflow tract. The lateral film should confirm the location of the mass in the anterior mediastinum (figure 3 a & b). Comparison with older films is useful to detect subtle changes in appearance. The tumors are usually well defined, rounded, or lobulated and vary in size (from 1 cm to >30 cm). One of the radiographic hallmarks of the disease is metastases to the pleura, which occurs more commonly than parenchymal pulmonary involvement.

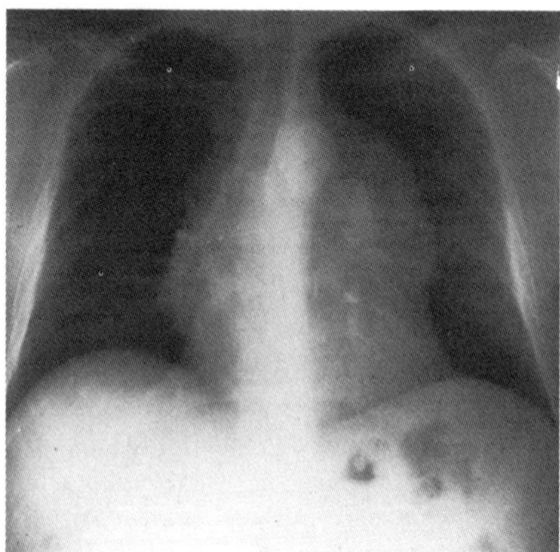

Figure 3a: Radiologic Findings of Thymoma. Chest radiograph of thymoma which demonstrate a mass overlying the hilum of the lung on posterior-anterior view (a). This mass is located in the anterior mediastinum which is appreciated best on the lateral chest film (b). Computerized tomograph scan demonstrates the anterior mediastinal mass and characteristic pleural-based metastasis (c).

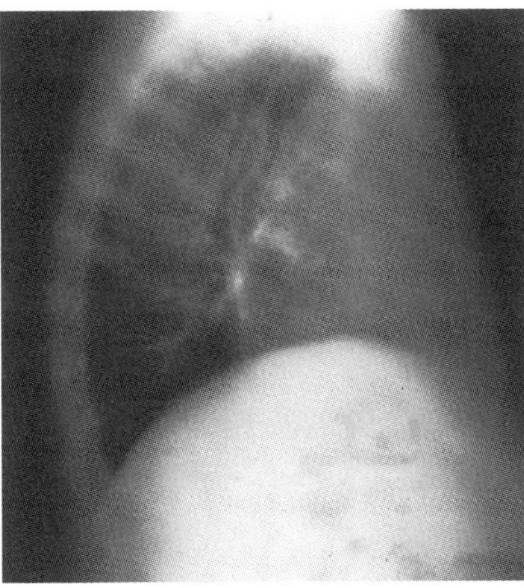

Figure 3b: Radiologic Findings of Thymoma.*Chest radiograph of thymoma which demonstrate a mass overlying the hilum of the lung on posterior-anterior view (a). This mass is located in the anterior mediastinum which is appreciated best on the lateral chest film (b). Computerized tomograph scan demonstrates the anterior mediastinal mass and characteristic pleural-based metastasis (c).*

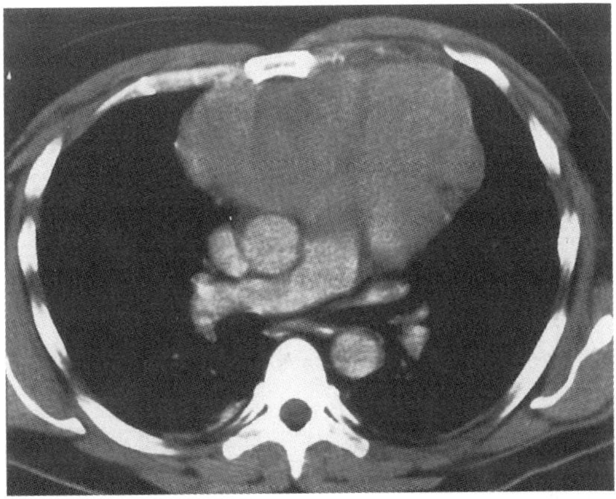

Figure 3c: Radiologic Findings of Thymoma.*Chest radiograph of thymoma which demonstrate a mass overlying the hilum of the lung on posterior-anterior view (a). This mass is located in the anterior mediastinum which is appreciated best on the lateral chest film (b). Computerized tomograph scan demonstrates the anterior mediastinal mass and characteristic pleural-based metastasis (c).*

Computerized axial tomography of the chest is useful to confirm the presence of a mass and may be useful to identify invasive disease (figure 3 c). Calcifications are present in approximately 10% of patients (71). Pleural involvement is common in advanced disease with occasional local invasion of the chest wall which may mimic mesothelioma. Metastases to the diaphragm and the retrocrural region can also be noted. Although secondary lesions in the liver, kidney, bones, and brain have been observed, more extensive radiographic imaging is generally not necessary in the absence of provocative symptoms and signs (63,64). Extrathoracic metastasis of thymoma is seen in less than 10% of cases.

Magnetic resonance imaging has special utility in some cases, especially to determine vascular invasion by the tumor. The signal enhancement is similar or slightly greater on T_1 weighted images and increased on T_2 weighted images (71). Thymomas are also particularly avid for certain isotopes used in nuclear medicine such as gallium and octreotide (72,73).

DIFFERENTIAL DIAGNOSIS

The differential diagnosis of anterior mediastinal masses includes germ cell tumors, lymphomas, thyroid proliferative disorders and thymic lesions. During initial evaluation, serum HCG and AFP should be measured to evaluate a possible primary mediastinal germ cell tumor (74,75). In the absence of an elevation of these markers, tissue confirmation is needed. Although percutaneous needle biopsy has a reported specificity of 94% and a sensitivity of 84%, the distinction between lymphoma and lymphoid predominant thymoma (cortical type) can be difficult using this technique. This drawback supports the need for large tumor samples via core biopsy, mediastinoscopy or limited thoracotomy (75,76,77). Some authors have expressed concern in breeching the capsule via incisional biopsy because of the potential to spill tumor cells (78,79).

Thymic carcinomas may be indistinguishable from metastatic tumors from other sites, although recent reports indicate that immunoreactivity for CD5 tends to support a thymic origin. Therefore, it is prudent to exclude an occult malignancy, particularly lung cancer, elsewhere before a final diagnosis is rendered.

STAGING

Several different clinical staging systems have been published (Table 3) of which the most clinically useful are the Masaoka and the GETT classifications (13,80,81). Distinctions between noninvasive (stage I), invasive (stage II-III), and disseminated disease (stage IV) have clear implications for prognosis and treatment recommendations. Some of the descriptions noted in these staging systems are somewhat vague. For example, the term, "tumor invasion", is ambiguous ("into" rather than "through" the capsule) and for stage IV_B tumors, intrathoracic and extrathoracic lymph node involvement are not distinguished. These areas of uncertainty cause some confusion in only a minority of patients but they have prompted modifications by some investigators (82,83).

Table 3: Staging Systems for Thymomas

Masaoka Staging (13)

I	Macroscopically completely encapsulated and microscopically no capsular invasion
II	1) Macroscopic invasion into surrounding fatty tissue, mediastinal pleura or both
	2) Microscopic invasion into capsule
III	Macroscopic invasion into neighboring organ, such as pericardium, great vessels, lung
IV_a	Pleural or pericardial dissemination
IV_b	Lymphogenous or hematogenous metastasis

GETT Classification (Groupe d'Etudes des Tumeurs Thymiques) (75)

Stage I

	I_A	Encapsulated tumor, totally resected
	I_B	Macroscopically encapsulated tumor, totally resected, but the surgeon suspects mediastinal adhesions and potential capsular invasion
Stage II		Invasive tumor, totally resected
Stage III		
	III_A	Invasive tumor subtotally resected
	III_B	Invasive tumor, biopsy
Stage IV		
	IV_A	Supraclavicular metastasis or distant pleural implants
	IV_B	Distant metastasis

Another more simplistic clinical classification separates patients with unresectable disease in the fashion used for small cell carcinoma of the lung, as limited or extensive disease. The former is defined as that in which all disease can be encompassed in a single radiotherapy portal; extensive disease pertains to all other patients. As combined modality therapy for locally advanced and metastatic disease becomes more accepted, this latter approach affords practical guidance for the clinician in determining treatment strategies.

As mentioned previously, the histologic classification of thymoma is not sufficient in distinguishing biologically benign from malignant tumors. The level of invasion remains the most important prognostic indicator. Besides invasion, prognostic factors which appear to adversely impact survival include metastasis, large size of the primary tumor (>10 cm), tracheal or vascular compromise, and age < 30 (88,90). Other factors such as myasthenia gravis and tumor cell DNA content have both been advocated and disputed as important prognostic indicators (17,20,86,87).

THERAPY

Surgery

Surgery remains the cornerstone of treatment for patients with low-stage thymoma. Fortunately most patients with thymoma will present with stage I or early stage II disease and thus should be curable with complete surgical resection. Several series report that over 90% of patients with stage I disease should be alive in five years and 80% at 10 years (84,85,86,87).

Excision should be accomplished by complete en-bloc resection of the tumor with the entire thymus gland. As ectopic thymic tissue may be present, a working knowledge of the anatomy of the thymus gland and possible extensions need to be known by the surgeon. Complete excision of the tumor is the goal of operative management (81,85,88). Although somewhat debatable (90,91), debulking procedures appear to confer no obvious survival advantage over biopsy alone (81,85,86,88). The median sternotomy produces optimal exposure to the thymus gland and is the preferred surgical procedure for most patients. In some patients in whom the tumor predominately lies within one hemithorax, a posteriolateral thoracotomy can be performed (87). extended resection may be required to remove portions of the pleura, pericardium, lung parenchyma and neurovascular structures in order to completely extirpate the tumor, but if this extensive approach is predicted, preoperative chemotherapy may be useful to downsize the tumor.
As expected, the complete resection rate varies with stage of disease (95-100% for stage II, 50-60% for stage III, and < 10% for stage IV). In many patients, particularly with this usually indolent malignancy, subsequent surgical resection of localized recurrences is associated with prolonged disease free survival. In some of these latter patients, preoperative chemotherapy or radiation therapy may facilitate surgery (84,89,92,93).

Radiation Therapy

For patients with incomplete surgical resection or invasive disease, radiotherapy is advocated (81,95). In one retrospective review, local recurrences were noted in 20 of 78 (26%) patients who had resected stage II or III thymoma and did not receive postoperative radiotherapy (90). These data contrasted with a local relapse rate of only 2 of 43 (5%) in similarly staged patients who had received postoperative radiation therapy. It should be noted that no prospective trial has evaluated the efficacy of radiation therapy as adjuvant treatment to date.

Until recently, most patients with locally advanced tumor (stage III and stage IV$_A$) have received radiation as monotherapy. Radiation produces approximately 65% local control and is associated with a five year survival rate of 40-50% (95). Patients with gross tumor resection prior to radiation appear to have substantially better local control and five year survival compared to those undergoing biopsy alone or minimal tumor resection (81,85,86,88).

A variety of dosages and schedules for radiotherapy have been reported. In general, dosages of 40-50 Gy (2 Gy/day fractions) have been used in the adjuvant setting. One retrospective analysis reported comparable local control rates for patients receiving ≤ 48 Gy or > 48 Gy, others feel that at least 50 Gy is indicated for maximal control (96,81). Dosages greater than 60 Gy used as primary therapy for patients with gross disease are associated with higher complication rates (e.g., pericarditis and radiation-induced myelitis) (91). Three dimensional treatment planning may minimize toxicity to adjacent non-involved structures and allow higher dosages to be delivered to the tumor. Although supraclavicular nodes have been reported as a site of recurrence (94), prophylactic irradiation of the supraclavicular fossa does not appear to confer any therapeutic advantage (84).

Chemotherapy

Chemotherapy has been reserved for those patients with metastatic disease, and more recently, it has been included as part of multiple modality therapy in patients with locally advanced disease. A variety of case reports or small series have suggested activity for many agents alone or as part of combination regimens. Only a few prospective clinical trials have been conducted to date in thymic malignancies.

Single Agent Data

Data for single agent therapy in thymoma are sparse. Based upon case reports suggesting clinical activity for cisplatin, one of the first prospective trials conducted for advanced thymoma evaluated this agent. Of 20 fully evaluable patients treated with cisplatin at a dose of 50 mg/m^2 every three weeks, only two patients (10%) had an objective response (97). In this trial, eligible patients were allowed to have had prior therapy, which may explain the lower than anticipated response rate.

Another case report was published in 1990 in which interleukin-2 produced a complete remission and reversal of immunologic abnormalities in a highly drug refractory patient with advanced thymoma (100). However, a subsequent prospective phase II trial of interleukin-2 in 14 patients with recurrent disease failed to confirm any activity for this drug in this disease(101).

In a multi-center trial conducted in Great Britain, single agent ifosfamide was associated with objective responses in 7 of 13 treated patients, making this perhaps one of the most active drugs in this disease (102). However, some of the patients who were designated as having a complete remission had undergone surgical resection of residual disease. Other agents which have produced responses include maytansine, paclitaxel, suramin and octreotide (plus prednisone) (73,103,104). The Eastern Cooperative Oncology Group is presently evaluating octreotide in patients with recurrent thymoma.

Corticosteroids have been associated with brief responses which are usually partial in nature (106,107,108). As a reminder, thymoma and thymic cancer are epithelial malignancies in which the lymphocyte population is considered reactive (non-neoplastic). The true effect of corticosteroids in thymoma is uncertain these drugs are lympholytic in nature and the majority of responses have been seen in lymphocyte predominant thymomas (109). Nonetheless, glucocorticoid receptors have been noted in murine thymoma cell lines which could suggest a possible direct effect by corticosteroids but these thymocytes are actually T-lymphocytes and not the epithelial cells of malignant potential in humans (98,99).

Combination Therapy

In the pre-cisplatin era, numerous regimens generally usually using lymphoma-based therapy were reported. Regimens which contain doxorubicin and cyclophosphamide appear to be among those with the most activity. After the suggestion of single agent activity for cisplatin, the Southeastern Cancer Study Group initiated a trial in 1983 for patients with locally advanced and metastatic thymoma (110,111). All patients received cisplatin, doxorubicin, and cyclophosphamide (or PAC). Patients with limited disease received involved field radiotherapy following 2-4 cycles of chemotherapy, while those patients with extensive disease (or prior radiation therapy) received 6 cycles of PAC chemotherapy only. In 30 patients with extensive thymoma or thymic carcinoma, three complete and 12 partial responses were observed (50% overall response rate). The time to treatment failure was 18.4 months (range 0.8 - 92+ months) and a median survival time was 38 months (2 - 92+ months). The five-year survival was 32%.

In limited stage patients, the above cited trial was subsequently completed by the Eastern Cooperative Oncology Group (111). This trial demonstrated five complete and 11 partial responses to PAC chemotherapy prior to radiation therapy in 23 evaluable patients (70% overall response rate) with a median time to treatment failure of 93 months (3 - 99+ months) and a median survival time of 93 months (1 - 110 months). The five-year survival was 52%.

Forniserro and colleagues reported a 43% complete and 92% overall objective rate in 37 patients with stage III and IV disease using cisplatin, doxorubicin, cyclophosphamide and vincristine (ADOC) (112). Despite a high response rate, the median survival time was only 15 months, calling into question the importance of vincristine in this regimen when compared to the previously mentioned experience with the PAC regimen (without vincristine).

The European Organization for Research and Treatment of Cancer evaluated cisplatin and etoposide given every three weeks for patients with advanced thymoma (113). In 16 patients entered in this multi-institutional prospective trial, there were five complete and four partial responses (CR + PR = 56%). The median survival time was 4.3 years. In a multi-institutional intergroup trial recently completed in the United States, ifosfamide was added to the cisplatin and etoposide regimen in previously untreated patients with advanced disease, but preliminary results do not suggest that this addition is advantageous.

Besides the trial mentioned above, three other prospective trials have evaluated primary chemotherapy as part of multi-modality therapy for limited stage thymoma (114,115,116). Although the regimens differed (cisplatin, etoposide and epirubicin; ADOC; and PAC plus prednisone), 70% to 100% of patients have had an objective response to chemotherapy when administered prior to surgery and/or radiotherapy. In one trial, an association between Ki67 and tumor necrosis following chemotherapy was noted (106). Novel treatment approaches currently underway include trials looking at high dose chemotherapy with stem cell rescue as initial salvage therapy for patients with recurrent disease.

In sum, these data confirm that thymoma is a chemosensitive tumor. The high response rate and five year survival in 30-50% of patients with stage III/IV disease also seem to confirm the role of systemic therapy. Prospective randomized trials, however, have not and probably will not be done to confirm the impact of chemotherapy in thymoma patients because of the rarity of this tumor. In at least one review, multivariate analysis did demonstrate that chemotherapy was associated with an improvement in overall survival for patients with stage III and IV disease (91).

THYMIC CARCINOMA

Thymic carcinomas represent an uncommon group of neoplasms. They differ clinically from thymoma in that it is not associated with paraneoplastic syndromes such as myasthenia gravis or pure red blood cell aplasia (63). Like thymoma, these malignancies usually present with local complaints such as chest pain, dyspnea or cough, or they are detected incidentally by chest radiography. Patients with thymic carcinomas are characteristically middle-aged or elderly adults with only infrequent pediatric cases.

These tumors also occur in the anterior mediastinum but are pathologically distinct from thymoma. Some authors believe that thymic carcinomas merely represent one end of a pathologic spectrum of tumors with epithelial origin. As mentioned previously, well differentiated thymic carcinoma (WDTC) is, in our opinion, poorly named as it is more closely aligned clinically with cortical thymoma. For example, unlike typical thymic carcinoma, WDTC is often associated with myasthenias gravis. The role of chemotherapy in advanced thymic carcinoma is unclear at this point, but responses with the same drugs mentioned above for thymomas have been seen in these tumors.

SUMMARY

Thymomas and thymic carcinomas are unique tumors of the anterior mediastinum. The association of a variety of different paraneoplastic syndromes with such lesions has fascinated physicians and researchers for years. Most recently, it has been demonstrated by numerous authors that thymomas are chemosensitive tumors. Their indolent nature and relative rarity have made evaluation through prospective randomized clinical trials extremely difficult. Further information regarding the molecular nature of these neoplasms and immunologic aspects is needed in future investigation.

REFERENCES

1.   Schierling S. Where there is smoke: An analogy of the soul. Classical Bull 61:6-7, 1985.

2.   Miller JFAP. Thymus & Immunity-II. The last three decades. Eur J Cancer Clin Oncol 24:1257-62, 1988.

3.   Buckley RH. Immunodeficiency disease. JAMA 258:2841-2850, 1987.

4.   Rosen FS, Cooper MD, Wedgwood RJP. The primary immunodeficiencies. N Engl J Med 311:235-242; 300-310, 1985.

5.   Muller-Hermelink HK, Wilisch A, Schultz A, et al. Characterization of the human thymic microenvironment: lymphoepithelial interaction in normal thymus and thymoma. Arch Histol Cytol. 60: 9-28, 1997.

6.   Skandalakis JE, Gray SW, Todd NW. Pharynx and its derivatives. In Skandalakis J, Gray S, eds. Embryology for Surgeons 2nd edition Baltimore: Williams and Wilkins 1994.

7.   Marino M, Muller-Hermelink HK. Thymoma and thymic carcinoma: relation of thymoma epithelial cells to the cortical and medullary differentiation of thymus. Virchows Arch [A] (Pathol Anat). 407:119-149, 1985.

8.   van de Wijngaert FP, Kendall MD, Schuurman H-J, et al. Heterogeneity of epithelial cells in the human thymus. An ultrastructural study. Cell Tissue Res 237:227-237, 1984.

9.   Davis RD, Oldham HN, Sabiston DC. Primary cysts and neoplasms of the mediastinum: Recent changes in clinical presentation, methods of diagnosis, management and results. Ann Thorac Surg. 44:229-237, 1987.

10.   Mullen B, Richardson JD. Primary anterior mediastinal tumors in children and adults. Ann Thorac Surg 42:338-345, 1986.

11.   National Cancer Institute: Surveillance Epidemiology and End Results Program 1990.

12.   dos Santos-Silua I, Swerdlow AJ. Thymus cancer epidemiologyin England and Wales. Br J Cancer 61:899-902, 1990.

13.   Masaoka A, Monden Y, Nakahara K et al. Follow-up study of thymomas with special reference to their clinical stages. Cancer 48:2485-2492, 1981.

14.   Bernatz PE, Khonsari S, Harrison EG et al. Thymoma: factors influencing prognosis. Surg Clin North Am 53:885-893, 1973.

15.   LeGolvan DP, Abell MR. Thymomas. Cancer 39:2142-2157, 1977.

16.   Legg MA, Brady WJ. Pathology and clinical behaviour of thymomas: a survey of 51 cases. Cancer 18:1131-1144, 1965.

17.   Lewis JE, Wick MR, Scheithauer BW et al. Thymoma: a clinicopathologic review. Cancer 60:2727-2743, 1987.

18.   Verley JM, Hollman KH. Thymoma: a comparative study of clinical features, histologic features and survival in 200 cases. Cancer 55:1074-1086, 1985.

19.   Batata MA, Martini N, Huvos AG et al. Thymomas: clinicopathologic features, therapy and prognosis. Cancer 34:389-396, 1974.

20.   Salyer WR, Eggleston JC. Thymoma: a clinical and pathological study of 65 cases. Cancer 37:229-249, 1976.

21.   Leyvraz S, Henle W, Chahinian A, Perlmann C, Klein G, Gordon R, Rosenblum M, Holland J. Association of Epstein-Barr virus with thymic carcinoma. N Engl J Med 312:1296-1299, 1985.

22. Wu T, Kuo T. Study of Epstein-Barr virus early RNA 1 (EBER 1) expression by in situ hybridization in thymic epithelial tumors of chinese patients in Taiwan. Hum Pathol 24:235-238, 1993.

23. Wu TC, Kuo TT. Study of Epstein-Barr virus early RNA 1 (EBER 1) expression by in situ hybridization in thymic epithelial tumors of chinese patients in Taiwan. Hum Pathol 24:235-238, 1993.

24. Rosai J. "Lymphoepthelioma-like" thymic carcinoma: Another tumor related to Epstein-Barr virus? N Engl J Med 312:1320-22, 1985.

25. Patton DP, Ribeiro RC, Jenkins JJ et al. Thymic carcinoma with a defective Epstein-Barr virus encoding the BZLF1 trans-activator. J Infect Dis 170:7-12, 1994.

26. Teoh R, McGuire L, Wong K et al. Increased incidence of thymoma in Chinese myesthenia gravis: possible relationship to Epstein Barr virus. Acta Neurol Scand 80:221-225, 1989.

27. Jensen MD, Antonenko D. Thyroid and thymic mnalignancies following childhood irradiation. J Surg Oncol 50:206-208, 1992.

28. Kubonishi I, Takehara N, Iwata J, Sonobe H, Ohtsuki Y, Abe T, Miyoshi I. Novel t(15;19)(q15;p13) chromosome abnormality in a thymic carcinoma. Cancer Res 51:3327-3327, 1991.

29. Matani A, Dristas C. Familial occurence of thymoma. Arch Path 95:90-91, 1973.

30. Lam WWM, Chan FL, Lau LY, Chau MT, Mok CK. Paediatric thymoma: Unusual occurence in wtwo siblings. Pediastr Radiol 23:124-126, 1993.

31. Wick MR, Scheithouer BWS, Dines DE. Thymic neoplasia in two male siblings. Mayo Clin Proc 57:653-656, 1982.

32. Kees UR, Mulcahy MT, Willoughby MLN. Intrathoracic carcioma in an 11-year-old girl showing a translocation t(15;19). Am J Pediatr Hematol Oncol 13:459-464, 1991.

33. Lee ACW, Kwong Y, Fu KH et al. Disseminated mediastinal carcinoma with chromosomal translocation (15;19). Cancer 72:2273-2276, 1993.

34. Shier KJ. The morphology of the epithelial thymus: observations on lymphocyte-depleted & fetal thymus. Lab Invest 12:315-326, 1963.

35. Clark SL. The intrathymic environment. In: Contemporary Topics in Immunobiology, Vol. 2 [Davies AJS, Carter RL, Eds], New York, Plenum Press, 1973; pp. 77-79.

36. Schier KJ. The thymus according to Schambacher: medullary ducts & reticular epithelium of thymus and thymomas. Cancer 48:1183-1199, 1981.

37. Wick MR. Mediastinum. In: Diagnostic Surgical Pathology, Ed. 2, Vol. 1 (Sternberg SS, Ed), Raven Press, New York, 1994; pp. 1125-1182.

38. Suster S, Rosai J. Cystic thymomas: a clinicopathologic study of 10 cases. Cancer 69:92-97, 1992.

39. Rosai J, Limas C, Husband EM. Ectopic hamartomatous thymoma: a distinctive benign lesion of the lower neck. Am J Surg Pathol 8:501-513, 1984.

40. Yeoh CB, Ford JM, Lattes R, et al. Intrapulmonary thymoma. J Thorac Cardiovasc Surg 51:131-136, 1966.

41.   Moran CA, Travis WD, Rosado-de-Christenson M, et al. Thymoma presenting as pleural tumors: report of eight cases. Am J Surg Pathol 16:138-144, 1992.

42.   Kirchner T, Schalke B, Buchwald J, et al. Well differentiated thymic carcinoma: an organotypical low grade carcinoma with realtionship to cortical thymoma. Am J Surg Pathol 16:1153-1169, 1992.

43.   Suster S, Rosai J. Thymic carcinoma: a clinicopathologic study of 60 cases. Cancer 67:1025-1032, 1991.

44.   Snover DC, Levine GD, Rosai J. Thymic carcinoma: five distinctive histological variants. Am J Surg Pathol 6:451-470, 1982.

45.   Walker AN, Mills SE, Fechner RE. Thymomas and thymic carcinomas. Semin Diagn Pathol 7:250-265, 1990.

46.   Engel P, Pilsgaard B, Francis D. Thymomas & thymic carcinomas: a retrospective investigation with histological reclassification. APMIS 103:671-678, 1995.

47.   Shimuzu J, Hayashi Y, Morita K. Primary thymic carcinoma: a clinicopathological and immunohistochemical study. J Surg Oncol 56:159-164, 1994.

48.   Bernatz PE, Harrison EG Jr, Clagett OT. Thymoma: a clinicopathologic study. J Thorac Cardiovasc Surg 42:424-444, 1961.

49.   Shimosato Y, Mukai K. Tumors of the Thymus & Mediastinum. In: Atlas of Tumor Pathology, Fascicle 21, Series 3, Armed Forces Institute of Pathology, Washington, DC, 1997; pp. 33-273.

50.   Pan CC, Wu HP, Yang CG, Chen WYK, Chiang H. The clinicopathological correlation of epithelial subtyping in thymoma: A study of 112 consecutive cases. Hum Pathol 25:893-899, 1994.

51.   Quintanilla-Matinez L, Wilkins EW et al. Thymoma. histologic subclassification is an independent prognostic factor. Cancer 74:606-617, 1994.

52.   Dawson A, Ibrahim NB, Gibbs AR. Observer variation in the histopathological classification of thymomas: correlation with prognosis. J Clin Pathol 47: 519-523, 1994.

53.   Ho FC, Fu KH, Lam SY, et al. Evaluation of a histogenetic classification for thymic epithelial tumors. Histopathology 25:21-29, 1994.

54.   Souadjian JV, Enriquez P, Silverstein MN et al. The spectrum of diseases associated with thymoma: coincidence or syndrome. Arch Int Med 134:374-379, 1974.

55.   Drachman DB. Myasthenia gravis. N Engl J Med 330:1797-1810, 1994.

56.   Hopper HH. Ein Beitrag zur Kenntnis der Bulbarparalyse. 1892. Berl. Klin. Wschr 29:332-36.

57.   Blossom GR, Ernstoff RM, Howellls GA et al. Thymectomy for Myasthenia Gravis. Arch Surg 128:855-862, 1993.

58.   Berrih-Aknin S, Morel E, Raimond F et al. The role of the thymus in myasthenia gravis: immunohistological and immunological studies in 115 cases. Ann N Y Acad Sci 505:50-70, 1987.

59.   Marx A, Wilisch A, Schultz A, Gattenlohner S, Nenninger R, Muller-Hermelink HK. Pathogenesis of myasthenia gravis. Virchows Arc 430:355-364, 1997.

60.   Williams CL, Hay JE, Huitt TW et al. Paraneoplastic IgG striational autoantibodies produced by clonal thymic B cells and in serum of patients with myastenia gravis and thymoma react with titan. Lab Invest 66:331-336, 1992.

61.   Skinnider LF, Alexander S. Concurrent thymoma and lymphoma: A report of two cases. Hum Pathol 13:163-166, 1982.

62.   Kao I, Drachman DB. Thymic muscle cells bear acetylcholene receptors: Possible relation to myasthenia gravis. Science 195:74-75, 1997.

63.   Morgentaler TI, Brown LR, Colby TV, Harper CM, Coles DT. Thymoma. Mayo Clin Proc 68:1110-1123, 1993.

64.   Zeok JV, Todd EP, Dillon M et al. The role of thymectomy in red cell aplasia. Ann Thorac Surg 28:257-260, 1979.

65.   Masaoka A, Hashimoto T, Shibata K et al. Thymomas associated with pure red cell aplasia: histologic and follow-up studies. Cancer 64: 1872-1878, 1989.

66.   Yip D, Rasko JE, Lee C et al. Thymoma and agranulocytosis: two case reports and literature review. Br J Haematol 65:52-56, 1996.

67.   Casadevall N, Dupuy E, Molho-Sabatier P et al. Brief report: autoantibodies against erythropoetin in a patient with pure red cell aplasia. N Eng J Med 334:630-33, 1996.

68.   Masuda M, Arai Y, Okamura T, Mizoguchi H. Pure red cell aplasia with thymoma: evidence of T-cell clonal disorder. Am J Hematol 54:324-328, 1997.

69.   Scully RE, Mark EJ, McNeely WF, McNeely BV. Case records of the Massachusetts General Hospital. N Engl Med Jnl 316:35-42, 1987.

70.   Loehrer PJ, Perez CA, Roth LM, Greco FA, Livingston RB, et al. Chemotherapy for advanced thymoma: Preliminary results of an intergroup study. Annals of Internal Medicine 113:520-524, 1990.

71.   Batra P, Brown K, Collins JD et al. Mediastinal masses: magnetic resonance imaging in comparison with computed tomography. J Natl Med Assoc 83: 969-974, 1991.

72.   Loehrer PJ, Bonomi P, Goldman S et al. Remission of invasive thymoma due to chemotherapy. Chest 87:377-380, 1985.

73.   Palmieri G, Lastoria S, Colao A et al. Successful treatment of a patient with a thymoma and pure red cell aplasia with octreotide and prednisone. N Engl J Med 336:263-265, 1997.

74.   Hoffman OA, Gillespie DJ, Aughenbaugh GL, Brown LR. Primary mediastinal neoplasms (other than thymoma). May Clin Proc 68:880-891, 1993.

75.   Dahlgren S, Sandstedt B, Sundstrom C. Fine needle aspiration cytology of thymic tumors. Acta Cytologica 27:1-6, 1983.

76.   Herman SJ, Holub RV, Weisbrod GL et al Anterior mediastinal masses: utility of transthoracic needle biopsy. Radiology 180:167-170, 1991.

77.   Morrisey B, Adams H, Gibbs AR et al. Percutaneous needle biopsy of the mediastinum: review of 94 procedures. Thorax 48:632-637, 1993.

78.   Moran CA, Travis WD, Rosado-de-Christensen M, Koss MN, Rosai J. Thyomas presenting as pleural tumors. Am J Surg Path 16:138-144, 1992.

79.   Shih DF, Wang JS, Tseng HH, Tiao WM: Primary pleural thymoma. Arch Pathol Lab Med 121:79-82, 1997.

80. Yamakawa Y, Masaoka A, Hashimoto T et al. A tentative tumor-node-metastasis classification of thymoma. Cancer 68:1984-1987, 1991.

81. Mornex F, Resbeut M, Richard P et al. Radiotherapy and chemotherapy for invasive thymoma: a multicentric retrospective review of 90 cases. Int J Radiat Oncol Biol Phys 32:651-659, 1995.

82. Kornstein MJ, Curran WJ, Turrisi AT et al. Cortical versus medullary thymomas; a useful morphologic distinction. Hum Pathol 19:1335-1339, 1988.

83. Haniunda M, Morimoto M, Nishimura H et al Adjuvant radiotherapy after complete resection of thymoma. Ann Thor Sur 54:311-315, 1992.

84. Ruffini E, Mancusco M, Oliarao A et al. Recurrence of thymoma: Analysis of clinicopathologic faetures, treatment and outcome. J Thorac Cardiovasc Surg 113:55-63, 1997.

85. Nakahara K, Ohno K, Hashimoto J et al. Thymoma: results with complete resection and adjuvant postoperative irradiation in 141 consecutive patients. J Thorac Cardiovasc Surg 95:1041-1047, 1988.

86. Maggi G, Casadio C, Cavallo A et al. Thymoma: results of 241 operated cases. Ann Thorac Surg 51:152-166, 1991.

87. Wilkins EW, Grillo HC, Scannell G et al. Role of staging in prognosis and management of thymoma. Ann Thorac Surg 51:888-892, 1991.

88. Cowen D, Richaud P, Mornex F et al Thymoma results of a multicentric retrospective review of 149 non-metastatic irradiated patients and review of the literature. Radiother Oncol 34:9-16, 1995.

89. Urgesi A, Monetti V, Rossi G et al. Aggressive treatment of intrathoracic recurrences of thymoma. Radiother Oncol 24:221-225, 1992.

90. Curran WJ, Kornstein MJ, Brooks JJ et al. Invasive thymoma: the role of mediastinal irradiation following complete or incomplete surgical resection. J Clin Oncol 6:1722-1727, 1988.

91. Ciernik IF, Meier U, Lutalf UM. Prognostic factors and outcome of incompletely resected invasive thymoma following radiation therapy. J Clin Oncol 12:1484-1490, 1994.

92. Jaretzki A, Wolff M. "Maximal" thymectomy for myasthenia gravis. J Thorac Cardiovasc Surg 96:711-716, 1993.

93. Kirchner PA. Reoperation for thymoma: report of 23 cases. Ann Thorac Surg 49:550-555, 1990.

94. Chahinian AP, Bhardwaj S, Meyer RJ. Treatment of invasive thymoma. Cancer 47:1752-1761, 1981.

95. Koh WJ, Loehrer PJ, Thomas C. Thymoma: Radiation and chemotherapy. In Mediastinal Tumors: Update 1995. Ed. Wood D, Thomas C. New York: Springer-Verlag 1995, 19-25.

96. Arriagada R, Bretel JJ, Caillaud JM et al. Invasive carcinoma of the thymus. A multicenter retrospective review of 56 cases. Eur J Clin Oncol 20:69-74, 1984.

97. Bonomi PD, Finkelstein D, Aisner S et al. EST 2582 phase II trial of cisplatin in metastatic or recurrent thymoma. Am J Clin Oncol 16:342-345, 1993.

98.   Chapman MS, Askew DJ, Juscuoglu V, Miesfelo RL. Transcriptional control of steroid-regulated apoptosis in murine thymoma cells. Molec Endocrin 10:967-78, 1996.

99.   Holbrook NJ, Bodwell JE, Munck A. Nonactivated and activated glucocorticoid-receptor complexes in WEHI-7 and rat thymus cells. J Steroid Biochem 20:19-22, 1984.

100. Berthaud P, le Chevalier T, Tursz T. Effective Interleukin-2 in invasive lymphoepithelial thymoma (letter). Lancet 335:1590, 1990.

101. Gordon MS, Battiato LA, Gonin R et al. A phase II trial of subcutaneously administered recombinant human interleukin-2 in patients with relapsed/refractory thymoma. J Immunother 18:179-184, 1995.

102. Harper PG, Addis B. Unusual tumors of the mediastinum. In Textbook of Uncommon Cancer. Williams C, Krikorian J, Green M, Ragahvan D eds. John Wiley & Sons 1988.

103. La Rocca R, Cooper M, Danesi R et al. Suramin therapy for malignant thymoma: a case report. Eur J Cancer 30A:718-719, 1994.

104. Boston B. Chemotherapy of invasive thymoma. Cancer 38:49-52, 1976.

105. Jaffrey L. Response to maytansine in a patient with malignant thymoma. Cancer Treat Reports 64:193-194, 1980.

106. Haussen S, Nibbelink D, Hackett E. Effect of adrenocorticosteroid therapy of myasthenia gravis on associated malignant thymomas [abstract] Neurology 25:347, 1975.

107. Hu E, Levine J. Chemotherapy of malignant thymoma. Cancer 57:1101-1104, 1986.

108. Kirkove C, Berghmans J, Noel H et al. Dramatic response of recurrent invasive thymoma to high doses corticosteroid. Clin Oncol (R Coll Radiol) 4:64-66, 1992.

109. Oldroyd K, Spiers A, Hussain M. Invasive thymoma: unique presentation as an anterior chest wall mass. Clin Oncol (R Coll Radiol) 9:169-176, 1983.

110. Loehrer PJ, Kim KM, Aisner SC et al. Cisplatin plus doxorubicin plus cyclophosphamide in metastatic or recurrent thymoma: Final results of an intergroup trial. J Clin Oncol 12:1164-1168, 1994.

111. Loehrer PJ, Chen M, Kim KM et al. Cisplatin, doxorubicin and cyclophosphamide plus thoracic radiation therapy for limited stage, unresectable thymoma: an intergroup trial. J Clin Oncol 15:3093-3099, 1997.

112. Forniasiero A, Daniele O, Ghiotto C et al. Chemotherapy for invasive thymoma: a 13 year experience. Cancer 68:30-33, 1991.

113. Giaccone G, Ardizzoni A, Kirkpatrick A et al. Cisplatin and etoposide combination chemotherapy for locally advanced or metastatic thymoma: A phase II study of the European Organization for Research and Treatment of Cancer Lung Cancer Cooperative Group J Clin Oncol 14:814-820, 1996.

114. Macchiarini P, Chella A, Ducci F et al. Neoadjuvant chemotherapy, surgery, and postoperative radiation therapy for invasive thymoma. Cancer 68:706-713, 1991.

115. Rea F, Sartori F, Loy M et al Chemotherapy and operation for invasive thymoma. J Thorac Cardiovasc Surg 106:543-549, 1993.

 Thymic Malignancies

116. Shin DM, Komaki R, Putnam JB et al. Induction chemotherapy (IC) followed by surgical resection (SR), radiotherapy and consolidative chemotherapy may cure the advanced stages of unresectable invasive thymoma. Proc ASCO 16: 1639, 1997.
117. Levine GD, Rosai J. Thymic hyperplasia and neoplasia: a review of current concepts. Human Pathology 9:495-419, 1978.
118. Muller-Hermelink HK, Marino M, Palestro G: Pathology of thymic epithelial tumors. Curr Topics Pathol 75:207-268, 1986.
119. Wick MR, Weiland LH, Scheithauer BW et al. Primary thymic carcinomas. Am J Surg Pathol 6:613-630, 1982.
120. Rosai J, Levine GD: Tumors of the thymus. In: Atlas of Tumor Pathology, Fascicle 13, Series 2, Armed Forces Institute of Pathology, Washington, DC, 1976; pp. 10-150.

GERM CELL NEOPLASMS AND OTHER MALIGNANCIES OF THE MEDIASTINUM

John D. Hainsworth, M.D.
Sarah Cannon Cancer Center Centennial Medical Center, Nashville, TN 37203 USA

F. Anthony Greco, M.D.
Sarah Cannon Cancer Center Centennial Medical Center, Nashville, TN 37203 USA

INTRODUCTION

The mediastinum is commonly involved by malignant tumors; however, the large majority of patients have metastatic involvement of mediastinal lymph nodes rather than a malignancy arising in the mediastinum. Approximately two-thirds of all primary mediastinal tumors are arising, and surgical removal is usually curative (1,2). The malignant tumors occurring in the mediastinum are an interesting and important group even though they are uncommon, since effective treatment is available for most of these tumors. Examples of treatable tumors arising in the mediastinum include extragonadal germ cell tumors, malignant thymoma, Hodgkin's disease, non-Hodgkin's lymphoma, and poorly differentiated carcinoma. The majority of this chapter is devoted to a discussion of primary mediastinal germ cell tumors, a unique and important group of highly treatable neoplasms. Brief sections on mediastinal lymphoma and various primary sarcomas are also included, although complete discussion of these neoplasms is beyond the scope of this chapter.

DIAGNOSTIC EVALUATION OF THE PATIENT WITH SUSPECTED MEDIASTINAL MALIGNANCY

Most patients with primary mediastinal tumors seek medical attention either because of development of local symptoms, or as a result of the finding of an asymptomatic mediastinal mass on routine chest radiography. Local symptoms are usually caused by compression or invasion of adjacent structures and can include substernal chest pain, dyspnea, cough, and dysphagia. Less common local symptoms include hemoptysis, hoarseness, and superior vena cava syndrome.

The initial evaluation should narrow the differential diagnosis and determine the most appropriate biopsy approach. Computerized tomography of the chest is essential in delineating the extent and location of the mediastinal tumor and in evaluating the lung fields. Most primary mediastinal tumors, including germ cell tumors, thymic neoplasms, and lymphomas, arise in the anterior mediastinum. The tumors arising in the middle and posterior mediastinum include mesenchymal and neurogenic neoplasms, as well as occasional lymphomas.

Initial evaluation should also include a staging evaluation to detect distant metastases. Physical examination should rule out the presence of peripheral adenopathy. All patients should have computerized tomography of the abdomen, as well as radiologic evaluation of any other symptomatic sites. Fiberoptic bronchoscopy should be considered in patients at risk for lung cancer. In young men, serum levels of α-fetoprotein and human chorionic gonadatrophin (HCG) should be measured. If staging evaluation reveals metastatic tumor, biopsy should be performed from the most accessible tumor site.

Options for biopsy of mediastinal tumors include fine needle aspiration, mediastinoscopy, limited thoracotomy, and full thoracotomy with resection. The biopsy technique should depend on the location of the mediastinal tumor as well as the suspected diagnosis based on pre-biopsy evaluation. Fine needle aspiration biopsy is the least invasive and best tolerated procedure; however, the small amount of tissue obtained often limits optimal pathologic evaluation of poorly differentiated tumors. This consideration is particularly relevant to primary mediastinal tumor types (e.g. germ cell tumor, lymphoma, carcinoma), which often have poorly differentiated histology. Definitive diagnosis of these tumors often requires open biopsy. In patients with tumors that are obviously unresectable, biopsy should be achieved with the least invasive technique, usually mediastinoscopy or limited parasternal exploration. However, in patients with small tumors that are potentially resectable, the most appropriate approach is usually a median sternotomy or a full thoracotomy, with complete tumor resection.

MALIGNANT MEDIASTINAL GERM CELL TUMORS

The biology, clinical characteristics, and treatment of mediastinal germ cell tumors have been defined during the last 25 years. Although these neoplasms are rare, they are of particular interest and importance because they affect predominantly young males, and because curative therapy is available in many cases. Patients with malignant mediastinal germ cell tumors are conveniently grouped into two subsets, those with pure seminoma and those with elements of nonseminomatous germ cell tumor. Treatment of patients in these two groups differs, and is discussed separately.

Etiology

Malignant mediastinal germ cell tumors of various histologies were first described as a clinical entity 50 years ago (3,4). Initially, mediastinal germ cell tumors were thought to represent isolated metastases from an occult gonadal primary site. Postmortem examination occasionally identified small unrecognized tumors in the testes, or fibrous scars thought to represent sites of regressed primary tumors (5,6). However, neither of these findings can be identified in most patients with mediastinal germ cell tumors, either at the time of testicular biopsy or at autopsy (7,8). In addition, large numbers of patients with mediastinal germ cell tumors are now long-term survivors following mediastinal irradiation for pure seminoma, or combination chemotherapy for nonseminomatous tumors. Testicular recurrences have not been observed in these patients. Therefore, there is now general acceptance that germ cell tumors can arise in a variety of locations including the mediastinum, retroperitoneum, and pineal area. Some investigators have suggested that this distribution arises as a consequence of abnormal migration of germ cells during embryogenesis (4,9). Others have hypothesized a widespread distribution of germ cells to multiple sites during normal embryogenesis, with these cells conveying genetic information or providing regulatory functions at somatic sites (10).

Incidence and Epidemiology

Malignant germ cell tumors of the mediastinum represent only 3 to 10% of tumors originating in the mediastinum (11-13). They are much less common than testicular germ cell tumors and account for only 1 to 5% of all germ cell neoplasms (14,15). These incidence figures may underestimate the true incidence of mediastinal germ cell tumors, since the histology of these tumors may be mistaken for other poorly differentiated tumors arising in the mediastinum. Other tumor types occasionally mistaken for germ cell tumors include malignant thymoma and aggressive non-Hodgkin's lymphoma. Some young men initially diagnosed with "poorly differentiated neoplasm" or "poorly differentiated carcinoma" actually have germ cell tumors, and display the pathognomonic i(12p) chromosomal abnormality (16,17). Some of the patients diagnosed with "poorly differentiated carcinoma" involving the mediastinum have excellent responses when treated with chemotherapy effective against germ cell tumors. Increased awareness of these tumors by clinicians and pathologists will probably result in an increased recognition and diagnosis of mediastinal germ cell tumors.

The great majority of mediastinal germ cell tumors occur in males between the ages of 20 and 35 years. For unknown reasons, extragonadal germ cell tumors are extremely rare in women, and are more common in Caucasian men than in men of other races.

Histopathology

Mediastinal germ cell tumors exhibit the same spectrum of histopathology that is seen in testicular germ cell tumors; however, there are several differences in the relative incidence of the nonseminomatous histologies (Table 1). In a recent review of 229 malignant mediastinal germ cell tumors seen between 1960 and 1994 at the Armed Forces Institute of Pathology, pure seminoma was the most common histology and accounted for 52% of cases (18). Nonseminomatous histologies included teratocarcinoma (20%), yolk sac tumor (17%), choriocarcinoma (3%), embryonal carcinoma (3%), and mixed nonseminomatous histologies (5%). The incidence of tumors with pure yolk sac histology is higher in mediastinal germ cell tumors than in the testicular cancer, whereas the incidence of embryonal carcinoma seems less common in the mediastinum than in the testis.

Table 1. Histology of Germ Cell Tumors Arising in the Testis and the Mediastinum

		Incidence (%)
Histology	Testis	Mediastinum [18]
Seminoma	50	52
Nonseminoma		
Teratocarcinoma	20	20
Embryonal carcinoma	15	3
Yolk sac tumor	-	17
Choriocarcinoma	2	3
Mixed histologies	13	5

Clinical Characteristics

Most malignant mediastinal germ cell tumors are large and symptomatic at the time of diagnosis. Local symptoms are common, and are caused by compression or invasion of local mediastinal structures including the lungs, pleura, pericardium, and chest wall. Pure seminomas are somewhat slower growing and have less potential for early metastasis than do tumors with nonseminomatous elements. Since clinical presentations vary to some extent, clinical features of pure seminomas and nonseminomatous tumors are discussed separately.

Seminoma

Seminomas grow relatively slowly and often become very large before causing symptoms. Tumors as large as 20 to 30 cm in diameter can exist with minimal local symptomatology. Approximately 20 to 30% of mediastinal seminomas are detected by chest radiography while still asymptomatic (19). The most common initial symptom is a sensation of pressure or dull retrosternal chest pain. Additional local symptoms include cough, exertional dyspnea, hoarseness, and dysphagia. Approximately 10% of patients develop superior vena cava syndrome. Systemic symptoms related to distant metastases are uncommon at presentation.

With careful initial staging, only 40% of patients with pure mediastinal seminoma have localized disease, while the remainder have one or more sites of distant metastases (20,21). The lungs and other intrathoracic structures are the most common sites for metastases; the skeletal system is the most frequently involved extrathoracic site. Approximately 10% of patients with mediastinal seminoma have elevated serum levels of HCG at the time of diagnosis (20). This incidence is similar to that reported in advanced testicular seminoma. Usually serum HCG levels are less than 100ng/ml; higher levels suggest the presence of nonseminomatous elements. Serum α-fetoprotein levels are always normal in pure seminoma; any elevation of α-fetoprotein indicates the presence of nonseminomatous elements. Serum lactate dehydrogenase (LDH) is elevated in the majority of patients with mediastinal seminoma (20).

On chest radiography, pure seminoma appears as a large noncalcified anterior mediastinal mass, often compressing or deviating the trachea or bronchi. Computerized tomography usually shows a large homogeneous mass that obliterates the fat planes surrounding mediastinal vascular structures (22). These radiographic findings are not specific enough to allow distinction of pure mediastinal seminoma from other mediastinal tumors.

Nonseminomatous Tumors
Almost all patients with mediastinal nonseminomatous germ cell tumors are symptomatic at the time of diagnosis. Local symptoms are similar to those seen in patients with mediastinal seminoma. In addition, symptoms due to distant metastases are more common in this group, since 85 to 95% of these patients have at least one metastatic site at time of diagnosis (23-26). Common metastatic sites include the lungs, pleura, lymph nodes (particularly supraclavicular and retroperitoneal), and liver. Multiple other sites are less frequently involved. Constitutional symptoms including weakness, weight loss, and fever are more common in these patients than in patients with pure seminoma. Patients with predominantly choriocarcinoma histology have a marked hemorrhagic tendency. These patients may have catastrophic events related to uncontrolled hemorrhage at a metastatic site (eg. massive hemoptysis, intracranial hemorrhage); such symptoms can be spontaneous or can follow a biopsy procedure (26). Gynecomastia is a presenting sign in a small percentage of patients who have high serum HCG levels.

The large majority of patients with mediastinal nonseminomatous germ cell tumors have elevations of either serum α-fetoprotein or HCG. Alpha-fetoprotein is elevated in approximately 80% of patients, while serum HCG is elevated in 30 to 35% (27,28). This pattern of tumor marker elevation differs somewhat from germ cell tumors of the testis, where α-fetoprotein and HCG are elevated in approximately the same percentage of patients. Serum LDH is also elevated in 80 to 90% of patients with mediastinal nonseminomatous germ cell tumors (24).

Chest radiographic features of mediastinal nonseminomatous germ cell tumors are similar to those described in mediastinal seminomas. The chest CT scan frequently shows a large anterior mediastinal mass with multiple areas of hemorrhage and necrosis, differing from the homogeneous appearance of mediastinal seminoma (22).

Syndromes Associated with Mediastinal Nonseminomatous Germ Cell Tumors

Klinefelter's Syndrome

Klinefelter's syndrome is caused by a relatively common chromosomal abnormality, and is characterized by hypogonadism, azoospermia, and elevated gonadotropin levels in association with an extra chromosome X. Men with this syndrome may have a slightly increased incidence of breast cancer, but a general predisposition to develop other cancers has not been observed (29). However, the association of Klinefelter's syndrome and mediastinal nonseminomatous germ cell tumors is now well recognized (30-32). In a group of 22 consecutive patients with mediastinal germ cell tumors seen at Indiana University, four (18%) had karyotypic confirmation of Klinefelter's syndrome and an additional patient had typical clinical features. Patients with Klinefelter's syndrome who developed mediastinal germ cell tumors had a median age of 18 years, 10 years younger than the median age of other patients developing these tumors. Klinefelter's syndrome has not been associated with testicular germ cell tumors of any histology.

The explanation for this association is unknown, but it is likely that the chromosomal abnormality plays a role. Many young men who develop germ cell tumors have underlying germ cell defects, and many have a history of infertility. Testicular biopsy in these men frequently shows abnormalities, including decreased spermatogenesis, peritubular fibrosis, or interstitial edema (33). It is likely that these patients have either a congenital or acquired germ cell defect that affects spermatogenesis and also contributes to the development of testicular or extragonadal germ cell tumors.

Hematologic Neoplasia

An unusual association between mediastinal nonseminomatous germ cell tumors and a variety of hematologic malignancies is now well recognized. Associated hematologic neoplasms have included acute myeloid leukemia, acute lymphocytic leukemia, erythroleukemia, acute megakaryocytic leukemia, myelodysplastic syndrome, and malignant histiocytosis (20, 34-39). In one large review of patients with germ cell tumors, 3 of 34 patients (9%) with primary mediastinal nonseminomatous tumors developed hematologic neoplasia, while none of 654 patients with testicular germ cell tumors developed such tumors (37). In most patients, the diagnosis of hematologic neoplasia has been made within the 24 months following the diagnosis of germ cell tumor, but in a few cases the two diagnoses were made concurrently.

Recent evidence indicates that hematologic neoplasia in this setting arises from clones of malignant lymphoblasts or myeloblasts contained within the mediastinal germ cell tumor. Occasionally, foci of malignant lymphoblasts can be recognized histologically within nonseminomatous germ cell tumors (40,41). In addition, molecular genetic analysis in several patients has revealed the i(12p) chromosomal abnormality, pathognomonic of germ cell tumors, in both the germ cell tumor and the hematologic neoplasm (41,42). This shared chromosomal abnormality provides strong evidence for the common origin of the two malignancies in these patients. However, hematologic neoplasia seems uniquely associated with mediastinal nonseminomatous germ cell tumors, and has not been described in tumors with similar histology arising in the testis or other extragonadal locations. The specificity of this association is unexplained.

Other hematologic abnormalities have also been rarely described in conjunction with nonseminomatous mediastinal germ cell tumors. Several cases of idiopathic thrombocytopenia have been described; the mechanism of thrombocytopenia was undefined in these patients, since normal numbers of megakariocytes were seen in the bone marrow and no evidence of immune destruction was obvious (43,44). Prednisone and splenectomy were unsuccessful in alleviating the thrombocytopenia, and treatment was unsuccessful in these patients. A single case of hemophagocytic syndrome has also been described in association with a mediastinal yolk sac tumor (45). The etiology of this association was also unexplained.

Pretreatment Evaluation and Staging

The diagnosis of a mediastinal germ cell tumor should be considered in all young men with an anterior mediastinal mass. Initial evaluation should include computerized tomography of the chest and abdomen as well as determination of serum levels of HCG and alpha-fetoprotein. Symptoms suggestive of distant metastases should be evaluated with appropriate radiologic studies.

Most patients with mediastinal germ cell tumors have either obvious evidence of distant metastases or large, unresectable intrathoracic tumors. In these patients, histologic diagnosis should be made using the least invasive approach, since surgical therapy will not play a role in the initial treatment. In patients with smaller tumors that seem localized to the mediastinum, exploration via thoracotomy or median sternotomy, with an attempt at complete tumor resection, is sometimes appropriate. Such an approach should not be considered in patients who have tumors invading mediastinal structures, or in whom complete tumor resection is not considered feasible. Surgical resection should also be avoided in patients with high serum levels of HCG or any elevation of alpha-fetoprotein, since these patients have nonseminomatous tumors and should proceed immediately to definitive systemic therapy.

Treatment of Seminoma

The large majority of patients with pure mediastinal seminoma are curable with appropriate therapy, and all of these patients should be approached with curative intent. Mediastinal seminomas are very sensitive to both radiation therapy and combination chemotherapy; selection of initial therapy therefore depends on disease stage and size of the primary tumor.

A minority of patients with pure mediastinal seminoma (approximately 20%) are asymptomatic at the time of diagnosis, and have an anterior mediastinal mass detected on incidental chest radiograph. Some of these patients have relatively small tumors, and complete surgical resection is easily accomplished at the time of surgical biopsy for diagnosis. Such patients should always receive a course of mediastinal irradiation after complete surgical resection; such treatment is curative in almost 100% of patients.

Most patients with mediastinal seminoma are not candidates for initial surgical resection, due to the large size of the mediastinal primary tumor. Even when primary tumors are large, the exquisite radiosensitivity of this neoplasm allows cure rates of approximately 60% in patients without evidence of distant metastases (20,46-48). A dose of 4,000 to 5,000 cGy is recommended, delivered to a shaped mediastinal field including bilateral supraclavicular areas (47,49). Routine irradiation of the retroperitoneum is not necessary. Most treatment failures are due to the appearance of distant metastases, rather than inadequate local tumor control. The benefits of surgical debulking prior to definitive radiation therapy are doubtful, and extensive surgical procedures should be avoided unless complete resection can be accomplished.

Combination chemotherapy is also highly effective in the treatment of pure mediastinal seminoma. Treatment with the intensive cisplatin-based regimens developed for nonseminomatous germ cell tumors is also the optimal treatment for pure mediastinal seminoma, and is even more effective against seminoma than nonseminomatous tumors. Results of treatment with modern cisplatin-based chemotherapy regimens in mediastinal seminoma are summarized in Table 2. Even though most patients had bulky primary tumors and/or distant metastases, the large majority were cured with initial cisplatin-based chemotherapy. As data accumulate, it is now clear that the cure rate with initial cisplatin-based chemotherapy is superior to initial radiation therapy. In one nonrandomized study comparing initial treatments, 5 of 9 patients treated with initial radiation therapy remained disease free, compared with 10 of 11 patients receiving initial chemotherapy (20). These cure rates are reflective of the comparative cure rates reported in multiple other series. Therefore, current data favor the treatment of most patients with initial chemotherapy rather than with mediastinal radiation therapy.

Patients with bulky mediastinal seminomas frequently have residual radiographic abnormalities after completing treatment with chemotherapy. In most patients, these residual masses represent scirrhous reaction or necrotic tumor, rather than residual viable seminoma (50-52). Residual benign teratoma are also rare in this group of patients. The management of residual lesions in these patients has been a matter of some debate, and recommendations for treating mediastinal seminoma are based on experience with bulky retroperitoneal involvement with seminoma from testicular primaries. In a large experience at the Memorial Sloan-Kettering Cancer Center, a substantial percentage of residual masses > 3cm in diameter harbored residual viable seminoma (59). Therefore, a biopsy of large residual lesions should be considered, so that patients with residual viable seminoma can proceed immediately to further therapy. If immediate biopsy is not performed, patients should be followed very closely, with early biopsy of any enlarging mass on chest X-ray or chest CT scan.

In summary, curative therapy is available for almost all patients with mediastinal seminoma. In patients with small tumors, usually asymptomatic at diagnosis, complete

Table 2. Mediastinal Seminoma: Treatment with Cisplatin-Based Combination Chemotherapy

Author, (ref)	Number of patients	Treatment regimen	Number of complete responses (%)	Number of long-term disease-free survivors (%)
Hainsworth [23]	4	PVB	3 (75%)	3 (75%)
Jain [20]	11	VAB-6, PVB, DDP/CTX	10 (91%)	10 (91%)
Logethetis [25]	4	DDP/CTX, $CISCA_2$	4 (100%)	4 (100%)
Loehrer [50]	9	PVB $\pm$ A or BEP	8 (89%)	7 (78%)
Bukowski [51]	8	PVB/EBAP	5 (63%)	4 (50%)
Delgado [52]	6	VAP-6, PVB, BEP	5 (83%)	5 (83%)
Goss [53]	8	BEP, BEP + RT, VAB-6	8 (100%)	8 (100%)
Mencel [54]	19	VAB-6, EP	19 (100%)	19 (100%)
Gerl [55]	4	VIOP, EIP	4 (100%)	4 (100%)
Total	73		66 (90%)	64 (88%)

Key: DDP = cisplatin; A = Adriamycin; CTX = cyclophosphamide; PVB (Einhorn regimen) = cisplatin 20mg/m² IV x 5 days, vinblastine 0.15 mg/kg D 1,2, bleomycin 30 units weekly, cycle repeated q 3 weeks; VAB-6 = multidrug regimen developed at Sloan-kettering; CISCA2 = multidrug regimen developed at M.D. Anderson; BEP = bleomycin 30 units weekly, etoposide 100mg/m² IV x 5 days, cisplatin 20mg/m² IV x 5 days, cycles repeated q 3 weeks; EBAP = etoposide, bleomycin, cisplatin; EP = etoposide, cisplatin; VIOP = vinblastine, ifosfamide, vincristine, cisplatin; EIP = etoposide, ifosfamide, cisplatin.

surgical resection followed by radiation therapy (4000 to 4500 cGy) is curative in almost all patients and is the treatment of choice. All other patients should receive initial cisplatin-based chemotherapy, unless they have a specific medical contraindication to such therapy. Optimal chemotherapy should follow guidelines for poor prognosis nonseminomatous germ cell tumors, and should include four courses of cisplatin, etoposide, and bleomycin (60). In patients who are not considered good candidates for combination chemotherapy and who have tumors localized to the mediastinum, radiation therapy is an acceptable initial treatment. Patients who relapse after initial radiation therapy can often be cured with four courses of chemotherapy, administered at the time of relapse.

Treatment of Nonseminomatous Tumors

Unlike pure mediastinal seminomas, germ cell tumors with nonseminomatous histologies are essentially incurable with local treatment modalities. In a review of the literature in 1975, prior to the development of cisplatin-based chemotherapy regimens, Cox found no reported survivors among 85 patients with mediastinal teratocarcinoma (61).

With the use of intensive cisplatin-based chemotherapy, a sizeable minority of patients with nonseminomatous mediastinal germ cell tumors can now be cured with treatment. Although overall cure rates remain lower than those achieved in the treatment of advanced testicular cancer, recent series using modern regimens document a potential cure rate of approximately 40% (Table 3). The relatively poor cure rates in patients with mediastinal nonseminomatous germ cell tumors are partially explained by the large tumor bulk usually present at diagnosis, as well as the high frequency of distant metastases. Treatment results in these patients are comparable to the 40 to 50% cure rates achieved in the worst group of patients with testicular cancer, who have far advanced, bulky metastases at visceral sites (64). However, it is likely that mediastinal nonseminomatous germ cell tumors have additional biologic differences that may also play a role in determining the relatively low cure rate (65).

Table 3. Mediastinal Nonseminomatous Germ Cell Tumors: Treatment with Cisplatin-Based Chemotherapy

Author (ref)	Number of evaluable patients	Chemotherapy regimen	Number of complete responders (%)	Number of long-term (>24 months) disease-free survivors (%)
Funes [62]	13	PVB	6 (46%)	5 (38%)
Hainsworth [23]	12	PVB ± A	7 (58%)	7 (58%)
Logothetis [25]	11	CISCA II CISCA/VBIV	NA	4 (36%)
Kay [27]	11	PVB, BEP	7 (64%)	5 (45%)
Nichols [28]	31	PVB ± A, BEP	18 (58%)	13 (42%)
Bukowski [51]	16	PVB/EBAP	13 (81%)	9 (56%)
Delgado [52]	40	VAB-6, PVB, BEP	15 (38%)	14 (35%)
Gerl [55]	12	PVB, BEP, ECBC	8 (67%)	6 (50%)
Fizazi [63]	29	VAB-6, PveVB, PVB, BEP	19 (60%)	10 (34%)
Total	175		89 (54%)	69 (39%)

Key: PVB = cisplatin 20mg/m^2 IV x 5 days, vinblastine 0.15 mg/kg D1, 2, bleomycin 30 units weekly; VAB-6 = multidrug regimen developed at Sloan-Kettering; A = Adriamycin; CISCAII, CISCA/VBIV = multidrug regimens developed at M.D. Anderson; BEP = bleomycin 30 units weekly, etoposide 100mg/m^2 IV x 5 days, cisplatin 20mg/m^2 IV x 5 days, cycles repeated q 3 weeks; EBAP = etoposide, bleomycin, doxorubicin, cisplatin; ECBC = etoposide, cisplatin, bleomycin, cyclophosphamide; PveVB = cisplatin, etoposide, vinblastine, bleomycin; NA = not available.

The treatment of mediastinal nonseminomatous germ cell tumors should follow guidelines for poor prognosis testicular cancer. Treatment with four courses of cisplatin, etoposide, and bleomycin is considered standard therapy (60). Although a number of modifications with similar efficacy have been described, the standard regimen includes: cisplatin 20mg/m^2 IV days 1-5; etoposide 100mg/m^2 IV days 1-5; bleomycin 30 units IV days 1, 8, and 15; courses repeated every 21 days. Administration of chemotherapy at full doses and on schedule is important in obtaining optimal results. At present, identical chemotherapy is recommended for the various nonseminomatous histologic subtypes. It is likely that patients with pure choriocarcinoma have relatively poor prognosis, although experience is limited with this rare tumor (23). Early reports suggested a worse prognosis for patients with pure yolk sac tumors (66), but more recent reports have documented an outcome in these patients similar to other nonseminomatous histologies (25,67).

Following completion of chemotherapy, patients should be completely restaged with CT scans and repeat serum tumor marker determinations. Subsequent management is determined by the response to initial chemotherapy as diagrammed in Figure 1. Patients with normal CT scans and normal serum levels of HCG and alpha-fetoprotein should receive no further therapy. These patients should be followed with monthly physical examination, chest radiographs and serum tumor marker determinations during the first year following therapy, and with similar evaluations every two months during the second year. Approximately 20% of these patients will relapse, with almost all relapses occurring during the first 24 months after completing therapy.

Patients with persistent elevations of either serum HCG or alpha-fetoprotein following four courses of chemotherapy have residual active carcinoma and a very poor prognosis. Results with standard salvage regimens, such as VIP (etoposide or vinblastine, ifosfamide, and cisplatin) have been poor, in spite of the 20 to 30% salvage rate seen with these regimens in patients with refractory testicular cancer. In a retrospective evaluation, only 5 of 73 patients (7%) with refractory extragonadal germ cell tumors treated with a cisplatin-containing regimen at Indiana University between 1976 and 1993 were long-term survivors (68). High dose chemotherapy with autologous bone marrow or peripheral stem cell hematopoietic support has also been ineffective in patients with highly refractory tumors, but may offer more promise as a second-line therapy. In one report, 5 of 16 patients with extragonadal germ cell tumors had complete response after second-line treatment with high dose carboplatin, etoposide, and ifosfamide (69). High dose therapy as part of the initial treatment is also being evaluated in patients with poor prognosis germ cell tumors.

A substantial percentage of patients with mediastinal nonseminomatous germ cell tumors have residual radiographic abnormalities following treatment, in spite of normalization of serum tumor markers. In this setting, approximately 75% of patients have either residual benign teratoma or necrotic non-viable tumor rather than residual carcinoma. Patients with components of teratocarcinoma in the original biopsy have a higher risk

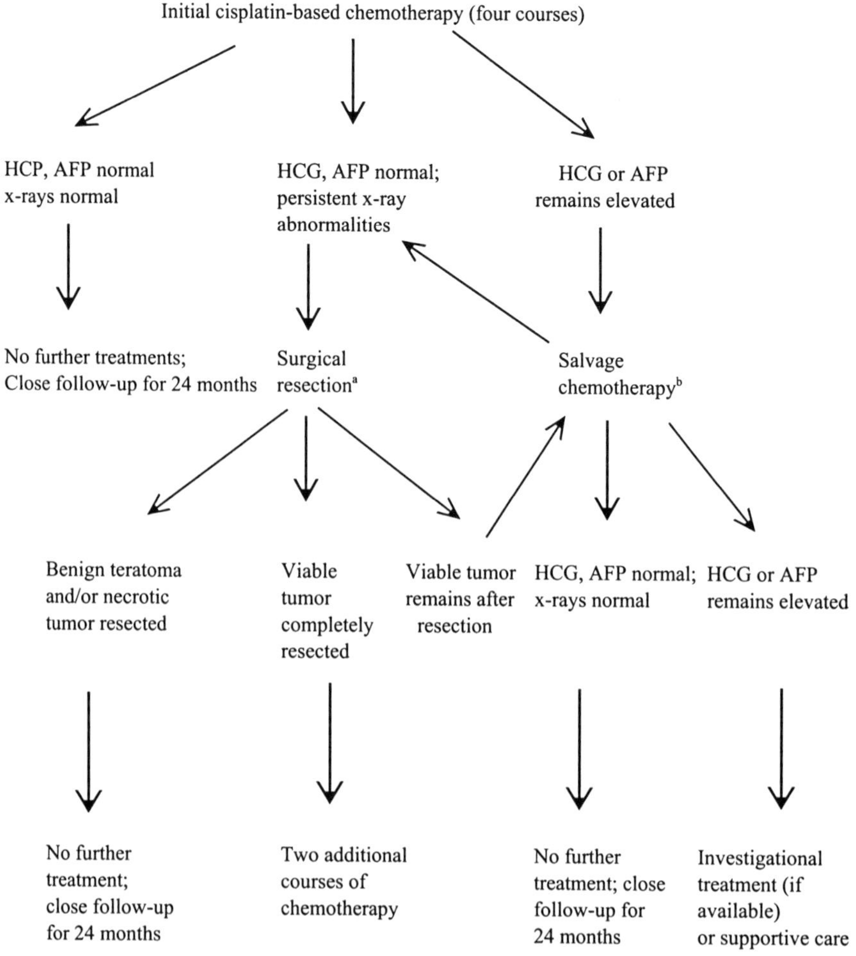

[a] Timing of resection depends on tumor response, initial histology (see text).
[b] No standard salvage regimen established; high-dose therapy appears promising (see text).

Figure 1 – Management of mediastinal nonseminomatous germ cell tumors after completion of initial chemotherapy.

of harboring residual benign teratoma after completion of initial chemotherapy. Surgical resection of residual radiographic abnormalities should be considered in these patients, since removal of residual benign teratoma successfully prevents subsequent local growth or malignant degeneration of these tumors. However, a delay in surgical resection of residual radiographic abnormalities is sometimes reasonable in patients who have experienced marked tumor shrinkage (> 80%) during initial chemotherapy. In such patients, serial scans often demonstrate progressive decrease in the size of residual radiographic abnormalities, and surgical resection can sometimes be avoided. However, tumors that fail to decrease in size should be resected. Patients who have no viable tumor found at the time of surgical resection, or who have only residual benign teratoma resected, have the same low risk for subsequent relapse as do patients achieving complete remission with chemotherapy alone. These patients should be followed without further therapy. If residual viable carcinoma is successfully resected, two additional courses of combination chemotherapy should be administered postoperatively (70).

Although treatment outcome for patients with nonseminomatous mediastinal germ cell tumors has improved markedly with the development of effective combination chemotherapy, more than half of these patients still die as a result of resistant first-line therapy have extremely poor prognosis, and should be considered for investigational treatment. Early use of high dose therapy may be of benefit in the future. Gemcitabine and paclitaxel have shown activity in patients refractory to cisplatin and etoposide, and may improve the efficacy of salvage regimens (71,72). Others of the newer chemotherapeutic agents have not been adequately investigated in refractory germ cell tumors, and trials are ongoing. Continued improvement in therapy will probably parallel the development of more effective treatment for patients with poor prognosis testicular germ cell tumors.

POORLY DIFFERENTIATED CARCINOMA OF THE MEDIASTINUM

In occasional patients with mediastinal tumors, biopsy yields the diagnosis of "poorly differentiated carcinoma". Staging evaluation in some of these patients fails to reveal evidence of metastatic cancer at other sites. Although some of these patients may have a non-small cell lung cancer with an inapparent primary site, palliative treatment of these patients for this presumed diagnosis is inappropriate. All such patients require further pathologic and clinical evaluation, since some patients have carcinomas with specific therapeutic implications. Even when no specific diagnosis can be made, some patients with poorly differentiated carcinoma in the mediastinum have tumors that are highly responsive to platinum-based chemotherapy.

Pathologic Evaluation

Several neoplasms arising in the mediastinum exhibit poorly differentiated histology, including mediastinal germ cell tumors, lymphoma, and thymoma. Differential diagnosis of these neoplasms often requires specialized pathologic evaluation. Cytologic examination from a needle biopsy specimen is often inadequate for optimum evaluation of these tumors. If light microscopic examination is inconclusive, immunoperoxidase staining and, at times, electron microscopy are useful in distinguishing between the various neoplasms occurring in the mediastinum. Immuperoxidase staining usually allows identification of lymphoma and neuroendocrine tumors, both of which have specific treatment implications. In young men with clinical features suggestive of mediastinal germ cell tumor, molecular genetic analysis can sometimes identify the i(12 p) chromosomal abnormality diagnostic of a germ cell tumor (16,17).

Diagnostic Evaluation

All patients who have poorly differentiated carcinoma involving the mediastinum should be evaluated with computerized tomography of the chest and abdomen; serum levels of alpha-fetoprotein and HCG should be determined in all male patients. Patients with substantial smoking history should undergo fiberoptic bronchoscopy. Patients with poorly differentiated carcinoma who have neuroendocrine features detected either by immunoperoxidase staining or electron microscopy are a distinct subset and require special evaluation and treatment. Small cell lung cancer should be suspected in patients with a smoking history, and fiberoptic bronchoscopy should be considered. In patients with no smoking history, the diagnosis of small cell lung cancer is unlikely even when neuroendocrine features are identified. Although the origin or these neuroendocrine tumors is not well defined, they are usually of high grade biology and usually respond to treatment with platinum- or paclitaxel-based chemotherapy (73).

Treatment

Appropriate diagnostic evaluation defines specific therapy for some patients in this group. Young men with elevated serum tumor markers or other clinical features suggestive of extragonadal germ cell tumors should be treated according to guidelines for these tumors, even if this diagnosis is not made by histologic examination. Patients who have an endobronchial lesion identified at bronchoscopy probably have lung cancer; those with neuroendocrine features should receive therapy for small cell lung cancer, while those lacking these features should be treated for non-small cell lung cancer. In the uncommon patient with poorly differentiated carcinoma limited to the mediastinum, an attempt at total tumor resection should be considered if there is no extensive invasion of local structures.

In some patients, no specific diagnosis can be obtained, and the extent of local or metastatic tumor makes surgical resection impossible. All such patients should receive an empiric trial of chemotherapy with a platinum/etoposide-based regimen. In a group of 43 such patients with poorly differentiated carcinoma or poorly differentiated adenocarcinoma located predominantly in the mediastinum, we achieved a complete response rate of 30% with cisplatin-based chemotherapy, and 16% of patients were long-term disease-free survivors (74).

Patients with poorly differentiated carcinoma of the mediastinum are therefore a heterogeneous group. Some of these patients actually have well defined tumor types which can be identified with appropriate additional pathological or clinical evaluation. Such patients should be treatment according to guidelines for their specific tumor type. Some of the remaining patients have tumors that are highly sensitive to treatment, and a trial of platinum-based chemotherapy is appropriate in these patients.

LYMPHOMAS INVOLVING THE MEDIASTINUM

Involvement of mediastinal lymph nodes by lymphoma is common, and usually occurs in conjunction with other areas of nodal and/or extranodal involvement. A full discussion of the management of lymphoma is beyond the scope of this chapter. However, brief mention is made of several lymphomas that typically arise in the mediastinum and can involve this area exclusively. Since the non-Hodgkin's lymphomas involving predominantly the mediastinum are of aggressive histology, they should always be considered when biopsy of a mediastinal mass shows a poorly differentiated neoplasm. Appropriate special stains allow accurate diagnosis in almost all cases.

Non-Hodgkin's Lymphoma
Lymphoblastic Lymphoma
Lymphoblastic lymphoma is a disease of children and young adults, and shares many clinical and biologic features with acute lymphoblastic leukemia (75). These lymphomas arise from T-cells typical of the middle or late stage of thymocyte maturation (76). The T-cells express various combinations of the CD1, CD2, CD5, and CD7 antigens, and in many cases express both CD 4 and CD8. Patients with this high-grade lymphoma usually develop rapidly enlarging anterior mediastinal masses, often in conjunction with involvement of cervical lymph nodes. The bone marrow is usually involved; when more than 25% of the bone marrow is replaced, the illness is arbitrarily defined as acute lymphoblastic leukemia rather than lymphoblastic lymphoma.

Curative therapy of this high grade neoplasm requires intensive combination chemotherapy, following treatment guidelines established for patients with high-risk acute lymphoblastic leukemia. Successful regimens have involved intensive, multi-drug induction therapy followed by subsequent intensification and maintenance therapy (77-79). Central nervous system prophylaxis is also a critical part of these regimens (80). In recent years, cure has been accomplished in 65 to 75% of children with this illness.

Primary Mediastinal B-Cell Lymphoma with Sclerosis
Primary mediastinal B-cell lymphoma with sclerosis is a distinctive subset of intermediate-grade lymphoma that usually occurs in young adults. Patients usually present with local symptoms from a large anterior mediastinal mass; systemic symptoms (fever, sweats, weight loss) are also common. In some series, over 50% of patients had superior vena cava syndrome at the time of diagnosis (81). Staging evaluation frequently reveals no additional areas of involvement. Pathologic examination shows features typical of large cell lymphoma; however, a dominant feature in most cases is the presence of massive sclerosis, appearing in either a diffuse interstitial pattern, or in broad bands dividing the tumor into large nodules. These lymphomas are of B-cell origin, and stain with various pan B-cell antibodies.

Although some controversy exists in the literature, treatment should follow established guidelines for intermediate grade lymphomas (81-85). Due to the large tumor bulk and frequent systemic symptoms, patients with primary mediastinal B-cell lymphoma are often in the poor prognosis category as defined by IWF criteria. Recent reports document a long-term disease-free survival rate of approximately 50% following treatment with combination chemotherapy. Residual mediastinal mass is frequent in these patients, and makes clinical reassessment after therapy difficult. The value of mediastinal radiation therapy is unclear.

Hodgkin's Disease

Mediastinal involvement is common in Hodgkin's disease, but occurs in the large majority of patients in conjunction with other adenopathy. In approximately 5% of patients with nodular sclerosing Hodgkin's disease, the mediastinal mass is the only abnormality found on clinical staging. Mediastinal masses measuring greater than one-third of the transverse diameter of the thoracic cavity have been identified as a poor prognostic factor by multiple investigators (86,87).

The optimum treatment for patients with Hodgkin's disease and large mediastinal mass is still the subject of debate. Combination chemotherapy is now considered a critical component of optimal therapy, with a variety of combined modality programs yielding superior responses than radiation therapy alone (88-90). Several current trials are evaluating the efficacy of combined modality regimens using less toxic regimens (short-course chemotherapy, involved field radiation therapy) (91-93).

TUMORS OF THE POSTERIOR MEDIASTINUM

Most primary tumors of the posterior mediastinum are neurogenic in origin, arising from the sympathetic and intercostal nerves in this area. Approximately 80% of these tumors are benign, and as a group they comprise up to 24% of all mediastinal tumors (94). Neurogenic tumors are usually found in the posterior costovertebral gutter and are usually asymptomatic when detected by routine chest radiography. However, some tumors cause symptoms by compression of adjacent nerves or by invasion into adjacent pleura or vetebral bodies. Neurologic symptoms occasionally arise when these tumors extend through intervetebral foramina. Prompt evaluation of neurologic symptoms with magnetic resonance imaging is important to prevent or minimize neurologic complications.

Neurofibroma

Neurofibromas are almost always benign and typically surround all of the nerve components (axon, sheath cell, and connective tissue). Neurofibromas can occur in all age groups, and occur with equal frequency in men and women. On chest radiograph, these tumors appear to have a narrow base and usually form an acute angle with the mediastinum. The treatment of choice is complete resection, and prognosis after surgical excision is excellent even if the tumor is incompletely removed. The removal of tumors extending through the intervetebral foramina ("dumb-bell" tumors) requires a combined procedure, with resection of the intraspinal portion of the tumor first. Radiation therapy and chemotherapy are not indicated.

Schwannoma (Neurilemoma)

Schwannoma is the most common neurogenic tumor, arising from nerve sheath cells, and is usually benign. Most patients are asymptomatic, but a few have back pain or mild osteoarthropathy. Chest radiograph sometimes reveals intratumoral calcification, but this finding is not indicative of invasiveness, and is not prognostically significant. Most tumors are solitary and encapsulated; treatment involves surgical resection as described for neurofibromas. The prognosis is excellent, with only rare recurrences. Radiation therapy and chemotherapy are not indicated.

Malignant Schwannoma (Neurosarcoma)

Microscopically, malignant schwannomas have similarities to benign schwannomas and neurofibromas, and may represent malignant "degeneration" of these tumors. These neoplasms usually occur in patients more than 50 years old, and are usually symptomatic at presentation. The most frequent symptom is pain caused by invasion of adjacent structures. Occasionally, these tumors have been associated with symptomatic hypoglycemia. Surgical excision is usually difficult, and local recurrence is common. The prognosis of patients with recurrent local tumor or metastatic disease is poor, and treatment guidelines should follow those described for soft tissue sarcomas.

Ganglioneuroma

Ganglioneuromas are benign, and arise from the sympathetic chain. These tumors are the most common neurogenic tumor in children, where they are usually asymptomatic at diagnosis. When they rarely present in adults, hypertension secondary to catecholamine production is a frequent accompaniment. Surgical excision is the treatment of choice, and is usually easily accomplished with a low recurrence rate.

Neuroblastoma

Occasional neuroblastomas arise in the chest, and the prognosis for these neoplasms seems better than for neuroblastomas arising in the abdomen. Treatment for these aggressive tumors includes intensive combination chemotherapy in addition to local modalities, and should follow the treatment guidelines outlined for the more common intra-abdominal neuroblastoma.

Neural Crest Tumors (pheochromocytoma, paraganglioma, chemodectoma, aortic body tumor)

Each of these rare tumors occasionally occurs in the posterior mediastinum. Surgical excision is the treatment of choice, and is curative in the large majority of patients.

REFERENCES

1.　　Davis RD, et al: Primary cysts and neoplasms of the mediastinum: recent changes in the clinical presentation, method of diagnosis, management, and results. Ann Thorac Surg 44:229-237, 1987.

2. Rubush JL, Gardner IR, Boyd WC, et al: Mediastinal tumors: Review of 186 cases. J. Thorac Cardiovasc Surg 65:216-223, 1973.

3. Friedman NB. The comparative morphogenesis of extragenital and gonadal teratoid tumors. Cancer 4:265, 1951.

4. Schlumberger HG. Teratoma of anterior mediastinum in group of military age: study of 16 cases and review of theories of genesis. Arch Pathol 41:398, 1946.

5. Azzopardi JG, Mostofi FK, Theiss EA. Lesions of testes observed in certain patients with widespread choriocarcinoma and related tumors. Am J Pathol 38:207, 1961.

6. Rather LJ, Gardiner WR, Frericks JB. Regression and maturation of primary testicular tumors with progressive growth of metastases: report of six new cases and review of literature. Stanford Med Bull 12:12, 1954.

7. Johnson DE, Laneri JP, Mountain CF, Luna M. Extragonadal germ-cell tumors. Surgery 73:85, 1973.

8. Luna MA, Valenzuela-Tamariz J. Germ-cell tumors of the mediastinum, postmortem findings. Am J Clin Pathol 65:450, 1976.

9. Willis RA. Borderland of Embryology and Pathology, 2nd ed. Washington: Butterworth, p 442, 1962.

10. Friedman NB. The function of the primordial germ-cell in extragonadal tissues. Int J Androl 10:43, 1987.

11. Boyd DP, Midell AI. Mediastinal cysts and tumors: an analysis of 96 cases. Surg Clin North Am 48:493, 1968.

12. Hodge J, Aponte G, McLauglin E. Primary mediastinal tumors. J Thorac Surg 37:730, 1959.

13. Ringertz N, Lidholm SO. Mediastinal tumors and cysts. J Thorac Surg 31:458, 1956.

14. Collins DH, Pugh RCB. Classification and frequency of testicular tumors. Br J Urol 36:1, 1984.

15. Einhorn LH, Williams SD. Management of disseminated testicular cancer. In Testicular Tumors: Management and treatment. Edited by LH Einhorn. New York: Mason, pp 117-151, 1980.

16. Motzer RJ, Rodriguez E, Reuter VE, Bosl GJ, Mazumdar M, Chaganti RSK. Molecular and cytogenetic studies in the diagnosis of patients with midline carcinomas of unknown primary site. J Clin Oncol 13:274, 1995.

17. Motzer RJ, Rodriguez E, Reuter VE, Samaniego F, Dmitrovsky E, Bajorin DF, et al. Genetic analysis as an aid in diagnosis for patients with poorly differentiated carcinomas of uncertain histologies. JNCI 83:341, 1991.

18. Moran CA, Suster S. Primary germ-cell tumors of the mediastinum – I. Analysis of 322 cases with special emphasis on teratomatous lesions and a proposal for histopathologic classification and clinical staging. Cancer 80:681, 1997.

19. Polansky SM, Barwick KW, Ravin CE. Primary mediastinal seminoma. Am J Radiology 132:17, 1979.

20. Jain KK, Bosl GJ, Bains MS, Whitmore WF, Golbey RB. The treatment of extragonadal seminoma. J Clin Oncol 2:820, 1984.

21. Knapp RH, Hurt RD, Payne WS, Farrow GM, Lewis BD, Hahn RG, Muhm JR, Earle JD. Malignant germ-cell tumors of the mediastinum. J Thorac Cardiovasc Surg 89:82, 1985.

22. Levitt RH, Husband JE, Glazer HS. CT of primary germ-cell tumors of the mediastinum. AJR 142:73, 1984.

23. Hainsworth JD, Einhorn LH, Williams SD, Stewart M, Greco FA. Advanced extragonadal germ-cell tumors. Successful treatment with combination chemotherapy. Ann Intern Med 97:7, 1982.

24. Israel A, Bosl GJ, Golbey RB, Whitmore W, Jr, Martini N. The results of chemotherapy for extragonadal germ-cell tumors in the cisplatin era: the Memorial Sloan-Kettering Cancer Center experience (1975 to 1982). J Clin Oncol 3:1073, 1985.

25. Logothetis CJ, Samuels ML, Selig DE, Dexeus FH, Johnson DE, Swanson DA, von Eschenbach AC. Chemotherapy of extragonadal germ-cell tumors. J Clin Oncol 3:316, 1985.

26. Sickles EA, Belliveau RF, Wiernik PH. Primary mediastinal choriocarcinoma in the male. Cancer 33:1196, 1974.

27. Kay PH, Wells FC, Goldstraw P. A multidisciplinary approach to primary nonseminomatous germ-cell tumors of the mediastinum. Ann Thorac Surg 44:578, 1987.

28. Nichols CR, Saxman S, Williams SD, Loehrer PJ, Miller ME, Wright C. Primary mediastinal nonseminomatous germ-cell tumors: a modern single institution experience. Cancer 65:1641, 1990.

29. Scheike D, Visfeldt J, Petersen B. Male breast cancer. 3. Breast carcinoma in association with the Klinefelter syndrome. Acta Path Michrobiol Scand 81:352, 1973.

30. Curry WA, McKay CE, Richardson RL, Greco FA. Klinefelter's syndrome and mediastinal germ cell neoplasms. J Urol 125:127, 1981.

31. Turner AR, MacDonald RN. Mediastinal germ-cell cancers in Klinefelter's syndrome. Ann Intern Med 94:279, 1981.

32. Nichols CR, Heerema NA, Palmer C, Loehrer PJ, Williams SD, Einhorn LH. Klinefelter's syndrome associated with mediastinal germ-cell neoplasms. J Clin Oncol 5:1290, 1987.

33. Carroll PR, Whitmore WF, Jr, Richardson M, Bajorunas D, Herr HW, Williams RD, Fair WR, Chaganti RSK. Testicular failure in patients with extragonadal germ-cell tumors. Cancer 60:108, 1987.

34. DeMent SH, Eggleston JC, Spivak JL. Association between mediastinal germ-cell tumors and hematologic malignancies: report of two cases and review of the literature. Am J Surg Pathol 9:23, 1985.

35. Hoekman K, ten Bokkel Huinink WW, Egbers-Bogaards MA, McVie JG, Somers R. Acute leukemia following therapy for teratoma. Eur J Cancer Clin Oncol 20:501, 1984.

36. Landanyi M, Roy I. Mediastinal germ-cell tumor and histiocytosis. Human Pathol 19:586, 1988.

37. Nichols CR, Hoffman R, Einhorn LH, Williams SD, Wheeler LA, Garnick MB. Hematologic malignancies associated with primary mediastinal germ-cell tumors. Ann Intern Med 102:603, 1985.

38. Nichols CR, Roth BJ, Heerema N, Griep J, Tricot G. Hematologic neoplasia associated with primary mediastinal germ-cell tumors. N Engl J Med 322:1425, 1990.

39. Sales LM, Vontz FK. Teratoma and diGuglielmo syndrome. South Med J 63:448, 1970.

40. Larsen M, Evans WK, Shepherd FA, Phillips MJ, Bailey D, Messner H. Acute lymphoblastic leukemia: possible origin from a mediastinal germ-cell tumor. 53:441, 1984.

41. Orazi A, Neiman RS, Ulbright TM, Heerema NA, John K, Nichols CR. Hematopoietic precursor cells within the yolk sac tumor component are the source of secondary hematopoietic malignancies in patients with mediastinal germ-cell tumors. Cancer 71:3873, 1993.

42. Chaganti RSK, Landanyi M, Samaniego F. Leukemic differentiation of a mediastinal germ-cell tumor. Genes Chromosomes Cancer 1:83, 1989.

43. Garnick MB, Griffin JD. Idiopathic thrombocytopenia in association with extragonadal germ-cell cancer. Ann Intern Med 98:926, 1983.

44. Helman LJ, Ozols RF, Longo DL. Thrombocytopenia and extragonadal germ-cell neoplasm. Ann Intern Med 101:280, 1984.

45. Myers TJ, Kessimian N, Schwartz S. Mediastinal germ-cell tumor associated with the hemophagocytic syndrome. Ann Intern Med 109:504, 1988.

46. Dulmet EM, Macchiarini P, Suc B, Verley JM. Germ-cell tumors of the mediastinum: a 30-year experience. Cancer 72:1894, 1993.

47. Hurt RD, Bruckman JE, Farrow GM, Bernatz PE, Hahn RG, Earle JD. Primary anterior mediastinal seminoma. Cancer 49:1658, 1982.

48. Martini N, Golbey RB, Hajdu SI, Whitmore WF, Beattie EJ, Jr. Primary mediastinal germ-cell tumors. Cancer 33:763, 1974.

49. Bush SE, Martinez A, Bagshaw MA. Primary mediastinal seminoma. Cancer 48:1877, 1981.

50. Loehrer PJ, Birch R, Williams SD, Greco FA, Einhorn LH. Chemotherapy of metastatic seminoma. The Southeastern Cancer Study Group experience. J Clin Oncol 5:1212. 1987.

51. Bukowski RM, Wolf M, Kulander BG, Montie J, Crawford ED, Blumenstein B. Alternating combination chemotherapy in patients with extragonadal germ cell tumors. Cancer 71:2631, 1993.

52. Delgado FG, Tjulandin SA, Gavin AM. Long-term results of treatment in patients with extragonadal germ cell tumours. Eur J Cancer 29A:1002, 1993.

53. Goss PE, Schwertfeger L, Blackstein ME, Iscoe NA, Ginsberg RJ, Simpson WJ, Jones DP, Shepherd FA. Extragonadal germ cell tumors: a 14-year Toronto experience. Cancer 73:1971, 1994.

54. Mencel PJ, Motzer RJ, Mazumdar M, Vlamis V, Bajorin DF, Bosl GJ. Advanced seminoma: treatment results, survival, and prognostic factors in 142 patients. J Clin Oncol 12:120, 1994.

55. Gerl A, Clemm C, Lamerz R, Wilmanns W: Cisplatin-based chemotherapy of primary extragonadal germ cell tumors: a single institution experience. Cancer 77:526, 1996.

56. Peckham MJ, Horwich A, Hendry WF. Advanced seminoma: treatment with cisplatin-based combination chemotherapy or carboplatin. Br J Cancer 52:7, 1985.

57. Schultz SM, Einhorn LH, Conces DJ, Williams SD, Loehrer PJ. Management of postchemotherapy residual mass in patients with advanced seminoma: Indiana University experience. J Clin Oncol 7:1497, 1989.

58. Puc HS, Heelan R, Mazumdar M, Herr H, Scheinfeld J, Vlamis V, Bajorin DF, Bosl GJ, Mencel P, Motzer RJ: Management of residual mass in advanced seminoma: results and recommendations from the Memorial Sloan-Kettering Cancer Center. J Clin Oncol 14:454, 1996.

59. Motzer R, Bosl G, Heclan R, Fair W, Whitmore W, Sagani P, Herr H, Morse M. Residual mass: an indication for further therapy in patients with advanced seminoma following systemic chemotherapy. J Clin Oncol 5:1064, 1987.

60. Williams SD, Birch R, Einhorn LH, Irwin L, Greco FA, Loehrer PJ. Treatment of disseminated germ-cell tumors with cisplatin, bleomycin, and either vinblastine or etoposide. N Engl J Med 316:1435, 1987.

61. Cox JD. Primary malignant germinal tumors of the mediastinum. Cancer 36:1162, 1975.

62. Funes HC, Mendez M, Alonso E, Oiben R, Manas A, Mendiola C. Mediastinal germ cell tumors treated with cisplatin, bleomycin and vinblastine (PVB). Proc Am Assoc Cancer Res 22:474 (Abstract), 1981.

63. Fizazi K, Culine S, Droz JP, Kramar A, Theodore C, Ruffie P, LeChavalier T. Primary mediastinal nonseminomatous germ cell tumors: results of modern therapy including cisplatin-based chemotherapy. J Clin Oncol 16:725, 1998.

64. Einhorn LH. Testicular cancer as a model for a curable neoplasm. The Richard and Hilda Rosenthal Foundation Award Lecture. Cancer Res 41:3275, 1981.

65. Toner GC, Geller NL, Lin S-Y, Bosl GJ. Extragonadal and poor risk nonseminomatous germ-cell tumors: survival and prognostic features. Cancer 67:2049, 1991.

66. Kuzur ME, Cobleigh MA, Greco FA, Einhorn LH, Oldham RK. Endodermal sinus tumor of the mediastinum. Cancer 50:766, 1982.

67. Chong CDK, Logothetis CJ, von Eschenbach AC, Ayala AG, Samuels ML. Successful treatment of pure endodermal sinus tumors in adult men. J Clin Oncol 6:303, 1988.

68. Saxman SB, Nichols CR, Einhorn LH. Salvage chemotherapy in patients with extragonadal nonseminomatous germ-cell tumors: the Indiana University experience. J Clin Oncol 12:1390, 1994.

69. Siegert W, Beyer J, Strohscheer I, Baurmann H, Oettle H, Zingsem J, Zimmermann R, Bakemeyer C, Schmoll HJ, Huhn D. High-dose treatment with carboplatin, etoposide, and ifosfamide followed by autologous stem-cell transplantation in relapsed or refractory germ-cell cancer: a phase I/II study. J Clin Oncol 12:1223, 1994.

70.   Fox EP, Weathers RD, Williams SD, Loehrer PJ, Ulbright TM, Donohue JP, Einhorn LH. Outcome analysis for patients with persistent nonteratomatous germ-cell tumor in post-chemotherapy retroperitoneal lymph node dissections. J Clin Oncol 11:1294, 1993.

71.   Einhorn LH, Stender MJ, Williams SD: Phase II trial of gemcitabine in refractory germ cell tumors. J Clin Oncol 17:509, 1999.

72.   Motzer RJ, Bajorin DF, Schwartz LH, Hutter HS, Bosl GJ, Scher HI, Lyn P, Fischer P: Phase II trial of paclitaxel shows antitumor activity in patients with previously treated germ cell tumors. J Clin Oncol 12:2277, 1994.

73.   Hainsworth JD, Johnson DH, Greco FA. Poorly differentiated neuroendocrine carcinoma of unknown primary site: a newly recognized clinicopathologic entity. Ann Intern Med 109:364, 1988.

74.   Hainsworth JD, Johnson DH, Greco FA.   Cisplatin-based combination chemotherapy in the treatment of poorly differentiated carcinoma and poorly differentiated adenocarcinoma of unknown primary site: results of a twelve-year experience at a single institution. J Clin Oncol 10:912, 1992.

75.   Weiss L, Bindl J, Picozzi V, et al: Lymphoblastic lymphoma: an immunophenotype study of 26 cases with comparison to T-cell acute lymphoblastic leukemia. Blood 67:474, 1986.

76.   Bernard A, Boumsell L, Reinherz E, et al: Cell surface characterization of malignant T-cells from lymphoblastic lymphoma using monoclonal antibodies: evidence for phenotype differences between malignant T-cells from patients with acute lymphoblastic leukemia and lymphoblastic lymphoma. Blood 57:1105, 1981.

77.   Reiter A, Schrappe M, Parwasesch R, et al: Non-Hodgkin's lymphomas of childhood and adolescence: results of a treatment stratified for biologic subtypes and stage. A report of The Berlin-Frankfort-Munster Group. J Clin Oncol 13:359, 1995.

78.   Weinstein WJ, Cassady JR, Levey R: Long-term results of the APO protocol (vincristine, doxorubicin, and prednisone) for the treatment of mediastinal lymphoblastic lymphoma. J Clin Oncol 1:537, 1983.

79.   Dahl GV, et al: A novel treatment of childhood lymphoblastic non-Hodgkin's lymphoma: Early and intermittent use of teniposide and cytarabine. Blood 66:1110, 1985.

80.   Anderson J, Jenkin D, Wilson J, et al: Long-term follow-up of patients treated with COMP or LSA2-L2 therapy for childhood NHL: a report of CCG-551 from the CCG. J Clin Oncol 11:1024, 1993.

81.   Lazzarino M, Orlando E, Paulli M, et al: Primary mediastinal B-cell lymphoma with sclerosis: an aggressive tumor with distinctive clinical and pathologic features. J Clin Oncol 11:2306-2313, 1983.

82.   Kirn D, Mauch P, Shaffer K, et al: Large-cell and immunoblastic lymphoma of the mediastinum: prognostic features and treatment outcome in 57 patients. J Clin Oncol 11:1336-1343, 1993.

83.   Todeschini G, Ambrosetti A, Meneghini V, et al: Mediastinal large-B-cell lymphoma with sclerosis: a clinical study of 21 patients. J Clin Oncol 8:804-808, 1990.

84.   Jacobson JO, Aisenberg AC, Lamarre L, et al: Mediastinal large cell lymphoma: an uncommon subset of adult lymphoma curable with combined modality therapy. Cancer 62:1893-1898, 1988.

85.   Lavabre-Bertrand T, Donadio D, Fegueux N, et al: A study of 15 cases of primary mediastinal lymphoma of B-cell type. Cancer 69:2561-2566, 1992.

86.   Lee CKK, Bloomfield CD, Goldman AI, Levitt SH: Prognostic significance of mediastinal involvement in Hodgkin's disease treated with curative radiotherapy. Cancer 46:2403-2409, 1980.

87.   Schomberg PJ, Evans RG, O'Connell MJ, et al: Prognostic significance of mediastinal mass in adult Hodgkin's disease. Cancer 53:324-328, 1984.

88.   Crnkovich MJ, Hoppe RT, Rosenberg SA: Stage IIB Hodgkin's disease: the Stanford experience. J Clin Oncol 4:472-479, 1986.

89.   Leopold KA, Canellos GP, Rosenthal D, et al: Stage IA-IIB Hodgkin's disease: staging and treatment of patients with large mediastinal adenopathy. J Clin Oncol 7:1059-1065, 1989.

90.   Specht L, Gray RG, Clarke MJ, et al: Influence of more extensive radiotherapy and adjuvant chemotherapy on long-term outcome of early-stage Hodgkin's disease: a meta-analysis of 23 randomized trials involving 3,888 patients. J Clin Oncol 16:830-843, 1998.

91.   Bartlett NL, Rosenberg SA, Hoppe RT, et al: Brief chemotherapy, Stanford V, and adjuvant radiotherapy for bulky or advanced-stage Hodgkin's disease: a preliminary report. J Clin Oncol 13:1080-1088, 1995.

92.   Noordijk EM, Kluin-Nelemans JL: Stage I or II Hodgkin's disease: more chemotherapy and less irradiation. Ned Tijdschr Genaeskd 141:1281-1284, 1997.

93.   Tebbi C, Leventhal B, Chauvenlt A, et al: Treatment of stage I, II, IIIA1 pediatric Hodgkin's disease with adriamycin, bleomycin, vincristine, and etoposide and low-dose radiation with option to eliminate laparotomy. Proc Am Soc Clin Oncol 13:1335A, 1994 (Abstract).

94.   Silverman NA, Sabiston DC Jr: Primary tumors and cysts of the mediastinum. Curr Probl Cancer 2:1-55, 1977.

MALIGNANT PLEURAL MESOTHELIOMA

Linus Ho, M.D., Ph.D.
M.D. Anderson Cancer Center, Houston, TX 77030

David J. Sugarbaker, M.D.
Brigham and Women's Hospital, Boston, MA 02115

Arthur T. Skarin, M.D.
Dana-Farber Cancer Institute, Boston, MA 02115

INTRODUCTION

Mesotheliomas are neoplasms originating from the thin layer of mesothelial cells lining the serosal surfaces of the pleural, pericardial and peritoneal cavities. This fact accounts for the otherwise curious reports of mesotheliomas arising from the tunica vaginalis testis (1), which represents a diverticular remnant of the peritoneum carried with the testes into the scrotum during their embryonic descent from the abdominal cavity. However, the vast majority of mesotheliomas (80%) originate within the pleural space (2), and this review will focus on recent advances in our understanding of malignant pleural mesotheliomas (MPMs) and on practical aspects of their management.

Epidemiology

An estimated 2000 to 3000 new cases of MPM are diagnosed in the United States each year. Unfortunately, precise numbers are lacking because of diagnostic difficulties and ambiguities inherent to the disease-coding system. The incidence of MPM is believed to have steadily increased since its first clinical description in 1931 (3) and will probably remain substantial for the next three decades (4,5).

The most frequently identified and best known risk factor for mesothelioma is asbestos exposure (although by far the most common malignancies following asbestos exposure are primary lung carcinomas). Persons working with insulation, brake linings, textiles, fireproofing, and tiling, those involved in shipbuilding and gas mask manufacturing, as well as custodians, firefighters and electricians are at particular risk. A population-based case-control study in France has established a clear dose-response relationship between cumulative asbestos exposure and MPM. It revealed significantly increased risk for the disease at levels of cumulative exposure far below the limits adopted in most industrial countries during the 1980's (6). With detailed questioning, a history of direct asbestos exposure can be elicited in 50% to 80% of patients. Because of other suspected risk factors (see below) and the fact that brief yet intense exposure to asbestos may be sufficient to predispose to MPM, the absence of an exposure history should not be taken as *prima facie* evidence against the diagnosis.

Asbestos fibers can be broadly classified into two groups which differ in their carcinogenicity. The carcinogenic risk associated with the serpentine chrysotile, a curly fiber which constitutes 90% to 95% of the asbestos found in the United States, is considerably less than that of the rod-like amphiboles (crocidolite, amosite, anthophyllite, termolite, and actinolyte) (7,8). Even among the amphiboles, crocidolite is regarded as the most carcinogenic. However, since the amphiboles are typically found as contaminants in chrysotile deposits, it is often difficult to separate the tumorigenic contribution of each in epidemiologic studies. Research suggests that physical characteristics of the fibers, rather than their chemical composition, are the critical factors in determining their relative carcinogenicity. The long, thin geometry of the amphibole fibers likely contributes to evasion of the normal pulmonary clearance mechanisms and to injury to phagocytosing cells, causing the release of free radicals and other reactive compounds. Inflammation and fibrosis may ensue, and some evidence suggests that such processes may predispose to MPM (9). (Mossman *et al* (7) provides a more detailed discussion of the possible carcinogenic mechanisms of asbestos.)

The latency period between initial exposure to asbestos and the development of MPM is long and averages 30 to 40 years (10) with a range as great as 14 to 72 years (11). The intervening stages in the evolution of MPM are unclear although the role of asbestosis (pulmonary fibrosis due to asbestos) and pleural plaques has been investigated. The evidence in support of a correlative relationship between lung cancer and pleural plaques is weak (12), but the lack of sensitivity in detecting pleural plaques may be a significant reason for this. For example, the sensitivity of chest radiographs for detecting pleural plaques is only 20% and is even worse (10%) for detecting calcification within plaques. On the other hand, pleural calcifications may be seen in approximately 50% of computed tomography (CT) scans (13) and up to 87% of post-mortem examinations.

Radiation has been hypothesized to be another risk factor for MPM. Approximately 25 cases of mesothelioma have been reported (14) following therapeutic radiation (15), thorium dioxide (Thorotrast) exposure, or atomic bomb exposure (16). However, these reports remain anecdotal, and one large retrospective cohort study found no evidence for a causal relationship between therapeutic radiation and MPM (17).

A third suspected etiologic factor is the SV40 virus (simian virus 40, a virus native to African macaque monkeys that causes tumors in rodents and transforms human cells in tissue culture. Presumably, its oncogenic activity is mediated by the SV40 large T antigen, which has been shown to bind and inactivate growth-suppressive proteins such as the retinoblastoma (Rb) and p53 proteins. Polio vaccines contaminated by live SV40 between 1959 and 1961 potentially exposed a large cohort of people to this virus. The timing of this exposure would coincide with the current increase in the incidence of mesothelioma when the expected latency period is taken into account. However, retrospective cohort studies conducted independently in the U.S (18) and Sweden (19) have failed to establish a relationship between these polio vaccines and the incidence of malignancies, including MPM. Several case-control studies have examined archival pathologic specimens for the presence of SV40-specific sequences, but results have been mixed. For example, one study by Galateau-Salle *et al.* (20) failed to demonstrate a statistically significant difference in the incidence of SV40 large T antigen sequences between pathologic samples from mesotheliomas (48%) and bronchogenic carcinomas (29%) although benign samples (16%) were significantly less likely to harbor such sequences compared with MPMs. Strickler *et al.* (21), using both a serologic test for anti-SV40 antibodies and a sensitive polymerase chain reaction (PCR) assay, found no correlation between MPM and the presence of anti-SV40 antibodies or SV40 DNA. The non-specificity of detecting SV40 sequences is further illustrated by their presence in tuberculous lesions (22). On the other hand, Carbone *et al.* (23) and Pepper *et al.* (24) have specifically detected SV40-like sequences and/or large T antigen expression in samples from mesotheliomas but not in normal tissue, reactive pleura or other tumors (including adenocarcinomas). Generally speaking, however, the function and/or expression of detected SV40 sequences must be considered in the interpretation of these data as well as the fact that PCR primer selection can critically influence the sensitivity and specificity of PCR assays (25,26). The most compelling data in favor of SV40's role in MPM pathogenesis may be those demonstrating the presence of large T antigen itself in MPM tissue (23,27) and work demonstrating a 100% induction rate of mesothelioma in hamsters receiving intrapleural infections of SV40 (28).

Finally, while tobacco smoke and asbestos are clearly synergistic in the etiology of bronchogenic carcinoma, there is no definitive evidence supporting a similar role for tobacco in the etiology of MPM.

Clinical Presentation and Diagnostic Workup

MPM is typically diagnosed in the fifth to seventh decades of life with a patient median age of 60. There is a strong male predominance (male:female ratio = 5:1) reflecting the historical bias in occupational exposure. Common symptoms include shortness of breath (80%) and non-pleuritic chest pain or discomfort (50-60%); physical examination and chest radiographs reveal the presence of a unilateral or, less commonly, asymmetric bilateral pleural effusions. There is a slight right-sided predominance of involvement by MPM (60%) that may be due to the straighter and more downward path taken by the right main-stem bronchus relative to the left; this geometry would presumably favor the passage of particulate matter such as asbestos fibers into the right lung.

The natural history of MPM is generally one of local progression and invasion with only late symptomatic distant metastases. Tumor infiltration along biopsy and surgical tracts is relatively common (10-20%), but sometimes can be prevented with local radiation

(29). Shortness of breath and chest pain or discomfort, as mentioned above, are the most common presenting symptoms and tend to steadily worsen as the pleural space becomes obliterated with fluid and tumor. The shortness of breath may seem out of proportion to the radiologic findings as a result of the functional shunting of blood through poorly ventilated lung parenchyma (30). Invasion into the lung parenchyma, chest wall, mediastinum, and diaphragm are common. Involvement of critical local structures such as the esophagus, vertebrae, nerves (31), and blood vessels will lead to specific syndromes such as dysphagia, paralysis, numbness, or the superior vena cava (SVC) syndrome. Symptomatic distant metastases occur late in the disease, if at all, despite the fact that post-mortem examinations typically reveal hematogenous spread in a majority of patients (14). Involvement of sites such as the brain, bone, and liver are generally more common, but metastases to such sites as skin (32), skeletal muscle (33), and the orbit (34) have also been reported.

Following documentation of a pleural effusion by routine chest radiographs, diagnostic thoracentesis with chemical, microbiologic, and cytologic evaluation of the fluid is usually indicated unless the etiology is patently obvious. The traditional distinction between transudates and exudates may help discriminate between benign and malignant entities, and a bloody effusion may suggest the presence of adenocarcinoma. Some pleural fluid characteristics may even provide prognostic information in cases of MPM (see below). Cytologic examination is notoriously difficult and inaccurate; however many a case of MPM has eluded cytologic diagnosis despite repeated attempts at thoracentesis because reactive mesothelial cells may be quite difficult to distinguish from malignant mesothelial cells (35). Thus, a negative cytologic examination in a patient with a significant pre-test probability of MPM should be followed by a biopsy procedure that can be performed blindly, under CT guidance, or thoracoscopically. The main drawback of a blind biopsy procedure is sampling error, and the estimated sensitivity of the combination of a blind pleural biopsy and fluid cytology is surprisingly low (<40%) (36). CT guidance may improve the yield to 60% with a single attempt and perhaps as high as 85% with repeated biopsies, but any closed biopsy procedure carries with it the risks of a pneumothorax (10%) and tract seeding with tumor (22%) (37). Thoracoscopy is the primary diagnostic modality for mesothelioma with a diagnostic yield in excess of 90% (38) and a tolerable complication rate of approximately 10% that includes tumor seeding, persistent air leaks, infection, hemorrhage, and subcutaneous emphysema (39). (A formal distinction should be made between "medical" thoracoscopy and "surgical" thoracoscopy, the latter being more properly encompassed by the term video-assisted thoracic surgery or VATS. The former is a less invasive and less costly procedure that can be performed in an endoscopy suite under local anesthesia or conscious sedation. It is a viable option for diagnostic purposes but is less applicable for treatment (40,41) Failing thoracoscopy, the only remaining option is an open thoracotomy; however, isolated cases of missed diagnoses have been reported with this procedure as well (2).

Staging
Once a definitive diagnosis has been obtained, staging is required. Radiologic studies are essential though not sufficient in the rigorous staging of MPM. Routine chest

radiography with postero-anterior and lateral views and CT and/or magnetic resonance imaging (MRI) scans of the chest and upper abdomen constitute the most commonly used modalities. Routine chest radiography is severely lacking in sensitivity and specificity and has little role in staging.(Figure 1A & 1B) Its use is largely relegated to the initial workup although some have also suggested its use in following patients for radiation-induced lung injury following hemi-thorax radiation (42). CT scan represent a significant improvement over chest radiography although its sensitivity and specificity for predicting the malignant nature of diffuse pleural lesions based upon morphologic criteria are only 72% and 83%, respectively (43). Furthermore, CT lacks sensitivity for detecting miliary pleural seeding and critical invasion into the mediastinum or through the diaphragm (44). MRI is probably the most accurate of the commonly available modalities because of its superior definition of tissue planes and its ability to provide sagittal and coronal views, thereby allowing better evaluation of the diaphragmatic and apical regions (45). (Figure 1B) The main drawbacks of MRI include patient discomfort and movement artifact. A recent study by Falaschi *et al.* has suggested a sensitivity as high as 100% with a specificity of 87% using certain criteria such as low signal intensity on long repetition time images to distinguish benign lesions from malignant lesions (46). For these reasons, we routinely use MRI scans in the pre-operative evaluation of patients prior to extrapleural pneumonectomy (see below).

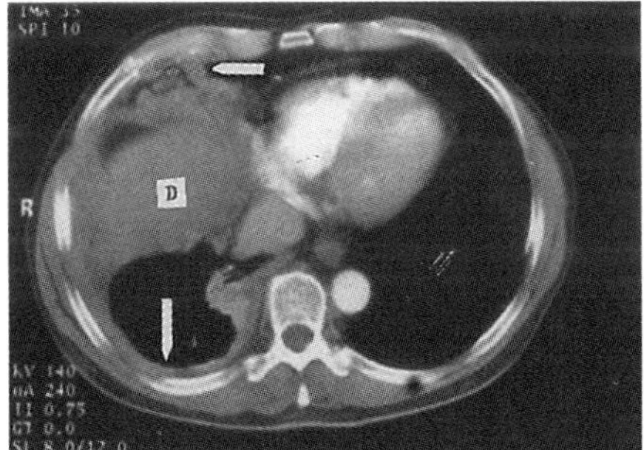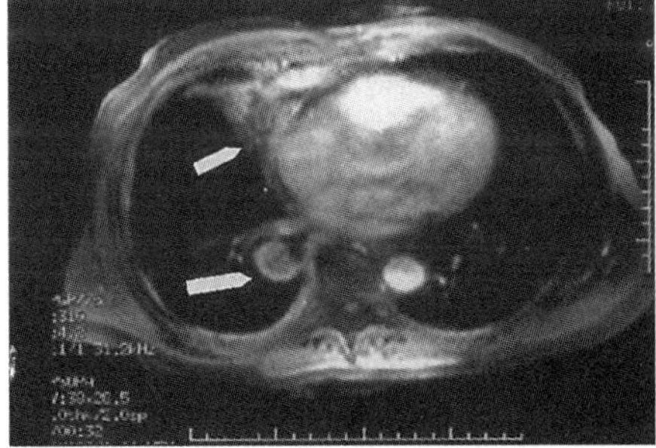

Figure 1A-B. A) Axial CT scan in a patient with early malignant mesothelioma (MM) shows nodular pleural involvement (arrows) possibly involving the dome of the diaphragm (D). B) MRI scan of same patient details the nodular clusters of MM in the anterior sulcus (upper arrow) along with a solid round MM mass in the posterior sulcus (lower arrow).

                                    Malignant Pleural Mesothelioma

One very promising modality under investigation is positron emission tomography (PET) scanning with the label ^{18}F-fluorodeoxyglucose (FDG), a metabolically active derivative of glucose. Because it distinguishes between degrees of tissue metabolic activity, PET scanning cannot necessarily differentiate between malignant processes (*e.g.*, MPM and metastatic implants from adenocarcinoma) or between malignant and certain benign processes (*e.g.*, granulomatous or infectious diseases); however, with a diagnosis in hand, its accuracy in determining the extent of disease is quite good. A recent report by Benard *et al.* described 28 consecutive patients with suspected MPM who underwent PET imaging (2). PET images correlated well with thoracoscopic assessments of primary tumor extent in 16 of 18 patients who underwent the latter procedure, but underestimated primary disease in the remaining two patients. Evaluation of nodal staging was sub-optimal because only 10 of the 24 patients with confirmed MPM underwent pathologic lymph node sampling; however, only 1 of 6 positive results (a case of granulomatous lymphadenitis) and 1 of 4 negative results (pathology performed at thoracotomy 3 months after the PET scan) were erroneous. Using a standardized uptake value (SUV) discriminant of 2.0, PET scanning was able to distinguish between benign and malignant disease with a sensitivity of 91% and a specificity of 100%. Thus, PET scanning may prove to be a useful adjunct to MRI in pre-operative staging protocols.(Figure 1C & 1D).

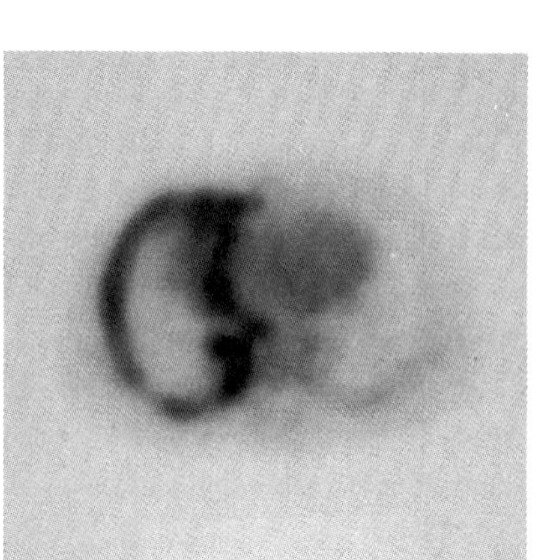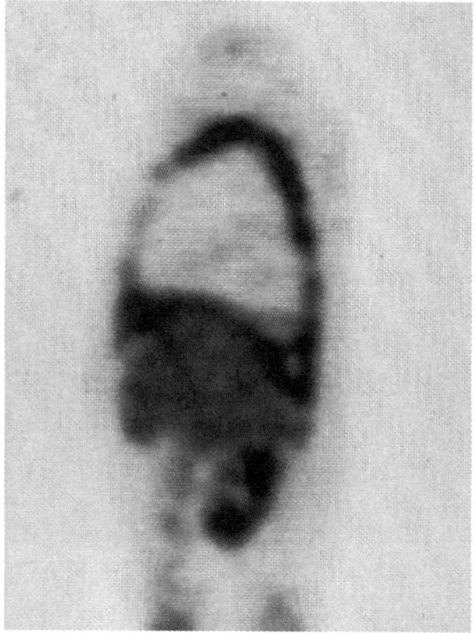

Figure 1C-D. C) Transaxial PET scan in same patient shows the pleural rind of MM surrounding the lung but without invasion of the chest wall, mediastinum or lung parenchyma. D) No invasion of the diaphragm was present on sagittal PET scan or coronal views (not shown). The patient had complete resection of the MM by an extrapleural pneumonectomy with mediastinal lymph node dissection. Surgical margins were free of tumor.

Despite the advances in radiology described above, surgical staging remains critically important in those patients being considered for aggressive surgical resection. As discussed elsewhere, extension through the diaphragm or into critical mediastinal structures renders curative surgical resection an impossibility, and extrapleural nodal involvement carries with it such a poor prognosis that radical resection such as extrapleural pneumonectomy, while technically feasible, probably does not offer sufficient benefit to warrant the morbidity and possible mortality associated with surgery (47,48). Thus, groups pursuing aggressive surgical approaches such as ours at Dana-Farber Cancer Institute and Rusch and her colleagues at Memorial Sloan-Kettering (49), have emphasized the importance of surgical staging. The results reported by Rusch and Venkatraman underscore the insensitivity of CT scans (49). In this study, 131 patients with "potentially resectable" disease by CT scan underwent exploratory thoracotomy. By the IMIG staging system, 32 patients (24%) had T4 (technically unresectable) disease and 46 patients (35%) had N2 or N3 (extrapleural) nodal disease. We currently use VATS and mediastinoscopy to assess pre-operative tumor and nodal status, respectively, both of which are important in almost any staging system and which correlate with prognosis.

The median survival for MPM varies widely but ranges between 4 and 18 months from the time of diagnosis (14). Without treatment, median survival is only 4-12 months (average = 8.7 months) (50). While death most frequently follows respiratory failure due to locally progressive disease or superimposed infection, up to one-third of patients may die from small bowel obstruction as a result of direct tumor extension through the diaphragm, and 10% die from cardiac complications resulting from pericardial or myocardial involvement (14).

Pathology
MPMs can exhibit great histological heterogeneity but are generally classified into three main types: epithelial, mixed (biphasic), and sarcomatoid. The epithelial class, accounting for 50% of all cases (51), can be further sub-divided into subtypes (*e.g.*, tubular, papillary, solid or epithelioid, large/giant cell, small cell, clear cell, signet cell, glandular, microcystic, myxoid, and adenoid cystic) (52) which reflect their histologic similarity to carcinomas arising from other sites. The sarcomatoid class is characterized by ovoid- to spindle-shaped cells reminiscent of those seen in fibrosarcomas and comprise approximately 15% (51). Most of the remaining cases are of the mixed type which, as suggested by its name, is composed of both epithelial and sarcomatoid elements, a combination which is virtually pathognomonic of mesothelioma. This histologic classification is of prognostic importance since the sarcomatoid component correlates negatively with predicted survival.

The pathologic diagnosis of MPM is understandably difficult given the gross histologic similarity to other types of neoplasms listed above. In particular, distinguishing between adenocarcinomas (especially of lung origin) and MPMs is the most commonly encountered pathologic dilemma. Thus, the concomitant use of conventional histochemical, immunohistochemical, and electron microscopic techniques has proven indispensable in the diagnosis of MPM (52). Since detection is not so much the issue as distinguishing among a list of possible malignancies, specificity is of principal concern in using a technique. Conventional histochemical stains include diastase-periodic acid-Schiff (D-PAS), Alcian blue or colloidal iron followed by hyaluronidase, and mucicarmine. The mucicarmine stain reveals the presence of neutral and weakly acidic mucopolysaccharides which are found frequently in adenocarcinomas but rarely in MPMs; this pattern is also seen with PAS following diastase treatment, which stains for neutral mucopolysaccharides only. Acidic mucopolysaccharides, a feature of both adenocarcinomas and MPMs, are detected by either Alcian blue or colloidal iron stains, but the disappearance of intracellular staining following treatment with hyaluronidase suggests the presence of hyaluronic acid, a fairly specific though relatively insensitive marker for MPM. However, a cautionary note must be made against overinterpreting the presence of extracellular hyaluronic acid, which is a non-specific finding) (14). IL-6 has been found to be secreted by mesothelioma cells, and high concentrations of IL-6 in pleural fluid argue for a diagnosis of MPM over adenocarcinoma, although this criterion alone is not specific (53).

Immunohistochemical assays, on the other hand, have gained ascendancy over the past decade and make use of antibodies to such antigens as CEA, CD15 (Leu-M1), cytokeratins, and EMA (epithelial membrane antigen) (Table 1). Except for EMA, these antigens are typically absent in MPMs but present in adenocarcinomas. In the case of EMA, MPMs can be distinguished from adenocarcinomas with moderate specificity on the basis of their membrane-associated staining pattern; adenocarcinomas, on the other hand, stain in a diffuse cytoplasmic pattern (54). (Wolanski *et al.* have suggested that quantitation of the average area of silver-stained nucleolar organizer regions (AgNORs) may improve upon the specificity of EMA alone (55). Cytokeratins, while generally ubiquitous, can sometimes be discriminating based upon their intracellular distribution (52), (see Table 1) but this problem can be circumvented by examining particular cytokeratin subtypes, especially cytokeratins 5 and 6, which are reasonably specific for MPM (56,57). Another promising marker is the calcium-binding protein, calretinin. When used alone (58,59) but perhaps preferably when used in combination with E-cadherin (60), calretinin has demonstrated good specificity for mesothelial cells. Other markers which have been touted but lack extensive track records include the transcription factor TTF-1 (61) and the antigens recognized by the monoclonal antibodies CA19-9 (62) and MOC-31(63). A recently described monoclonal antibody, Ber-EP4, which recognizes an epitope common to a pair of glycoproteins expressed by the MCF-7 breast carcinoma cell line, may be helpful in certain cases since staining is focal and sporadic in MPMs but diffuse in pulmonary adenocarcinomas, but its general utility is limited by its inconsistency when compared among adenocarcinomas arising from various primary sites (64).

In difficult cases, electron microscopy (EM) may play an important role (65). For example, epithelial MPMs often possess large numbers of desmosomes, tonofilaments, and long, slender, branching microvilli while adenocarcinomas have much fewer desmosomes and tonofilaments and short, stubby, unbranched microvilli. Some have attempted to quantify these differences between microvilli by calculating their length:diameter ratio (LDR) (66). Thus, an LDR $\geq$15 is suggestive of a mesothelioma whereas adenocarcinoma microvilli typically have an LDR $\leq$10. However, none of these assays demonstrate sufficient accuracy to stand alone, and a panel of representative tests is usually performed to arrive at a definitive diagnosis. Atomic force microscopy may be a simpler, though less accurate, substitute for EM in the analysis of ultrastructural features (67).

A distinction should be made between MPMs, which are diffuse in nature, and "localized" or "benign" mesotheliomas, which are more correctly known as localized fibrous tumors of the pleura (68). The latter are solitary, well-demarcated tumors originating not from pleural mesothelial cells but from submesothelial mesenchymal cells, are not strongly associated with asbestos exposure, and can usually be resected for cure without the need for pulmonary resection. Their (immuno)histochemical staining profile and electron microscopic appearance also differ considerably from MPMs as shown in Table 1.

Table 1. Staining and microscopical profiles of MPMs, adenocarcinomas (AC), and localized fibrous tumors of the pleura (LFTP)

Marker	MPM	AC	LFTP
Diastase-PAS	-	+ (50%)	-
Hyaluronic acid	+++	+/-	-
Mucicarmine	-	+ (50%)	-
CD34	-	-	+ (80%)
CEA	+/- (10%)	+ (>75%)	-
Cytokeratins	Diffuse cytoplasmic or perinuclear	Peripheral cyto-plasmic or mem-brane-associated	-
EMA	Membrane	Diffuse, cytoplasmic	-
Leu-M1 (CD15)	-	+ (60-70%)	
Desmosomes/ tonofilaments	Abundant	-	Few
Secretory granules, glycocalyceal bodies	-	+	
Villi	Long, thin, curved, branched (LDR >15)	Short, thick, straight, sparse (LDR <10)	Absent
Vimentin	-	-	++

CEA - carcinoembryonic antigen, EMA - epithelial membrane antigen, HMFG - human milk fat globule, PAS - periodic acid/Schiff.

Genetic analyses of MPMs have yielded a wide range of chromosomal abnormalities. Most series report the predominance of genetic loss over gain though this impression is by no means unanimous (69). The relatively small number of cases involved undoubtedly contributes to much of the variability reported in the literature, but, by one reckoning, the most frequently reported losses involve the regions 1p, 3p, 6q, 9p, 15q and 22q (70). Positional candidate gene approaches have identified tumor suppressor genes within two of these regions (p16/CDKN2A at 9p21 and NF2 at 22q12), and both of these genes are frequently involved in MPMs. Homozygous deletions appear to be the major mechanism affecting p16/CDKN2A (71), whereas inactivating mutations coupled with allelic loss occur at the NF2 locus (72,73). Duplication of chromosomal regions localized to 5p, 7p, and 15q have also been reported (74), but not yet linked with the amplification of specific genes. Incidentally, aneuploidy has been recommended by some as a criterion for malignancy in effusion cytology although it is clearly not specific for MPM.(75,76).

Staging Systems
The pre-operative staging of MPM remains problematic due to the sampling error of blind biopsies, the diffuse nature of MPM, the frequent absence of measurable disease, and the lack of accurate non-invasive staging methods for measuring disease. Furthermore, the lack of a universally accepted staging system has hampered interpretation of the literature and inter-study comparisons.

Several staging systems have been proposed although none has yet achieved universal acceptance. The oldest, simplest, and perhaps most commonly used staging system is that introduced by Butchart *et al.* in 1976 (Table 2), (77) but it suffers from imprecision (involvement of the opposite pleura is listed under both stage II and stage III) and predates both technical advances in surgery and the recognition of important prognostic factors (see below). In a prospective study of 188 consecutive patients evaluated by thoracoscopic biopsies, Boutin *et al.* found that involvement of the parietal pleura could distinguish between two groups within Butchart's stage I classification with widely disparate prognoses: patients with parietal pleural involvement had a median survival of 7 months compared with 32.7 months for those without parietal pleural involvement (78) Mattson, (79) Chahinian, (80) Sugarbaker *et al.* (Table 3), (48) and the Union Internationale Contre Cancer (UICC) (81,82) have proposed alternative staging systems, of which the Chahinian and UICC systems are TNM-based. The Mattson staging system shares many of the same drawbacks as the Butchart system, but also contradicts most of the other systems in considering contralateral pleura involvement as being relatively early stage (stage II) instead of advanced-stage disease (stage IV under the other three systems). The UICC system is limited by its failure to distinguish between types of pleural involvement because patients with parietal and diaphragmatic pleural involvement survive longer than those with visceral pleural involvement (median survival 31.2 months vs. 6.75 months, respectively) (83).

Recently, the International Mesothelioma Interest Group (IMIG) has tried to incorporate our current understanding of the impact of tumor (T) and nodal (N) status into a TNM-based staging system (Table 4) (81,82). It incorporates features of previous mesothelioma staging systems into the general TNM framework used in the staging of almost every other solid tumor and familiar to all oncologists. For example, T1 tumors have been subdivided into stages IA and IB on the basis of the work of Boutin *et al* (78), T2 tumors require an extrapleural pneumonectomy for complete tumor debulking, T3 tumors are locally advanced but technically resectable, and T4 tumors are technically unresectable. The nodal staging is identical to that used in the staging of non-small cell lung cancer. The tumor staging is somewhat complicated compared to some other systems such as that proposed by Sugarbaker *et al.* (48), but validation of either system in an independent patient population is still pending.

Table 2. The Butchart Staging System[77]

Stage	Definition
I	Tumor is confined to the capsule of the parietal pleura (*i.e.*, involves only the ipsilateral lung, pleura, pericardium, and/or diaphragm)
II	Tumor invades the chest wall or mediastinal structures (*e.g.*, esophagus, heart, and/or contralateral pleura), or Tumor involves intrathoracic lymph nodes
III	Tumor penetrates the diaphragm to involve peritoneum, or Tumor involves the contralateral pleura, or Tumor involves extrathoracic lymph nodes
IV	Distant blood-borne metastases

Reprinted with permission.[77]

Table 3. Revised staging system proposed by Sugarbaker et al.[48]

Stage	Definition
I	Disease completely resected within the capsule of the parietal pleura without adenopathy: ipsilateral pleura, lung, pericardium, diaphragm, or chest-wall disease limited to previous biopsy sites
II	All of stage I with positive resection margins and/or intrapleural adenopathy
III	Local extension (1) into the chest wall or mediastinum; into the heart or through the diaphragm or peritoneum; or with extrapleural lymph node involvement
IV	Distant metastatic disease

Reprinted with permission.[48]

Prognostic Factors
In thirteen multivariate analyses of prognostic factors in MPM, stage (7 of the 13 studies), histology (7/13), age (6/13), performance status (5/13), and prior treatment (4/13) emerge as the most consistently identified prognostic factors in MPM; other less consistently reported variables include gender, pleural site, presence of chest pain, race, asbestos exposure, duration of symptoms, delay in diagnosis, weight loss, type of treatment, platelet count, and geographic location. However, included within "stage" are several variables which, individually, could be important prognostic determinants. Not surprisingly, pre-operative tumor volume has been positively correlated with stage and lymph node status and inversely correlated with median survival (84). However, our experience suggests that extrapleural lymph node status is also a powerful prognostic factor, particularly if aggressive multimodality therapy is to be considered (47,48). For example, in our cohort of 183 patients treated with trimodality therapy between 1980 and 1997, those patients with negative extrapleural lymph nodes experienced 2- and 5-year overall survival rates of 42% and 17%, respectively, in contrast with those with positive nodes, whose survival rates were 23% and 0%, respectively (odds ratio of 2.0 by the Cox proportional hazards method) (48).

Two of the largest and most recent studies to examine prognostic factors in MPM were reported by the CALGB (Cancer and Leukemia Group B) and EORTC (European Organization for Research and Treatment of Cancer). The former group conducted a retrospective, multivariate analysis of 337 patients randomized to CALGB trials between 1984 and 1994 and found, in order of decreasing relative risk, that pleural involvement, LDH >500 IU/L, poor performance status (PS), chest pain, platelet count >400,000/?L, non-epithelial histology, and age >75 years were all predictive of poor survival. Similarly, the EORTC analyzed their 9-year experience (1984-1993) involving 204 patients with MPM enrolled in EORTC phase II trials (85). Thirteen parameters were included in a multivariate analysis. Poor median survival was associated with a high WBC count ($\geq 8.3 \times 10^3$/?L), poor performance status, uncertainty in the histologic diagnosis, sarcomatoid histology, and male gender (in order of decreasing statistical significance). The EORTC also stratified these same patients into low- and high-risk categories and observed significant differences in median survival and in 1- and 2-year rates of overall survival, but the significance of such model validation using the original patient set is highly questionable.

Increasingly, biological and molecular correlates have been examined as potential prognostic factors. For example, a low pleural fluid pH and a low pleural fluid:serum glucose ratio may be poor prognostic features, likely reflecting pleural tumor burden (86). Tumor proliferative potential, as reflected by MIB-1 index (87) or PCNA expression (particularly a PCNA index >20%) (88), DNA aneuploidy (89), S-phase fraction (90,91), and "intratumoral microvascular density" (92) have all been reported to be negative prognostic factors. However, most of these variables have yet to be validated in independent series or in multivariate analyses.

***Table 4. Staging system proposed by the International Mesothelioma Interest Group (IMIG)*[81,82]**

<u>Tumor (T) staging:</u>

T1a   Tumor limited to the ipsilateral parietal pleura, including the mediastinal and diaphragmatic pleura, without involvement of the visceral pleura

T1b   T1a + scattered foci of tumor involving the visceral pleura

T2   Tumor involving each of the ipsilateral pleural surfaces (parietal, mediastinal, diaphragmatic, and visceral pleura) with at least one of the following features:involvement of diaphragmatic muscle confluent visceral pleural tumor (including the fissures) or extension of tumor from the visceral pleura into the underlying pulmonary parenchyma

T3   Locally advanced but potentially resectable tumor. The tumor involves all of the ipsilateral pleural surfaces with at least one of the following features: involvement of the endothoracic fascia extension into the mediastinal fat a solitary, completely resectable focus of tumor extending into the soft tissues of the chest wall non-transmural involvement of the pericardium

T4   Locally advanced, technically unresectable tumor. The tumor involves all of the ipsilateral pleural surfaces with at least one of the following features: diffuse extension or metastatic spread to the chest wall with or without rib destruction direct trans-diaphragmatic extension to the peritoneum direct extension to the contralateral pleura direct extension to any mediastinal organ direct extension to the spine

<u>Lymph node (N) staging</u>

Nx   Regional lymph nodes (LNs) cannot be assessed
N0   No regional LN metastases
N1   Involvement of ipsilateral bronchopulmonary or hilar LNs
N2   Involvement of subcarinal or ipsilateral mediastinal LNs (including the internal mammary LNs)
N3   Involvement of the contralateral mediastinal or internal mammary LNs or any supraclavicular LNs

<u>Metastases (M) staging</u>

Mx   Presence of distant metastases cannot be assessed
M0   No distant metastases
M1   Distant metastases present

<u>Overall staging</u>

Stage I
      Ia   T1a N0 M0
      Ib   T1b N0 M0

Stage II   T2 N0 M0

Stage III   Any T3 M0
              Any N1 M0
              Any N2 M0

Stage IV   Any T4
              Any N3
              Any M1

Reprinted with permission.[81]

Radiation Therapy
Although the radiosensitivity of mesothelioma cell lines is intermediate between that of non-small cell and small cell lung cancer cell lines (93) the role of radiation therapy in the definitive treatment of MPM is problematic because of the large radiation field required to treat the entire ipsilateral pleura at tumoricidal doses (probably >40 Gy; see below) and the proximity of dose-limiting thoracic structures: lung (20 Gy), liver (30 Gy), spinal cord (45 Gy), heart (45 Gy), and esophagus (45-50 Gy). Radiation pneumonitis is a frequent complication of hemithorax radiation (94) and myelitis and fatal hepatitis have also been reported (95). Earlier studies devoid of reports of complications from radiation may have enrolled patients with short survival times or used inadequate radiation fields or doses.

Interpretation of and extrapolation from the literature is difficult because of the small numbers of patients, the non-uniformity of radiation techniques, and the variable natural history of MPM itself. For instance, even the optimal dose of radiation has yet to be established. A minimum effective dose of 40 Gy is suggested by a report from the Joint Center for Radiation Therapy in Boston (96). In this retrospective review of patients treated over a 12-year period (1968-1980), only 1 of 23 patients (4%) treated with doses <40 Gy achieved palliation while 4 of 6 patients (67%) treated with doses >40 Gy achieved palliation. However, this dose represents a minimum for radical radiotherapy since the treatment outcome in this study was only symptomatic relief, and doses of 60-70 Gy may be necessary to control masses $\geq$3 cm in size. In addition, larger fractions of radiation ($\geq$4 Gy) may be more efficacious (97). Thus, experiences such as that reported by Lindén *et al.* (a response rate of 3% in 31 patients given 40 Gy hemithorax irradiation over 20 fractions) (98) may be at least partially explained by a suboptimal radiotherapy schedule. Nonetheless, radiation therapy as a single modality is unlikely to impact significantly upon overall survival. For example, one large South African series compared four different treatment strategies (chemotherapy, radiation therapy, chemotherapy + radiation therapy, and decortication + chemotherapy + radiation therapy) and found no difference in median survival among the four groups (99).

Boutin *et al.* (29) have conducted a prospective randomized trial testing the role of local radiotherapy in decreasing malignant seeding after invasive diagnostic procedures. Forty patients who had undergone needle biopsy followed by thoracoscopy were randomized to receive 21 Gy over 3 days (*i.e.*, 700 cGy fractions) to all sites of previous invasive procedures. None of the 20 irradiated patients (0%) developed entry tract metastases while 8 of the 20 control patients (40%) developed entry tract metastases. Although this latter figure is somewhat higher than the average incidence of malignant seeding (19%) (29), the absence of such spread in irradiated patients is notable. The authors emphasize the importance of early treatment (within 10-15 days of the invasive procedure) and treatment of all entry sites.

The role of intrapleural colloidal radioisotopes (*e.g.*, P^{32} or Au^{198}) has been poorly studied. Since both radioisotopes are primarily beta emitters, tissue penetration is limited (<8 mm for P^{32} and <5 mm for Au^{192}), and their utility would presumably be limited to low-volume disease. Furthermore, there is the issue of distribution of the radioisotope within the pleural cavity, which may harbor loculated regions inaccessible to the colloid. For this reason, test instillation of a contrast agent or radioactive tracer should be performed prior to definitive intrapleural therapy.

Surgery
There are three surgical options available in the treatment of MPM: thoracoscopy with sclerosis, pleurectomy/decortication (P/D), and extrapleural pneumonectomy. The first procedure is primarily palliative in intent. The latter two options represent radical operations intended to prolong survival.

Thoracoscopy with sclerosis is a palliative technique designed to relieve the dyspneic symptoms frequently experienced by patients with recurrent pleural effusions. In this procedure, a sclerosant such as talc, bleomycin, doxycycline or tetracycline is instilled into the pleural space via thoracoscope or chest tube, where it creates an intense inflammatory reaction with subsequent scarring and forced apposition of the visceral and parietal pleurae. Randomized trials have compared talc with bleomycin (100), tetracycline with bleomycin (101) and doxycycline with bleomycin (102) and found no significant differences in efficacy or tolerability. Thus, the lower cost of talc and the current unavailability of tetracycline for pleurodesis in the United States has made the former the current sclerosant of choice. One randomized trial has suggested the equivalence of talc insufflation via thoracoscope and instillation of a talc slurry via tube thoracostomy (103), again, cost considerations make the latter option preferable in most cases. A large retrospective review of 327 patients with MPM or pleural metastases reported a 90% success rate in controlling pleural effusions at 1 month and 82% over the patients' lifetimes (104) making pleurodesis a highly effective palliative procedure.

The primary factor to be considered prior to pleurodesis is the eligibility of the patient for a more radical surgical approach because pleurodesis considerably complicates or may even obviate pleurectomy or extrapleural pneumonectomy.

Pleurectomy/decortication (P/D) is performed with curative intent. The procedure, described in detail by Rusch (105), involves removal of the pericardium and the visceral and parietal pleura from the apex of the lung to the diaphragm. A clean separation of lung and visceral pleura may be difficult because tumor often grows from the pleura into adjacent tissues and lung (30). Compared with extrapleural pneumonectomy, P/D demonstrates somewhat lower rates of morbidity and mortality (1-5-5.0%) (105), but it has drawbacks: (1) complete resection is usually possible only in patients with lower-stage disease, (2) deliverable post-operative radiation doses are necessarily lower because of the retained lung, and (3) disease recurrence occurs more rapidly.

Extrapleural pneumonectomy (EPP) resects *en bloc* the parietal and visceral pleura, the contained lung, the pericardium, and the ipsilateral diaphragm. Both the pericardium and the diaphragmatic defect are repaired, the latter to prevent herniation of the abdominal contents (106). Complications include bronchial leaks, empyema, vocal cord paralysis, chylothorax, arrhythmias, and respiratory insufficiency (30). Median survival following EPP as single-modality therapy has been estimated at 11.1 months (83); however, the studies included in this review are somewhat dated. Ours is perhaps the most extensive single-institution experience with EPP. We consistently perform EPP within the context of multimodality treatment for mesothelioma. A recent update of 183 patients treated with trimodality therapy including EPP revealed a peri-operative mortality rate (within 30 days of surgery) of 3.8% and a major morbidity rate (an untoward event resulting in prolonged hospitalization) of 24.5% (48). These rates are likely the result of improvements in operative techniques and perioperative care at a center with extensive experience in the treatment of mesothelioma.

There is considerable debate regarding the merits of P/D and EPP. The median survivals cited above would suggest a slight advantage to P/D, but there have been no randomized trials to confirm this. A recent report by Rusch and Venkatraman is revealing (49). They describe 131 patients undergoing open thoracotomy; 51 underwent P/D and 50 EPP. A univariate analysis suggested improved survival with P/D (median survival: 18.3 months vs. 9.9 months; p=0.00054), but a multivariate analysis found the difference to be less significant (p=0.022). Furthermore, patients treated with EPP had more advanced-stage disease than those who underwent P/D, a not unexpected fact since the decision to perform P/D or EPP was based upon the extent of visceral pleural tumor found at thoracotomy. Thus, as reported in the literature, EPP has probably been used to treat patients with more advanced-stage disease, thereby negatively biasing the survival data.

At our institutions, routine pre-operative testing prior to extrapleural pneumonectomy includes an echocardiogram, an MRI scan of the chest and upper abdomen (for reasons previously discussed), and an evaluation of pulmonary function with dynamic spirometry, arterial blood gases (ABGs), and functional oximetry. An echocardiogram is useful for two reasons: (1) it provides a quantitative evaluation of baseline cardiac function, which has prognostic implications for the peri-operative period and may impact upon the choice of future chemotherapeutic agents such as anthracyclines, and (2) it serves as a staging adjunct by assessing potential pericardial involvement. Pulmonary function tests are important in evaluating the tolerability of pneumonectomy in each patient, and a predicted post-operative FEV_1 >1L is generally required. In borderline cases (*e.g.*, the baseline FEV_1 is <2L or the predicted post-operative FEV_1 is <1.2L), a quantitative ventilation-perfusion (V/Q) scan is then obtained. We generally consider any of the following results to be a physiologic exclusionary criterion: (1) a predicted post-operative FEV_1 <1L, (2) an ejection fraction <45%, (3) a room-air arterial carbon dioxide partial pressure (P_aCO_2) >45 mm Hg, or (4) a room-air oxygen partial pressure (P_aO_2) <65 mm Hg.

Chemotherapy

The relative benefit of chemotherapeutic agents in the treatment of MPM has been difficult to evaluate because of small patient numbers and a lack of randomized trials. In addition, responses to chemotherapy are difficult to assess because of the location and distribution of the predominant tumor burden (within the pleural space, often obscured by effusions that may be loculated) and its diffuse distribution. We have reviewed all trials with 15 or more evaluable patients and discuss herein the main points derived from these studies, referring the reader to other reviews for more detailed discussions of older trials (Ong and Vogelzang, 1996 (107); Taub and Antman, 1997(108); Ryan *et al.*, 1998 (109).

Conventional single-agent chemotherapy has generally been ineffective. The scant available data on single-agent trials are summarized in Table 5. By class, only the anti-metabolites, platinum compounds, anthracyclines, and biologic agents appear to have any significant activity against MPM (see later section for the last group). Notably, the plant alkaloids (*e.g.*, the vinca alkaloids, taxanes, and epipodophyllotoxins) appear to be inactive although irinotecan, which has demonstrated activity *in vitro*, is currently being tested by the CALGB in a phase II study. Gemcitabine has also shown some promise, demonstrating a response rate of 31% in a single-agent trial (1 complete response (CR) and 4 partial responses (PR) out of 16 evaluable patients with Butchart stage I/II disease) (110). However, the true activity of these drugs and the superiority of any single agent over another remain uncertain. For example, neither cyclophosphamide nor doxorubicin provided responses in any of 30 evaluable patients when evaluated in a randomized setting (111), and the addition of either doxorubicin or mitomycin C to cisplatin seemed to make no difference in time to treatment failure or survival (112).

Unfortunately, combination chemotherapy has not yielded significantly better results compared with single agents (Table 6). A European trial testing the combination of three active single agents (cisplatin, doxorubicin, and mitomycin C) reported a response rate of only 21% (5 partial responses/23 evaluable patients) (113); this is equivalent to the response rate to mitomycin C alone in a similarly sized trial. Similarly, Middleton *et al.* reported a response rate of 21% (8 PRs/39 evaluable patients) with MVP (mitomycin C, vinblastine, and cisplatin) although a considerably higher rate of symptom palliation (62%) was claimed (114). The CAP regimen (cyclophosphamide, doxorubicin, and cisplatin), used extensively in the past for non-small cell lung cancer, has been applied to MPM with moderate success. While Shin and his colleagues at M. D. Anderson have tested CAP up-front in previously untreated patients with unresectable MPM, reporting a 30% partial response rate in 23 patients, our group has used CAP in the adjuvant setting following extrapleural pneumonectomy and prior to radiotherapy (see below). In this subset of patients treated between 1987 and 1993, the median time to relapse was approximately 20 months, but it is impossible to separate the relative contribution of any single treatment modality to outcome. Finally, in an Australian phase II trial (115), the combination of gemcitabine and cisplatin did yield a remarkable response rate of 48%, albeit only partial responses (10/21 patients), thus recommending gemcitabine for consideration in future novel therapeutic combinations.

Intrathoracic chemotherapy (Table 7) has gained support over the past several years for several reasons. First, it is intellectually appealing because drugs can be delivered directly and effectively to an area of the body where the tumor is concentrated and that is otherwise poorly exposed to systemic chemotherapy. This has been demonstrated pharmacokinetically for cisplatin and mitomycin C (116), each of which is concentrated 3- to 5-fold and exhibits a 50-fold greater AUC in the pleural space relative to plasma. Second, intrathoracic chemotherapy may decrease the systemic toxicity to the patient. Third, response rates following intrathoracic chemotherapy may be slightly superior to those seen with systemic chemotherapy although no randomized comparison has yet been reported. The group at UCLA found no difference in survival between patients receiving intrapleural chemotherapy (cisplatin + cytosine arabinoside) and those who did not receive chemotherapy following incomplete resections (117), but the small population size and the lack of randomization preclude drawing definite conclusions. Nonetheless, it is unlikely that intracavitary therapy will be useful in cases of extensive or bulky disease. This suspicion is borne out by the results of Boutin *et al.*, who report a response rate of 45% in Butchart stage I patients but an overall response rate of only 20% with intrapleural interferon-γ (118). However, a group from M. D. Anderson has reported surprisingly high CR rates (11/15 patients, or 73%) with the liposome-entrapped platinum compound L-NDDP as demonstrated by cytology and thoracoscopic biopsies (119), and such new agents may yet prove useful in the adjuvant or minimal residual disease settings.

Thus, the role of systemic chemotherapy remains unclear. There are no studies demonstrating either the superiority of chemotherapy to best supportive care or of combination chemotherapy to single-agent chemotherapy. Therefore, patients ineligible for a prospective study should be treated symptomatically or with single-agent chemotherapy. Similarly, the role of intracavitary chemotherapy remains undefined. It holds potential promise in the adjuvant and combined modality settings and in the treatment of low-volume disease, but these and other hypotheses should be rigorously tested in prospective cooperative trials with randomization when patient numbers allow.

Multimodality Therapy

The apparent failure of surgery, radiation, and chemotherapy individually to impact significantly on survival has led to attempts to combine modalities. Since surgery is the most effective modality for local control in this locally invasive disease, multimodality protocols have typically combined surgery with adjuvant radiation and/or chemotherapy, depending upon the predominant pattern of relapse. Efforts have focused largely on local control, and chemotherapy administered into the pleural space or used as radiosensitizing agents offers ways of enhancing local control.

The use of chemotherapeutic agents as radiation sensitizers in the treatment of limited-stage small cell lung cancer and locally advanced non-small cell lung cancer is well established, but its applicability to MPM has not been intensively studied. To date, doxorubicin (120) and paclitaxel (121) have been the only agents studied as radiosensitizers in trials primarily focused on MPM. Herscher *et al.* (121) reported a recent phase I trial using paclitaxel as a radiosensitizer in patients with MPM and non-small cell lung cancer. Twenty-seven of the 30 patients had unresectable MPM. Paclitaxel was administered as a 5-day continuous infusion every 3 weeks during radiation treatment to a total dose of 5760-6300 cGy. However, overall median survival after the completion of treatment was only 5 months.

We first began treating patients on a trimodality protocol in 1980, using sequential chemotherapy and radiation (30 Gy to the involved hemithorax and boosts to involved areas to 50-55 Gy) following EPP. Prior to 1985, chemotherapy consisted of AC (Adriamycin and cyclophosphamide), but cisplatin was added to the regimen (CAP) in 1985. More recently, we have switched to a "sandwich" schedule of adjuvant therapy consisting of 2 cycles of carboplatin and paclitaxel followed by 5 to 6 weeks of radiation with concomitant weekly paclitaxel followed in turn by 2 additional cycles of carboplatin and paclitaxel. Through 1997, 183 patients had received trimodality therapy. The 2- and 5-year overall survival rates for the 176 patients surviving the peri-operative period are 38% and 15%, respectively (Figure 2) (48). Histologic subtype, lymph node involvement, and resection margins were found to be significant prognostic factors. The 31 patients with an epithelial subtype, negative lymph nodes, and negative margins experienced 51-month median survival with 2- and 5-year survivals of 68% and 46%, respectively.

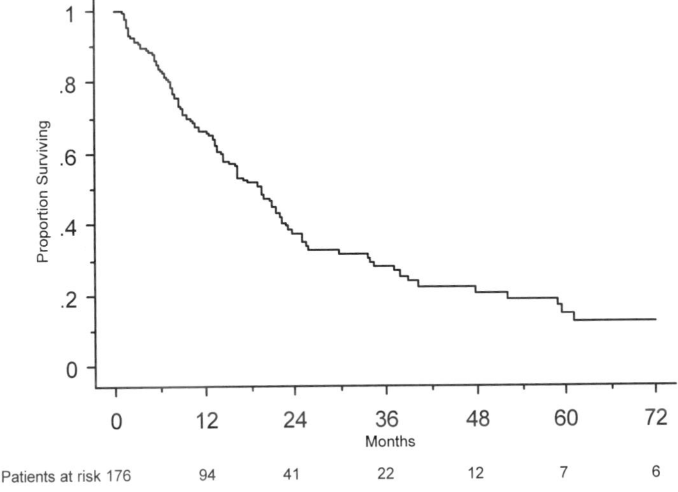

Figure 2. Kaplan-Meier survival curve for all patients surviving surgery (n=176). Reprinted with permission.[48]

Several important points are raised by this work. First, in agreement with results from Memorial Sloan-Kettering (49), an analysis of the subset of patients treated between 1987 and 1993 demonstrated that sites of relapse were more likely to be outside the ipsilateral pleura (122). Thus, more effective systemic therapy might prolong survival. Second, prognosis was more accurately predicted by the staging system proposed by Sugarbaker *et al.* (p=0.0011) (48) than by either the Butchart system (p=0.09) or the IMIG system (p=0.31). However, since the first system was derived using a subset of these same patients (47), it has yet to be fully and independently validated. The data do suggest that a carefully selected subset of patients can experience prolonged survival with an aggressive approach.

In comparison, the group at Memorial Sloan-Kettering has treated patients with P/D and intraoperative brachytherapy followed by external-beam radiation (105). Brachytherapy was delivered with (125) I seeds or (192) Ir implants to areas with gross residual disease, and external beam radiation was administered to the ipsilateral hemithorax to a total dose of 4500 cGy. One hundred and five patients were treated between 1976 and 1988, with a median survival of 12.5 months and 1- and 2-year overall survival rates of 52% and 23%, respectively. However, the 27 patients with pure epithelial history and minimal residual disease experienced a median survival of 15 months and 1- and 2-year survival rates of 68% and 35%, respectively. Local recurrence was noted to be the predominant site of treatment failure in this trial (64/105 patients), supporting the notion that P/D may be inferior to EPP as a local extirpative procedure. In addition, while the survival data suggest a modest improvement over supportive care, comparison of survival in the groups of patients with good prognosis treated on this protocol versus our trimodality approach does suggest a benefit for the latter group. However, a true randomized comparison is lacking, and patient selection and other factors remain possible explanations for the differences.

Adjuvant chemotherapy has also been tested. Patients at Memorial Sloan-Kettering (123) and the Cleveland Clinic (124) were treated with both intrapleural and systemic cisplatin and mitomycin C following radical surgery (P/D at Memorial and either P/D or EPP at the Cleveland Clinic). Systemic chemotherapy was poorly tolerated in both cases, and local recurrence was again the most common site of relapse. The survival data were insufficiently impressive (median survival of 17 and 13 months, respectively) to warrant pursuit of this combination (105). Adjuvant cisplatin, interferon-α, and tamoxifen (CIT) did not result in much better survival (median survival only 12 months) (125), but direct comparisons are difficult because of the more advanced-stage patient population in this study.

In summary, these heterogeneous data suggest avenues for further research. EPP seems to offer better local control than P/D, but surgery at an institution with considerable experience in these complicated and morbid procedures is required for optimal results. Aggressive adjuvant therapy with radiation and chemotherapy may be necessary to address both local and distant sites of occult disease, but the shift of predominant disease recurrence to distant sites noted in our experience with trimodality therapy suggests that much work is needed in identifying improved systemic treatments. However, all of these concepts await rigorous testing in a randomized setting.

Novel Therapeutic Approaches
Hyperthermia
One approach that we and others are testing to address local disease in MPM is hyperthermic chemotherapy. Hyperthermia by itself is capable of inducing cell death

through a variety of mechanisms (including apoptosis, rapid cell necrosis without cell cycle progression, and a third mechanism which is cell cycle-dependent (126). Intracavitary chemotherapy also demonstrates promise as an adjuvant modality. For example, a French group treated 54 patients with abdominal carcinomatosis from various primary sites with intraperitoneal chemotherapy (either mitomycin C + 5-fluorouracil or doxorubicin + platinum) following complete resection of gross disease and reported only a 30% recurrence rate at 2 years. On the down side, these outcomes were associated with a high morbidity rate (65%), including a 35% incidence of intra-abdominal complications (requiring surgery in 13%) (127).

One might reasonably expect the combination of hyperthermia and chemotherapy to have additive tumoricidal effects, and this has been verified in preclinical studies (128,129). Animal studies also suggest that hyperthermic chemotherapy may enhance the therapeutic ratio of subsequent fractionated radiation therapy (130). As a cautionary note, the interaction of hyperthermia with drugs may be complex and unpredictable, and on occasion, hyperthermia may even interact antagonistically with some drugs (*e.g.*, cytosine arabinoside and amsacrine) (126). However, hyperthermia seems to interact supra-additively with cisplatin and mitomycin C. These combinations have formed the basis for several trials of intracavitary hyperthermic chemotherapy, including an on-going trial at Brigham and Women's Hospital using intraoperative heated cisplatin applied intrapleurally for MPM. Doxorubicin has also been used intraperitoneally (131) although its interaction with hyperthermia is more problematic (126).

The published experience with intrapleural hyperthermic chemotherapy is extremely limited. For example, Matsuzaki *et al.* (132) treated lung cancer patients with malignant pleural implants (12 patients) or effusions (7 patients) for 2 hours with cisplatin heated to 43°C. All 7 cases involving pleural effusions were adequately controlled without thoracotomy, and the 12 patients with disseminated pleural implants experienced a 20-month median survival, in contrast with a 7-month median survival in 7 matched case controls. However, the usual caveats about small, non-randomized trials apply here.
On the other hand, the experience with intraperitoneal hyperthermic chemotherapy is much more extensive, particularly in Japan. Ma *et al.* (133) treated 10 patients (9 with malignant peritoneal mesothelioma and 1 with recurrent benign peritoneal mesothelioma) with continuous hyperthermic peritoneal perfusion (CHPP) with cisplatin following optimal debulking. Seven patients with symptomatic ascites were completely palliated, and 8 of the 10 patients remained disease-free after a median follow-up of 10 months. One randomized trial of adjuvant CHPP has been conducted. Eighty-two patients with gastric carcinoma invading the serosa but without gross peritoneal metastases were randomized to receive CHPP with mitomycin C. A trend towards improved 5-year overall survival rate and decreased specific mortality from peritoneal recurrence was noted for patients receiving CHPP (64.2% compared with 52.5% for those not receiving CHPP) (134). Fujimoto and colleagues (135) have also reported significantly improved survival in gastric cancer patients with peritoneal carcinomatosis following CHPP with mitomycin C, although, as might be expected, this benefit was

limited to patients with decreased tumor burden ("countable metastases"). Patients were not randomized between the experimental and control groups.

Complications of intraperitoneal thermochemotherapy (136) include scald injuries, anastomotic leaks, perforations, pancreatitis, and even thoracic complications (137) such as atelectasis, pleural effusions, pulmonary edema, and pneumothoraces. The risk of intra-abdominal complications may be correlated with the number of previous surgical procedures and high intraperitoneal temperatures (136).

Photodynamic Therapy
Photodynamic therapy (PDT) would seem to be an ideal treatment modality for a diffuse, superficial tumor such as MPM. A photosensitizer (typically a porphyrin derivative) is administered systemically, preferentially retained by neoplastic tissues, and subsequently activated to an excited state *in situ* by light of appropriate wavelength. The activated photosensitizer can then react either with the substrate or solvent (a type I reaction) or directly with oxygen (a type II reaction). The former involves hydrogen atom or electron transfer and yields radicals or radical ions that act as oxidizing agents whereas the latter, via direct energy transfer, produces singlet oxygen, which is the suspected ultimate cytotoxic agent.

Initial feasibility studies in animals were complicated by dose-limiting parenchymal damage to internal organs (138,139), but more modest light doses following debulking surgery proved tolerable in a preliminary human feasibility study (140). Other than expected systemic photosensitivity and risks associated with any invasive procedure, the major complication reported to date has been fistula formation (141,142). To date, only a handful of anecdotal "trials" of PDT for MPM have been reported (143), none of which allow any conclusions to be drawn regarding the efficacy of PDT.

Many fundamental questions still remain, including selection of the optimal photosensitizer, the role of carrier systems for photosensitizers, the maximally tolerated doses of light and photosensitizer, the optimal treatment schedule, the optimal setting in which to use PDT (*e.g.*, after pleurectomy vs. extrapleural pneumonectomy), and the effects of PDT on survival, both overall and disease-free. A recent NCI-sponsored phase III trial randomized 48 patients to intra-operative PDT or not in conjunction with optimal surgical debulking (residual disease of <5-mm thickness) and post-operative CIT (cisplatin/interferon-α/tamoxifen) chemotherapy (142). The study suggested an absence of survival benefit (median survival was approximately 14 months for each treatment arm) or even local control with the first-generation photosensitizer Photofrin II, but 40 of the 48 patients had advanced (stage III or IV) disease. A non-randomized trial conducted at Roswell Park Cancer Institute treated similarly debulked patients with intracavitary PDT using Photofrin, but had a slightly higher percentage of early-stage (stage I or II) disease (13/40 patients) (144). Overall median survival was only 15 months, but those patients with stage I/II disease had a median survival of 36 months and an estimated 2-year survival rate of 61%. *A priori*, PDT is most likely to benefit patients with early-stage, optimally resected disease, and subsequent improvements in technology require that further trials be performed before this approach is abandoned.

Cytokines

The presence of tumor-infiltrating lymphocytes in animal models of mesothelioma strongly suggests that an anti-tumor response can be mounted against mesothelioma; however, mesothelioma cells themselves may sometimes produce factors that antagonize such responses (145). For example, transforming growth factor-beta (TGF-β), which has anti-proliferative effects on multiple hematologic cell types (*e.g.*, B and T cells, NK cells, phagocytes, and lymphokine-activated killer cells) (146), is secreted by mesotheliomas (147,148). Other cytokines and growth factors such as interleukin-6 (IL-6) (149,150), insulin-like growth factor-1 (IGF-1) and platelet-derived growth factors A and B (PDGF-A/B) (151) are also produced by mesothelioma cells, and some of these factors (particularly IL-6) may mediate signs and constitutional symptoms described in MPM such as thrombocytosis (53).

In an effort to boost the endogenous anti-tumor response, many groups have tested immunomodulatory cytokines as treatments for MPM. The interferons, for example, demonstrate several potential anti-tumor effects, only some of which are immunologically mediated. Direct anti-proliferative effects of interferons include induction of differentiation, prolongation of the cell cycle, and modulation of oncogene expression, while indirect effects include the up-regulation of immune effector cells (*e.g.*, natural killer cells, macrophages, and both cytotoxic and helper subsets of T lymphocytes) (152).

Using mesothelioma xenografts in nude mice, Ohnuma *et al.* (153) reported that IFN-α, in contrast to TNF-α, exhibited strong anti-proliferative effects against all three cell lines tested. However, an Australian group reported "suboptimal" results with IFN-α using a different murine model (154). In clinical trials, results with single-agent IFN-α have been generally disappointing. For example, combining the results reported by Ardizzoni *et al.*(155) and Christmas *et al.* (156), only 4 responses were seen in 38 evaluable patients (response rate 11%).

Interferon-beta (IFN-β) has warranted little excitement in either pre-clinical or clinical studies though these are few in number. For example, the Southwest Oncology Group (SWOG) has treated 14 patients with refractory MPM and noted no responses (157). Though IFN-β may have some utility in the palliation of malignant pleural effusions (158), reasons to recommend it over more conventional agents are lacking.

Of the three subtypes of interferons, interferon-gamma (IFN-γ) has shown perhaps the greatest promise in MPM. *In vitro* testing of 32 mesothelioma cell lines found eleven (34%) to be sensitive to IFN-γ (159). Boutin and his colleagues have reported an overall response rate of 19% in a cohort of 89 patients treated intrapleurally with IFN-γ (118), but several points need to be considered. First, the exclusion of previously treated patients and patients with later-stage disease (only patients with Butchart stage I and II disease were eligible) would favor an improved response rate. However, the prospective and multi-institutional design of this trial strengthens its findings. Second, a strong correlation between stage and response rate was noted. Eleven of the 13 responses were seen in patients with stage I disease (response rate 45%), and in patients with disease confined to the parietal or diaphragmatic pleura (stage IA), 5 CRs and 3 PRs (response rate 61%) were seen. These data suggest that IFN-γ may be optimally administered in the adjuvant setting. Third, the demonstration of 8 thoracoscopically confirmed CRs is, in and of itself, quite noteworthy. The significance of these points is underscored by a comparison with Hasturk *et al.* (160) in which IFN-α was administered in combination with cisplatin and mitomycin C to pleurectomized (and presumably debulked) patients. In this setting, none of 20 patients exhibited even a partial response.

The interferons have also been tested in combination with conventional chemotherapeutic agents. Pre-clinical tests with mesothelioma cell lines have yielded mixed results, with IFN-α and IFN-γ demonstrating increased cytotoxicity in tissue culture when combined with methotrexate (161) but not with etoposide, cisplatin, mitoxantrone, 4-epirubicin, and vindesine (162). However, using xenografts in nude mice, Sklarin *et al.* (163) demonstrated significantly improved responses against specific cell lines without apparent additional toxicity after adding IFN-α to either cisplatin or mitomycin C. In clinical trials, IFN-α has been the most extensively tested of the interferons, but as seen in Table 6, it has generally provided little in the way of improved response rates. The sole exception is the study by Soulie *et al.*, which reports a 35% response rate (all PRs) in previously untreated patients with MPM (164). Noteworthy in this study are the dependence of response rates on histologic subtype (6/12 responses in epithelial-type tumors but only 2/11 responses in biphasic or sarcomatous tumors) and the toxicity of the weekly regimen. In fact, the latter was of sufficient magnitude to warrant a modification of the original treatment plan from 5 weeks on/3 weeks off to 4 weeks on/4 weeks off.

Interleukin-2 (IL-2) has attracted considerable attention for its ability to stimulate immune effector cells, including T cells and NK cells. In fact, IL-2-stimulated NK cells are responsible for the lymphokine-activated killer (LAK) cell activity which has been harnessed to treat autologous tumors in individual patients. The importance of IL-2 in the host response against mesothelioma has been suggested by *in vitro* studies which demonstrate cytotoxicity against six otherwise NK cell-insensitive patient-derived cell lines upon the addition of IL-2 (165). Two of the larger studies have administered single-agent IL-2 into the intrapleural space (166,167) yielding very high intracavitary concentrations of IL-2 while minimizing systemic levels and hence toxicity. These phase I trials have yielded a combined response rate of 37% with the dose-limiting side effects being fluid retention and flu-like symptoms. An interesting observation made by Astoul *et al.* (168) in a series of 9 patients with MPM or adenocarcinoma was that the extent of pleural invasion may affect the concentration and duration of intrapleural IL-2 levels. Two patients in this small series had undetectable intrapleural IL-2 levels and exhibited no response to continuously administered IL-2, whereas 4 of the remaining 7 patients did.

One of the few randomized studies evaluating the role of cytokines in the treatment of MPM was conducted by Lissoni *et al.*, who randomized 70 patients with malignant effusions (pleural, pericardial, or peritoneal) arising from MPM and other tumors to receive intracavitary IFN-α, IFN-β, or IL-2 (169). In the subset of patients with MPM treated with IL-2 compared with either subtype of interferon, both a superior response rate and a prolonged period during which fluid drainage was avoided were noted.

Gene therapy
A detailed discussion of the science and technology behind gene therapy is beyond the scope of this paper. The reader is referred to several recent reviews (170,171). In brief, the goal of gene therapy is to introduce into target cells (*e.g.*, hematopoietic stem cells or tumor cells) DNA sequences coding for new proteins that can alter the biologic phenotype of the target cells for intended therapeutic benefit. The means by which DNA can be introduced into target cells is highly variable and may involve physical methods (*e.g.*, liposomal delivery, DNA precipitates with calcium phosphate, electroporation, ballistic techniques, and direct microinjection) or viral vectors. In addition, treatment of the target cells may occur within (*in vivo*) or outside (*ex vivo*) the human body. *Ex vivo* treatment offers a number of advantages such as greater efficiency and selectivity, the ability to use techniques generally not feasible *in vivo* (*e.g.*, electroporation and microinjection), the ability to select for cells expressing the gene of interest, and the ability to expand the target cell population prior to re-introduction into the body. However, in cases such as cancer therapy, *in vivo* treatment is often required because of the need to target spatially dispersed cells.

Selection of the gene(s) to be introduced into target cells is obviously of critical importance. While cancer cells are well-documented to have loss-of-function mutations and deletions, the strategy of replacing such lost functions with exogenous DNA is quite difficult to carry out for several reasons. First, such a strategy requires that the DNA be taken up by the vast majority (if not all) of the tumor cells, a degree of efficiency that is currently unattainable. Second, tumors often accumulate multiple genetic abnormalities, making single-gene replacement less efficacious. Third, both qualitative (*e.g.*, cell-type specificity) and quantitative control of gene expression remain central problems because ectopic expression and overexpression could cause undesirable side effects and underexpression leaves the tumor effectively untreated. For these reasons, many researchers have taken the alternative strategy of introducing "suicide" genes or immune-enhancing genes into tumor cells. Unfortunately, this approach addresses only the second point adequately although a "bystander" effect has been described following the expression of "suicide" (172) or cytokine (173) genes in target cell populations.
In studies directed at mesothelioma, the favorite strategy has employed adenoviral vectors expressing "suicide" or cytokine genes. Adenoviruses are preferred for several reasons: (1) their general efficiency of infection, (2) their ability to infect non-dividing cells, (3) the relative ease with which large quantities of virus at high titers can be produced, and (4) the decreased risk of insertional mutagenesis because of the episomal propagation of adenovirus (171). Furthermore, based upon the multiplicity of infection, adenoviral vectors appear to infect mesothelioma and squamous cell lung cancer cell

more effectively than adenocarcinoma cells, presumably on the basis of the cells' relative binding affinities for the adenoviral fiber knob (174). The herpes simplex virus (HSV) thymidine kinase (tk) gene is a commonly used effector gene because it renders cells expressing the protein susceptible to drugs such as acyclovir and ganciclovir. (These drugs are inactive prodrugs and require intracellular phosphorylation to the monophosphate form for activation, a process that cannot normally take place in human cells. The specificity of the HSV-tk protein for such drugs makes them such specific and relatively non-toxic anti-herpetic agents.) Other genes have been studied, and these include p16 (175), p53, (176) and IL-2 (177).

In pre-clinical studies, rodent models, both immunosuppressed and immunocompetent, have been used primarily. Although one might consider the host anti-tumor immune response to be of critical importance, data suggest that the efficacy of gene therapy is enhanced by immunosuppression (178) This enhancement may be a consequence of adverse effects of host immune responses on transgene persistence (179). Fortunately, considerable *in vitro* (179,180) and *in vivo* (181) evidence exists for a bystander effect whereby non-infected cells may be killed; this effect may be mediated by the transfer of toxic metabolites from infected to non-infected cells through gap junctions (172). In fact, studies have suggested that a 10% infection rate may be sufficient to achieve optimal tumor cytotoxicity (180,182). However, a report by Schwarzenberger and colleagues using mesothelioma cells expressing the HSV-tk gene (PA-1-STK cells) casts some doubt on these optimistic figures (183). In this study, PA-1-STK cells were introduced into the peritoneal cavities of mice bearing mesotheliomas. While animal survival was enhanced when PA-1-STK cells comprised 70% of tumor cells, no such survival was noted when this percentage was decreased to 30%. More recently, adenovirus-mediated transfection of $p14^{ARF}$ into mesothelioma cells led to the overexpression of $p14^{ARF}$ resulting in G1-arrest and apoptotic cell death (184).

Another promising development in pre-clinical studies has been the detection of adenoviral infection deep within bulky tumor masses and of corresponding responses in animals with bulky disease (184,185). This is in contradistinction to all of the previously mentioned intracavitary modalities (e.g., intracavitary colloidal radioisotopes, intrapleural chemotherapy, PDT, and hyperthermia), which are severely limited by their inability to treat bulky disease.

Unfortunately, clinical gene therapy trials for MPM are few in number, and conclusive data on efficacy are lacking. Robinson *et al.* have injected an IL-2-expressing vaccinia vector directly into the tumors of 6 patients at a tri-weekly intervals, but failed to detect any objective response (177). Kaiser and his colleagues at the University of Pennsylvania recently issued an interim report on a phase I dose-escalation study in which they introduced replication-incompetent adenoviral vectors carrying an HSV-tk gene into the pleural cavities of 21 previously untreated patients with MPM (186,187). Doses of virus ranging from 10^9 to 10^{12} pfu (plaque-forming units) were administered on day 2 via chest tube, followed by intravenous ganciclovir at 10 mg/kg/d in divided doses on days 6 to 20. Thoracoscopic pleural biopsies performed on days 1 and 5 revealed strong intrapleural and intratumoral immune responses, and viral HSV-tk gene expression was detected in 12/20 patients in a dose-dependent fashion. No dose-limiting toxicities were noted although patients invariably developed a transient fever on day 2 (following administration of the virus), and transient LFT abnormalities were noted in 2 patients. No objective responses have yet been observed, and at last report, 12 of 21 patients had died of progressive disease (median follow-up of 12 months) (171,187).

Chemoprevention?

A handful of trials have been conducted to identify possible prophylactic agents against asbestos-induced cancers, but results have been generally disappointing. A non-randomized Australian trial comparing 1203 occupationally exposed workers receiving β-carotene or retinol with 996 controls who chose not to enroll in the study reported a decrease in the risk of MPM and lung cancer in treated patients, a disparity which increased with time (188). However, the relative risk for overall mortality for the treated group was noted to increase with time and, in fact, slightly exceeded 1.0 for those patients enrolled the longest (approaching 5 years). Unfortunately, imbalances between the groups consisting of additional medical interventions (assistance with smoking cessation and diet) and a longer average duration of asbestos exposure for the treatment group make interpretation of these data difficult. Within the intervention group, eligible patients were randomized to receive β-carotene or retinol, and analysis of these adequately matched subsets revealed a lower relative risk of MPM (RR=0.24) and "all other deaths" (RR=0.46) in the retinol group although lung cancer risk was unchanged (189).

In a major randomized multi-institutional study, the CARET (β-Carotene and Retinal Efficacy Trial) trial tested the combination of β-carotene and retinyl palmitate in reducing the risk of lung cancer in a high-risk population of smokers and asbestos-exposed workers (190). Paradoxically, however, the incidence of lung cancer was increased in the intervention group, leading to premature termination of the study (191). Later analysis revealed an increased incidence of mesothelioma and ischemic heart disease, as well as increased all-cause mortality, in the intervention group (190).

These and other studies are quite thought-provoking and suggest several avenues for further research. The first study raises the possibility that retinol may play a role in preventing mesothelioma. More intriguing are the consistently detrimental effects demonstrated by β-carotene (consider also the large Finnish Alpha-Tocopherol, Beta-Carotene Cancer Prevention trial, which reported increased overall and lung cancer mortality in people randomized to receive β-carotene (192). Frequent mention has been made of the fact that synthetic β-carotene, which consists entirely of the *trans* isomer, was used in each of these trials, whereas dietary β-carotene is a mixture of *cis* and *trans* isomers. Finally, given the long latency periods required for clinical tumor development, it is notable that any differences at all in cancer incidence are discernible within the relatively short follow-up times of these trials. This suggests a role for retinoids in later stages of tumorigenesis and may provide clues for further basic research.

SUMMARY

Malignant pleural mesothelioma remains a difficult tumor to treat, much less cure. Currently, the best chance for long-term survival lies with early diagnosis and aggressive surgical extirpation, but given the typically long delay between the onset of symptoms and diagnosis, this is only possible with a high index of suspicion and an aggressive diagnostic workup. Early referral to a tertiary center experienced in the treatment of MPM may be important for several reasons: (1) decreased risk of tumor spread along multiple thoracentesis/biopsy tracts, (2) the availability of specialized pathologic assays for definitive diagnosis, (3) the availability of critical staging modalities (aggressive mediastinoscopy $\pm$ thoracoscopy, MRI scans performed according to specific mesothelioma protocols, and perhaps PET scans), (4) surgical experience with pleurectomy/decortication and/or extrapleural pneumonectomy, that may decrease morbidity and mortality, and (5) the availability of novel adjuvant protocols.

Single-modality therapy is unlikely to result in long-term survival. Aggressive surgery is required for optimal debulking, and extrapleural pneumonectomy may offer better local control compared with pleurectomy/decortication. Delivery of optimal radiation schedules, which may involve large fractions as well as large total doses, is limited by the presence of nearby dose-limiting structures. Current chemotherapy is severely lacking in producing objective responses and improved survival although gemcitabine and IL-2 may be active agents to be combined with radiation and/or other agents. Hyperthermia, photodynamic therapy, intracavitary therapy, and gene therapy are all relatively new techniques under active investigation that should be supported by enrollment in on-going protocols. Predictably, many of these techniques provide greater benefit when used in the setting of adjuvant protocols or minimal residual disease, emphasizing the importance of multimodality therapy.

Table 5. Results of single-agent chemotherapy trials with >15 evaluable patients.

Agent	No. of studies	No. of patients	Overall RR, %	Reference(s)
Anti-metabolites				
DHAC	1	41	17	[193]
Dideazafolic acid (CB3717)	1	18	6	[194]
Edatrexate	1	37	22	[195]
5-Fluorouracil	1	20	5	[196]
Methotrexate	1	60	37	[197]
Trimetrexate	1	51	12	[198]
Platinum compounds				
Carboplatin	3	88	11	[199] [200] [201]
Cisplatin	2	59	14	[202] [203]
Anthracyclines/ DNA intercalators				
Amsacrine	1	19	5	[204]
Detorubicin	1	35	26	[205]
Diaziquone	1	20	0	[206]
Doxorubicin	2	66	11	[207] [111]
Epirubicin	2	69	12	[208] [209]
Menogaril	1	22	5	[210]
Mitoxantrone	2	62	5	[211] [212]
Pirarubicin	2	50	16	[213] [214]
Alkylating agents				
Cyclophosphamide	1	16	0	[111]
Ifosfamide	4	104	12	[215] [216] [217] [218] [219]
Mitomycin C	1	19	21	[220]
PCNU	1	34	0	
Miscellaneous cytotoxic agents				
Docetaxel	1	19	5	[221]
Etoposide	1	23	4	[222]
Gemcitabine	1	16	31	[110]
Paclitaxel	1	35	9	[223]
Topotecan	1	22	0	[224]
Vinblastine	1	20	0	[225]
Vincristine	1	23	0	[226]
Vindesine	2	38	3	[227] [228]
Vinorelbine	1	19	21	[229]
Cytokines and miscellaneous biological response modifiers				
BCG	1	30	0	[230]
Interferon-α-2a	1	25	12	[156]
Interferon-γ	1	89	19	[118]
Interleukin-2	2	43	37	[167] [166]
P30 protein	1	15	13	[231]

RR = response rate; DHAC = dihydro-5-azacytidine. Adapted from Ryan et al. (1998)[109].

Table 6. Results of combination chemotherapy trials with ≥15 patients.

Combination	No. of studies	No. of patients	Overall RR, %	Reference(s)
Doxorubicin-based:				
+ 5-azacytidine	1	36	22	232
+ CDDP	2	59	19	233 112
+ CDDP, + CTX	1	23	26	234
+ CDDP, + MMC	1	23	21	235
+ CDDP, + MMC, + bleomycin	1	25	44	236
+ CTX	1	52	12	237 98
+ CTX, + DTIC	2	60	17	238 237
+ IFF	2	38	24	239 240
+ Interferon-α	1	25	16	241
Cisplatin-based:				
+ DHAC	1	29	17	242
+ Etoposide	2	51	18	243 244
+ IFN-α	1	23	35	164
+ IFN-α, + tamoxifen	2	61	16	245 125
+ IFN-α, + MMC	3	60	10	246 247 160
+ MMC	1	35	26	112
+ MMC, + vinblastine	1	39	21	114
+ Pirarubicin	1	38	13	248
+ Vinblastine	1	20	25	249
Other agents				
Carboplatin + IFN-α	1			250
CDDP + gemcitabine	1	21	48	115
Epirubicin + IFF	1	17	6	251
Epirubicin + IL-2	1	21	5	252
Mitoxantrone + MTX + MMC	1	20	30	253
Raltitrexed + oxaliplatin	1	22	23	254
Rubidazone + DTIC	1	23	0	255

RR = response rate; CTX = cyclophosphamide; IFF = ifosfamide; CDDP = cisplatin; MMC = mitomycin C; MTX = methotrexate.

Table 7. Results of trials of intrapleural chemotherapy with $\geq$15 patients.

Agent(s)	No. of trials	No. of patients	Response rate, %	Reference(s)
CDDP + araC	1	37	49	256
Interferon-γ	1	89	20	118
Interleukin-2	2	36	31	257 166
L-NDDP	1	15	73	119

CDDP = cisplatin; ara
C = cytosine arabinoside.

REFERENCES

1. Plas E, Riedl CR, Pflüger H. Malignant mesothelioma of the tunica vaginalis testis: review of the literature and assessment of prognostic parameters. Cancer 83:2437-46, 1998.

2. Benard F, Sterman D, Smith RJ, et al. Metabolic imaging of malignant pleural mesothelioma with fluorodeoxyglucose positron emission tomography [see comments]. Chest 114:713-22, 1998.

3. Klemperer P, Rabin CB. Primary neoplasms of the pleura: a report of five cases. Arch. Pathol. 11:385-412, 1931.

4. Nicholson W, Perkel G, Selikoff I. Occupational exposure to asbestos: population at risk and projected mortality: 1980-2030. Am. J. Ind. Med. 3:259-311, 1982.

5. Peto J, Decarli A, La Vecchia C, et al. The European mesothelioma epidemic. Br J Cancer 79:666-72, 1999.

6. Iwatsubo Y, Pairon JC, Boutin C, et al. Pleural mesothelioma: dose-response relation at low levels of asbestos exposure in a French population-based case-control study [see comments]. Am J Epidemiol 148:133-42, 1998.

7. Mossman BT, Kamp DW, Weitzman SA. Mechanisms of carcinogenesis and clinical features of asbestos-associated cancers. Cancer Invest. 14:466-480, 1996.

8. Camus M, Siemiatycki J, Meek B. Nonoccupational exposure to chrysotile asbestos and the risk of lung cancer [see comments]. N Engl J Med 338:1565-71, 1998.

9. Rovia GC, Sartori F, Calabro F, et al. The association of pleural mesothelioma and tuberculosis. Am. Rev. Respir. Dis. 126:569-571, 1982.

10. Mossman BT, Gee JB. Asbestos-related diseases. N. Engl. J. Med. 320:1721-1730, 1989.

11. Bianchi C, Giarelli L, Grandi G, et al. Latency periods in asbestos-related mesothelioma of the pleura. Eur J Cancer Prev 6:162-6, 1997.

12. Smith TR. Malignant peritoneal mesothelioma: marked variability of CT findings. Abdom Imaging 19:27-9, 1994.

13. Grant DC, Seltzer SE, Antman KH, et al. Computed tomography of malignant pleural mesothelioma. J Comput Assist Tomogr 7:626-32, 1983.

14. Antman KH, Pass HI, Schiff PB. Benign and malignant mesothelioma, in DeVita VT, Hellman S, Rosenberg SA (eds): Cancer: principles and practice of oncology (ed 5th). Philadelphia, Lippincott-Raven, 1997, pp 1853-1878.

15. Weissmann LB, Corson JM, Neugut AI, et al. Malignant mesothelioma following treatment for Hodgkin's disease. J Clin Oncol 14:2098-100, 1996.

16. Mizuki M, Yukishige K, Abe Y, et al. A case of malignant pleural mesothelioma following exposure to atomic radiation in Nagasaki. Respirology 2:201-5, 1997.

17. Neugut AI, Ahsan H, Antman KH. Incidence of malignant pleural mesothelioma after thoracic radiotherapy. Cancer 80:948-50, 1997.

18. Strickler HD, Rosenberg PS, Devesa SS, et al.   Contamination of poliovirus vaccines with simian virus 40 (1955-1963) and subsequent cancer rates [see comments]. Jama 279:292-5, 1998.

19. Olin P, Giesecke J. Potential exposure to SV40 in polio vaccines used in Sweden during 1957: no impact on cancer incidence rates 1960 to 1993. Dev Biol Stand 94:227-33, 1998.

20. Galateau-Salle F, Bidet P, Iwatsubo Y, et al. SV40-like DNA sequences in pleural mesothelioma, bronchopulmonary carcinoma, and non-malignant pulmonary diseases. J Pathol 184:252-7, 1998.

21. Strickler HD, Goedert JJ, Fleming M, et al. Simian virus 40 and pleural mesothelioma in humans. Cancer Epidemiol Biomarkers Prev 5:473-5, 1996.

22. Procopio A, Marinacci R, Marinetti MR, et al.   SV40 expression in human neoplastic and non-neoplastic tissues: perspectives on diagnosis, prognosis and therapy of human malignant mesothelioma. Dev Biol Stand 94:361-7, 1998.

23. Carbone M, Pass HI, Rizzo P, et al.   Simian virus 40-like DNA sequences in human pleural mesothelioma. Oncogene 9:1781-90, 1994.

24. Pepper C, Jasani B, Navabi H, et al: Simian virus 40 large T antigen (SV40LTAg) primer specific DNA amplification in human pleural mesothelioma tissue. Thorax 51:1074-6, 1996.

25. Gibbs AR, Jasani B, Pepper C, et al.   SV40 DNA sequences in mesotheliomas. Dev Biol Stand 94:41-5, 1998.

26. Griffiths DJ, Nicholson AG, Weiss RA. Detection of SV40 sequences in human mesothelioma. Dev Biol Stand 94:127-36, 1998.

27. Testa JR, Carbone M, Hirvonen A, et al. A multi-institutional study confirms the presence and expression of simian virus 40 in human malignant mesotheliomas. Cancer Res 58:4505-9, 1998.

28. Carbone M, Stach R, Di Resta I, et al. Simian virus 40 oncogenesis in hamsters. Dev Biol Stand 94:273-9, 1998.

29. Boutin C, Rey F, Viallat JR. Prevention of malignant seeding after invasive diagnostic procedures in patients with pleural mesothelioma. A randomized trial of local radiotherapy [see comments]. Chest 108:754-8, 1995.

30. Aisner J. Current approach to malignant mesothelioma of the pleura. Chest 107:332S-344S, 1995.

31. Steel TR, Allibone J, Revesz T, et al. Intradural neurotropic spread of malignant mesothelioma. Case report and review of the literature. J Neurosurg 88:122-5, 1998.

32. Prieto VG, Kenet BJ, Varghese M. Malignant mesothelioma metastatic to the skin, presenting as inflammatory carcinoma. Am J Dermatopathol 19:261-5, 1997.

33. Grellner W, Staak M: Multiple skeletal muscle metastases from malignant pleural mesothelioma. Pathol Res Pract 191:456-60; discussion 461-2, 1995.

34. Kubota K, Furuse K, Kawahara M, et al. A case of malignant pleural mesothelioma with metastasis to the orbit. Jpn J Clin Oncol 26:469-71, 1996.

35. Henderson DW, Shilkin KB, Whitaker D. Reactive mesothelial hyperplasia vs mesothelioma, including mesothelioma in situ: a brief review. Am J Clin Pathol 110:397-404, 1998.

36. Boutin C, Loddenkemper R, Astoul P. Diagnostic and therapeutic thoracoscopy: techniques and indications in pulmonary medicine. Tuber. Lung Dis. 74:225-239, 1993.

37. Metintas M, Ozdemir N, Isiksoy S, et al. CT-guided pleural needle biopsy in the diagnosis of malignant mesothelioma. J Comput Assist Tomogr 19:370-4, 1995.

38. Boutin C, Rey F. Thoracoscopy in pleural malignant mesothelioma: a prospective study of 188 consecutive patients. Part 1: Diagnosis. Cancer 72:389-93, 1993.

39. Kaiser L, Bavaria J. Complications of thoracoscopy. Ann. Thorac. Surg. 56:431-451, 1993.

40. Loddenkemper R. Thoracoscopy--state of the art. Eur Respir J 11:213-21, 1998.

41. Wilsher ML, Veale AG. Medical thoracoscopy in the diagnosis of unexplained pleural effusion. Respirology 3:77-80, 1998.

42. Maasilta P, Vehmas T, Kivisaari L, et al. Correlations between findings at computed tomography (CT) and at thoracoscopy/thoracotomy/autopsy in pleural mesothelioma. Eur Respir J 4:952-4, 1991.

43. Leung AN, Muller NL, Miller RR. CT in differential diagnosis of diffuse pleural disease. AJR Am J Roentgenol 154:487-92, 1990.

44. Rusch VW, Godwin JD, Shuman WP. The role of computed tomography scanning in the initial assessment and the follow-up of malignant pleural mesothelioma. J Thorac Cardiovasc Surg 96:171-7, 1988.

45. McLoud TC. CT and MR in pleural disease. Clin Chest Med 19:261-76, 1998.

46. Falaschi F, Battolla L, Mascalchi M, et al. Usefulness of MR signal intensity in distinguishing benign from malignant pleural disease. AJR Am. J. Roentgenol. 166:963-968, 1996.

47. Sugarbaker DJ, Strauss GM, Lynch TJ, et al. Node status has prognostic significance in the multimodality therapy of diffuse, malignant mesothelioma. J Clin Oncol 11:1172-8, 1993.

48. Sugarbaker DJ, Flores RM, Jaklitsch MT, et al. Resection margins, extrapleural nodal status, and cell type determine postoperative long-term survival in trimodality therapy of malignant pleural mesothelioma: results in 183 patients. J Thorac Cardiovasc Surg 117:54-63; discussion 63-5, 1999.

49. Rusch VW, Venkatraman E. The importance of surgical staging in the treatment of malignant pleural mesothelioma. J Thorac Cardiovasc Surg 111:815-25; discussion 825-6, 1996.

50. Sugarbaker DJ, Jaklitsch MT, Liptay MJ. Mesothelioma and radical multimodality therapy: who benefits? Chest 107:345S-350S, 1995.

51. Hillerdahl G. Malignant mesothelioma 1982: review of 4710 published cases. Br. J. Dis. Chest 77:321-343, 1983.

52. Corson JM. Pathology of diffuse malignant pleural mesothelioma. Semin Thorac Cardiovasc Surg 9:347-55, 1997.

53. Nakano T, Chahinian AP, Shinjo M, et al. Interleukin 6 and its relationship to clinical parameters in patients with malignant pleural mesothelioma. Br J Cancer 77:907-12, 1998.

54. King JA, Tucker JA. Evaluation of membranous staining of mesothelioma. Cell Vis 5:24-7, 1998.

55. Wolanski KD, Whitaker D, Shilkin KB, et al. The use of epithelial membrane antigen and silver-stained nucleolar organizer regions testing in the differential diagnosis of mesothelioma from benign reactive mesothelioses. Cancer 82:583-90, 1998.

56. Clover J, Oates J, Edwards C. Anti-cytokeratin 5/6: a positive marker for epithelioid mesothelioma. Histopathology 31:140-3, 1997.

57. Ordóñez NG. Value of cytokeratin 5/6 immunostaining in distinguishing epithelial mesothelioma of the pleura from lung adenocarcinoma. Am J Surg Pathol 22:1215-21, 1998.

58. Nagel H, Hemmerlein B, Ruschenburg I, et al. The value of anti-calretinin antibody in the differential diagnosis of normal and reactive mesothelia versus metastatic tumors in effusion cytology. Pathol Res Pract 194:759-64, 1998.

59. Ordóñez NG. Value of calretinin immunostaining in differentiating epithelial mesothelioma from lung adenocarcinoma. Mod Pathol 11:929-33, 1998.

60. Leers MP, Aarts MM, Theunissen PH. E-cadherin and calretinin: a useful combination of immunochemical markers for differentiation between mesothelioma and metastatic adenocarcinoma. Histopathology 32:209-16, 1998.

61. Di Loreto C, Puglisi F, Di Lauro V, et al. TTF-1 protein expression in pleural malignant mesotheliomas and adenocarcinomas of the lung. Cancer Lett 124:73-8, 1998.

62. Fetsch PA, Abati A, Hijazi YM. Utility of the antibodies CA 19-9, HBME-1, and thrombomodulin in the diagnosis of malignant mesothelioma and adenocarcinoma in cytology. Cancer 84:101-8, 1998.

63. Ordóñez NG. Value of the MOC-31 monoclonal antibody in differentiating epithelial pleural mesothelioma from lung adenocarcinoma. Hum Pathol 29:166-9, 1998.

64. Ordonez NG. Value of the Ber-EP4 antibody in differentiating epithelial pleural mesothelioma from adenocarcinoma. The M.D. Anderson experience and a critical review of the literature. Am J Clin Pathol 109:85-9, 1998.

65. Oury TD, Hammar SP, Roggli VL. Ultrastructural features of diffuse malignant mesotheliomas. Hum Pathol 29:1382-92, 1998.

66. Warhol M, Hickey WF, Corson JM. Malignant mesothelioma: ultrastructural distinction from adenocarcinoma. Am. J. Surg. Pathol. 6:307-314, 1982.

67. Ross B, Motherby H, Saurenbach F, et al. Atomic force microscopy in effusion cytology. Anal Quant Cytol Histol 20:97-104, 1998.

68. Suter M, Gebhard S, Boumghar M, et al. Localized fibrous tumours of the pleura: 15 new cases and review of the literature. Eur J Cardiothorac Surg 14:453-9, 1998.

69. Björkqvist AM, Tammilehto L, Nordling S, et al. Comparison of DNA copy number changes in malignant mesothelioma, adenocarcinoma and large-cell anaplastic carcinoma of the lung. Br J Cancer 77:260-9, 1998.

70. Lee WC, Testa JR. Somatic genetic alterations in human malignant mesothelioma (review). Int J Oncol 14:181-8, 1999.

71. Prins JB, Williamson KA, Kamp MM, et al. The gene for the cyclin-dependent-kinase-4 inhibitor, CDKN2A, is preferentially deleted in malignant mesothelioma. Int J Cancer 75:649-53, 1998.

72. Bianchi AB, Mitsunaga SI, Cheng JQ, et al. High frequency of inactivating mutations in the neurofibromatosis type 2 gene (NF2) in primary malignant mesotheliomas [see comments]. Proc Natl Acad Sci U S A 92:10854-8, 1995.

73. Deguen B, Goutebroze L, Giovannini M, et al. Heterogeneity of mesothelioma cell lines as defined by altered genomic structure and expression of the NF2 gene. Int J Cancer 77:554-60, 1998.

74. Balsara BR, Bell DW, Sonoda G, et al. Comparative genomic hybridization and loss of heterozygosity analyses identify a common region of deletion at 15q11. 1-15 in human malignant mesothelioma. Cancer Res 59:450-4, 1999.

75. Motherby H, Marcy T, Hecker M, et al. Static DNA cytometry as a diagnostic aid in effusion cytology: I. DNA aneuploidy for identification and differentiation of primary and secondary tumors of the serous membranes. Anal Quant Cytol Histol 20:153-61, 1998.

76. Motherby H, Nadjari B, Remmerbach T, et al. Static DNA cytometry as a diagnostic aid in effusion cytology: II. DNA aneuploidy for identification of neoplastic cells in equivocal effusions. Anal Quant Cytol Histol 20:162-8, 1998.

77. Butchart EG, Ashcroft T, Barnsley WC, et al. Pleuropneumonectomy in the management of diffuse malignant mesothelioma of the pleura: experience with 29 patients. Thorax 31:15-24, 1976.

78. Boutin C, Rey F, Gouvernet J, et al. Thoracoscopy in pleural malignant mesothelioma: a prospective study of 188 consecutive patients. Part 2: Prognosis and staging. Cancer 72:394-404, 1993.

79. Mattson K. Natural history and clinical staging of malignant mesothelioma. Eur. J. Respir. Dis. 63:87 (abstract), 1982.

80. Chahinian AP. Therapeutic modalities in malignant pleural mesothelioma, in Chretien J, Hirsch A (eds): Diseases of the Pleura. New York, Masson, 1983, pp 224-236.

81. Rusch VW. A proposed new international TNM staging system for malignant pleural mesothelioma. From the International Mesothelioma Interest Group [see comments]. Chest 108:1122-8, 1995.

82. Rusch VW. A proposed new international TNM staging system for malignant pleural mesothelioma from the International Mesothelioma Interest Group. Lung Cancer 14:1-12, 1996.

83. Mew D, Pass HI. Malignant mesotheliomas: a clinical challenge. Contemp Oncol :50-54, 62, 63, 66, 67, 1993.

84. Pass HI, Temeck BK, Kranda K, et al. Preoperative tumor volume is associated with outcome in malignant pleural mesothelioma. J Thorac Cardiovasc Surg 115:310-7; discussion 317-8, 1998.

85. Curran D, Sahmoud T, Therasse P, et al. Prognostic factors in patients with pleural mesothelioma: the European Organization for Research and Treatment of Cancer experience. J Clin Oncol 16:145-52, 1998.

86. Gottehrer A, Taryle DA, Reed CE, et al. Pleural fluid analysis in malignant mesothelioma. Prognostic implications. Chest 100:1003-6, 1991.

87. Beer TW, Buchanan R, Matthews AW, et al. Prognosis in malignant mesothelioma related to MIB 1 proliferation index and histological subtype. Hum Pathol 29:246-51, 1998.

88. Bethwaite PB, Delahunt B, Holloway LJ, et al. Comparison of silver-staining nucleolar organizer region (AgNOR) counts and proliferating cell nuclear antigen (PCNA) expression in reactive mesothelial hyperplasia and malignant mesothelioma. Pathology 27:1-4, 1995.

89. Isobe H, Sridhar KS, Doria R, et al. Prognostic significance of DNA aneuploidy in diffuse malignant mesothelioma. Cytometry 19:86-91, 1995.

90. Dazzi H, Thatcher N, Hasleton PS, et al. DNA analysis by flow cytometry in malignant pleural mesothelioma: relationship to histology and survival. J Pathol 162:51-5, 1990.

91. Pyrhonen S, Laasonen A, Lammilehto L, et al. Diploid predominance and prognostic significance of S-phase cells in malignant mesothelioma. Eur J Cancer 27:197, 1991.

92. Kumar Singh S, Vermeulen PB, Weyler J, et al. Evaluation of tumour angiogenesis as a prognostic marker in malignant mesothelioma. J Pathol 182:211-6, 1997.

93. Carmichael J, Degraff WG, Gamson J, et al. Radiation sensitivity of human lung cancer cell lines. Eur. J. Cancer Clin. Oncol. 25:527, 1989.

94. Maasilta P. Deterioration in lung function following hemithorax irradiation for pleural mesothelioma. Int J Radiat Oncol Biol Phys 20:433-8, 1991.

95. Ball DL, Druickhawk DG. The treatment of malignant mesothelioma of the pleura: review of a 5-year experience with special reference to radiotherapy. J. Clin. Oncol. 13:4-9, 1990.

96. Gordon W, Antman K, Breenberger J, et al: Radiation therapy in the management of patients with mesothelioma. Int J Radiat Oncol Biol Phys 8:19, 1982.

97. de Graaf Strukowska L, van der Zee J, van Putten W, et al. Factors influencing the outcome of radiotherapy in malignant mesothelioma of the pleura--a single-institution experience with 189 patients. Int J Radiat Oncol Biol Phys 43:511-6, 1999.

98. Lindén CJ, Mercke C, Albrechtsson U, et al. Effect of hemithorax irradiation alone or combined with doxorubicin and cyclophosphamide in 47 pleural mesotheliomas: a nonrandomized phase II study. Eur Respir J 9:2565-72, 1996.

99. Alberts AS, Falkson G, Goedhals L, et al. Malignant pleural mesothelioma: a disease unaffected by current therapeutic maneuvers. J Clin Oncol 6:527, 1988.

100. Noppen M, Degreve J, Mignolet M, et al. A prospective, randomised study comparing the efficacy of talc slurry and bleomycin in the treatment of malignant pleural effusions. Acta Clin Belg 52:258-62, 1997.

101. Martinez-Moragon E, Aparicio J, Rogado MC, et al. Pleurodesis in malignant pleural effusions: a randomized study of tetracycline versus bleomycin. Eur Respir J 10:2380-3, 1997.

102. Patz EF Jr, McAdams HP, Erasmus JJ, et al. Sclerotherapy for malignant pleural effusions: a prospective randomized trial of bleomycin vs doxycycline with small-bore catheter drainage. Chest 113:1305-11, 1998.

103. Yim AP, Chan AT, Lee TW, et al. Thoracoscopic talc insufflation versus talc slurry for symptomatic malignant pleural effusion. Ann Thorac Surg 62:1655-8, 1996.

104. Viallat JR, Rey F, Astoul P, et al. Thoracoscopic talc poudrage pleurodesis for malignant effusions. A review of 360 cases. Chest 110:1387-93, 1996.

105. Rusch VW. Pleurectomy/decortication in the setting of multimodality treatment for diffuse malignant pleural mesothelioma. Semin Thorac Cardiovasc Surg 9:367-72, 1997.

106. Sugarbaker DJ, Richards WG, Garcia JP. Extrapleural pneumonectomy for malignant mesothelioma. Adv Surg 31:253-71, 1997.

107. Ong ST, Vogelzang NJ. Chemotherapy in malignant pleural mesothelioma. A review. J Clin Oncol 14:1007-17, 1996.

108. Taub RN, Antman KH. Chemotherapy for malignant mesothelioma. Semin Thorac Cardiovasc Surg 9:361-6, 1997.

109. Ryan CW, Herndon J, Vogelzang NJ. A review of chemotherapy trials for malignant mesothelioma. Chest 113:66S-73S, 1998.

110. Bischoff HG, Manegold C, Knopp M, et al. Gemcitabine (Gemzar) may reduce tumor load and tumor-associated symptoms in malignant pleural mesothelioma [abstract 1784], Proc. Am. Soc. Clin. Oncol. Los Angeles, CA, 1998, pp 464.

111. Sorensen PG, Bach F, Bork E, et al. Randomized trial of doxorubicin versus cyclophosphamide in diffuse malignant pleural mesothelioma. Cancer Treat Rep 69:1431-2, 1985.

112. Chahinian AP, Antman K, Goutsou M, et al. Randomized phase II trial of cisplatin with mitomycin or doxorubicin for malignant mesothelioma by the Cancer and Leukemia Group B. J Clin Oncol 11:1559-65, 1993.

113. Pennucci MC, Ardizzoni A, Pronzato P, et al. Combined cisplatin, doxorubicin, and mitomycin for the treatment of advanced pleural mesothelioma: a phase II FONICAP trial. Italian Lung Cancer Task Force. Cancer 79:1897-902, 1997.

114. Middleton GW, Smith IE, ME OB, et al. Good symptom relief with palliative MVP (mitomycin-C, vinblastine and cisplatin) chemotherapy in malignant mesothelioma. Ann Oncol 9:269-73, 1998.

115. Byrne MJ, Davidson JA, Musk AW, et al. Cisplatin and gemcitabine treatment for malignant mesothelioma: a phase II study. J. Clin. Oncol. 17:25-30, 1999.

116. Rusch VW, Niedzwiecki D, Tao Y, et al. Intrapleural cisplatin and mitomycin for malignant mesothelioma following pleurectomy: pharmacokinetic studies. J Clin Oncol 10:1001-6, 1992.

117. Lee JD, Perez S, Wang HJ, et al. Intrapleural chemotherapy for patients with incompletely resected malignant mesothelioma: the UCLA experience. J Surg Oncol 60:262-7, 1995.

118. Boutin C, Nussbaum E, Monnet I, et al. Intrapleural treatment with recombinant gamma-interferon in early stage malignant pleural mesothelioma. Cancer 74:2460-7, 1994.

119. Perez-Soler R, Walsh GL, Swisher SG, et al. Phase II study of a liposome-entrapped cisplatin analog (L-NDDP) administered intrapleurally in patients (PTS) with malignant pleural mesothelioma (MPM). Proc Am Soc Clin Oncol 18:#1626, 1999.

120. Sinoff C, Falkson G, Sandison AG, et al. Combined doxorubicin and radiation therapy in malignant pleural mesothelioma. Cancer Treat. Rep. 66:1605-1607, 1982.

121. Herscher LL, Hahn SM, Kroog G, et al. Phase I study of paclitaxel as a radiation sensitizer in the treatment of mesothelioma and non-small-cell lung cancer. J Clin Oncol 16:635-41, 1998.

122. Baldini EH, Recht A, Strauss GM, et al. Patterns of failure after trimodality therapy for malignant pleural mesothelioma. Ann Thorac Surg 63:334-8, 1997.

123. Rusch V, Saltz L, Venkatraman E, et al. A phase II trial of pleurectomy/decortication followed by intrapleural and systemic chemotherapy for malignant pleural mesothelioma. J Clin Oncol 12:1156-63, 1994.

124. Rice TW, Adelstein DJ, Kirby TJ, et al. Aggressive multimodality therapy for malignant pleural mesothelioma. Ann Thorac Surg 58:24-9, 1994.

125. Pass HW, Temeck BK, Kranda K, et al. A phase II trial investigating primary immunochemotherapy for malignant pleural mesothelioma and the feasibility of adjuvant immunochemotherapy after maximal cytoreduction. Ann Surg Oncol 2:214-20, 1995.

126. Myerson RJ, Moros E, Roti Roti JL. Hyperthermia, in Perez CA, Brady LW (eds): Principles and practice of radiation oncology (ed 3rd). Philadelphia, Lippincott-Raven Publishers, Inc., 1997, pp 637-683.

127. Elias D, Gachot B, Bonvallot S, et al. [Peritoneal carcinosis treated by complete excision and immediate postoperative intra-peritoneal chemotherapy. Phase II study in 54 patients]. Gastroenterol Clin Biol 21:181-7, 1997.

128. Los G, van Vugt MJ, Pinedo HM. Response of peritoneal solid tumours after intraperitoneal chemohyperthermia treatment with cisplatin or carboplatin. Br J Cancer 69:235-41, 1994.

129. van de Vaart PJ, van der Vange N, Zoetmulder FA, et al. Intraperitoneal cisplatin with regional hyperthermia in advanced ovarian cancer: pharmacokinetics and cisplatin-DNA adduct formation in patients and ovarian cancer cell lines. Eur J Cancer 34:148-54, 1998.

130. Kuroda M, Urano M, Nishimura Y, et al. Induction thermochemotherapy increases therapeutic gain factor for the fractionated radiotherapy given to a mouse fibrosarcoma. Int J Radiat Oncol Biol Phys 38:411-7, 1997.

131. Jacquet P, Averbach A, Stuart OA, et al. Hyperthermic intraperitoneal doxorubicin: pharmacokinetics, metabolism, and tissue distribution in a rat model. Cancer Chemother Pharmacol 41:147-54, 1998.

132. Matsuzaki Y, Shibata K, Yoshioka M, et al. Intrapleural perfusion hyperthermochemotherapy for malignant pleural dissemination and effusion. Ann Thorac Surg 59:127-31, 1995.

133. Ma GY, Bartlett DL, Reed E, et al. Continuous hyperthermic peritoneal perfusion with cisplatin for the treatment of peritoneal mesothelioma. Cancer J Sci Am 3:174-9, 1997.

134. Hamazoe R, Maeta M, Kaibara N. Intraperitoneal thermochemotherapy for prevention of peritoneal recurrence of gastric cancer. Final results of a randomized controlled study. Cancer 73:2048-52, 1994.

135. Fujimoto S, Takahashi M, Mutou T, et al. Improved mortality rate of gastric carcinoma patients with peritoneal carcinomatosis treated with intraperitoneal hyperthermic chemoperfusion combined with surgery. Cancer 79:884-91, 1997.

136. Jacquet P, Stephens AD, Averbach AM, et al. Analysis of morbidity and mortality in 60 patients with peritoneal carcinomatosis treated by cytoreductive surgery and heated intraoperative intraperitoneal chemotherapy. Cancer 77:2622-9, 1996.

137. Chen MY, Chiles C, Loggie BW, et al. Thoracic complications in patients undergoing intraperitoneal heated chemotherapy with mitomycin following cytoreductive surgery. J Surg Oncol 66:19-23, 1997.

138. Pelton JJ, Kowalyshyn MJ, Keller SM. Intrathoracic organ injury associated with photodynamic therapy. J Thorac Cardiovasc Surg 103:1218-23, 1992.

139. Tochner ZA, Pass HI, Smith PD, et al. Intrathoracic photodynamic therapy: a canine normal tissue tolerance study and early clinical experience. Lasers Surg Med 14:118-23, 1994.

140. Pass HI, Pogrebniak H. Photodynamic therapy for thoracic malignancies. Semin Surg Oncol 8:217-25, 1992.

141. Luketich JD, Westkaemper J, Sommers KE, et al. Bronchoesophagopleural fistula after photodynamic therapy for malignant mesothelioma. Ann Thorac Surg 62:283-4, 1996.

142. Pass HI, Temeck BK, Kranda K, et al. Phase III randomized trial of surgery with or without intraoperative photodynamic therapy and postoperative immunochemotherapy for malignant pleural mesothelioma. Ann Surg Oncol 4:628-33, 1997.

143. Pass HI, Donington JS. Use of photodynamic therapy for the management of pleural malignancies. Semin Surg Oncol 11:360-7, 1995.

144. Moskal TL, Dougherty TJ, Urschel JD, et al. Operation and photodynamic therapy for pleural mesothelioma: 6-year follow-up. Ann Thorac Surg 66:1128-33, 1998.

145. Bielefeldt-Ohmann H, Fitzpatrick DR, Marzo AL, et al. Patho- and immunobiology of malignant mesothelioma: characterization of tumor-infiltrating leukocytes and cytokine production in a murine model. Cancer Immunol Immunother 39:347-359, 1994.
146. Casciari JJ, Sato H, Durum SK, et al. Tabular lexicon of cytokine structure and function, in Chabner BA, Longo DL (eds): Cancer Chemotherapy and Biotherapy (ed 2nd). Philadelphia, Lippincott-Raven Publishers, 1996, pp 787-810.
147. Jagirdar J, Lee TC, Reibman J, et al. Immunohistochemical localization of transforming growth factor beta isoforms in asbestos-related diseases. Environ Health Perspect 105 Suppl 5:1197-203, 1997.
148. Maeda J, Ueki N, Ohkawa T, et al. Transforming growth factor-beta 1 (TGF-beta 1)- and beta 2-like activities in malignant pleural effusions caused by malignant mesothelioma or primary lung cancer. Clin Exp Immunol 98:319-22, 1994.
149. Schmitter D, Lauber B, Fagg B, et al. Hematopoietic growth factors secreted by seven human pleural mesothelioma cell lines: interleukin-6 production as a common feature. Int J Cancer 51:296-301, 1992.
150. Monti G, Jaurand MC, Monnet I, et al. Intrapleural production of interleukin 6 during mesothelioma and its modulation by gamma-interferon treatment. Cancer Res 54:4419-23, 1994.
151. Garlepp MJ, Leong CC. Biological and immunological aspects of malignant mesothelioma. Eur Respir J 8:643-50, 1995.
152. Witt PL, Lindner DJ, D'Cunha J, et al. Pharmacology of interferons: induced proteins, cell activation, and antitumor activity, in Chabner BA, Longo DL (eds): Cancer Chemotherapy and Biotherapy (ed 2nd). Philadelphia, Lippincott-Raven Publishers, 1996, pp 585-607.
153. Ohnuma T, Szrajer L, Holland JF, et al. Effects of natural interferon alpha, natural tumor necrosis factor alpha and their combination on human mesothelioma xenografts in nude mice. Cancer Immunol Immunother 36:31-6, 1993.
154. Bielefeldt-Ohmann H, Fitzpatrick DR, Marzo AL, et al. Potential for interferon-alpha-based therapy in mesothelioma: assessment in a murine model. J Interferon Cytokine Res 15:213-23, 1995.
155. Ardizzoni A, Pennucci MC, Castagneto B, et al. Recombinant interferon alpha-2b in the treatment of diffuse malignant pleural mesothelioma. Am J Clin Oncol 17:80-2, 1994.
156. Christmas TI, Manning LS, Garlepp MJ, et al. Effect of interferon-alpha 2a on malignant mesothelioma. J. Interferon Res. 13:9-12, 1993.
157. Von Hoff DD, Metch B, Lucas JG, et al. Phase II evaluation of recombinant interferon-beta (IFN-beta ser) in patients with diffuse mesothelioma: a Southwest Oncology Group study. J Interferon Res 10:531-4, 1990.
158. Rosso R, Rimoldi R, Salvati F, et al. Intrapleural natural beta interferon in the treatment of malignant pleural effusions. Oncology 45:253-6, 1988.
159. Zeng L, Buard A, Monnet I, et al. In vitro effects of recombinant human interferon gamma on human mesothelioma cell lines. Int J Cancer 55:515-20, 1993.

160. Hasturk S, Tastepe I, Unlu M, et al. Combined chemotherapy in pleurectomized malignant pleural mesothelioma patients. J Chemother 8:159-64, 1996.

161. Hand A, Pelin K, Mattson K, et al. Interferon (IFN)-alpha and IFN-gamma in combination with methotrexate: in vitro sensitivity studies in four human mesothelioma cell lines. Anticancer Drugs 6:77-82, 1995.

162. Hand AM, Husgafvel-Pursiainen K, Pelin K, et al. Interferon-alpha and -gamma in combination with chemotherapeutic drugs: in vitro sensitivity studies in four human mesothelioma cell lines. Anticancer Drugs 3:687-94, 1992.

163. Sklarin NT, Chahinian AP, Feuer EJ, et al. Augmentation of activity of cis-diamminedichloroplatinum(II) and mitomycin C by interferon in human malignant mesothelioma xenografts in nude mice. Cancer Res 48:64-7, 1988.

164. Soulie P, Ruffie P, Trandafir L, et al. Combined systemic chemoimmunotherapy in advanced diffuse malignant mesothelioma. Report of a phase I-II study of weekly cisplatin/interferon alfa-2a. J Clin Oncol 14:878-85, 1996.

165. Manning LS, Bowman RV, Darby SB, et al. Lysis of human malignant mesothelioma cells by natural killer (NK) and lymphokine-activated killer (LAK) cells. Am Rev Respir Dis 139:1369-74, 1989.

166. Goey SH, Eggermont AM, Punt CJ, et al. Intrapleural administration of interleukin 2 in pleural mesothelioma: a phase I-II study. Br J Cancer 72:1283-8, 1995.

167. Astoul P, Picat Joossen D, Viallat JR, et al. Intrapleural administration of interleukin-2 for the treatment of patients with malignant pleural mesothelioma: a Phase II study. Cancer 83:2099-104, 1998.

168. Astoul P, Bertault-Peres P, Durand A, et al. Pharmacokinetics of intrapleural recombinant interleukin-2 in immunotherapy for malignant pleural effusion. Cancer 73:308-13, 1994.

169. Lissoni P, Barni S, Tancini G, et al. Intracavitary therapy of neoplastic effusions with cytokines: comparison among interferon alpha, beta and interleukin-2. Support Care Cancer 3:78-80, 1995.

170. Curiel DT, Pilewski JM, Albelda SM. Gene therapy approaches for inherited and acquired lung diseases. Am J Respir Cell Mol Biol 14:1-18, 1996.

171. Sterman DH, Kaiser LR, Albelda SM. Gene therapy for malignant pleural mesothelioma. Hematol Oncol Clin North Am 12:553-68, 1998.

172. Elshami AA, Saavedra A, Zhang H, et al. Gap junctions play a role in the 'bystander effect' of the herpes simplex virus thymidine kinase/ganciclovir system in vitro. Gene Ther 3:85-92, 1996.

173. Russell SJ, Eccles SA, Flemming C, et al. Decreased tumorigenicity of a transplantable rat sarcoma following transfer and expression of an IL-2 cDNA. Int. J. Cancer 47:244, 1991.

174. Batra RK, Olsen JC, Pickles RJ, et al. Transduction of non-small cell lung cancer cells by adenoviral and retroviral vectors. Am J Respir Cell Mol Biol 18:402-10, 1998.

175. Frizelle SP, Grim J, Zhou J, et al. Re-expression of p16INK4a in mesothelioma cells results in cell cycle arrest, cell death, tumor suppression and tumor regression. Oncogene 16:3087-95, 1998.

176. Procopio A, Strizzi L, Giuffrida A, et al. Human malignant mesothelioma of the pleura: new perspectives for diagnosis and therapy. Monaldi Arch Chest Dis 53:241-3, 1998.

177. Robinson BW, Mukherjee SA, Davidson A, et al. Cytokine gene therapy or infusion as treatment for solid human cancer. J Immunother 21:211-7, 1998.

178. Elshami AA, Kucharczuk JC, Sterman DH, et al. The role of immunosuppression in the efficacy of cancer gene therapy using adenovirus transfer of the herpes simplex thymidine kinase gene. Ann Surg 222:298-307; 307-10, 1995.

179. Elshami AA, Kucharczuk JC, Zhang HB, et al. Treatment of pleural mesothelioma in an immunocompetent rat model utilizing adenoviral transfer of the herpes simplex virus thymidine kinase gene. Hum Gene Ther 7:141-8, 1996.

180. Smythe WR, Hwang HC, Amin KM, et al. Use of recombinant adenovirus to transfer the herpes simplex virus thymidine kinase (HSVtk) gene to thoracic neoplasms: an effective in vitro drug sensitization system. Cancer Res 54:2055-9, 1994.

181. Esandi MC, van Someren GD, Vincent AJ, et al. Gene therapy of experimental malignant mesothelioma using adenovirus vectors encoding the HSVtk gene. Gene Ther 4:280-7, 1997.

182. Smythe WR, Hwang HC, Elshami AA, et al. Treatment of experimental human mesothelioma using adenovirus transfer of the herpes simplex thymidine kinase gene. Ann Surg 222:78-86, 1995.

183. Schwarzenberger P, Lei D, Freeman SM, et al. Antitumor activity with the HSV-tk-gene-modified cell line PA-1-STK in malignant mesothelioma. Am J Respir Cell Mol Biol 19:333-7, 1998.

184. Yang CT, You L, Yeh CC, et al. Adenovirus-mediated p14[ARF] gene transfer I in human mesothelioma cells. J Natl Cancer Inst 92:636-41, 2000.

185. Hwang HC, Smythe WR, Elshami AA, et al. Gene therapy using adenovirus carrying the herpes simplex-thymidine kinase gene to treat in vivo models of human malignant mesothelioma and lung cancer. Am J Respir Cell Mol Biol 13:7-16, 1995.

186. Kucharczuk JC, Elshami AA, Zhang HB, et al. Pleural-based mesothelioma in immune competent rats: a model to study adenoviral gene transfer. Ann Thorac Surg 60:593-7; discussion 597-8, 1995.

187. Kaiser LR. New therapies in the treatment of malignant pleural mesothelioma. Semin Thorac Cardiovasc Surg 9:383-90, 1997.

188. Sterman DH, Treat J, Litzky LA, et al. Adenovirus-mediated herpes simplex virus thymidine kinase/ganciclovir gene therapy in patients with localized malignancy: results of a phase I clinical trial in malignant mesothelioma. Hum Gene Ther 9:1083-92, 1998.

189. Musk AW, de Klerk NH, Ambrosini GL, et al. Vitamin A and cancer prevention I: observations in workers previously exposed to asbestos at Wittenoom, Western Australia. Int J Cancer 75:355-61, 1998.

190. de Klerk NH, Musk AW, Ambrosini GL, et al. Vitamin A and cancer prevention II: comparison of the effects of retinol and beta-carotene. Int J Cancer 75:362-7, 1998.

191. Omenn GS, Goodman GE, Thornquist MD, et al. Effects of a combination of beta carotene and vitamin A on lung cancer and cardiovascular disease [see comments]. N Engl J Med 334:1150-5, 1996.
192. Omenn GS, Goodman G, Thornquist M, et al. The β-Carotene and Retinol Efficacy Trial (CARET) for chemoprevention of lung cancer in high-risk populations: smokers and asbestos-exposed workers. Cancer Res. 54:2038-2043, 1994.
193. Goodman GE, Thornquist M, Kestin M, et al. The effect of vitamin E and beta carotene on the incidence of lung cancer and other cancers in male smokers. The Alpha- Tocopherol, Beta Carotene Cancer Prevention Study Group [see comments]. N Engl J Med 330:1029-35, 1994.
194. Harmon D, Vogelzang NJ, Roboz J, et al. Dihydro-5-azacytidine (DHAC) in malignant mesothelioma (Meso) using secrum hyaluronic acid (SHA) as a tumor marker: a phase II trial of the CALGB [abstract 1248], Proc Am Soc Clin Oncol pp 351, 1991.
195. Cantwell BMJ, Earnshaw M, Harris AL, et al. Phase II study of a novel antifolate, N^{10}-propargyl-5,8-dideazafolic acid (CB3717), in malignant mesothelioma. Cancer Treat Rep 70:1335-1336, 1986.
196. Belani CP, Herndon J, Vogelzang NJ, et al. Edatrexate with oral leucovorin rescue for malignant mesothelioma: a phase II study of the Cancer and Leukemia Group B-CALGB 9131 [abstract 1068]., Proc. Am. Soc. Clin. Oncol pp 352, 1995.
197. Harvey VJ, Slevin ML, Ponder BAJ, et al. Chemotherapy of diffuse malignant mesothelioma: phase II trials of single agent 5-fluorouracil and adriamycin. Cancer 54:961-964, 1984.
198. Solheim OP, Saeter G, Finnanger AM, et al. High-dose methotrexate in the treatment of malignant mesothelioma of the pleura. A phase II study. Br J Cancer 65:956-60, 1992.
199. Vogelzang NJ, Weissman LB, Herndon JE, et al. Trimetrexate in malignant mesothelioma: A Cancer and Leukemia Group B Phase II study. J Clin Oncol 12:1436-42, 1994.
200. Mbidde EK, Harland SJ, Cavert AH, et al. Phase II trial of carboplatin (JM8) in treatment of patients with malignant mesothelioma. Cancer Chemother. Pharmacol. 18:284-285, 1986.
201. Raghavan D, Gianoutsos P, Bishop J, et al. Phase II trial of carboplatin in the management of malignant mesothelioma. J Clin Oncol 8:151-4, 1990.
202. Vogelzang NJ, Goutsou M, Corson JM, et al. Carboplatin in malignant mesothelioma: a phase II study of the Cancer and Leukemia Group B. Cancer Chemother. Pharmacol. 27:239-242, 1990.
203. Mintzer DM, Kelsen D, Frimmer D, et al. Phase II trial of high-dose cisplatin in patients with malignant mesothelioma. Cancer Treat. Rep. 69:711-712, 1985.
204. Zidar BL, Green S, Pierce HI, et al. A phase II evaluation of cisplatin in unresectable diffuse malignant mesothelioma: a Southwest Oncology Group study. Invest. New Drugs 6:223-226, 1988.

205. Falkson G, Vorobiof DA, Lerner JH, et al. A phase II study of M-AMSA in patients with malignant mesothelioma. Cancer Chemother. Pharmacol. 11:94-97, 1983.
206. Colbert N, Vannetzel JM, Izrael V. A prospective study of detorubicin in malignant pleural mesothelioma. Cancer 56:2170-2174, 1985.
207. Eagan R, Frytak S, Richardson R, et al. Phase II trial of high-dose cisplatin in patients with malignant mesothelioma. Cancer Treat Rep 70:429, 1986.
208. Lerner HJ, Schoenfeld DA, Martin A, et al. Malignant mesothelioma, the Eastern Cooperative Oncology Group (ECOG) experience. Cancer 52:1981-1985, 1983.
209. Magri MD, Veronesi A, Foladore S, et al. Epirubicin in the treatment of malignant mesothelioma: a phase II cooperative study. Tumori 77:49-51, 1991.
210. Mattson K, Giaccone G, Kirkpatrick A, et al. Epirubicin in malignant mesothelioma: a phase II study of th European Organization for Research and Treatment of Cancer Lung Cancer Cooperative Group. J Clin Oncol 10:824-828, 1992.
211. Hudis CA, Kelsen DP. Menogaril in treatment of malignant mesothelioma: a phase II study. Invest. New Drugs 10:103-106, 1992.
212. Eisenhauer EA, Evans WK, Raghavan D, et al. Phase II study of mitoxantrone in patients with mesothelioma: a National Cancer Institute of Canada Clinical Trials Group study. Cancer Treat. Rep. 70:1029-1030, 1986.
213. van Breukelen FJ, Mattson K, Giaccone G, et al. Mitoxantrone in malignant pleural mesothelioma: a study by the EORTC Lung Cancer Cooperative Group. Eur J Cancer 27:1627-9, 1991.
214. Sridhar KS, Doria R, Hussein AM, et al. Activity and toxicity of 4'-o-tetrahydropyranyladriamycin (pirarubicin) in malignant mesothelioma [abstract 1225], Proc. Am. Soc. Clin. Oncol., pp 356, 1992.
215. Kaukel E, Koschel G, Gatzemeyer U, et al. A phase II study of pirarubicin in malignant pleural mesothelioma. Cancer 66:651-4, 1990.
216. Alberts AS, Falkson G, Zyl LV. Malignant pleural mesothelioma: phase II pilot study of ifosfamide and mesna. J. Natl. Cancer Inst. 80:968-970, 1988.
217. Falkson G, Hunt M, Borden EC, et al. An extended phase II trial of ifosfamide plus mesna in malignant mesothelioma. Invest. New Drugs 10:337-343, 1992.
218. Zidar BL, Metch B, Balcerzak SP, et al. A phase II evaluation of ifosfamide and mesna in unresectable diffuse malignant mesothelioma. A Southwest Oncology Group study. Cancer 70:2547-51, 1992.
219. Icli F, Karaoguz H, Dincol D, et al. A phase II study of ifosfamide (I) in unresectable diffuse malignant mesothelioma (MM) [abstract 1650], Proc. Am. Soc. Clin. Oncol., pp 472, 1993.
220. Bajorin D, Kelsen D, Mintzer DM. Phase II trial of mitomycin in malignant mesothelioma. Cancer Treat. Rep. 71:857-858, 1987.
221. Wasser L, Hunt M, Lerner H, et al. Phase II trial of PCNU in malignant mesothelioma: an ECOG trial, Proc. Am. Soc. Clin. Oncol., pp. 309, 1989.
222. Belani CP, Adak S, Aisner S, et al. Docetaxel for malignant mesothelioma: phase II study of the Eastern Cooperative Oncology Group (ECOG 2595). Proc Am Soc Clin Oncol 18:#1829, 1999.

223. Tammilehto L, Maasilta P, Mantyla M, et al. Oral etoposide in the treatment of malignant mesothelioma. A phase II study. Ann Oncol 5:949-50, 1994.

224. Vogelzang NJ, Herndon J, Clamon GH, et al. Paclitaxel (Taxol) for malignant mesothelioma (MM): a phase II study of the Cancer and Leukemia Group B (CALGB 9234) [abstract 1382], Proc. Am. Soc. Clin. Oncol., pp 405, 1994.

225. Maksymiuk AW, Marschke RF, Jr., Tazelaar HD, et al. Phase II trial of topotecan for the treatment of mesothelioma. Am J Clin Oncol 21:610-3, 1998.

226. Cowan JD, Green S, Lucas J, et al. Phase II trial of 5-day intravenous infusion of vinblastine sulfate in patients with diffuse malignant mesothelioma: a Southwest Oncology Group study [letter. Invest. New Drugs 6, 1988.

227. Martensson G, Sorenson S. A phase II study of vincristine in malignant mesothelioma--a negative report. Cancer Chemother Pharmacol 24:133-4, 1989.

228. Kelsen D, Gralla R, Cheng E, et al. Vindesine in the treatment of malignant mesothelioma: a phase II study. Cancer Treat. Rep. 67:821-822, 1983.

229. Boutin C, Irisson M, Guerin JC, et al. Phase II trial of vindesine in malignant pleural mesothelioma. Cancer Treat. Rep. 71:205-206, 1987.

230. Steele JPC, Evans MT, Tischkowitz MD, et al. Vinorelbine is an active and well-tolerated drug for the treatment of malignant mesothelioma: a phase II study. Proc Am Soc Clin Oncol 18:#1891, 1999.

231. Webster I, Cochrane JWC, Burkhardt KR, et al. Immunotherapy with BCG in 30 cases of mesothelioma. S. Afr. Med. J. 61:277-278, 1982.

232. Costanzi J, Darzynkiewicz Z, Chun H, et al. The use of Onconase (ONC) for patients (PTS) with advanced malignant mesothelioma (MM) [abstract 1414], Proc. Am. Soc. Clin. Oncol., pp 452, 1996.

233. Chahinian AP, Pajak TF, Holland JF, et al. Diffuse malignant mesothelioma. Prospective evaluation of 69 patients. Ann Intern Med 96:746-55, 1982.

234. Ardizzoni A, Rosso R, Salvati F, et al. Activity of doxorubicin and cisplatin combination chemotherapy in patients with diffuse malignant pleural mesothelioma. An Italian Lung Cancer Task Force (FONICAP) Phase II study. Cancer 67:2984-7, 1991.

235. Shin DM, Fossella FV, Umsawasdi T, et al. Prospective study of combination chemotherapy with cyclophosphamide, doxorubicin, and cisplatin for unresectable or metastatic malignant pleural mesothelioma [see comments]. Cancer 76:2230-6, 1995.

236. Pronzato P, Ardizzoni A, Pennucci MC, et al. Phase II FONICAP trial with cisplatin, doxorubicin, and mitomycin for advanced pleural mesothelioma patients [abstract 1209], Proc. Am. Soc. Clin. Oncol., pp 398, 1991.

237. Breau JL, Boaziz C, Morere JJF, et al. Combination chemotherapy with cisplatinum, Adriamycin, bleomycin, and mitomycin C plus systemic and intrapleural hyaluronidase in 25 consecutive cases of stage II and III pleural mesothelioma, First International Mesothelioma Conference. Paris, France, 1991.

238. Samson MK, Wasser LP, Borden EC, et al. Randomized comparison of cyclophosphamide, imidazole carboxamide, and adriamycin versus cyclophosphamide and adriamycin in patients with advanced stage malignant mesothelioma: a Sarcoma Intergroup Study. J Clin Oncol 5:86-91, 1987.

239. Dhingra H, Valdivieso M, Tannir N, et al. Combined modality treatment for mesothelioma with Cytoxan, Adriamycin, and DTIC (CYADIC) and adjuvant surgery [abstract C-800], Proc. Am. Soc. Clin. Oncol., pp 205, 1983.
240. Carmichael J, Cantwell BM, Harris AL. A phase II trial of ifosfamide/mesna with doxorubicin for malignant mesothelioma [see comments]. Eur J Cancer Clin Oncol 25:911-2, 1989.
241. Dirix LY, van Meerbeeck J, Schrijvers D, et al. A phase II trial of dose-escalated doxorubicin and ifosfamide/mesna in patients with malignant mesothelioma. Ann Oncol 5:653-5, 1994.
242. Upham JW, Musk AW, van Hazel G, et al. Interferon alpha and doxorubicin in malignant mesothelioma: a phase II study. Aust N Z J Med 23:683-7, 1993.
243. Samuels BL, Herndon JE, Harmon DC, et al. Dihydro-5-azacytidine and cisplatin in the treatment of malignant mesothelioma: a phase II study by the Cancer and Leukemia Group B. Cancer 82:1578-84, 1998.
244. Eisenhauer EA, Evans WK, Murray N, et al. A phase II study of VP-16 and cisplatin in patients with unresectable malignant mesothelioma: an NCI Canada Clinical Trials Group study. Invest. New Drugs 6:327-329, 1988.
245. Planting AS, van der Burg ME, Goey SH, et al. Phase II study of a short course of weekly high-dose cisplatin combined with long-term oral etoposide in pleural mesothelioma. Ann Oncol 6:613-5, 1995.
246. Pogrebniak H, Kranda K, Steinberg S, et al. Cisplatin, interferon-a, and tamoxifen (CIT) for malignant pleural mesothelioma [abstract 1363], Proc. Am. Soc. Clin. Oncol., pp 398, 1993.
247. Tansan S, Emri S, Selcuk T, et al. Treatment of malignant pleural mesothelioma with cisplatin, mitomycin C and alpha interferon. Oncology 51:348-51, 1994.
248. Rodier JM, Couteau C, Ruffie P, et al. Phase II study of a monthly combination of cisplatin, mitomycin, and interferon-alfa in malignant pleural mesothelioma [abstract 1174], Proc Am Soc Clin Oncol, pp 390, 1996.
249. Koschel G, Calavrezos A, Kaukel E, et al. Phase III randomized comparison of pirarubicin vs. pirarubicin and cisplatin for treatment of pleural mesotheliomas [abstract 1097]. Eur J Cancer 27:S180, 1991.
250. Tsavaris N, Mylonakis N, Karvounis N, et al. Combination chemotherapy with cisplatin-vinblastine in malignant mesothelioma [see comments]. Lung Cancer 11:299-303, 1994.
251. Ilson DH, Saltz L, Martin L, et al. A phase II trial of interferon alpha 2a (IFNα) and carboplatin in malignant mesothelioma [abstract], Proc. Am. Soc. Clin. Oncol., pp 456, 1996.
252. Magri MD, Foladore S, Veronis A, et al. Treatment of malignant mesothelioma with epirubicin and ifosfamide: a phase II comparative study. Ann Oncol 2:237-238, 1992.
253. Bretti S, Berruti A, Dogliotti L, et al. Combined epirubicin and interleukin-2 regimen in the treatment of malignant mesothelioma: a multicenter phase II study of the Italian Group on Rare Tumors. Tumori 84:558-61, 1998.

254. Pinto C, Melotti B, Piana E, et al. Phase II study of mitoxantrone, methotrexate, and mitomycin (MMM regimen) in malignant mesothelioma of the pleura. Proc Am Soc Clin Oncol 18:#2113, 1999.
255. Daniel C, Fizazi K, Fandi A, et al. 'Tomudex' (raltitrexed) and Eloxatine (oxaliplatin) is an active combination with acceptable toxicity in malignant mesothelioma. Proc Am Soc Clin Oncol 18:#1844, 1999.
256. Zidar BL, Benjamin RS, Frank J, et al. Combination chemotherapy for advanced sarcomas of bone and mesothelioma utilizing rubidazone and DTIC: a Southwest Oncology Group study. Am J Clin Oncol 6:71-74, 1983.
257. Rusch VW, Figlin R, Godwin D, et al. Intrapleural cisplatin and cytarabine in the management of malignant pleural effusions: a Lung Cancer Study Group trial. J Clin Oncol 9:313-9, 1991.
258. Astoul P, Viallat JR, Laurent JC, et al. Intrapleural recombinant IL-2 in passive immunotherapy for malignant pleural effusion. Chest 103:209-13, 1993.

EPIDEMIOLOGY, DIAGNOSIS, AND STAGING OF ESOPHAGEAL CANCER

Richard F. Heitmiller M.D.
Johns Hopkins Medical Institutions, Baltimore, MD 21287 USA

INTRODUCTION

Esophageal carcinoma is an uncommon gastrointestinal malignancy with a prevalence rate which is far less than the more common colo-rectal cancers. Whereas the overall incidence of esophageal cancer has risen only gradually with time, in the United States, Canada, and Western Europe, there has been a dramatic change in the distribution of esophageal cancer by cell type (figure 1). Currently esophageal adenocarcinoma has replaced squamous cell carcinoma as the most common tumor diagnosed (1-4). Although esophageal carcinoma, regardless of cell type, continues to be an aggressive malignancy that usually presents in a locally advanced stage, new treatment plans using combination therapies have made significant progress in improving survival for patients with these tumors. These new treatment options, the surge of new cases of adenocarcinoma, and the introduction of new diagnostic modalities, have altered the current approach to the diagnosis and staging of esophageal carcinoma.

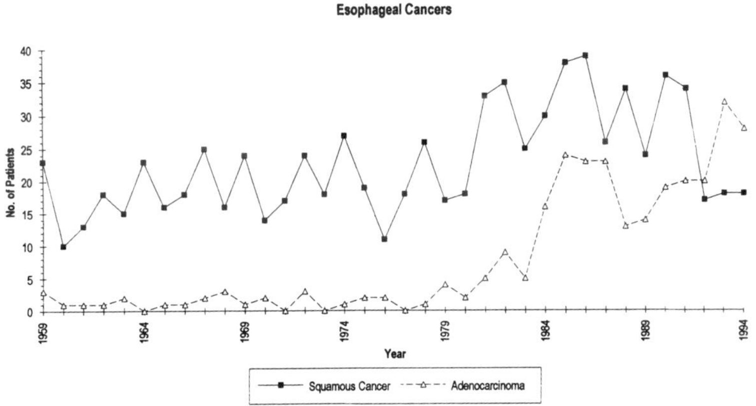

Figure 1. Prevalence of esophageal cancer by cell type at The Johns Hopkins Hospital 1959-1994. Squamous cell cancer=black square. Adenocarcinoma=open triangle. (From Heitmiller RF, Sharma R: Comparison of incidence and resection rates in patients with esophageal squamous cell carcinoma and adenocarcinoma. J Thorac Cardiovasc Surg 1996;112:130-6, with permission)

Epidemiology and Pathogenesis

The data support the hypothesis that esophageal squamous cell carcinoma and adenocarcinoma arise as a result of chronic mucosal irritation, and that the likelihood of developing cancer may be increased in immunocompromised patients. The most commonly identified mucosal irritants include tobacco, alcohol, dietary factors, lye, radiation, and refluxed gastric contents. The role of genetic predisposition in the development of esophageal cancer is suspected but not proven. Not surprisingly, the incidence and predominant cell type of esophageal cancer worldwide varies widely depending on geographic location, local cultural practices, and demographics.

Squamous cell carcinoma

Tobacco smoking is a proven etiologic factor in the development of esophageal squamous cell carcinoma for both men and women. Numerous studies have documented a dose- dependent effect of tobacco smoking and risk of developing squamous cancer. Choi and Kahyo (5) have demonstrated that the risk of squamous cancer decreases with smoking cessation. The use of smokeless tobacco products, such as snuff and chewing tobacco, also increases the risk of squamous tumors of the mouth, larynx, throat, and esophagus (6).

Alcohol consumption also independently increases the risk of developing esophageal squamous carcinoma. The type of alcohol consumed appears to affect the risk. Gronbaek et al (7) demonstrated a 'considerable' increase risk in developing esophageal squamous tumors in patients with a moderate intake of beer or spirits, however, no such increased risk was seen in patients with similar intake of wine. When tobacco smoking and alcohol consumption occur together, the risk of squamous cancer increases dramatically. Castellsague et al (8) noted only a slight increase in the risk of squamous tumors in South American men and women who smoked or drank in moderation. On the other hand, when moderate alcohol consumption and tobacco smoking were used together, the risk of cancer rose to 12 to 19 fold for men and women respectively.

Patients who have had a previous tumor of the head and neck have a risk of a developing a second malignancy of 4% per year of follow-up. According to Leon et al (9), the second neoplasms were located in the head and neck (40%), lungs (31%), and esophagus (9%). Whether this risk of second malignancy reflects an inherent 'field defect' of the oropharynx and aerodigestive tract squamous mucosa, or whether it is secondary to similar environmental exposure is unclear.

Human papillomavirus (HPV) has been implicated as a possible cause of esophageal squamous carcinoma, however, the data supporting this is conflicting. Sur and Cooper (10) speculate that infection with HPV may be an integral part in a multistep process leading to esophageal squamous cancer, and that regional susceptibility of populations to HPV may explain the observed geographic distribution of esophageal squamous tumors. In contrast, Lagergren et al (11), in a nationwide study in Sweden demonstrated no association between HPVinfection and esophageal squamous cell carcinoma or adenocarcinoma.

Ghardirian et al (12) reported that populations with the highest incidence of esophageal cancer shared similar diets and dietary habits. Many of the dishes served in these high-risk regions consisted of granular foods, or foods and beverages which are served very hot and which are consumed rapidly. The most common diets were high in starches with little or no fruits and vegetables. Block et al (13) reported that a diet rich in fruits and vegetables is protective against esophageal cancer. Kinjo et al (14) has reported that tobacco smoking, alcohol consumption, and dietary factors are all additive to the risk of developing esophageal squamous cancer.

Whether or not achalasia increases the risk of developing squamous tumors is still a debated issue. Aggestrup et al (15) emphasize that the time interval from diagnosis of achalasia to the diagnosis of squamous cancer may be quite long and that studies in which achalasia patients are followed for short intervals markedly underestimate the true risk. In their series 70% of achalasia patients who did develop esophageal cancer were males. All but one of the cancer patients developed squamous tumors.

Other factors which have been associated with an increased risk of esophageal squamous cell cancer include lye ingestion, radiation therapy, and Plummer-Vinson syndrome.

Adenocarcinoma
Historically, there is a proven clinical association between Barrett mucosa and esophageal adenocarcinoma. More recently, there is accumulating pathologic and molecular genetic data to confirm this relationship. Pera et al (16) identified Barrett mucosa in 63.6% of patients with esophageal adenocarcinoma. We noted similar findings at Hopkins where Barrett mucosa was identified in 62.5% of all esophageal specimens following esophagectomy for adenocarcinoma. Many believe that all cases of adenocarcinoma arise from Barrett mucosa and, when BE is not identified, it is because it has been replaced by the tumor. Accumulating molecular genetic data supports the theory that there is a single mechanism of origin for adenocarcinoma. Moskaluk et al (17) evaluated 98 adenocarinoma esophagectomy specimens for p53, an important gene in the regulation of cell-cycle control and apoptosis, and p21 WAF1 proteins, a gene which encodes a cyclin-dependent kinase inhibitor. The authors found that p53 and p21 WAF1 expression was the same regardless of whether BE was present or not. They conclude that the molecular mechanism of carcinogenesis of adenocarcinoma was the same for both groups.

There is increasing data demonstrating that dysplasia in BE is a precursor to esophageal adenocarcinoma. Miros et al (18) prospectively followed 81 patients with BE. Three patients developed adenocarcinoma. All were documented to have first developed at least low-grade dysplasia. No patient without dysplasia developed adenocarcinoma. Tygat et al (19) have provided graphic evidence (figure 2) that dysplasia is a prerequisite to adenocarcinoma, that low-grade dysplasia is potentially reversible, and that once the threshold of high grade dysplasia is reached, it always progresses to invasive adenocarcinoma. Molecular genetic data support these clinical findings. Wu et al (20) assayed DNA replication errors and allelic losses of chromosomes 17p, 18q, and 5q in BE with dysplasia, and in esophageal adenocarcinoma, with and without associated BE.

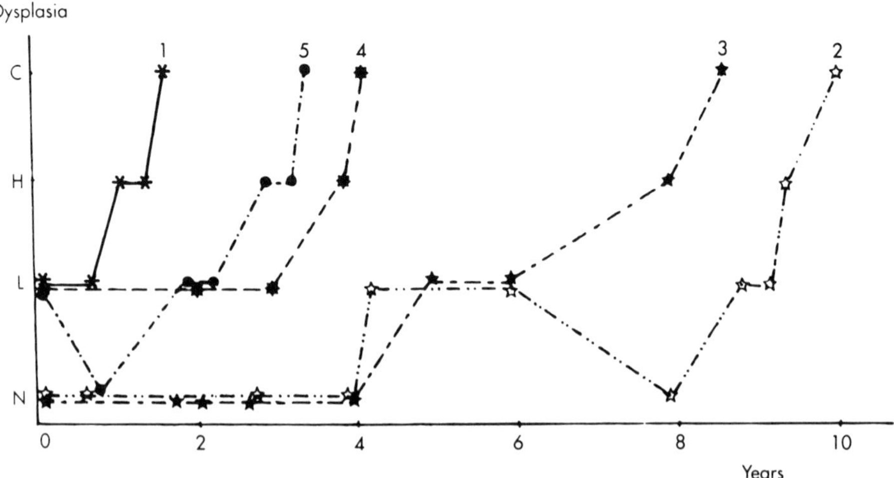

Figure 2. The pathologic progression of five patients from distinctive Barrett mucosa (N), to dysplasia (L=low grade, H=high grade), to invasive adenocarcinoma (C) is graphically displayed (From Tygat GNJ, HameetemanW: The neoplastic potential of colunar-lined (Barrett) esophagus. World J Surg 1992;16:302-12, with permission)

The authors found an increase in the prevalence of chromosomal losses paralleling the Barrett mucosa-BE with dysplasia-adenocarcinoma sequence.

Some evidence supports the hypothesis that impaired host defense increases the risk of developing esophageal cancer. Both vitamins and mineral deficiencies have been cited as explanations for the cancer rates seen in regions endemic for esophageal neoplasia.

Diagnosis
Clinical characteristics
The typical patient with esophageal carcinoma presents with a history of progressive solid food dysphagia and weight loss. The degree of weight loss often appears to be greater than would be expected for the amount of reported dysphagia. Less frequently, patients present with anemia or with hemocult positive stools who are then found to have an esophageal tumor on diagnostic work-up. Even less frequently, an esophageal tumor is identified serendipitously in a totally asymptomatic patient. Mid-scapular, or posterior lower chest pain not associated with swallowing is an ominous finding often suggesting local tumor invasion. Respiratory symptoms including cough, hemoptysis, and excess sputum production may signal airway invasion or the presence of a malignant tracheo-esophageal fistula. Hoarseness, from recurrent laryngeal nerve impairment, may result from either direct tumor invasion for more proximal tumors, or from cervical or mediastinal invasion. New onset headache or dizziness may signal brain metastases.

Likewise, new bone or joint aches or pains should alert the clinician to the possibility of bone metastases.

Regardless of cell type, esophageal cancer most commonly occurs in men aged 60-62 years. In our review of patients undergoing esophagectomy for carcinoma, a history of tobacco smoking was elicited in 71% and 91% for patients with adenocarcinoma and squamous cell carcinoma respectively (21). Patients with adenocarcinoma often have a history of hiatal hernia and gastroesophageal reflux. Some have been under surveillance for BE.

If esophageal carcinoma is suspected on clinical grounds, then a contrast esophagogram is often the next best screening test. It is safe, readily available, and reasonably inexpensive. Esophageal cancer classically appears as an "apple-core" lesion obstructing the flow of contrast. Other radiographic findings suggestive of cancer include a non-circumferential polypoid mass, or a segment of mucosal irregularity or ulceration. Contrast swallowing studies can identify associated esophagogastric pathology and provides an excellent overview of the esophagus and stomach to help with planning surgery should that be necessary.

Even if a "classic" appearing cancer lesion is identified on contrast esophagogram, esophagoscopy with biopsy is necessary to establish the diagnosis. Given the safety and accessibility of flexible endoscopic techniques, many proceed directly to esophagoscopy without swallowing radiographs. Endoscopic biopsies and brushings for cytology will yield the diagnosis of cancer in over 90% of cases. A diagnosis of in situ cancer when radiographic studies demonstrate a large lesion should not be accepted and deeper biopsies repeated to document invasive tumor. Regardless, in addition to obtaining tissue for diagnosis, the endoscopist should also determine the exact location of the tumor, its length, if there is any involvement of the stomach, if there is any other stomach pathology, and if there is associated esophageal pathology such as BE.

For proximal esophageal tumors which lie adjacent to the mainstem bronchi or trachea, or in any patient in which an esophago-respiratory fistula is suspected, flexible bronchoscopy is recommended. Bronchoscopy is more sensitive than esophagoscopy at identifying tracheo-esophageal fistulas (TEF), especially smaller ones. In a recent study, Reidel et al (22) have shown bronchoscopy to have an overall accuracy of 96% in diagnosing malignant TEF. If a tissue diagnosis of tumor has not otherwise been established, it can be obtained bronchoscopically.

Staging

The introduction of new treatment options for patients with esophageal cancer, and the accumulating data demonstrating improved survival for stage II and III tumors with neoadjuvant chemoradiation therapy protocols have made pre-treatment clinical staging of esophageal cancer essential in order to appropriately triage patients into appropriate care. There is currently a great deal of clinical interest in developing safe and accurate pre-treatment staging methods for patients with esophageal cancer. This work is on-going but results to date will be reviewed here.

Because the goal of pre-treatment staging tests are to determine the TNM status, the current American Joint Committee on Cancer Staging (AJCC) system (23) is included in table 1. Of note is that the most recent revision of the staging system acknowledges that adenocarcinomas of the esophagogastric junction are to be staged as esophageal tumors.

TABLE 1. American Joint Commission on Cancer TNM Staging (AJCC) for Esophageal Cancer

Primary tumor (T)

TX	Primary tumor cannot be assessed
T0	No evidence of primary tumor
Tis	Carcinoma in situ
T1	Tumor invades lamina propria or submucosa
T2	Tumor invades muscularis propria
T3	Tumor invades adventitia
T4	Tumor invades adjacent structures

Regional lymph nodes (N)

Cervical esophagus (cervical and supraclavicular nodes)

Nx	Regional lymph nodes cannot be assessed
N0	No regional lymph node metastasis
N1	Regional lymph node metastasis

Thoracic esophagus (nodes in the thorax not those in cervical supraclavicular or abdominal areas)

N0	No nodal involvement
N1	Nodal involvement

Distant metastasis (M)

MX	Distant metastasis cannot be assessed
M0	No evidence of distant metastasis
M1	Distant metastasis present

Stage grouping

Stage	T	N	M
Stage 0	Tis	N0	M0
Stage I	T1	N0	M0
Stage IIA	T2	N0	M0
	T3	N0	M0
Stage IIB	T1	N1	M0
	T2	N1	M0
Stage III	T3	N1	M0
	T4	Any N	M0
Stage IV	Any T	Any N	M1

American Joint Committee on Cancer Staging (AJCC) for esophageal cancer (23)
The best initial staging test for patients with esophageal cancer is computed tomography (CT) scanning of the chest and abdomen. CT scans are readily available, quick , and well tolerated by patients. In addition to visualizing the tumor site, it can screen for lymph nodal enlargement, and metastatic disease. Esophageal carcinoma tends to metastasize in a site-specific fashion to the lung parenchyma, liver, and celiac lymph nodes. All of these sites are included on the chest and abdominal CT scan. Whereas CT scanning has been shown to be accurate at identifying the presence of vertebral or mediastinal soft tissue invasion by bulky tumors (T4 tumors) and lung and liver metastases (M1 disease), it is notably inaccurate at differentiating between T1-3 tumors and in determining the presence or absence of nodal metastases (N status). Therefore, chest and abdominal CT scanning is an excellent initial staging test which can reliably identify advanced staged disease in which palliative therapy only is indicated. Magnetic resonance imaging (MRI) staging of esophageal tumors, like CT scanning, is most accurate at detecting T4 tumors and M1 disease but poor at determining earlier staged disease. It offers no specific advantage over CT scanning, is more costly, takes longer, and has poorer patient acceptance.

The gold standard test to determine T status is endoscopic ultrasound (EUS). EUS is recommended for all lesions in which a previous CT scan has ruled out T4 and M1 disease. In experienced hands, the depth of tumor invasion into the esophageal wall can be determined with an accuracy of 86-94% (26-31). Brugge et al (32) noted no difference in accuracy between radial or linear EUS. However, EUS requires expensive, specialized equipment which is not available at all medical centers. The accuracy of EUS is also very much dependent on the experience of the operator. In approximately 25% of patients, the exam is incomplete or can not be performed for technical reasons, most commonly inability to pass the endoscope beyond the obstructing tumor. Accuracy of determining T stage improves with increasing T stage. EUS is very accurate at determining extraesophageal extension of tumor (T4 tumors). Accuracy of T staging ranges from approximately 60% for T1 tumors to 98% for T4 tumors. Over-staging and under-staging occurs in 6% and 5% respectively. Periesophageal lymph node size, shape, and internal echogenicity are the criteria used to determine the probability of nodal metastatic disease. In addition, numerous studies have shown a direct correlation between the depth of tumor invasion and the probability of nodal metastasis (33, 34) as illustrated in figure 3. Using T stage, nodal size, and appearance, accuracy rates of assessing nodal involvement of 81% have been reported (sensitivity of 95%, specificity of 50%). More recently, real time ultrasound guided transesophageal biopsy techniques permit cytologic confirmation of nodal metastatic disease in many cases. Reed et al (35) have shown that adding transesophageal lymph node biopsy to EUS screening of regional nodal status confirmed regional lymph nodal involvement to 88%.

Esophageal adenocarcinomas are invariably located in the distal esophagus just proximal to the esophagogastric junction. Therefore these tumors, and their regional lymph nodes are accessible to visual inspection and biopsy using laparoscopic techniques. Krasna et al (36,37) make the point that minimal invasive staging of esophageal cancer with laparoscopy and thoracoscopy is analogous to staging lung cancer with mediastinoscopy.

In their experience, laparoscopy correctly identified the pathologic stage of esophageal tumor in 94% of cases. Stein et al (38) reported a sensitivity of 67% and a specificity of 92% using laparoscopic staging. In their experience with 127 patients, previously unidentified liver and peritoneal metastases were discovered in 22% and 25% of cases respectively. The authors make the point, however, that laparoscopy is best suited for distal esophageal adenocarcinomas. For more proximal squamous cell cancers, laparoscopy is a low-yield staging procedure. Several studies have demonstrated that

Figure 3. Percent N1 by T Status

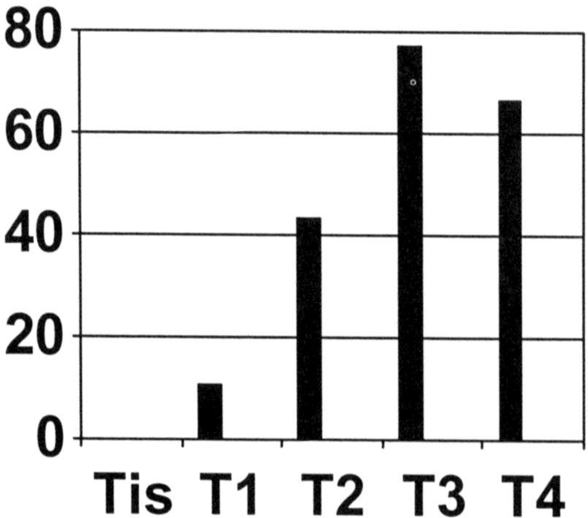

Figure 3. The percentage of regional lymph nodes (N1) with metastatic cancer by T status is shown. Tis=in-situ carcinoma. (Adapted from Rice TW, Zuccaro G Jr, Adelstein DJ, Rybicki LA, Blackstone EH, Goldblum JR: Esophageal carcinoma: depth of tumor invasion is predictive of regional lymph node status. Ann Thorac Surg 1998;65:787-92, with permission)

adding ultrasound to 'standard' laparoscopy increases the accuracy of the staging procedure (39,40).

Krasna et al (36,37) has advocated thoracoscopic staging of esophageal cancers. Thoracoscopy, generally performed through the right chest, does permit direct biopsy of regional lymph nodes and assessment of the tumor/mediastinal interface. In their experience, thoracoscopy accurately determined pathologic staging in 93% of cases. Most consider thoracoscopy unnecessary to stage distal esophageal cancers. Whether thoracoscopy adds significantly to non-operative staging methods is still under evaluation.

There are several studies which compare the accuracy of non-operative staging using EUS, with or without CT, and the minimally invasive staging techniques of laparoscopy and thoracoscopy (41,42). These studies show that adding minimal invasive staging to non-operative staging improves the overall staging accuracy, obtains pathologic determination of regional lymph nodal status. More importantly, laparoscopic findings have clinical significance in that they lead to a change in patient management in 10-15% of cases.

Positron emmision tomography (PET) is a new staging modality whose role in the work-up of patients with esophageal cancers is currently under investigation. Several studies have compared PET to CT scanning in staging patients with esophageal disease (43-47). Most studies demonstrate that PET and CT scan modalities have equivalent accuracy at imaging the primary tumor site and identifying regional lymph nodal metastasis. There is a variation in accuracy for both modalities based on primary tumor or regional lymph nodal size. PET scan has been shown to be effective at detecting distant metastatic disease. Luketich et al (44) reported that PET detection of distant metastases had a sensitivity of 88%, specificity of 93%, and an overall accuracy of 91%. These findings are consistent with reports from other centers. Kole et al (46) concluded that CT and PET imaging are complimentary staging techniques with a combined accuracy which exceeds the staging accuracy if either study was performed alone.

Bone metastases, more common in adenocarcinoma than squamous cell tumors, are nonetheless infrequent sites of early metastatic disease in patients with esophageal cancers. Routine screening bone scan staging for all esophageal cancer patients is, therefore, not recommended. A bone scan should be obtained to evaluate symptomatic patients, or patients with an elevated alkaline phosphatase.

Flexible bronchoscopy has already been discussed as a potential diagnostic method. All patients with tumors adjacent to the mainstem bronchi or trachea should undergo staging bronchoscopy to rule out airway invasion. The most subtle bronchoscopic finding suggestive of early invasion of the membranous wall of the airway is edema and loss of mucosal folds (from tumor invasion of the airway lymphatics).

In summary (table 2), once the diagnosis of esophageal cancer is made by endoscopy with biopsy, patients are best initially screened by chest and abdominal CT scan. If a T4 tumor is suspected, or if determination of lower T status (T1-3) will affect patient triage to protocol therapy, then EUS is recommended. For distal esophageal adenocarcinoma, laparoscopy yields the best pathologic pre-operative staging modality. Adding laparoscopy to non-operative staging methods changes the recommended treatment options in 10-15% of patients. For more proximal cancers, usually squamous cell carcinomas, it is still unproven whether thoracoscopy will be superior to EUS with transesophageal biopsy in staging patients. Bone scans are not routinely obtained, but are reserved for symptomatic patients, or patients in which the alkaline phosphatase is elevated. The role of PET scanning is under investigation. Early results indicate that it can accurately detect distant metastatic disease.

TABLE 2. Diagnosis and Staging Summary
Diagnosis
Contrast esophagogram, Esophagoscopy with biopsy, Bronchoscopy with biopsy for patients with suspected airway invasion or TEF
Staging
All patients: Chest and Abdominal CT scan, (PET scan)
For upper ½ tumors: Bronchoscopy, EUS, (Thoracoscopy)
For lower ½ tumors: EUS, Laparoscopy

Esophageal cancer diagnosis and staging: summary

REFERENCES

1. Heitmiller RF, Sharma R: Comparison of incidence and resection rates in patients with esophageal squamous cell carcinoma and adenocarcinoma. J Thorac Cardiovasc Surgery 112:130-6, 1996.
2. Blot J, DeVessa SS, Kneller RW, Fraumen JF: Increasing incidence of adenocarcinoma of the esophagus and gastric cardia. JAMA 265:1287-9, 1991.
3. Powell J, McConkey CC: Increasing incidence of adenocarcinoma of the gastric cardia and adjacent sites. Br J Cancer 62:440-43, 1990.
4. Reed PI: Changing pattern of oesophageal cancer. Lancet 338:178, 1991.
5. Choi SY, Kahyo H: Effect of cigarette smoking and alcohol consumption in the etiology of cancers of the digestive tract. Int J Cancer 49:381-6, 1991.
6. Christen AG, McDonald JL Jr, Olsen BL, Christen JA: Smokeless tobacco addiction: a threat to the oral and systemic health of the child and adolescent. Pediatrician 16:170-77, 1989.
7. Gronbaek M, Becker U, Johansen D, Tonnesen H, Jensen G, Sorensen TI: Population based cohort study of the association between alcohol intake and cancer of the upper digestive tract. BMJ 317:844-7, 1998.
8. Castellsague X, Munoz N, De Stefani E, Victora CG, Castelletto R, Rolon PA, Quintana MJ: Independent and joint effects of tobacco smoking and alcohol drinking on the risk of esophageal cancer in men and women. Int J Cancer 82:657-64, 1999.
9. Leon X, Quer M, Diez S, Orus C, Lopez-Pousa A, Burgues J: Second neoplasm in patients with head and neck cancer. Head Neck 21:204-10, 1999.
10. Sur M, Cooper K: The role of the human papilloma virus in esophageal cancer. Pathology 30:348-54, 1998.
11. Lagergren J, Wang Z, Bergstrom R, Dillner J, Nyren O: Human papillomavirus infection and esophageal cancer: a nationwide seroepidemiologic case-control study in Sweden. J Natl Cancer Inst 91:156-62, 1999.
12. Ghardirian P, Ekoe JM, Thouez JP: Food habits and esophageal cancer: an overview. Cancer Detect Prev 16:163-68, 1992.
13. Block G, Patterson B, Subar A: Fruit, vegetables, and cancer prevention:a review of the epidemiologic evidence. Nutr Cancer 18:1-29, 1992.
14. Kinjo Y, Cui Y, Akiba S, Watanabe S, Yamaguchi N, Sobue T, Mizuno S, Beral V: Mortality risks of oesophageal cancer associated with hot tea, alcohol, tobacco, and diet in Japan. J Epidemiol 8:235-43, 1998.

15. Aggestrup S, Holm JC, Sorensen HR: Does achalasia predispose to cancer of the esophagus? Chest 102:1013-1016, 1992.

16. Pera M, Cameron AJ, Trastek VF, et al: Increasing incidence of adenocarcinoma of the esophagus and gastric cardia. JAMA 265:1287-89, 1991.

17. Moskaluk CA, Heitmiller RF, Zuharak M, Scwab D, Sidransky D, Hamilton SR: p53 and p21 WAF1/CIP1/SDI1 gene products in Barrett esophagus and adenocarcinoma of the esophagus and esophagogastric junction . Human Pathol 27:1211-20, 1996.

18. Miros M, Kerlin P, Walker N: Only patients with dysplasia progress to adenocarcinoma in Barrett's oesophagus. Gut 32:1441-46, 1991.

19. Tygat GNJ, Hameeteman W: The neoplastic potential of columnar-lined (Barrett) esophagus. World J Surg 16:302-12, 1992.

20. Wu TT, Watanabe T, Heitmiller RF, Zaharak M, Forastiere AA, Hamilton SR: Genetic alterations in Barrett esophagus and adenocarcinoma of the esophagus and esophagogastric junction region. Am J Pathol 153:287-94, 1998.

21. Salazar JD, Doty JR, Lin JW, Dyke MC, Roberts J, Heitmiller ES, Heitmiller RF: Does cell type influence post-esophagectomy survival in patients with esophageal cancer? Diseases of the Esophagus 11:168-71, 1998.

22. Reidel M, Hauck RW, Stein HJ, et al: Preoperative brochoscopic assessment of airway invasion by esophageal cancer. Chest 113:687-95, 1998.

23. American Joint Committee on Cancer: AJCC Cancer Staging Manual (5th edition). Philadelphia, Lippincott/Williams&Wilkins, 1997, pgs 65-68.

24. Takashima S, Takeuchi N, Shiozaki H, et al: Carcinoma of the esophagus: CT vs MR imaging in determining resectability. AJR 156:297-302, 1991.

25. Quint LE, Glazer GM, Orringer MB: Esophageal imaging by MR and CT: study of normal anatomy and neoplasms. Radiology 156:727-31, 1985.

26. Botet JF, Lightdale CJ, Zauber AG, Gerdes H, Urmacher C, Brennan MF: Preoperative staging of esophageal cancer: comparison of endoscopic US and dynamic CT. Radiology 181:419-25, 1991.

27. Dittler HJ, Siewert JR: Role of endoscopic ultrasonography in esophageal carcinoma. Endoscopy 25:156-61, 1993.

28. Wiersema M, Vilmann P, Giovannini G, et al: Endosonography-guided fine-needle aspiration biopsy: diagnostic accuracy and complication assessment. Gastrointest Endosc 112:1087-95, 1996.

29. Tio TL, Coene PP, den Hartog Jager FCA, Tygat GNJ: Preoperative TNM classification of the esophageal carcinoma by endosonography. Hepatogastroenterology 37:376, 1990.

30. Tio TL, Cohen P, Coene PP: Endosonography and computed tomography of esophageal carcinoma. Gastroenterology 96:1478, 1989.

31. Rice TW, Boyce GA, Sivall MV: Esophageal ultrasound and the preoperative staging of carcinoma of the esophagus. J Thorac Cardiovasc Surg 101:536-44, 1991.

32. Brugge WR, Lee MJ, Carey RW, Mathisen DJ: Endoscopic ultrasound staging criteria for esophageal cancer. Gastrointest Endosc 45:147-52, 1997.

33. Nigro JJ, Hagen JA, DeMeester TR, DeMeester SR, Peters JH, Oberg S, Theisen J, Kiyabu M, Crookes PF, Bremner CG: J Thorac Cardiovasc Surg 117:16-23, 1999.

34. Rice TW, Zuccaro G Jr, Adelstein DJ, Rybicki LA, Blackstone EH, Goldblum JR: Esophageal carcinoma: depth of tumor invasion is predictive of regional lymph node status. Ann Thorac Surg 65:787-92, 1998.

35. Reed CE, Mishra G, Sahai AV, Hoffman BJ, Hawes RH: Esophageal cancer staging: improved accuracy by endoscopic ultrasound of celiac lymph nodes. Ann Thorac Surg 67:319-21, 1999.

36. Krasna MJ, Flowers JL, Attar S, McLaughlin J:Combined thoracoscopic/laparoscopic staging of esophageal cancer. J Thorac Cardiovasc Surg 111:800-6, 1996.

37. Krasna MJ: The role of thoracoscopic lymph node staging in esophageal cancer. Int Surg 82:7-11, 1997.

38. Stein HJ, Kraemer SJ, Feussner H, Fink U, Siewert JR: Clinical value of diagnostic laparoscopy with laparoscopic ultrasound in patients with cancer of the esophagus or cardia. J Gastrointest Surg 1:167-73, 1997.

39. Smith A, John TG, Garden OJ, Brown SP: Role of laparoscopic ultrasonography in the management of patients with oesophageal cancer. Br J Surg 86:1083-7, 1999.

40. Finch MD, John TG, Garden OJ, Allan PL, Paterson-Brown S: Laparoscopic ultrasonography for staging gastroesophageal cancer. Surgery 121:10-17, 1997.

41. Bonavina L, Incarbone R, Lattuada E, Segalin A, Cesana B, Peracchia A: Preoperative laparoscopy in management of patients with carcinoma of the esophagus and of the esophagogastric junction. J Surg Oncol 65:171-4, 1997.

42. Luketich JD, Schauer P, Landreneau R, Nguyen N, Urso K, Ferson P, Keenan R, Kim R: Minimally invasive surgical staging is superior to endoscopic ultrasound in detecting lymph node metastases in esophageal cancer. J Thorac Cardiovasc Surg 114:817-21, 1997.

43. Flanagan FL, Dehdashti F, Siegel BA, Trask DD, Sundaresan SR, Patterson GA, Cooper JD: Staging of esophageal cancer with 18F-fluorodeoxyglucose positron emission tomography. Am J Roentgenol 168:417-24, 1997.

44. Luketich JD, Schauer PR, Meltzer CC, Landreneau RJ, Urso GK, Townsend DW, Ferson PF, Keenan RJ, Belani CP: Role of positron emission tomography in staging esophageal cancer. Ann Thorac Surg 64:765-69, 1997.

45. Block MI, Patterson GA, Sundaresan RS, Bailey MS, Flanagan FL, Dehdashti F, Siegel BA, Cooper JD: Improvement in staging of esophageal cancer with the addition of positron emission tomography. Ann Thorac Surg 64:770-6, 1997.

46. Kole AC, Plukker JT, Nieweg OE, Vaalburg W: Positron emission tomography for staging of oesophageal and gastroesophageal malignancy. Br J Surg 78:521-7, 1998.

47. Rankin SC, Taylor H, Cook GJ, Mason R: Computed tomography and positron emission tomography in the pre-operative staging of oesophageal carcinoma. Clin Radiol 53:659-65, 1998.

THERAPY FOR ESOPHAGEAL CANCER

Elisabeth I. Heath, M.D.
Johns Hopkins Oncology Center, Baltimore, MD 21287 USA

Arlene A. Forastiere, M.D.
Johns Hopkins Oncology Center, Baltimore, MD 21287 USA

INTRODUCTION

There are three traditional therapeutic modalities employed in the treatment of esophageal cancer; surgery, radiation therapy, and chemotherapy. These modalities have been utilized, either in combination or alone, as primary or adjuvant therapy for locally advanced disease as well as palliative therapy for metastatic disease. A thorough review of the incidence, risk factors and clinical presentation of esophageal cancer is described elsewhere in this book. However, it remains critically important to emphasize the changing epidemiology of this disease. The incidence of adenocarcinoma of the esophagus and gastric cardia in the United States and parts of Western Europe is rising, while squamous cell carcinoma of the esophagus remains the dominant histologic type in Asia and Africa (1,2). Although there are current efforts to stratify therapy based on histology, the existing studies are not adequate to support histology-specific therapeutic recommendations. Therefore, the treatment modalities discussed in this chapter are for both types of esophageal cancer.

SURGICAL THERAPY

For patients with locally advanced esophageal cancer, surgery represents the gold standard for curative therapy. Patients with carcinoma-in-situ or stage I disease are frequently recommended surgical resection and may have prolonged survival regardless of the extent or type of resection. For patients with metastatic disease, surgery is rarely recommended as a means of restoring swallowing function. The morbidity and mortality of the procedure have to be carefully accounted for when assessing patient risks and benefits. The operative mortality is often less than 5%, but the operative morbidity is usually higher at 30%. As with any complicated surgical procedure, the expertise of the operating surgeon is proportionally correlated with the outcome. Another important factor is determining appropriate candidates for surgery. Esophageal cancer patients who are considered for surgery have cleared many of the pre-operative requirements, including having no major medical contraindications and having adequate performance status. One of the more frequently used pre-operative criteria is age. Recently, there have been two studies that evaluated the role of esophagectomy in the elderly patient. Ellis et al. stratified patients into two groups; patients older than 70 years of age (147) versus those younger than 70 (358) (3). The surgical complication rate was similar in both groups (28% vs 31%), the short and long term mortality rate was similar as were the actuarial 5-year survival rates. Alexiou et al. stratified patients into three groups; younger than 70, 70-79 and older than 80 (4). Although the post-operative complication rate was higher in the greater than 80 years of age group (36%) versus the younger than 70 group (25%), there were no significant differences in median survival or actuarial 5-year survival rates. These two studies and previous publications support esophagectomy being performed in the elderly patient. Therefore, surgical recommendations should be based on the stage of disease and other pre-operative criteria.

The surgery performed is the esophagogastrectomy with regional lymphadenectomy. Historically, multiple incisional strategies included the Ivor Lewis esophagogastrectomy, the transhiatal esophagectomy, and the left thoracoabdominal approach. Experience has shown that all strategies have equal morbidity, mortality, and stage-related survival rates. All stages post surgery 5-year survival is approximately 20%. Current surgical strategies are focusing on optimizing safety, decreasing hospital length of stay and decreasing cost.

RADIATION THERAPY

Definitive radiation therapy
Radiation therapy alone has been evaluated in several trials. In general, radiation therapy as the sole treatment modality is reserved for patients with poor performance status or for palliation of advanced disease. The standard of care for definitive non-surgical therapy is the combination of chemotherapy and radiation therapy (discussed later). The recommended total dose for definitive treatment ranges from 5,000 cGy to 6,500 cGy, in fractions of 200 cGy per day. Sykes et al. reported a 5-year survival rate of 20% in patients with a < 5cm squamous cell carcinoma (6). However, other studies support a more dismal 5-year survival rate of 0-10% (7,8). Complications from irradiation, such as strictures, fistula formation, pneumonitis, pericarditis, and myocarditis, can be significant and may impact on a patient's quality of life. For palliative purposes, radiation therapy used for rapid improvement of obstructive symptoms is quite effective.

Pre-operative radiation therapy
The use of pre-operative radiation therapy is based on the hypothesis that tumor shrinkage and field sterilization may translate into an increased resectability rate. At least six randomized trials evaluating the role of pre-operative radiation therapy, mostly in patients with squamous cell carcinoma of the esophagus, have been performed. In general, the trials reported a decrease in the rate of local failure, but there was no difference in the rate of resectability or survival. The were two trials which reported an improvement in overall survival. Nygaard et al. reported a four arm study, in which one of the arms evaluated pre-operative radiation therapy (9). The group which received radiation therapy had a significantly better survival rate than the groups that did not.

However, the authors did acknowledge that although their protracted treatment schedule may have been successful in terms of improving survival, the long term survival data may not be as successful. Other explanations as to the positive trial results include criticism in the statistical analysis. The study was an intention-to-treat trial, but only 82% of the patients were evaluable for therapy and only 62% of those patients were operable. Huang et al. reported a randomized study evaluating pre-operative radiation therapy versus surgery alone in 160 patients. Although the 5-year survival rate was higher with combined therapy (45.5% versus 25%), this was not a statistically significant difference (10). At the present, pre-operative radiation therapy alone is not indicated.

Post-operative radiation therapy

The intent of post-operative radiation therapy is to decrease the local recurrence rate after surgery and thereby improve overall survival. This approach is associated with high morbidity since large volumes of normal tissue are irradiated, particularly in patients who undergo gastric pull-up or intestinal interposition. Three randomized trials have evaluated adjuvant radiation therapy versus observation. All trials reported no significant improvement in overall survival. In one trial by Fok et al., there was no decrease in the local recurrence rate (11). In this trial, 350 cGy per fraction was used instead of the lower conventional doses of 180 -200 cGy. In another trial by Teniere et al., there was again no improvement in overall survival (12). This particular trial did show a positive effect in decreasing local recurrence rates in patients with negative lymph nodes. This is counterintuitive, since the expectation is that radiation therapy will be most beneficial in patients with positive lymph nodes. However, it was noted that the incidence of anastomotic strictures was increased and post-operative recovery of function was delayed. This meant poor quality of life in the radiation treated patients compared to non-treated patients.

In patients who did not have a complete resection and are left with a positive margin, there are data to support the role of adjuvant therapy. However, this is usually with combined modality therapy, using chemotherapy and radiation therapy.

CHEMOTHERAPY

Definitive chemotherapy

There have been no randomized or non-randomized trials evaluating the role of chemotherapy alone in the treatment of locally advanced esophageal cancer. The role of chemotherapy alone is in the setting of metastatic disease, with the obvious objective of delivering systemic treatment to a disease that has already become widespread. The experience with chemotherapy to date has been primarily in patients with squamous cell carcinoma of the esophagus. The more recent clinical trials have included both histologies. There have been many trials performed evaluating single agents. In general, the response rate for single agent therapy is in the range of 15-30% and there is no significant survival benefit. Chemotherapeutic agents that were studied from the early 1970's to late 1980's include 5-fluorouracil, mitomycin, cisplatin, and bleomycin. More recently, clinical trials have evaluated the efficacy of newer agents, such as taxanes (paclitaxel). The trial evaluating the role of paclitaxel was performed in patients with adenocarcinoma and squamous cell carcinoma of the esophagus. A 34% response rate was observed in patients with adenocarcinoma and a 28% response rate in those with squamous cell carcinoma of the esophagus (using a dose of 250 mg/m^2 over 24 hours every 3 weeks) (13).

Combination chemotherapy with two or three drugs have been evaluated and provide a higher response rate than single agent chemotherapy. The standard first line treatment for patients with either type of esophageal cancer is 5-fluorouracil and cisplatin. In a randomized trial by the EORTC comparing single agent cisplatin at 100 mg/m^2 versus cisplatin and 5-fluorouracil at 1000 mg/m^2/day infused for 5 days, the overall response rate for the combination arm was 38% (14). Another trial by Iizuka et al. reported a 34% response rate with the combination therapy, but it was mainly in patients with squamous cell carcinoma of the esophagus (15). Newer trials evaluating the role of taxanes in combination with cisplatin and/or 5-fluorouracil have reported response rates of 50% in patients with esophageal cancer, both types (16). More recently, a phase I trial studying increasing doses of paclitaxel along with weekly cisplatin has reported a tolerable dosing combination with a response rate of 52%(17). Another phase II study recently reported a 44% response rate with paclitaxel and carboplatin (18). Other compounds under evaluation include CPT-11 (irinotecan), docetaxel and gemcitabine. The reportedly higher response rates have to be weighed against the toxicities, such as neutropenia, myalgias, neuropathy and fatigue. Thus, these newer agents are being tested in a variety of doses and schedules to improve efficacy while minimizing toxicities.

Pre-operative chemotherapy

The potential benefits from adding pre-operative chemotherapy include increased resectability rates, improved local control and the eradication of micrometastatic disease. In addition, at the time of surgery, the direct effects of chemotherapy may be assessed. Identifying patients who respond to chemotherapy is beneficial in selecting the appropriate patient population for post-operative chemotherapy. One disadvantage of pre-operative chemotherapy is the delay in definitive surgical treatment. If the tumor is chemotherapy resistant, then the risk of further spread of disease is increased. The risk unfortunately is a real one as approximately 50% of patients will not respond to the most widely used combination chemotherapy of cisplatin and 5-fluorouracil.

There have been multiple phase II trials, both in squamous cell carcinoma and adenocarcinoma of the esophagus evaluating pre-operative chemotherapy. In general, the response rates were encouraging enough to proceed to randomized trials. To date there have been at least three randomized trials evaluating the role of pre-operative chemotherapy versus surgery alone. In a large intergroup trial (INT 0113) comparing pre-operative chemotherapy versus surgery alone no differences in median survival, overall survival, or local failure rates between the two groups were observed (19). There was also no difference in the survival outcome when comparisons were made between histologies. However, another trial reported better success rate with respect to increased median survival (19 versus 11 months, p=0.002) when comparing two cycles of pre-operative cisplatin and etoposide versus surgery alone (20). Another trial evaluated two cycles of pre-operative vindesine, cisplatin, and bleomycin versus surgery alone (21). The median survival for both groups was 9 months, but the median survival in patients who responded to chemotherapy was 20 months compared to 6.2 months in the group who did not. Overall, it remains difficult to recommend pre-operative chemotherapy outside of a clinical trial.

Post-operative chemotherapy

The data evaluating the role of post-operative chemotherapy are few. The objective of post-operative chemotherapy is to eradicate any possible micrometastatic disease. When chemotherapy has been administered post-operatively in phase II trials, it was feasible in only half of the patients. In one randomized trial performed in patients with squamous cell carcinoma of the esophagus, the administration of two cycles of adjuvant cisplatin and vindesine did not result in a survival benefit compared to observation (22). Similar to the pre-operative chemotherapy recommendation, post-operative chemotherapy should be administered in the context of a clinical trial.

COMBINED MODALITY THERAPY

Definitive chemotherapy and radiation therapy

Patients who are not surgical candidates or have locally advanced unresectable disease are considered for definitive treatment with chemotherapy and radiation therapy. This approach addresses both issues of local and systemic disease. There have been numerous single-institution and multi-institution phase II trials evaluating chemotherapy and radiation therapy in squamous cell carcinoma and adenocarcinoma of the esophagus (23-26). In general, the chemotherapy included 5-fluorouracil, cisplatin, and MMC and the radiation dose was in range of 4,000 cGy to 6,000 cGy. Median survival was in the order of 11-22 months and the 2-year overall survival rate in the range of 29-39%. Encouraging results have led to several phase III randomized trials comparing chemotherapy and radiation therapy versus radiation therapy alone.

To date, there are six randomized trials that have been performed (27-32). Unfortunately, all but one trial was criticized for suboptimal doses of radiation therapy or chemotherapy. The one well- defined study testing non-surgical combined modality treatment in patients with squamous cell carcinoma of the esophagus was initially reported by Herskovic et al.(32). Patients were randomized to receive four cycles of 5-fluorouracil (1000 mg/m^2/day) for 4 days and cisplatin (75 mg/m^2) on the first day along with concomitant radiation therapy (5,000 cGy) or to the radiotherapy alone arm (6,400 cGy). In the combined modality arm, patients received two cycles of chemotherapy concurrent with radiation followed by two additional cycles of chemotherapy. The results showed a significantly improved 5-year survival rates for the combined modality arm (26%) versus the radiation only arm (0%) (33).

Table 1.   **Summary   of   Randomized   Trials   of Combined-Modality Treatment**

Chemotherapy followed by Surgery

Author[ref]	Chemotherapy	Radiation (cGy)	# Pts.	Median Survival	Survival (3 yr)
Kelsen [19]	cisp/5-FU	----	213	14.9	23
	surgery	----	227	16.1	26
Schlag [45]	cisp/5-FU	----	22	10	----
	surgery	----	24	10	----
Kok [20]	cisp/etoposide	----	74	18.5*	----
	surgery	----	74	11	----

Chemotherapy/Radiation Therapy followed by Surgery

Author[ref]	Chemotherapy	Radiation (cGy)	# Pts.	Median Survival	Survival (3yr)
Urba [38]	cisp/vinb/5-FU	4500	50	1.41	32
	surgery	----	50	1.46	15
Walsh[40]	cisp/5-FU	4000	58	16	32*
	surgery	----	55	11	6
Bossett [41]	cisp/5-FU	3700	142	18.6	38
	surgery	----	139	18.6	38

Chemotherapy and Radiation Therapy as Definitive Treatment

Author[ref]	Chemotherapy	Radiation (cGy)	# Pts.	Median Survival	Survival
Araujo [31]	cisp/mmc/5-FU	5000	28	8	38 at 2 yrs
	control	5000	31	8	22
Cooper [33]	cisp/5-FU	5000	61	----	26% at 5 yrs
	control	6400	62	----	0%

NS= not stated
*= statistically significant

The issue of whether race influenced survival in this trial was studied by Streeter et al. (34). In an analysis limited to patients in the combined chemotherapy and radiation therapy treatment arm, the overall survival in the two groups was not significantly different (p= 0.2757). African-American patients had more advanced disease at presentation, all had squamous cell histology and were younger in age compared to white patients. It was also reported that the patients who were younger than 60, but older than 70 had a worse outcome. However, there were too few patients to determine if stratifying by age would have made a difference.

Another important finding in this trial was the high local failure rate of 44%, even though that is considerably lower than the radiation alone arm, which had a local failure rate of 68%. A follow-up trial intensifying both chemotherapy and radiation therapy in the combined modality arm was performed. In this trial (INT 0122), 5-fluorouracil and cisplatin were given for 5 cycles with concurrent radiation (6,480 cGy) during the last two cycles (35). The median survival time was 20 months and the 5-year actuarial survival rate was 20%. The lack of a higher survival rate and increased toxicities led the Intergroup to abandon this regimen. The subsequent phase III (INT 0123) intensified radiation therapy alone in the experimental arm. Patients with adenocarcinoma or squamous cell cancer were randomized to receive either 5-fluorouracil, cisplatin for four cycles and radiation therapy 5,040 cGy or the same chemotherapy with radiation therapy 6,480 cGy. The study was closed at the first interim analysis because of a worse survival rate in the experimental arm.

Pre-operative chemotherapy and radiation therapy

The rationale for the use of combination chemotherapy and radiation therapy prior to surgery is to maximize tumor reduction, improve resectability rate, improve local control and increase survival rate. There have been multiple phase II non-randomized trials in both squamous cell carcinoma and adenocarcinoma of the esophagus that have been performed. Overall, the numbers of patients on the trial ranges from 21 to 113 (36,37). The pathologic complete response rate is in the range of 25 - 30% with a median survival of approximately two years.

With respect to randomized trials, there have been three trials comparing chemotherapy and radiation therapy followed by surgery with surgery alone. One trial by Urba et al. evaluated 5-fluorouracil, cisplatin, and vinblastine with concurrent radiation therapy (4,500 cGy) followed by surgery versus surgery alone (38). The results showed no differences in median survival (1.46 vs 1.48 years, respectively) or in the estimated 2-year survival. An update in the trial with a median survival of 5.2 years still showed no improvement in median survival, but an improvement in the 3-year survival rate (32% vs 15%, p=0.07) (39). There was also a decrease in the local recurrence rate.

A second trial by Walsh et al. evaluated primarily patients with adenocarcinoma of the esophagus (40). Patients received either pre-operative chemotherapy with 5-fluorouracil with cisplatin and radiation therapy (4,000 cGy) followed by surgery or surgery alone. There was a statistically significant improvement in median survival (16 vs 11 months, p=0.01) as well as the 3-year survival rate (32% vs 6%, p=0.01) in the combined modality arm. This study has received criticism for the lower than average survival rate (6%) in the surgery only arm.

The third trial by Bossett et al. evaluated 282 patients with squamous cell carcinoma of the esophagus (41). Patients were randomized to receive cisplatin (80 mg/m2) along with split dose radiation therapy followed by surgery or surgery alone. Although there was a pathologic complete response rate of 26% in the combined modality arm, the median and 3-year survival rates were equal in both arms, 19 months and 36%, respectively. With the data being encouraging but controversial, a current intergroup trial (CALGB C9781) is underway. This trial is randomizing patients to combined modality therapy with 5-fluorouracil, cisplatin and radiation therapy (5,040 cGy) followed by surgery to surgery alone.

Other current phase I and II trials are evaluating newer agents such as paclitaxel and docetaxel (42,43). A different trial design utilizing induction chemotherapy prior to definitive chemotherapy and radiation therapy has also been studied. In this trial, patients received two cycles of paclitaxel and cisplatin followed by weekly paclitaxel and cisplatin and radiation therapy (5,040 cGy) (44). The regimen appears well tolerated and the trial is ongoing.

Post-operative chemotherapy and radiation therapy

As discussed in the section of post-operative chemotherapy, there have been no formal trials evaluating post-operative combined modality therapy. The toxicities in this setting are anticipated to be high and treatment should not be done outside of a clinical trial.

PALLIATIVE THERAPY

Patients with advanced disease are candidates for palliative therapy. There have been multiple trials evaluating the role of chemotherapy for this stage of disease (discussed earlier). In addition to systemic disease, local symptoms, such as dysphagia, odynophagia, and complete obstruction can be very debilitating and impact greatly on quality of life. Local therapy options include external-beam radiation, intraluminal brachytherapy, stent therapy, laser therapy, dilation therapy and photodynamic therapy (PDT). Photodynamic therapy utilizes the activation of photofrin in the tumor cells. The activation process produces a toxin which kills tumor cells. Several trials have been performed evaluating the role of PDT in the treatment of esophageal cancer. The results are encouraging, although the toxicities of this treatment, such as photosensitivity are not minimal. In general, the palliative therapy of choice is dependent on tumor location, size of tumor, expertise of the physician and patient wishes.

CONCLUSION

The options for treatment of esophageal cancer have increased in the past three decades. Such advancements are important because less than half of the patients with this disease are candidates for surgery. The role of chemotherapy, radiation therapy and the combination of the two modalities have offered patients other means of definitive treatment. There have been many clinical trials evaluating the efficacy of chemotherapy and radiation therapy in the pre-operative and post-operative setting. Although the survival rates are better with the incorporation of chemotherapy and radiation therapy, there is room for much more improvement. With incorporation of newer agents in future trials, further advancements are forthcoming.

REFERENCES

1. Blot WJ. Esophageal cancer trends and risk factors. Semin Oncol 21:403-410, 1994.
2. Blot WJ, Devessa SS, Kneller RW. Rising incidence of adenocarcinoma of the esophagus and gastric cardia. JAMA 265:1287-1289, 1991.
3. Ellis FH, Williamson WA, Heatley GJ. Cancer of the esophagus and cardia: does age influence treatment selection and surgical outcomes? J Am Coll Surg 187:345-51, 1998.
4. Alexiou C, Beggs D, Salama FD, et al. Surgery for esophageal cancer in elderly patients: the view from Nottingham. J Thorac Cardiovasc Surg 116:545-53, 1998.
5. Pommier RF, Vetto JT, Ferris BL, et al. Relationships between operative approaches and outcomes in esophageal surgery. Am J Surg 175:422-425, 1998.
6. Sykes AJ, Burt PA, Slevin NJ, et al. Radical radiotherapy for carcinoma of the oesophagus: An effective alternative to surgery. Radiother Oncol 48:15-21, 1998.
7. De-Ren S. Ten-year follow-up of esophageal cancer treated by radical radiation therapy: Analysis of 869 patients. Int J Radiat Oncol Biol Phys 16:329-334, 1989.
8. Okawa T, Kita M, Tanaka M, et al: Results of radiotherapy for inoperable locally advanced esophageal cancer. Int J Radiat Oncol Biol Phys 17:49-54, 1989.
9. Nygaard K, Hagen S, Hansen HS, et al. Pre-operative radiotherapy prolongs survival in operable esophageal carcinoma: A randomized, multicenter study of pre-operative radiotherapy and chemotherapy: the second Scandinavian trial in esophageal cancer. World J Surg 16:1104-1110, 1992.
10. Huang GJ, Gu XZ, Wang LJ, et al. Combined preoperative irradiation and surgery for esophageal carcinoma, in Deluarue NC (ed): International Trends in General Thoracic Surgery, 1st ed, 315-318. St. Louis, CV Mosby, 1988.
11. Fok M, Sham JST, Choy D, et al. Postoperative radiotherapy for carcinoma of the esophagus: A prospective, randomized controlled trial. Surgery 113:138-147, 1993.
12. Teniere P, Hay J-M, Fingerhut A, et al. Postoperative radiation therapy does not increase survival after curative resection for squamous cell carcinoma of the middle and lower esophagus as shown by a multicenter controlled trial. Surg Gynecol Obstet 173:123-130, 1991.
13. Ajani JA, Ilson DH, Daugherty K, et al. Activity of taxol in patients with squamous cell and adenocarcinoma of the esophagus. J Natl Cancer Inst 86:1086-1091, 1994
14. Bleiberg H, Jacob JH, Bedennne L, et al. Randomized phase II trial of 5-fluorouracil (5FU) and cisplatin (DDP) versus DDP alone in advanced oesophageal cancer. Proc Am Soc Clin Oncol 10:447, 1991.

15. Iizuka T, Kakegawa T, Ide H, et al. Phase II study of CDDP + 5FU for squamous esophageal carcinoma. JEOG Co-operative Study results. Proc Am Soc Clin Oncol 10:496, 1991.

16. Kelsen D, Ginsberg R, Bains, M, et al. A phase II trial of paclitaxel and cisplatin in patients with locally advanced metastatic esophageal cancer: A preliminary report. Seminars in Oncology 24:suppl 19, 1997.

17. Van der Gaast A, Polee M, Kok TC, et al. Phase I study of a biweekly schedule of a fixed dose of cisplatin with increasing doses of paclitaxel in patients with advanced oesophageal cancer. British Journal of Cancer 80:1052-1057, 1999.

18. Philip PA, Gadgeel S, Hussain M, et al. Phase II study of paclitaxel and carboplatin in patients with advanced gastric and esophageal cancers. Proc Am Soc Clin Oncol 17:1001, 1999.

19. Kelsen DP, Ginsberg R, Pajak T, et al. Chemotherapy followed by surgery compared with surgery alone for localized esophageal cancer. N Engl J Med 339:1979-1984, 1998.

20. Kok TC, Lanschott JV, Siersema PD, et al. Neoadjuvant chemotherapy in operable esophageal squamous cell cancer: Final report of a phase III multicenter randomized trial. Proc Am Soc Clin Oncol 16:984, 1997.

21. Roth JA, Pass HU, Flanagan MM, et al. Randomized clinical trials of preoperative and postoperative adjuvant chemotherapy with cisplatin, vindesine, and bleomycin for carcinoma of the esophagus. J Thorac Cardiovasc Surg 96:242, 1998.

22. Ando N, Iizuka T, Kakegawa T, et al. A randomized trial of surgery with and without chemotherapy for localized squamous carcinoma of the thoracic esophagus: the Japan Clinical Oncology Group Study. J Thorac Cardiovasc Surgery 114:205-9, 1997.

23. Chan A, Wong A, Arthur K. Concomitant 5-fluorouracil infusion, mitomycin C and radical therapy in esophageal squamous cell carcinoma. Int J Radiat Oncol Biol Phys 16:59-65, 1998.

24. John M, Flam M, Mowry P, et al. Radiotherapy alone and chemoradiation for non-metastatic esophageal carcinoma: A critical review of chemoradiation. Cancer 63:2397-2403, 1989.

25. Leichman L, Herskovic A, Leichman P, et al. Nonoperative therapy for squamous cell cancer of the esophagus. J Clin Oncol 5:365-370, 1987.

26. Seitz J, Giovannini M, Padaut-Casana J, et al. Inoperable nonmetastatic squamous cell carcinoma of the esophagus managed by concomitant chemotherapy (5-fluorouracil and cisplatin) and radiation therapy. Cancer 66: 214-219, 1990.

27. Smith TJ, Ryan LM, Douglass HO, et al. Combined chemoradiotherapy vs radiotherapy alone for early stage squamous cell carcinoma of the esophagus: A study of the Eastern Cooperative Oncology Group. Int J Radiat Oncol Biol Phys 42: 269-276, 1998.

28. Slabber CF, Nel JS, Schoeman L, et al. A randomized study of radiotherapy alone vs radiotherapy plus 5-fluorouracil and platinum in patients with inoperable, locally advanced squamous cell cancer of the esophagus. Am J Clin Oncol (CCT) 21:462-465, 1998.

29. Nygaard K, Hagen S, Hansen HS, et al. Pre-operative radiotherapy prolongs survival in operable esophageal carcinoma: A randomized, multicenter study of pre-operative radiotherapy and chemotherapy: The second Scandinavian trial in esophageal cancer. World J Surg 16:1104-1110, 1992.

30. Roussel A, Jacob JH, Jung GM, et al. Controlled clinical trial for the treatment of patients with inoperable esophageal carcinoma: A study of the EORTC gastrointestinal tract cancer cooperative group. Schlag P (ed). Recent Results in Cancer Research, 1st ed, 21-30. Berlin, Springer-Verlag, 1988.

31. Arajuo CM, Souhami L, Gil RA, et al. A randomized trial comparing radiation therapy vs concomitant radiation therapy and chemotherapy in carcinoma of the thoracic esophagus. Cancer 67:2258-2261, 1991.

32. Herskovic A, Martz LK, Al-Sarraf M, et al. Combined chemotherapy and radiotherapy compared with radiotherapy alone in patients with cancer of the esophagus. N Engl J Med 326:1593-1598, 1992.

33. Cooper JS, Guo MD, Herskovic, MD, et al. Chemoradiotherapy of locally advanced esopahgeal cancer. JAMA 281:1623-1627, 1999.

34. Streeter OE, Martz KL, Gaspar LE, et al. Does race influence survival for esophageal cancer patients treated on the radiation and chemotherapy arm of RTOG #85-01? Int J Radiat Oncol Biol Phys 44:1047-1052, 1999.

35. Minsky BD, Neuberg D, Kelsen DP, et al. Final report of intergroup trial 0122 (ECOG PE-289, RTOG 90-12): Phase II trial of neoadjuvant chemotherapy plus concurrent chemotherapy and high-dose radiation for squamous cell carcinoma of the esophagus. Int J Radiat Oncol Biol Phys 43:517-523, 1999.

36. Leichman L, Steiger Z, Seydel HG, et al. Preoperative chemotherapy and radiation therapy for patients with cancer of the esophagus: A potentially curative approach. J Clin Oncol 2:75-79, 1984.

37. Poplin E, Fleming T, Leichman L, et al. Combined therapies for squamous-cell carcinoma of the esophagus, a Southwest Oncology Group study (SWOG-8037). J Clin Oncol 5:622-628, 1987.

38. Urba S, Orringer M, Turrisi A, et al. A randomized trial comparing transhiatal esophagectomy (THE) to preoperative concurrent chemoradiation (CT/SRT) followed by esophagectomy in locoregional esophageal carcinoma. Proc Am Soc Clin Oncol 14:199, 1995.

39. Urba S, Orringer M, Turrisi A, et al. A randomized trial comparing surgery (S) to preoperative concomitant chemoradiation plus surgery in patients (pts) with resectable esophageal cancer. Proc Am Soc Clin Oncol 16:277, 1997.

40. Walsh TN, Noonan N, Hollywood D, et al. A comparison of multimodality therapy and surgery for esophageal adenocarcinoma. N Engl J Med 335:462-467, 1996.

41. Bosset JF, Gignoux M, Triboulet JP, et al. Chemoradiotherapy followed by surgery compared with surgery alone in squamous cell cancer of the esophagus. N Engl J Med 337:161-167, 1997.

42. Lampert C, Colarusso P, Goldberg M, et al. Survival following intensive preoperative combined modality therapy with paclitaxel, cisplatin and 5-fluorouracil and radiation in resectable esophageal carcinoma. Proc Am Soc Clin Oncol 17:962, 1999.

43.   Kelsen D, Ilson D, Lipton, R, et al. A phase I trial of radiation therapy (RT) plus concurrent fixed dose cisplatin (C) with escalating doses of paclitaxel (P) as a 96 hour continuous infusion in patients (pts) with localized esophageal cancer (EC). Proc Am Soc Clin Oncol 17:1039, 1999.

44.   Enziger P, Ilson D, Minsky B, et al. Phase I/II neoadjuvant concurrent 96 hour taxol, cisplatin, and radiation therapy: promising toxicity profile an response in localized esophageal cancer. Proc Am Soc Clin Oncol 17:1038, 1999.

45.   Schlag PM. Randomized trial of preoperative chemotherapy for squamous cell cancer of the esophagus: The Chirurgische Arbeitsgemeinschaft fur Onkologie der Deutschen Gesellschaft fur Chirurgie Study Group. Arch Surg 127:1446-1450, 1992.

INDEX

C

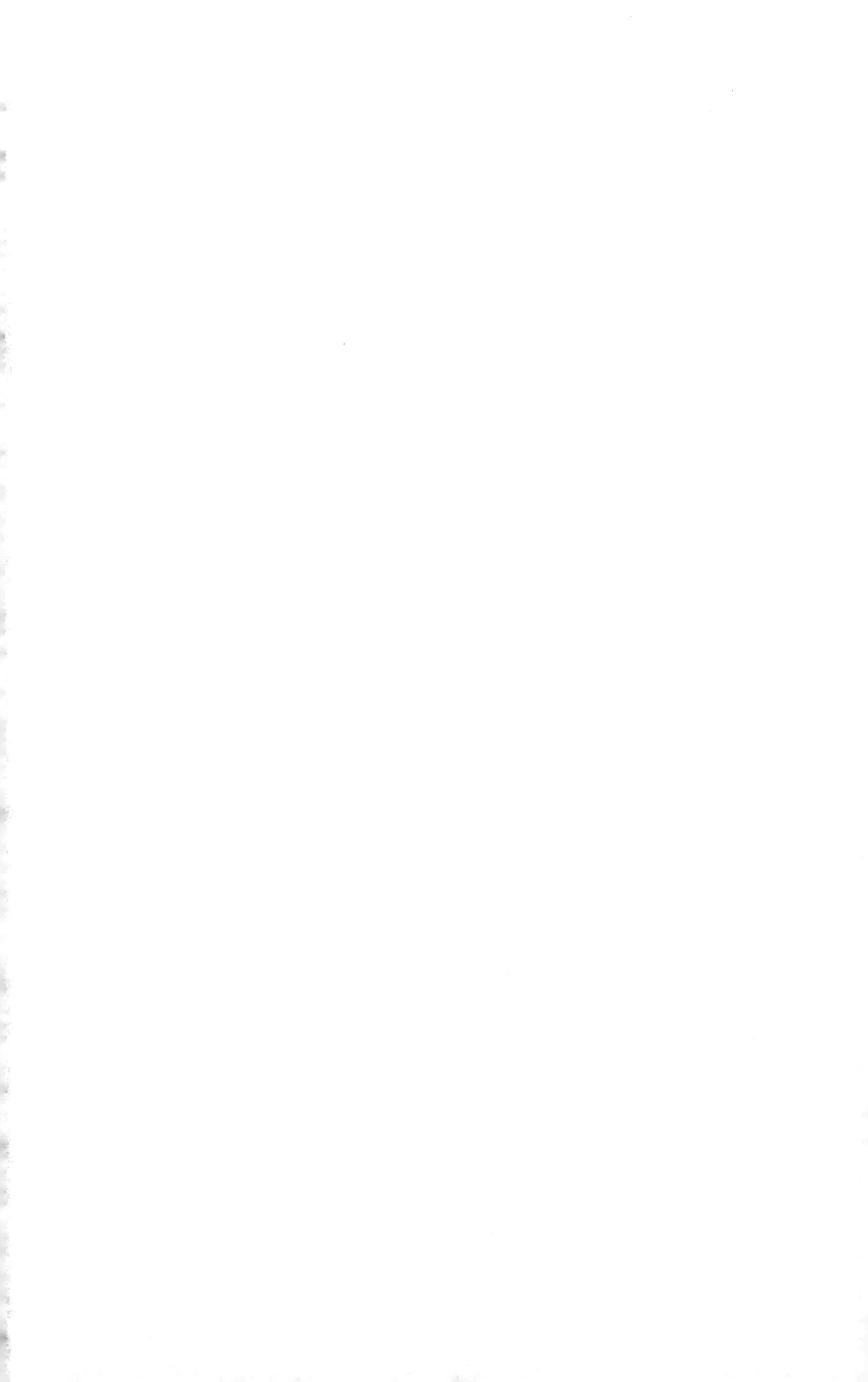